Principles of Animal Behavior

SECOND EDITION

Lee Alan Dugatkin

UNIVERSITY OF LOUISVILLE

W. W. NORTON & COMPANY | NEW YORK | LONDON

W. W. Norton & Company has been independent since its founding in 1923, when
William Warder Norton and Mary D. Herter Norton first published lectures delivered at
the People's Institute, the adult education division of New York City's Cooper Union.
The Nortons soon expanded their program beyond the Institute, publishing books
by celebrated academics from America and abroad. By mid-century, the two major
pillars of Norton's publishing program—trade books and college texts—were firmly
established. In the 1950s, the Norton family transferred control of the company to
its employees, and today—with a staff of four hundred and a comparable number of
trade, college, and professional titles published each year—W. W. Norton & Company
stands as the largest and oldest publishing house owned wholly by its employees.

Editor: Michael Wright
Developmental editor: Sandy Lifland
Editorial assistant: Jennifer Cantelmi
Senior Production Manager: Christopher Granville
Design Director: Rubina Yeh
Photo Researchers: Kelly Mitchell and Rae Grant
Marketing manager: Betsy Twitchell
Managing editor, College: Marian Johnson
Illustrations by Penumbra Design, Inc., and John McAusland
Composition by TSI Graphics
Manufacturing by Courier Companies
Cover design: Andrew Newman Design/newmandesign.com
Cover photograph: Kitchin & Hurst/leesonphoto.com.

Library of Congress Cataloging-in-Publication Data
Dugatkin, Lee Alan, 1962–
  Principles of animal behavior / Lee Alan Dugatkin. — 2nd ed.
    p. cm.
  Includes bibliographical references and index.
  ISBN 13-978-0-393-93169-3 (hardcover)
    1. Animal behavior. I. Title.
  QL751.D748 2009
  591.5—dc22   2008021360

W. W. Norton & Company, Inc., 500 Fifth Avenue, New York, N.Y. 10110
                    www.wwnorton.com
W. W. Norton & Company Ltd., Castle House, 75/76 Wells Street, London W1T 3QT
    2   3   4   5   6   7   8   9   0

For Dana, My True Helpmate

Contents in Brief

Contents

Preface

Much has happened in the field of animal behavior since the initial publication of this book in 2004. In this second edition, I have tried to capture the exciting advances that have occurred in ethology and ecology over the last five years. Recent research findings have given me ample opportunity not only to update and expand on the studies presented in the book, but also to reinforce the first edition's focus on ultimate and proximate causation, as well as its unique emphasis on natural selection, learning, and cultural transmission.

The heart of this book continues to be an examination of the empirical, theoretical, and conceptual foundations upon which the field of animal behavior rests. This examination, by necessity, involves a thorough integration of ultimate and proximate perspectives on ethology. Throughout the book, I analyze the extent and manner in which natural selection, learning, and cultural transmission shape behavior. I delve deeply into the neurobiology, physiology, endocrinology, molecular genetics, and development influences underlying animal behavior. I also emphasize in all the chapters how it is the *interaction* of all these forces that is important, as the tapestry of animal behavior is created from weaving all of its components into a beautiful whole.

My aim is to explain underlying concepts in a way that is scientifically rigorous but, at the same time, accessible to students. Each chapter in the book has a sound theoretical and conceptual basis upon which the empirical studies rest. The presentation of theory, sometimes in the form if mathematical models, is not meant to intimidate students but rather to mesh with the glorious examples of animal behavior that surround it. The goal is to produce a book that instructors can use in their courses as well as in their research programs. My hope is to have a written book that students will actually enjoy and will recommend to their friends as a "keeper."

MAJOR FEATURES

The book is written both for the student of biology and for the psychology student. Its core strengths are:

▸ **A BALANCED TREATMENT OF PROXIMATE AND ULTIMATE FACTORS.** A comprehensive understanding of animal behavior requires a balanced and integrated approach to proximate and ultimate causation. Each of these perspectives informs the other, and both are necessary to understand animal behavior. This book weaves together these two perspectives in ways that other books do not. In Chapter 3, for example, I use Geoff Hill's elegant work on coloration in finches to show how proximate explanations of what causes differences in coloration can also point the way to ultimate explanations for why there are such color differences, and how studies about coloration and fitness shed light on what sort of proximate work should follow.

▸ **LEARNING AND CULTURAL TRANSMISSION PRESENTED ALONGSIDE NATURAL SELECTION AND PHYLOGENY.** Historically, ethology books written by biologists have tended to concentrate on how natural selection has shaped animal behavior and relegated learning to a separate chapter that was specifically on that topic, rarely even touching on cultural transmission. Psychologists have generally devoted the vast majority of their textbooks on animal behavior to learning per se, with only a chapter or two on the evolutionary underpinnings of the behaviors they were describing. A unique aspect of this book is that it integrates learning, cultural transmission, natural selection, and phylogeny throughout the book, and brings together behavioral perspectives and examples of animal behavior research from various subdisciplines in biology, psychology, and anthropology. For example, the discussion of foraging in Chapter 10 includes an examination of the evolution of spatial memory and foraging, cultural transmission of information about foraging sites, and a section on phylogeny and caching ability.

▸ **A THOROUGH INTEGRATION OF PROXIMATE FACTORS, INCLUDING NEUROBIOLOGY, ENDOCRINOLOGY, DEVELOPMENT, AND MOLECULAR GENETICS.** The tools and techniques available for undertaking proximate analyses have increased exponentially in recent years, and the text employs them often to test hypotheses. For example, in Chapter 3, I introduce students to each proximate approach individually, so that they can gain a basic understanding of how each one works. Afterwards, I integrate all of the approaches so that students will learn about proximate factors as ethologists understand them: as a complex interaction of each type of causation. In Chapter 3, I do this by providing a detailed examination of the work coming out of Gene Robinson's laboratory, work that beautifully integrates the effects of neural structures, genes, development, and hormones on honeybee social behavior. I use this approach throughout the book, integrating all of the approaches ethologists use to understand the many proximate influences on specific animal behaviors.

▶ **AN EXTENSIVE DISCUSSION OF PHYLOGENY.** Darwin spoke of two "great laws," one centered on natural selection and the other on phylogeny. An emphasis on phylogeny has become more evident in animal behavior research in the last few years, and so this edition delves more deeply into the role that phylogeny plays in understanding fundamental issues in animal behavior. Chapter 2 provides an overview of phylogenetic approaches to ethology, and later chapters include comprehensive discussions of the phylogeny of specific animal behaviors, including learning, parental care, cooperation, foraging, migratory behavior, and play. For example, the text covers how a complete understanding of the evolution of parental care in fish requires not only knowledge of the selective forces that have been operating, but also knowledge of the historical (evolutionary) relationship between the species being studied.

▶ **INTERVIEWS OF PROMINENT RESEARCHERS AT THE END OF EVERY CHAPTER.** As with the first edition, each chapter ends with a two-page interview of a leader in the field. These interviews are meant to engage students by giving a human face to current and exciting research. They also serve a pedagogical purpose because the researchers being interviewed explain *why* they came up with the hypotheses they did, and *how* they went about testing these hypotheses, providing students with valuable lessons in critical thinking. New interviewees are Alan Grafen, Cecilia Heyes, Geoffrey Hill, Karen Hollis, Anne Houde, Rufus Johnstone, Anne Magurran, and Francis Ratnieks. I am also delighted to use interviews of the following people for a second time: Nick Davies, Bernd Heinrich, Jerome Kagan, John Krebs, Hudson Kern Reeve, Sara Shettleworth, Judy Stamps, E. O. Wilson, and Richard Wrangham. I am grateful to each and every one of these very busy people for taking the time to answer questions about the foundations of animal behavior.

▶ **THE NORTON ANIMAL BEHAVIOR DVD.** To illustrate animal behavior in its entirety and to show students the behaviors they are learning about, the text includes hundreds of beautiful photos and line drawings. But that isn't enough. Students in the twenty-first century have been weaned on videos, and they expect to see animals in action. They will not be disappointed. In addition to the photos and line art in the text, we are providing instructors who adopt this book with a collection of nearly 200 wonderful *videos* that capture the beauty of studying animal behavior. We hope that providing this resource will help professors share with students the awe and excitement that animal behaviorists experience when studying behavior in action, whether in the lab or in the field.

INSTRUCTOR RESOURCES

THE NORTON ANIMAL BEHAVIOR DVD

Available to instructors who adopt *Principles of Animal Behavior*, Second Edition. A resource of nearly 200 video clips accompanied by a booklet written by Jim Hare of the University of Manitoba, in which he provides short descriptions of each clip. The footage is drawn from three sources:

1. RESEARCHERS CITED IN THE TEXT. Numerous adopters of the first edition of this book expressed a desire to show their students the studies described in the text. Many researchers generously provided their lab and field videos to make this desire a reality.

2. BBC. Most people who are familiar with the BBC's offerings rank their collection of animal behavior videos as among the best in the world. In reviewing the clips that are included on *The Norton Animal Behavior DVD*, I am inclined to agree. We are fortunate to be able to offer so many BBC video clips of animal behavior in this book.

3. CORNELL LAB OF ORNITHOLOGY. The Cornell Lab of Ornithology has an unparalleled collection of footage done by animal behavior researchers. The quality of both the production and the science in the CLO's collection is remarkable.

INSTRUCTOR'S MANUAL

Ryan Earley of the University of Alabama has updated the *Instructor's Manual* to reflect changes in the second edition of the text. This resource includes in-depth answers to end-of-chapter discussion questions in the text. It also includes a bank of multiple-choice questions, as well as review and challenge questions, from which instructors can draw when creating tests.

NORTON MEDIA LIBRARY

A CD-ROM including digital files of all drawn art and most photographs is available to adopters of the text.

ACKNOWLEDGMENTS

I wish to thank my editor, Michael Wright, for shaping this second edition. His editorial skills helped to make the book what it is. I also would like to thank Jack Repcheck, my editor on the first edition of this book, for all the time and effort that he invested in this project. Sandy Lifland has remained the developmental editor across the first and second editions, and I could not be more pleased; her work is fantastic. Sandy's eye for detail and her sense of what makes for a good book have been invaluable.

My thanks also go to Ryan Earley, who has been involved in both editions of this book, producing a wonderful *Instructor's Manual* for each edition. I would also like to thank Jim Hare for his outstanding work on *The Norton Animal Behavior DVD*. Jim not only selected each and every clip on the DVD, but he also wrote useful and succinct descriptions for each clip that will aid instructors in presenting the clips in their lectures. Jim's extensive field experience, and his deep understanding of the conceptual underpinnings of animal behavior, are evident in every description. I also extend my thanks to electronic media editor Sally Whiting for helping us all turn the idea of a DVD into a reality.

The production of the text itself has benefited from the artistic skills of Kelly Paralis Keenan of Penumbra Design, Inc., who created the new schematics for the book, and of John McAusland, who produced the graphs and flowcharts for the book. The keen eyes of my photo editors, Kelly Mitchell and Rae Grant, have taken the text and brought it to life through the beautiful new photos that they found. Production manager Chris Granville deserves thanks for managing the transformation of the manuscript files into a beautiful book and for coordinating the many aspects of the book's production. I am also grateful to Jennifer Cantelmi for her assistance in helping us keep track of all the important details of the project. And all of this—the whole book—might have turned out differently had it not been for my remarkable agent, Susan Rabiner.

Literally dozens of my colleagues have read all or parts of *Principles of Animal Behavior*, and I extend my thanks to them all. The manuscript of the first edition of the book was reviewed by Marc Bekoff, Samuel Beshers, Anne Clark, Fred Dyer, Susan Foster, Nick Fuzessery, Deborah Gordon, Ann Hedrick, Geoff Hill, Anne Houde, Rudolph Jandler, Curt Lively, Anne Magurran, Michael Mesterton-Gibbons, Manfred Milinski, Allen Moore, Dan Papaj, Geoff Parker, David Pfennig, Naomi Pierce, Locke Rowe, Michelle Scott, Max Terman, and Jerry Wilkinson. Reviewers for the second edition of the book were Andrea Aspbury, Marc Bekoff, Thore Bergman, Richard Buchholz, Terry Christenson, Anne Clark, Reuven Dukas, George Gamboa, Harold Gouzoules, David Gray, Douglas Grimsley, Teresa Horton, Melissa Hughes, Eileen Lacey, John Maerz, Jill Mateo, Jennifer Mather, Kevin McGraw, Roger Mellgren, Peter Nonacs, Shawn Nordell, Dan Papaj, Aras Petrulis, Stephen Pruett-Jones, Rick Relyea, Christoph Richter, Bruce Schulte, Con Slobodchikoff, Jeanette Thomas, Kaci Thompson, Sean Veney, Stim Wilcox, and Sarah Wooley. The manuscript in each edition benefited from their close reading and sound advice. Please credit these folks with all that is good about this book, and assign any problems you have to my hand.

Lastly, special thanks go to my wife Dana, who helped with almost every aspect of this project, and to my son Aaron for being such a special young man, and for keeping me smiling. Also thanks to Red C., who knows who he is.

L.A.D.
June 2008

Principles of
Animal Behavior

SECOND EDITION

Principles of Animal Behavior

3

FIGURE 1.1. American cockroach.
Almost everyone is familiar with the roach, often a pest in households around the world. *(Photo credit: Bates Littlehales/ Animals Animals—Earth Scenes)*

I grew up in the heart of New York City. Metropolitan New York may be a melting pot of human diversity, but it is anything but a hotbed of animal diversity. One animal that my family and I did encounter on a fairly regular basis, however, was the American cockroach (Figure 1.1). Much to my mother's chagrin, we seemed locked in a never-ending battle with these creatures— a battle, I might add, that we usually lost. And we probably lost because cockroaches have been subject to this sort of problem—other organisms trying to kill them—for tens of millions of years. As a result, they have evolved an exquisite set of antipredator behaviors, and this has had the side effect of long making them a thorn in the side of apartment dwellers.

Even as a young child I was able to draw some inferences and formulate some hypotheses about cockroach behavior by watching my mother put out the bug traps. First, it seemed to me that roaches liked to spend their time in dark places, and second, it appeared that most roaches agreed on what was a good place for roaches to be, as my mom kept putting the traps out in the same place. These two thoughts on cockroach behavior could easily be developed into the following hypotheses: (1) cockroaches will choose dark places over light places, and (2) roaches tend to return to the same places, rather than moving randomly through their environment. Of course, as a young boy, I didn't formally sit down and generate these hypotheses, and I surely didn't run the controlled experiments that a scientist studying animal behavior would run to test these ideas, but I was nonetheless dabbling with scientific hypotheses about animal behavior—a field technically known as **ethology**. Although ethology overlaps with **ecology**, they are different disciplines, with ecologists focusing on the interaction of organisms with their environment, and ethologists investigating all aspects of animal behavior.

There are many people who think like ethologists: from my mother, who understood roach behavior, to the farmer, who has detailed knowledge about pigs, cows, chickens, and other domesticated farm animals. What's more, people who also think like ethologists include the girl who works to train her dog, and the outdoorsman who, on his camping vacation, searches for some animals and tries to avoid others. Indeed, humans have always thought and acted like ethologists. If our hunter-gatherer ancestors had not thought like ethologists, and hadn't, for example, understood the prey they were trying to catch, as well as the behavior of the predators that were trying to catch them, we humans wouldn't be here today.

The study of animal behavior appears to have been so fundamental to human existence that the earliest cave paintings tended to depict animals. This was certainly not inevitable—early cave drawings might have focused on any number of things, but apparently understanding something about the other life forms surrounding our ancestors was fundamental enough that primitive man chose animals as the subjects for the first modern art. This focus on animals, and their behaviors, continued as humans began developing other types of art. For example, using artifacts from 4,000-year-old Minoan cultures, Marco Masseti argues that the Minoans had an advanced understanding of some aspects of animal behavior (Masseti, 2000). One fascinating example supporting this claim is a golden pendant from a Cretan cemetery that depicts two wasps transferring food to one another (Figure 1.2). Masseti hypothesizes that this kind of knowledge of insect food-sharing behavior could only have come from people who observed and studied the details of wasp life. A similar sort of argument is offered regarding a beautiful wall painting of "white antelopes."

FIGURE 1.2. Art captures animal behavior. This pendant from the Chrysolakkos funeral complex in Crete suggests that some members of the ancient culture had a detailed knowledge of bees and animal behavior in general. *(From Masseti, 2000, p. 90)*

This painting most likely depicts gazelles in the early stages of an aggressive interaction (Figure 1.3), and again it is the sort of art that is associated with an in-depth knowledge of the subject in question (Voultsiadou and Tatolas, 2005).

Spanning the millennia between ancient Cretan civilization and the present, there have been literally thousands of amateur and professional naturalists who have made some contribution to the study of animal behavior. These contributions have enabled ethologists to draw on a rich trove of information that has greatly expanded our understanding of animal behavior (Figure 1.4). Aristotle's work on animals, for example, though 2,500 years old, is a veritable treasure chest of ethological tidbits. Indeed, with Aristotle's books, *Physics* and *Natural History of Animals*, the field of natural history was born. In these and other works, Aristotle distinguished among 500 species of birds, mammals, and fish, and he wrote entire tracts on the behavior of animals.

This is a textbook about animal behavior and, in many ways, a course in animal behavior is where all the other biology and psychology classes that students have sat through up to this point in their academic career come together. Evolution, learning, genetics, molecular biology, development, neurobiology, and endocrinology congeal into one grand subject—animal behavior. The field of ethology is integrative in the true sense of the word, in that it combines the insights of biologists, psychologists, anthropologists, and even mathematicians and economists. To cover such a diverse array of topics is a daunting task, but in the case of ethology, the case studies, field studies, and experiments that drive the narrative in this book should make the learning enjoyable.

FIGURE 1.3. Wall paintings of "white antelopes." The drawing may depict a "lateral intimidation" during an aggressive encounter between antelopes. *(From Masseti, 2000)*

Types of Questions and Levels of Analysis

In this book, we shall see that ethologists have asked questions about almost every conceivable aspect of animal behavior—feeding, mating, fighting, and so on. At a broad level, however, we can talk about different *types of questions*

FIGURE 1.4. Fantastic images from a cave. A beautiful drawing of a herd of antelope found on the walls of a cave at Dunhuang, China. *(Photo credit: Pierre Colombel/Corbis)*

that ethologists pose. In a classic paper entitled "On the Aims and Methods of Ethology," Niko Tinbergen argued that animal behaviorists ask four types of questions (Tinbergen, 1963). These questions center on:

- Immediate stimuli—what stimuli elicit behavior? These stimuli can take many forms, including neurobiological, chemical, hormonal, and so on.
- Development—how does the behavior of interest change as an animal matures?
- Survival function—how does behavior affect survival and reproduction?
- Evolutionary history—how does behavior vary as a function of the evolutionary history, or **phylogeny**, of the animal being studied?

Literally thousands of studies have been undertaken on each of these four types of questions. Tinbergen's questions can be boiled down to two different kinds of analyses—proximate analysis and ultimate analysis (Alcock and Sherman, 1994; Dewsbury, 1992, 1994; Hailman, 1982; Hogan, 1994; Huxley, 1942; Mayr, 1961; Orians, 1962; Reeve and Sherman, 1993). **Proximate analysis** focuses on *immediate causes*, while **ultimate analysis** is defined in terms of the *evolutionary forces* that have shaped a trait over time. As such, proximate analysis incorporates Tinbergen's first two types of questions, while ultimate analysis covers the latter two types. We could ask, for example, the following question: Why do humans like sugar? A proximate explanation might center on the sequence of events that occurs between the moment that the sugar makes contact with the taste buds to the point where the section of the brain associated with rewards is stimulated. An ultimate explanation, on the other hand, would ask: What selective forces in our evolutionary past would have favored individuals who had strong preferences for sugary foods and liquids?

In each and every chapter of this book, we will be examining all aspects of animal behavior from both proximate and ultimate perspectives.

Three Foundations

Incredible tales and fascinating natural history make a textbook on animal behavior different from a textbook on organic chemistry or molecular genetics. What links animal behavior to all scientific endeavors, however, is a structured system for developing and testing hypotheses and a bedrock set of foundations on which such hypotheses can be built. Over and over again throughout this book, we shall see that the force of natural selection, the ability of animals to learn, and the power of transmitting learned information to others (cultural transmission) serve as the foundations upon which we shall build our approach to ethology.

Charles Robert Darwin accomplished many things in his classic book, *On the Origin of Species*—a text widely regarded as the most important biology book ever written. In this book, Darwin put forth his argument on evolution by natural selection (Darwin, 1859). In a nutshell, Darwin argued that any trait that provided an animal with some sort of reproductive advantage would be favored by a process that he dubbed natural selection. **Natural selection** is thus the process whereby traits that confer the highest relative reproductive success (that is, the greatest relative fitness) on their bearers and that can be passed down across generations increase in frequency over many generations (evolutionary time). Again and again, we shall turn to natural selection to understand animal behavior.

In addition to natural selection changing the frequency of different behaviors over the course of many generations, **individual learning** can alter the frequency of behaviors within the lifetime of an organism. Animals learn about everything from food and shelter to predators and familial relationships. If we study how learning affects behavior within the lifetime of an organism, we are studying learning from a proximate perspective. If we study how natural selection affects the *ability* of animals to learn, however, we are approaching learning from an ultimate perspective. Both approaches can shed light on animal behavior, and throughout the book we shall be employing these complementary approaches to learning.

Cultural transmission is a third major force affecting animal behavior. While definitions of cultural transmission vary across disciplines, when we speak of this phenomenon, we shall be referring to situations in which animals learn something by copying the behavior of others, through what is typically referred to as **social learning**. Cultural transmission can allow newly acquired traits to spread through populations at a very quick rate, as well as permit the rapid transmission of information across generations.

FOUNDATION 1—NATURAL SELECTION

Darwin recognized all too well that his theory of natural selection applied to behavioral traits as well as morphological, anatomical, and developmental traits. Indeed, morphological traits are often the physical underpinning for the production of behavior, and so morphology and behavior are often linked at many different levels. We shall go into more detail about this linkage below and throughout the book, but for the moment, the key point here is that Darwin's ideas on evolution, natural selection, and behavior were revolutionary, and ethology today would look very different were it not for the ideas that Darwin set forth in *On the Origin of Species*. To see how natural selection operates on animal behavior in the wild, we begin with a fascinating example involving mating and parasites in Hawaiian crickets.

In the evening on the Hawaiian Islands, male crickets sing to attract their mates. This "singing" results when the male cricket rapidly moves the smooth scraper on the front of one wing against the serrated file on the other wing. Females cue in on male songs, and they typically refuse to mate with males that do not produce songs. But as with many behavioral traits associated with attracting mates, male singing is not cost free. For just as females are attracted to male song, so are potentially very dangerous parasites (Zuk and Kolluru, 1998).

Marlene Zuk and her colleagues have been studying this trade-off in song production—between attracting females, on the one hand, and attracting parasites on the other—in the field cricket *Teleogryllus oceanicus* (Zuk et al., 2006). This North American species of crickets is parasitized by the fly *Ormia ochracea*, a species that is attracted to the singing male *T. oceanicus*. If a fly finds a singing cricket, it lays its eggs on the cricket, after which the fly larvae burrow their way into the cricket and grow. When the flies emerge from the larvae, they kill the cricket.

Parasitic flies are found on three Hawaiian Islands—Oahu, Hawaii, and Kauai—that are also home to *T. oceanicus*. The flies are most prevalent on the island of Kauai, however, where 30 percent of the crickets are parasitized. Zuk and her team have been studying the relationship between crickets and parasitic flies since 1991, and over time, they noted what appeared to be a significant decline in the cricket population on Kauai. Over the years, they heard fewer and fewer singing males on this heavily parasitized island, and they assumed that the parasitic fly was slowly causing the extinction of *T. oceanicus* on Kauai. Indeed, in 2003 they heard only a single male singing. Nonetheless, when they got down on their hands and knees and searched for crickets, Zuk and her team found *T. oceanicus* in abundance.

Surprisingly, the researchers found that most of the males on Kauai had modified wings that were not capable of producing song (Figure 1.5). The file section of the wings of these Kauai males (called "flatwing males") was significantly reduced compared to that of normal males, and its position on the wings changed, such that song production was no longer possible. These changes were likely the result of mutations of one, or possibly, a few genes associated with wing development and song production. Once such mutations arose, natural selection should strongly favor such flatwing males, who would virtually never be parasitized by very dangerous flies. Or should it?

While it is true that flatwing males have a huge survival advantage, they are also at a severe disadvantage with respect to attracting females, who hone in on singing males as potential mates. For flatwing males to be favored by natural selection, they must somehow still secure opportunities to mate. Zuk and her colleagues hypothesized that flatwing males do this by staying near the handful of singing males still on Kauai, and mating with females as they approach singers. To test this hypothesis, they collected 133 Kauai males—121 of which were flatwings, and 12 of which were singers. They then used "playback" experiments, in which male songs were broadcast over loudspeakers. What they

FIGURE 1.5. Natural selection in crickets. Marlene Zuk and her colleagues have been studying the field cricket *Teleogryllus oceanicus*. Pictured here are **(A)** a field cricket with normal wings (the arrow points to the file on its outstretched wing), **(B)** a field cricket with flat wings, in which the file section on the outstretched wing has evolved to a much smaller size and is visible only under a high-powered microscope, and **(C)** sandfly larvae in a parasitized cricket. *(Photo credits: Robin Tinghitella)*

found was that flatwing males were drawn to playbacks more strongly than normal males, suggesting that flatwing males stay near singer males in order to secure chances to mate with females drawn in by the singers. With both a huge survival advantage, and the continued ability to obtain matings, flatwing males should be strongly favored by natural selection. And indeed, Zuk and her colleagues suggest that the mutation leading to the loss of song occurred only fifteen to twenty generations ago, and has quickly increased in frequency, so that now most males on Kauai are flatwing males.

As a second example of natural selection acting on animal behavior, let's examine how individuals in social groups respond to strangers. For animals that live in stable groups, strangers—unknown individuals from outside one's group—represent a significant danger. Such individuals may compete for scarce resources, disrupt group dynamics that have long been in place, and so on. As such, ethologists are interested in whether animals from group-living species display a fear of strangers, a phenomenon technically known as **xenophobia**. In particular, ethologists hypothesize that xenophobia may be especially strong when resources are scarce, since competition for such resources will be intense under such a scenario, and keeping strangers away may have a strong impact on the lifetime reproductive success of group members.

To examine the effect of resource scarcity on the evolution of xenophobia, Andrew Spinks and his colleagues examined xenophobia in the common mole rat (*Cryptomys hottentotus*) (Spinks et al., 1998; Figure 1.6). Common mole rats live in South Africa in underground colonies made up of two to fourteen individuals. They are an ideal species in which to examine xenophobia and its possible connection to resource availability for two reasons: First, all populations of common mole rats are "tightly knit" in the sense that each group typically has a single pair of "reproductive individuals" who produce most of the offspring in a colony, which means that all group members tend to be genetic relatives (Bishop et al., 2004). Second, populations of common mole rats differ in terms of the amount of resources in their environments. Some common mole rat populations inhabit mesic (moderately moist) environments that present only mild resource limitations, while other populations live in arid environments and face intense limitations on their resources. This variation in resource availability is largely due to the fact that mesic environments have about four times as much rainfall as arid environments.

Spinks and his colleagues examined whether populations from arid areas were more xenophobic than those from mesic environments, as one might predict based on our above discussion of natural selection, resources, and xenophobia. To do this, they conducted 206 "aggression" trials. The protocol for these experiments was quite simple: Two mole rats—one from the arid and one from the mesic environment—were placed together, and any aggression that occurred between them was recorded. Results were clear-cut: When the pair of individuals were both males or both females, fear of strangers and aggression toward such strangers was much more pronounced in the common mole rats from the arid environment, where resources were limited, than it was in the common mole rats from the mesic environment. This result was not a function of individuals from arid populations just being more aggressive in general. Control experiments demonstrated that when two individuals who knew each other from the arid population were tested together, aggression disappeared—thus it was the identification of a stranger that initiated the aggression. This is precisely the sort of behavior that natural selection should favor.

FIGURE 1.6. Common mole rats. This xenophobic common mole rat (*Cryptomys hottentotus*) is showing an aggressive stance in response to a stranger. *(Photo credit: Graham Hickman)*

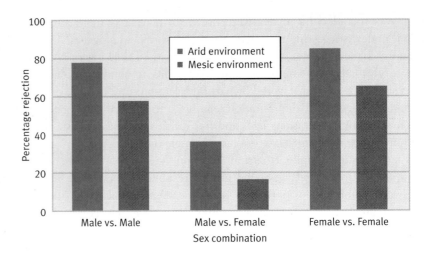

FIGURE 1.7. Xenophobia in common mole rats. Spinks and his colleagues found that individuals were more likely to reject a potential partner via aggression when both mole rats came from an arid environment (green bars) with few resources rather than from a more resource-rich mesic environment (orange bars). *(From Spinks et al., 1998, p. 357)*

Common mole rats that are lucky enough to end up reproducing almost always move from their home colony to find a mate. What this means is that some strangers that are encountered by members of a social group are potential mates, and hence perhaps worth tolerating. Natural selection then should not simply favor all xenophobia, but a xenophobia that is sensitive to the sex of the stranger. In support of this, in trials in which the two individuals tested were a male and a female, Spinks and his colleagues found that while aggression was still uncovered in the low-resource, arid population, the level of aggression decreased dramatically when compared to aggression in same-sex interactions (Figure 1.7). In other words, natural selection has produced common mole rats that temper their fear of strangers as a function of both where they live and the sex of the strangers.

FOUNDATION 2—INDIVIDUAL LEARNING

Individual learning can take many forms (see Chapter 4), but let us begin by considering a hypothetical case of learning in the context of mating. Let's imagine that we are studying a species in which female birds mate with numerous males throughout the course of their lifetime and are able to keep track of how many chicks fledged their nest when they mated with male 1, male 2, male 3, and so forth. Further suppose that older females prefer to mate with the males that fathered the most successful fledglings. We propose to examine the hypothesis that females change their mating behavior as a result of direct personal experience. If we found evidence supporting such a hypothesis, these results might lead us to conclude that learning had changed the behavior of an animal within the course of its lifetime (Figure 1.8).

The learning example above was chosen to emphasize an important relationship between learning and natural selection. In our example, females changed their preference for mates as a result of prior experience, and so learning affected mating behavior within a generation. But just because the frequency of a behavior is changing within the course of an individual's lifetime does not mean that natural selection is removed from the picture, for it is certainly possible for natural selection to operate on the *ability* to learn. That is, natural selection might very well favor the ability to learn about mates over, say, the lack of such an ability. If this were the case in the example above, learning would

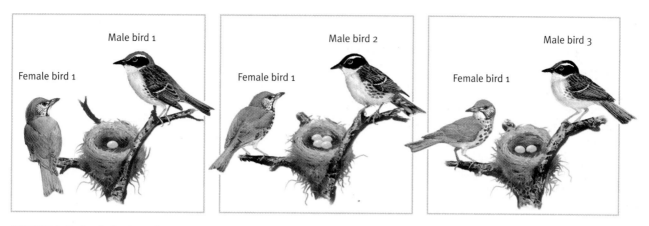

Male bird 1

Female bird 1

Male bird 2

Female bird 1

Male bird 3

Female bird 1

FIGURE 1.8. A role for learning. Imagine a female who mates with different males over the course of time. Such a female might learn which male is a good mate by keeping track of the number of eggs she laid when associated with each male. During future mating opportunities, female bird 1 (pictured here) would be likely to choose male bird 2 because she had learned that she lays the most eggs after mating with him.

change behaviors within a generation, but natural selection might be changing the frequency of different learning rules across generations.

As a good example of how learning and natural selection can be intimately tied together, we turn to Reuven Dukas and Elizabeth Bernays's ingenious experiment examining the fitness consequences of learning in insects (Dukas and Bernays, 2000). While learning in insects is well documented, pinning down the potential fitness-related benefits of learning has proved to be more difficult (Dukas, 2006). To tackle the question of benefits directly, Dukas and Bernays examined the potential fitness-related benefits of learning in the context of feeding behavior in grasshoppers (*Schistocerca americana*) (Figure 1.9).

In their experiment, Dukas and Bernays placed two food dishes in a grasshopper's cage. One dish contained food that provided a "balanced diet (b)" that included proteins and carbohydrates—a diet that promotes maximal growth rates in S. *americana*. The food in a second dish was labeled a "deficient diet (d)." This diet contained flavoring and protein, but no carbohydrates. The balanced and deficient diets had specific odors and specific colors associated with each of them. The diet was supplemented with either citral (odor 1) or coumarin (odor 2), and the food dish was placed near either a brown-colored card (color 1) or a green-colored card (color 2). This created an opportunity for

FIGURE 1.9. Some aspects of foraging in grasshoppers are learned. *Schistocerca americana* grasshoppers learned to associate various cues with food sources. *(Photo credit: © James Winfred Smith)*

FIGURE 1.10. Learning, foraging, and fitness in grasshoppers. (A) A photograph of the experimental set-up. *(Photo credit: R. Dukas)* **(B)** A schematic of the set-up showing the learning and random conditions. In the learning condition, the set-up consisted of a water dish in the center of the cage and a nutritionally balanced dish (b) on one side of the cage and a nutritionally deficient dish (d) on the other side of the cage. Each dish was paired with one odor (citral [cit] or coumarin [co]) and one colored card (brown or green). In the learning condition, when the dishes were removed and replaced by new dishes, the new balanced and deficient dishes were flavored in the same way as the old balanced and deficient dishes and were placed on the same sides of the cage and next to the same colored cards as the old dishes. In the random condition, location, colored card, and odor were all changed when the new dishes were put into the cage later in the day. *(Based on Dukas and Bernays, 2000)*

the grasshoppers to pair balanced and deficient diets with both odor cues and color cues.

Dukas and Bernays's experiment contained a "learning" treatment and what we will call a "random" treatment (Figure 1.10A). In the learning treatment, the balanced diet dish was always associated with one specific odor and one specific colored card. Twice a day, a grasshopper was presented with the two food dishes and allowed to choose one from which to forage. For example, grasshopper A might be placed in a cage in which the balanced diet was associated with the brown color and the odor of coumarin. In principle, grasshopper A could learn that together the cues coumarin and brown color meant that a food dish contained the balanced diet (Figure 1.10B). In contrast, in the random treatment, the odor and color cues associated with the balanced diet would be randomly assigned. For example, in the morning, grasshopper B might have the balanced diet dish paired with the color green and the odor of coumarin, but in the afternoon, the balanced diet dish might be paired with the color green and the odor of citral, while the next morning the balanced diet dish might be paired with the color brown and the odor of coumarin. As such, the grasshopper would be prevented from learning to associate the balanced diet with specific color and odor cues.

Major differences between the learning and random treatments were uncovered. Grasshoppers in the learning treatment ate from the balanced diet dish to a much greater extent than did the grasshoppers in the random treatment (Figure 1.11). That is, grasshoppers learned to pair diet type with color and odor cues when the situation allowed for such learning. Over the course of the experiment, individuals in both treatments increased the proportion of time they spent feeding on the balanced diet, but grasshoppers in the learning treatment

A

B

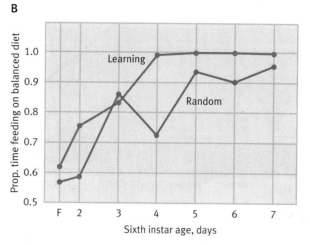

FIGURE 1.11. A balanced diet in grasshoppers. Grasshoppers in the instar stage of insect development were given a choice between a balanced diet or a deficient diet, and researchers recorded the proportion of visits and feeding times of those in a learning treatment and those in a random treatment. In the learning condition, the food was presented in a way in which grasshoppers could learn to associate colored background cards and odors with balanced and unbalanced diets, while this was not possible in the random condition. **(A)** Grasshoppers in the learning condition visited the balanced diet dish more often than those in the random condition. **(B)** Grasshoppers in the random condition eventually also ended up feeding more often on the balanced diet dish, but it took more trial and error for them to recognize and feed on the balanced diet. *(From Dukas and Bernays, 2000)*

did so more quickly than did those in the random treatment. This difference was most likely due to the fact that grasshoppers in the learning treatment went to the balanced diet dish almost immediately when feeding, while those in the random treatment ended up at the balanced diet dish, but only after much sampling of the deficient diet dish. Perhaps most important of all, the individuals in the learning treatment had a growth rate that was 20 percent higher than that of the grasshoppers in the random treatment (Figure 1.12).

Thus, the ability to learn about food in S. *americana* translated into important gains, with a significant increase in growth rate observed in individuals in the learning treatment. This difference in growth rate likely translates into greater fitness later in life, as growth rate is positively correlated with the number and size of eggs laid over the course of an individual's life (Atkinson and Begon, 1987; Slansky and Scriber, 1985).

FOUNDATION 3—CULTURAL TRANSMISSION

Recall that when we speak of cultural transmission, we are referring to situations in which animals learn something by copying the behavior of others through what is known as social learning. This is, by far, the least studied of our three foundations, but ethological work in this area is growing very quickly (Danchin et al., 2004; Galef and Laland, 2005; Galef et al., 2005; Kendal et al., 2005; Mesoudi et al., 2006).

For an interesting case study illustrating the importance of cultural transmission and social learning in animals, let's consider Jeff Galef's work on foraging in rats. Rats are scavengers, and they are often presented with

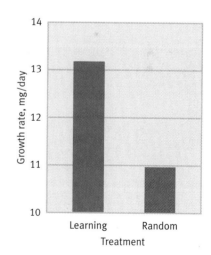

FIGURE 1.12. Fitness and foraging. Not only did grasshoppers in the learning condition approach the balanced diet dish more often, but this translated into quicker growth. Growth rate in grasshoppers is positively correlated with egg size and number. *(From Dukas and Bernays, 2000)*

A

B

FIGURE 1.13. Scavenging rats and cultural transmission. (A) When a rat scavenges in the trash, it may encounter new food items that are dangerous or spoiled and that can lead to illness or even death. **(B)** Smelling another rat provides olfactory cues about what it has eaten. This transfer of information from one rat to another about safe foods is a form of cultural transmission. *(Photo credits: Stephen Dalton/Mindon Pictures; Tom McHugh)*

opportunities to sample new foods (Figure 1.13A). This has probably been true for most of the rat's long evolutionary history, but it has been especially true over the last few thousand years, during which time humans and rats have had a close relationship. Scavenging presents a foraging dilemma. On the one hand, a new food source may be an unexpected bounty for rats. On the other hand, new foods may be dangerous, either because they contain elements inherently bad for rats, or because rats don't know how a new food should smell, and so it is difficult to tell if some piece of this new food type is fresh or spoiled. One possible way to get information about new food types, however, is through the cultural transmission of information.

Galef began his study of cultural transmission and food preferences in rats by testing what is known as the information-center hypothesis (Ward and Zahavi, 1973). This hypothesis posits that foragers may learn critical pieces of information about the location and identity of food by interacting with others who have recently returned from foraging (Figure 1.13B). Galef and his colleagues tested this hypothesis in the Norway rat, a species that often finds itself in this precise scenario (Galef and Wigmore, 1983). To test whether cultural transmission via social learning played a role in rat foraging, rats were divided into two groups—observers and demonstrators (also known as tutors). The critical question that Galef examined was whether observers could learn about a new, distant food source simply by interacting with a demonstrator that had recently encountered such a food source.

After living together in the same cage for a few days, a demonstrator rat was removed and taken to another experimental room, where it was given one of two new diets—either rat chow flavored with Hershey's cocoa (eight demonstrators) or rat chow mixed with ground cinnamon (eight demonstrators). The demonstrator was then brought back to its home cage and allowed to interact with the observer for fifteen minutes, at which time the demonstrator was removed from the cage. For the next two days, the observer rat was given two food bowls, one with rat chow and cocoa, the other with rat chow and cinnamon. Keep in mind that observers had no personal experience with either of the novel food mixes they were experiencing, nor had they ever seen their tutor eat these new food items. Galef's results were clear. Through the use of olfactory cues, observer rats were influenced by the food their tutors had eaten, and they were more likely to eat the food that their tutors had eaten (Figure 1.14).

As was the case for individual learning, it is certainly possible that if "copy the diet choice of others" is a genetically coded behavior in the animal, this behavior may increase in frequency across generations through natural selection. But cultural transmission is more complicated than individual learning. The reason for this is that what an animal learns via individual learning is lost when that animal dies. The actual information that one learns via individual learning never makes it across generations. This is not the case with cultural transmission. What a single animal does, if the behavior is copied, can affect individuals many generations down the road (see Chapter 5).

Suppose adult rat A (in generation 1) adopts a new, formerly uneaten, type of food into its diet because it smelled this food on a nestmate. Now suppose young individuals (generation 2) in the same colony as rat A add this new food to their diet because they smell it on rat A. When individual A eventually dies, the cultural transmission chain it began may still be in force, as the young individuals who copied rat A will still be around. In other words, a culturally learned preference in generation 1 may make it to generation 2 (Figure 1.15). If generation 3 individuals learn from generation 2 individuals, then our culturally derived preference will have been transmitted across two generations. And potentially so on down the generations (Mesoudi et al., 2006). Cultural transmission itself, in other words, has both within- and between-generation effects (see Chapter 5).

FIGURE 1.14. Social learning and foraging in the Norway rat. Observer rats had a "tutor" (demonstrator) who was trained to eat rat chow containing either cocoa (CO) or cinnamon (CIN) flavoring. Once the observer rats had time to interact with a demonstrator rat, the observer rats were much more likely to add their tutor's food preferences to their own. *(From Galef and Wigmore, 1983)*

FIGURE 1.15. A role for cultural transmission. In panel 1, a rat eats a new food type (hot dog). When this rat (D for demonstrator rat) returns to his nest (panel 2), observer rats (O1) smell him, and then are more likely to add hot dogs to their diet when they encounter such an item. Multigenerational cultural transmission occurs when rats from the next generation (O2) smell generation O1 rats after they have eaten hot dogs and subsequently add hot dogs to their own diet (panel 3).

It is important to note that we shall constantly be turning to natural selection, learning, and cultural transmission in our analysis of animal behavior, and that all of them are critical to any broad-based overview of ethology. Yet, by necessity, each chapter of this book does not give equal weight to each of these three forces; in fact, in some chapters, we will not even touch on all three. Historically, there have been many more studies on the role of natural selection on nonlearning-related behaviors (see Chapter 2), and hence this approach will often take up a significant proportion of most chapters. Conversely, while social psychologists have been studying social learning in humans for more than a century (see Chapter 5), it is only over the last few decades that animal behaviorists have seriously investigated social learning, or more generally cultural transmission, and this too is reflected in the text.

Conceptual, Theoretical, and Empirical Approaches

Every question in science can be studied using conceptual, theoretical, and empirical approaches (Dugatkin, 2001a, 2001b; Figure 1.16). This is true in ethology as well. In fact, the best studies in animal behavior tend to use all three of these approaches to one degree or another. In addition to focusing on natural selection, learning, and cultural transmission, the empirical/theoretical/conceptual axis will also play an important role in almost every chapter of this book.

CONCEPTUAL APPROACHES

Conceptual approaches to ethology typically involve integrating what were formerly disparate and unconnected ideas and combining such ideas in new, cohesive ways to make advances in the field. Generally speaking, natural history and experimentation play a role in concept generation, but a broad-based concept itself is not usually directly tied to any specific observation or experiment.

Major conceptual advances tend not only to generate new experimental work, but they also reshape the way that a discipline looks at itself. The clearest case for a conceptual advance that has made animal behaviorists rethink the basic way they approach their science is the late W. D. Hamilton's ideas on

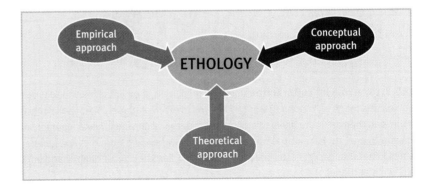

FIGURE 1.16. Different approaches to ethology. Ethology can be studied from a conceptual, theoretical, or empirical approach.

FIGURE 1.17. Kin selection and the mother-offspring bond. In many species, like the vervets shown here, mothers go to extreme lengths to provide for and protect their young offspring. W. D. Hamilton's kin selection ideas provided a conceptual framework for understanding the special relations that close genetic relatives share. *(Photo credit: Alissa Crandall/Corbis)*

kin selection, a theory that natural selection not only favors behaviors that increase the reproductive success of individuals expressing that behavior, but also favors behaviors that increase the reproductive success of their close genetic kin (Figure 1.17).

Hamilton hypothesized that an individual's total fitness, measured by its genetic contribution to the next generation, is not simply a function of the number of viable offspring that it produces (Hamilton, 1964; Figure 1.18). Rather, he made a conceptual breakthrough in recognizing that an individual's total fitness is composed of two parts, one of which is the number of viable offspring that it produces and the other of which are the viable offspring of close genetic relatives. Thus, he saw that when an individual increases the number of its close genetic kin that survive and reproduce, it is indirectly getting copies of its own genes into the next generation. Hamilton termed the sum of these two components the inclusive fitness of an individual.

FIGURE 1.18. Two components to fitness. Three vervet monkeys are pictured—a mother, her juvenile offspring, and her subadult female offspring. Direct fitness effects are a consequence of mother-offspring interactions, while the more mature offspring can increase her indirect fitness by helping her younger sibling. Direct effects are assigned to individuals that physically transmit their genes through their own sperm or eggs to the affected individual. Indirect effects do not require the transmission of gametes between affected individuals. *(Based on Brown, 1987)*

We will explore the logic of inclusive fitness in detail in Chapter 8, but the kernel of this powerful idea is that, evolutionarily speaking, close genetic relatives are important because of their shared genes—that is, genes held in common and inherited from some common ancestor. So, imagine for a moment a Mexican jay bird, a species that has been the subject of much work on inclusive fitness (Brown, 1987). A jay's inclusive fitness is a composite of the number of offspring it has, plus some fraction of the number of offspring it helps a relative raise. Let's say that a jay helps its parents raise an additional brood of two birds, above and beyond what its mother and father could have raised on their own. Our helper is related to its siblings by a value of 0.5 (see Chapter 8 for more on this calculation). By helping mother (and perhaps father) raise two additional offspring, it has contributed 2×0.5 or 1 offspring "equivalent" to its inclusive fitness. If this is the only help that it undertakes, our jay's inclusive fitness is calculated by adding its indirect fitness (from helping its parents to raise its siblings) to its direct fitness (measured by its success at raising its own offspring).

The concept of inclusive fitness has made ethologists and behavioral ecologists rethink their entire discipline (Dugatkin, 2001a). Now, one of the first things that ethologists consider when studying social behavior is whether the individuals involved are close genetic kin. This is a direct result of Hamilton's conceptual breakthrough.

The mathematical theory underlying kin selection is critical for specific predictions in any particular animal system. Kin selection's strength, however, lies not only in its predictive power in any given animal system, but in helping ethologists rethink the way to approach relatedness in ethology in general. The ability of ethologists to understand the concept of kin selection, even outside of the mathematics, is a sure sign that a conceptual idea has made its mark on the discipline.

THEORETICAL APPROACHES

In the late 1960s and early 1970s, ethologists' understanding of how natural selection operates on animal behavior was greatly advanced with the appearance of sophisticated, usually mathematical, models of the evolution of social behavior in animals and humans. This work is most closely associated with George C. Williams, John Krebs, William D. Hamilton, John Maynard Smith, Robert Trivers, E. O. Wilson, and Richard Alexander. As we shall see throughout this book, the models that were developed by these animal behaviorists in the 1960s and 1970s revolutionized the way that ethologists look at almost every type of behavior they study.

A **theoretical approach** to animal behavior entails the generation of some sort of mathematical model of the world. During the formative years of modern ethology, much theoretical work focused on animal foraging behaviors (Kamil et al., 1987; Stephens and Krebs, 1986). One foraging-related question of particular interest was: Given a list of potential edible items, which ones should an animal add to its diet, and under what conditions? To tackle this question, a mathematical tool called optimality theory was used (see Chapter 10). Optimality theory searches for the best (optimal) solution to a particular problem, given that certain constraints exist in a system. In terms of foraging,

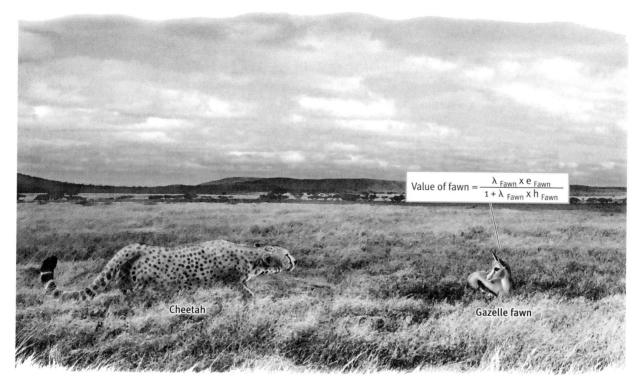

FIGURE 1.19. Mathematical optimality theory and foraging. Cheetahs can feed on many different prey items, including a gazelle fawn. Ethologists have constructed mathematical models of foraging that determine which potential prey items should be taken. The value assigned to each prey is a composite of energy value (e), handling time (h), and encounter rate (λ). We shall delve into the mathematical theory underlying foraging behavior in Chapter 10.

a constraint might be how quickly an area was being depleted of food, and the decision might be how long a forager should stay in a particular food patch it is depleting before moving on to another food patch.

An optimal foraging model might ask how the energy (e) provided by a prey type, the time it takes to handle (h) the prey (that is, to kill and then eat it), and the rate at which prey are encountered (λ) affect foraging decisions made by animals (Figure 1.19). These variables would be placed in a fairly complex algebraic inequality, and solving this inequality would produce numerous testable, and often counterintuitive, predictions (see Chapter 10). For example, the model predicts that the decision to add certain prey types into a forager's diet may not depend solely on how often a predator encounters that prey, but also on how often it encounters (or does not encounter) more preferred prey types. Without a mathematical model of foraging behavior, it is unlikely that anyone could have used intuition to come up with that hypothesis.

One final comment for now on how theoreticians, including those who work on ethological questions, operate. Theoreticians are not interested in mimicking the natural world in their models, but rather in condensing a difficult, complex topic to its barest ingredients in an attempt to make specific predictions. In that sense, the criticism that a particular theory doesn't match the details of any given system will often be true, but irrelevant. A good theory will whittle away the details of specific systems, but just enough to allow for general predictions that can apply to many systems.

EMPIRICAL APPROACHES

The lion's share of this book will be devoted to empirical studies and the **empirical approach**, which involves gathering data and drawing conclusions from that data. Empirical work in ethology can take many forms, but essentially it can be boiled down to one of two types—either observational or experimental studies. Both have been, and continue to be, extraordinarily important to the field of animal behavior.

While empirical studies in ethology preceded the work of Karl von Frisch, Niko Tinbergen, and Konrad Lorenz, modern ethological experimentation is often associated with these three Nobel Prize winners, each of whom was an extraordinary naturalist who had a fundamental understanding of the creatures with whom he worked and the world in which these creatures lived. Above and beyond this, they were able to ask fundamentally important questions about animal behavior—questions that could be addressed by a combination of observation and experimentation.

Observational work entails watching and recording what animals do, but making no attempt to manipulate or control any ethological or environmental variable. For example, I might go out into a marsh and record every action that I see red-winged blackbirds doing from 9 a.m. to 5 p.m. Thus, I might note foraging behavior, encounters with predators, the feeding of nestlings, and so forth, and be able to piece together how red-winged blackbirds in my study population spend their time. Next, from my observations, I might hypothesize that red-winged blackbirds, for example, seem to make few foraging bouts when predators are in the vicinity. To empirically examine the relationship between foraging and predation pressure, I might make detailed observations on how much food red-winged blackbirds eat and how many predators I can spot. I could then look for a relationship between these two variables, and test the notion that they are related (that is, that they are correlated).

Let's say that when I graph foraging behavior against predation pressure, I do in fact find that they are correlated. Redwings do increase and decrease their foraging behavior as a function of the number of predators in their environment. At times when lots of predators are around, redwings forage infrequently, but when predators are few and far between, redwings forage significantly more often. What then can I conclude? Is it fair to say that increased predation pressure causes decreased foraging? No, the data we have so far cannot be used to infer causation. We can say that predation and foraging are correlated, but from the data we have, we can't speak to the subject of what caused what—in other words, we cannot infer causation from correlation. It might be that some other variable is causing both greater predation pressure and less redwing foraging behavior. For example, it might be that when the temperature rises, redwing predators become more active, but redwings themselves become less active, and hence forage less frequently. Increased predation pressure and foraging would still be correlated, but now the former wouldn't be seen as causing the latter; rather, they would both be associated with changes in weather.

In order to examine causality, we must experimentally manipulate our system. We might, for example, experimentally increase the number of redwing predators in area 1, but not in area 2, and see how redwing foraging is affected in these populations (Figure 1.20). This could be done by using trained predators or by simulating increased predation pressure by flying realistic predator

FIGURE 1.20. Observation and experimentation. Imagine your observations led you to believe that red-winged blackbirds decrease foraging when under predation pressure. To experimentally examine causality, you could use a trained falcon to fly over a red-winged blackbird area and observe how this affected the amount of foraging.

models in area 1, but not in area 2. In either case, if we see redwing foraging behavior decrease in area 1, but not in area 2, we can feel much more confident that increased predation pressure causes decreased foraging in red-winged blackbirds.

Before completing this section on conceptual, theoretical, and empirical perspectives in ethology, let us touch on one more topic—the question of whether there is any natural ordering when it comes to the theoretical and empirical approaches. Does theory come before or after empirical work? The answer is, "It depends." Good theory can precede or postdate data collecting and hypothesis testing. On some occasions, an observation or experiment will suggest to a researcher that the results obtained beg for a mathematical model of behavior to be developed. Models of reciprocity and cooperation, for example, originally emerged from anecdotal evidence that many animals appeared to sacrifice something in order to help others. Given that natural selection should typically eliminate such unselfish actions, the anecdotes cried out for mathematical models to explain their existence. Mathematical models were then developed, and they provided some very useful insights on this question, as well as stimulating more empirical work.

On the other hand, the foraging models we discussed earlier in the chapter preceded the large number of empirical studies on foraging that ethologists and behavioral ecologists continue to undertake. While it is true that ethologists have long studied what and when animals eat, controlled experimental work

INTERVIEW WITH

Dr. E. O. Wilson

The 25th Anniversary edition of your classic book *Sociobiology*, a landmark book in the field of animal behavior, was published in 2000. What prompted you to write *Sociobiology*?

In the 1960s, as a young researcher working in the new field of population biology, which covers the genetics and ecology of populations of organisms, I saw the logic of applying the principles of making that discipline the foundation of the study of social behavior in animals. At that time a great deal was known about societies of bees, ants, fish, chimpanzees, and so forth, but the subject largely comprised descriptions of each kind of society in turn, and with few connections. There had been little effort to tie all that information together. I had the idea of analyzing animal societies as special kinds of populations, with their characteristics determined by the heredity of behavior of the individual members, the birth rates of the members, together with their death rates, tendency to emigrate or cluster, and so forth—in other words, all the properties we study and put together in analyzing ordinary, nonsocial populations.

Sociobiology as a discipline grew from this idea and was born, not in my 1975 book with that name (*Sociobiology: The New Synthesis*), but in my 1971 *The Insect Societies*. In this earlier work I synthesized available knowledge of the social insects (ants, termites, the social bees, and the social wasps) on the base of population biology. I defined

the term sociobiology that way, and predicted that if made a full unified discipline it would organize knowledge of all animal societies, from termites to chimpanzees. In *Sociobiology: The New Synthesis* I added the vertebrates to the social insects (and other invertebrates) to

substantiate this view, then in the opening and closing chapters, the human species. In the latter chapters, I suggested that sociobiology could (and eventually would) serve as a true scientific foundation for the social sciences. This was a very controversial notion then, but it is mainstream today.

What do you see as *Sociobiology's* legacy to date?

The legacy of *Sociobiology,* which took hold and generated interest and discussion as *The Insect Societies* never could, is indeed the discipline of

sociobiology, with journals and many new lines of research devoted to it. This advance was greatly enhanced by the rapid growth of studies on animal communication, behavioral ecology, and, in population genetics, kin selection. Of ultimately equal and probably even greater importance, it showed how to create a link of cause-and-effect explanation between the natural sciences, including especially the study of animal social behavior on the one side and the social sciences on the other.

What sort of debt do ethologists owe Charles Robert Darwin?

Ethologists owe an enormous debt to Darwin, by encouraging the deep and now well-established concept that instincts are biological traits that evolved by natural selection. A word on terminology is worth introducing here. Ethology is the systematic (i.e., scientific) study of the behavior of animals (including, by extension, humans) under natural conditions. Sociobiology is the sudy of the biological basis of all forms of social behavior and social organization in all kinds of organisms, including humans, and organized on a base of ethology and population biology. Evolutionary psychology is a spin-off of both ethology and sociobiology, including both social and nonsocial behavior with special links to traditional studies of psychology.

After Darwin, whose work has had the most profound impact on the scientific study of animal behavior?

22 | CHAPTER 1 | PRINCIPLES OF ANIMAL BEHAVIOR

In 1989 the Fellows of the International Animal Behavior Society voted *Sociobiology: The New Synthesis* the most influential book on animal behavior of all time. The most important individual discoveries of all time would have to include sign stimuli, ritualization, the multiple modalities of nonhuman communication, the neurological and endocrinological basis of many forms of behavior, and the amazingly diverse and precise manifestations of kin selection.

Why should a talented undergraduate studying biology care about animal behavior?

Animal behavior is of course a fundamental and extraordinarily interesting subject in its own right. But it is also basic to other disciplines of biology, all the way from neuroscience and behavioral genetics to ecology and conservation biology.

Why should social scientists pay attention to what is happening in the field of animal behavior? What can they gain by doing so?

The social sciences desperately need biology as their foundational discipline, in the same way and to the same degree as chemistry needed physics and biology needed chemistry. Without biology, and in particular genetics, the neurosciences, and sociobiology, the social sciences can never penetrate the deep wells of human behavior; they can never acquire the same solidity and explanatory power as biology and the other natural sciences.

You and Bert Hölldobler won a Pulitzer prize for *The Ants*. Why have you devoted so much time and effort to studying this taxa?

There are two kinds of biologists, those who select a scientific problem and then search for the ideal organism to solve it (such as bacteria for the problems of molecular genetics), and those who select a group of organisms for personal aesthetic reasons and then search for those scientific problems which their organisms are ideally suited to solve. Bert Hölldobler and I independently acquired a lifelong interest in ants as children, and added science to that fascination later.

> Sociobiology is the study of the biological basis of all forms of social behavior and social organization in all kinds of organisms, including humans, and organized on a base of ethology and population biology.

You have written much on the subject of conservation biology. How does work in animal behavior affect conservation biology studies, and vice versa?

The understanding of animal behavior is crucial to conservation biology and its applications. Consider how important to ecosystems and

species survival are the behaviors of mating, territorial defense, dispersal, pollination, resource searching, and predation. To be successfully grasped, these phenomena have to be studied in an organized, scientific manner, not just added haphazardly to conservation strategies.

What do you believe will be the most important advance in animal behavior in the next twenty-five years?

My prediction: the complete linkage of a number of complex behavior patterns from genes to proteonones to sensors and neuron circuits to whole patterns of behavior. Biologists will learn how to scan the whole range of levels of organization to account for each animal behavior in turn.

Will animal behavior be a discipline fifty years from now, or will it be subsumed by other disciplines?

Today the study of animal behavior is the broad gateway to a wide array of different modes of study. But in fifty years—who knows? It may well be subsumed by other disciplines, some as yet undefined.

Dr. E. O. Wilson is an emeritus professor at Harvard University and a member of the National Academy of Sciences. He is the recipient of two Pulitzer prizes, and his book Sociobiology *(Harvard University Press, 1975) is regarded as one of the most important books on evolution and behavior ever written.*

designed to test specific predictions about foraging were initially spurred on by the theoretical work in this area. Regardless of whether theoretical work predates or postdates empirical work, however, a very powerful feedback loop typically emerges wherein advances in one realm (theoretical or empirical) lead to advances in the other realm.

An Overview of What Is to Follow

Following this chapter, we shall work our way through four "primers" that provide an overview of natural selection and animal behavior (Chapter 2), proximate issues in animal behavior (Chapter 3), learning and animal behavior (Chapter 4), and cultural transmission from an ethological perspective (Chapter 5). The topics reviewed in the primer chapters will be intertwined in the remaining twelve chapters, which cover sexual selection (Chapter 6), mating systems (Chapter 7), kinship (Chapter 8), cooperation (Chapter 9), foraging (Chapter 10), antipredator behavior (Chapter 11), communication (Chapter 12), habitat selection and territoriality (Chapter 13), aggression (Chapter 14), play (Chapter 15), aging and disease (Chapter 16), and animal personalities (Chapter 17).

Textbooks on animal behavior often have a closing chapter devoted to one specific animal—our own species, *Homo sapiens*. Rather than adopting this segmented view of behavior, studies of human behavior (though in the minority in this book) will be woven into the fabric of each chapter. Only then can the reader receive a truly integrative view of animal (nonhuman and human) behavior.

As mentioned earlier in this chapter, ethologists need to be as clear as possible about whether a particular study of behavior is examining ultimate questions, proximate questions, or both. It is to the issue of ultimate and proximate approaches to ethology that we now turn in the first two primer chapters.

SUMMARY

1. The scientific study of animal behavior, which dates back hundreds, if not thousands of years, is called ethology.
2. The force of natural selection, the ability of animals to learn, and cultural transmission serve as the foundations upon which we shall build our approach to ethology.
3. Niko Tinbergen has suggested that ethologists ask four types of questions: What stimuli elicit behavior? How does behavior change as an animal develops and matures? How does behavior affect survival and reproduction? How does behavior vary as a function of evolutionary history?
4. Ethologists examine behavior from a proximate perspective—examining immediate causes of behavior—and from an ultimate perspective—examining evolutionary factors that lead to a behavior.
5. Work in ethology, like in all scientific fields, can be conceptual, theoretical, or empirical. Empirical work can be further subdivided into observational and experimental studies.

DISCUSSION QUESTIONS

1. Take a few hours one weekend day and focus on writing down all the behavioral observations you've made, as well as any, even indirect, behavioral hypotheses you have constructed. Think about your interaction with both humans and nonhumans. How has your very brief introduction into ethology reshaped the way you observe behavior?
2. Why do we need a science of ethology? What insights does this discipline provide both the scientist and the layperson?
3. Imagine that you are out in a forest, and you observe that squirrels there appear to cache their food only in the vicinity of certain species of plants. Construct a hypothesis for how this behavior may have been the result of (a) natural selection, (b) individual learning, and (c) social learning.
4. Why do you suppose that mathematical theories play such a large part in ethology? Couldn't hypotheses be derived in their absence? Why does mathematics force an investigator to be very explicit about his or her ethological hypotheses?

SUGGESTED READING

Alexander, R. D. (1974). The evolution of social behavior. *Annual Review of Ecology and Systematics, 5,* 325–383. This paper, published just before E. O. Wilson's *Sociobiology,* provides the reader with a good overview of how one approaches behavior using "natural selection thinking."

Dewsbury, D. (Ed.) (1985). *Studying animal behavior: Autobiographies of the founders.* Chicago: University of Chicago Press. A fascinating introduction to the lives of early ethologists.

Galef, B. G. (1996). Social enhancement of food preferences in Norway rats: A brief review. In C. M. Heyes & B. G. Galef (Eds.), *Social learning in animals: The roots of culture* (pp. 49–64). London: Academic Press. A short, but comprehensive account of one of the best long-term studies of social learning.

Heinrich, B. (1999). *Mind of the raven.* New York: HarperCollins. Heinrich is a top-notch writer who gives the reader a sense of both the science of animal behavior and the beauty of nature.

Tinbergen, N. (1963). On aims and methods of ethology. *Zeitschrift fur Tierpsychologie, 20,* 410–440. A classic paper that outlines Niko Tinbergen's approach to animal behavior.

The Evolution of Behavior

As an undergraduate with a burgeoning interest in evolution and animal behavior, I naturally asked my professors what books I should read to get a better feel for the subject. Every single one mentioned Charles Darwin's *On the Origin of Species*, and so I bought a copy—but not without a bit of trepidation. Even as a novice biologist I was aware that *On the Origin of Species* was considered one of, if not *the* greatest science book ever written, and so I was worried that it would simply be above me (Watson, 2005; Wilson, 2005). As it turns out, this book was not only readable, it was one of the best books that I have ever read.

What surprised me most about Darwin's book was not the ease with which it could be read, but rather the subject material of the first chapter. The opening chapter of the most significant book ever written in biology talks at some length about pigeon breeding in Victorian England. Victorians and others, Darwin noted, had bred many varieties of pigeons that looked and behaved dramatically differently from one another. Indeed, Darwin himself was a pigeon breeder, informing the readers of *On the Origin of Species,* "I have kept every breed [of pigeon] I could purchase or obtain. . . ." (p. 23). These various breeds have exquisite color and very elaborate tail feathers (Figure 2.1).

Darwin was fascinated by both the morphological and *behavioral varieties* of pigeons. "Tumbler" pigeons, for example, seem to somersault over themselves as they fly. Homing pigeons can be released long distances from home and somehow find their way back (Figure 2.2). All of these morphological and behavioral varieties of pigeons were the product of many generations of breeding, primarily by amateur pigeon breeders.

The reason for this seemingly odd subject matter for the opening chapter of *On the Origin of Species* was strategic—Darwin was bracing the reader for what was to come. He knew that his readers would feel at home with a discussion of pigeon breeding, a popular pastime in Victorian days. If Darwin could convince them that the process leading to the creation of extraordinary breeds of pigeons was similar to the process leading to *variation* in nature, his task would be a little simpler. The process leading to pigeon variation—tumbler pigeons, homing pigeons, and so on—is called **artificial selection**, which is defined as

A B

FIGURE 2.1. Natural and artificial selection. Both natural and artificial selection have produced many morphological varieties of the pigeon, including **(A)** bright colors, and **(B)** elaborate tail feathers. *(Photo credits: Brandon Borgelt; Rashad Zainal).*

A

B

FIGURE 2.2. Artificial selection on pigeon behavior. Pigeon breeders have selected for behavioral varieties of pigeons, including **(A)** tumbler pigeons (here we see one bird tumble as it flies), and **(B)** homing pigeons. *(Photo credits: James Whitmore/Time Life Pictures/Getty Images; Alamy Images)*

the process of humans choosing certain varieties of an organism over others by implementing breeding programs that favor one variety over another.

As opposed to artificial selection, the evolutionary process leading to the extraordinary variation—including behavioral variation—that we see in nature is called natural selection, which, you will recall from Chapter 1, is the process whereby traits conferring the highest reproductive success to their bearers increase in frequency over time. Chapter 2 will serve as an introduction or "primer" to the manner in which ethologists think about evolution and animal behavior.

Few concepts have had a more profound impact on the way that animal behaviorists operate than natural selection. Once Darwin's ideas were widely disseminated and integrated into the heart of biology during what is called "the modern synthesis" (Huxley, 1942), animal behaviorists possessed a theory that helped explain not only *what* animals do, but *why* they do it. These sorts of "why" questions—that is, questions that deal with how evolutionary processes shape traits—are often also labeled "ultimate" questions (see Chapter 1). The term "ultimate" does not infer a greater importance attached to such questions than to any other questions in animal behavior. Instead, the word ultimate simply refers to a focus on evolutionary forces per se.

Throughout this chapter, we shall be outlining, step-by-step, how one tackles ultimate questions. We begin this process by discussing how selection operates when humans, rather than "nature," are the selective force shaping behavior; that is, we begin with artificial selection. From there, we will move directly to the discussion of natural selection and animal behavior.

Artificial Selection

For close to 10,000 years, humans have been shaping the way that animals and plants look, as well as the way that animals behave, by the process of artificial selection (Denison et al., 2003). Ever since we selected some varieties of wheat, corn, and rice over others, and systematically planted their seeds, we have been involved in artificial selection. The question "Why do we see particular forms

FIGURE 2.3. Artificial selection on herding behavior. An example of how herding behavior might be selected in dogs. In each generation, the dogs that displayed the "herding" traits that a breeder was interested in would be allowed to breed, with preferential access to breeding given to the best herders. Over many generations, this can lead to dogs that are excellent herders—dogs that will circle around a flock of sheep, keeping the sheep together and also keeping predators away from the flock of sheep.

of grain today?" can only be understood in terms of the process of artificial selection. The same can be said of our systematic preference for breeding certain varieties of dogs over others, as well as hundreds of other examples.

Consider the case of dogs. Suppose we begin an artificial selection program with a group of collies, and we wish to create a variety of dog that is useful in herding sheep. What we want is a dog breed in which individuals will circle around our flock of sheep, keeping the sheep together, and also keeping predators away from our economically valuable flock. How would we go about this through artificial selection? First, we'd begin our breeding program by choosing the individuals that are already closest to our ideal herding dog—that is, those that behaved the way we wanted our dogs to behave. We could determine which male and female collies were best at herding sheep, and keeping flocks safe, and then preferentially breed those individuals. That is, in every generation we would sort the dogs we had, choose those that met our breeding criteria (herding ability) and allow them the chance to mate, while at the same time denying breeding opportunities to those dogs that failed to meet our criteria. With each new generation of dogs, we would repeat this process, producing individuals that were coming closer and closer to our ideal dog variety. Eventually we would recognize that we were as close as we were ever going to get to our ideal herding dog. As with the case of grains, we can answer our "why" question—why do we see the breeds of dog we see today—by referring to a selection process; in this case, artificial selection (Figure 2.3).

With a basic understanding of the nuts and bolts of artificial selection and behavior in hand, we, like Darwin's original readers, are ready to move on to natural selection and animal behavior.

Natural Selection

We will begin our analysis of natural selection at the broadest level possible, and then examine this process and its role in ethological studies in more detail. Given the monumental impact that Darwin's two greatest works, *On the Origin of Species* and *The Descent of Man and Selection in Relation to Sex* have had, it is often surprising to many that Darwin's ideas with respect to natural selection are very straightforward, particularly once artificial selection is understood (Bell, 1997; Darwin, 1859, 1871; Endler, 1986; Williams, 1966). Indeed, Darwin came up with his theory of natural selection before Mendel published his ideas on genetics. But Darwin didn't need to know about modern-day genetics for his theory to work; all he needed to realize was that somehow behavioral traits that affected reproductive success were passed from parents to offspring. Any Victorian naturalist worth his salt would know that offspring resemble their parents, and Darwin was more than a good naturalist—he was an excellent naturalist (Darwin, 1845).

SELECTIVE ADVANTAGE OF A TRAIT

Consider any trait—for example, height, weight, fur color, foraging behavior, mating preferences, and so on—and instead of imagining humans as the selective agent, allow the selective agent to be nature itself. When nature is the selective agent, traits, including behavioral traits, increase or decrease as a function of how well they suit organisms to their environments. If one variety of a trait helps individuals to survive and reproduce better in their environment than another variety of the same trait, and if the trait can be passed down across generations, then natural selection will operate to increase its frequency over time. To see this, let's examine how natural selection might have favored "pack hunting" behavior in wild dogs (*Lycaon pictus*). Modern wild dogs tend to hunt in packs of ten individuals, but let's walk through a hypothetical scenario for the evolution of the trait "hunt in packs" (Creel, 2001; Figure 2.4). We will begin by imagining a simplified scenario during the early stages of wild dog evolution, in which two types of foragers existed: one type that hunted in packs, and one type that hunted prey alone.

FIGURE 2.4. Group hunting in wild dogs. Wild dogs are ferocious predators, and often hunt in groups. Here they are shown capturing a wildebeest. *(Photo credit: © Bruce Davidson/naturepl. com/ARKive)*

Hunting behavior—alone or in groups—represents one component of a wild dog's **phenotype**, where a phenotype is typically defined as the observable properties of an organism. An individual's phenotype itself is the result of its **genotype**—that is, which genes it possesses—and the way that a particular genotype manifests itself in the environment. In our wild dogs hunting scenario, suppose that in the evolutionary past, individuals that hunted as part of a group got more meat, on average, than wild dogs that hunted alone, and that the more food a wild dog took in, the more offspring it could produce (Figure 2.5). When wild dogs that prefer to hunt in groups produce offspring that also like to hunt in groups, this behavioral variant will increase in frequency over time, helping us to understand why modern wild dogs display this behavior. This holds true even if group-hunting behavior produces only a very slight edge in terms of the number of offspring an individual raises. To see why, we need to think about the implication of small differences that are magnified over long periods of time; that is, we need to conceptualize natural selection in terms of an evolutionary time frame.

Even a selective advantage of 1 percent per generation is sufficient for one behavior to replace another over evolutionary time. For example, for the sake of simplicity, let's assume that hunting preference—alone or in groups—is controlled by a single gene. In reality, of course, there are probably dozens of genes that work together to control this trait. The logic we are invoking would work equally well for traits controlled by dozens of genes; it's just that the math would be more difficult, and so for our purposes, let's imagine a single gene at work.

If an **allele**—that is, a gene variant, one of two or more alternative forms of a gene—that codes for group hunting provides its possessors with an average of just 1 percent more offspring per generation than the allele associated with hunting alone, then all else being equal, the group-hunting allele will eventually increase in frequency to the point where virtually all dogs in the population have it. That is, as a result of natural selection, we will end up with a population of individuals that almost always hunt in groups. This is because the selective advantage conferred by group hunting makes those with our hypothetical group-

FIGURE 2.5. Natural selection for group hunting. A schematic of how natural selection could favor wild dogs that prefer to hunt in groups. If hunting in larger groups (up to some maximum group size) provides more food per dog than hunting in smaller groups (or alone), natural selection can favor group hunting.

TABLE 2.1. Fitness benefits and frequency of traits. When population size equals 100, the number of wild dogs that hunt in groups will increase in frequency, and they will eventually make up 100 percent of the population. In this model, we are assuming no mutation and no migration in or out of our population. The number of generations for group hunting to go to 100 percent is calculated as follows: (2/the selective advantage to group hunting) × the natural log of population size. *(Based on Carroll, 2007)*

FITNESS BENEFIT TO GROUP HUNTING	POPULATION SIZE	GENERATIONS BEFORE GROUP HUNTING REACHES 100% OF POPULATION
1%	100	1,060
5%	100	212
10%	100	106
20%	100	53

hunting allele more likely to survive and produce offspring. These offspring, who in turn will have the allele coding for hunting in groups, are more likely to survive and reproduce, and so on, down through the generations. Over evolutionary time, small differences in fitness can accumulate into large changes in gene frequencies. (To see how evolutionary time allows small differences in fitness to translate into large-scale changes in the frequency of traits, see Table 2.1.)

In a breeding population of about 100 wild dogs, if group hunting provided a fitness benefit of just 1 percent, it would increase to a frequency of 100 percent in 1,060 generations. If we assume an average generation time of about five years for a wild dog, that amounts to just 5,300 years. If the selective advantage were 5 percent—that is, if those who hunted in groups had reproductive success that was 5 percent higher than that of other individuals—in just 211 generations, or about 1,055 years, our entire hypothetical population of wild dogs would be composed of animals that hunted in groups. Even the longest time period mentioned—5,300 years—is tiny when we think of natural selection acting over evolutionary time.

HOW NATURAL SELECTION OPERATES

The above example was meant to give you a flavor for how natural selection operates on behavior. At this point, however, we need to delve a bit into the details. What exactly does it take for the process of natural selection to operate, and what is the end product of this process (Bell, 1997; Endler, 1986; Mousseau et al., 1999; Williams, 1966)?

To understand how natural selection operates, the first thing any ethologist must do is to be specific about which behavior is being studied. That is, we don't so much speak of "natural selection" as we do of "natural selection on foraging behavior," or "natural selection on fighting behavior," and so on. Once we have picked a trait, the process of natural selection requires three prerequisites to operate:

- ▸ Variation in the trait—that is, different forms of the trait.
- ▸ Fitness consequences for the trait—that is, the trait must affect reproductive success.
- ▸ A mode of inheritance for the trait—that is, a means to pass the trait on to future generations.

Technically speaking, a fourth requirement also exists, and that is that resources must be limited with respect to the trait being studied. So, if one is studying natural selection and foraging, food in some sense must be limited, while if one is studying natural selection and mating, there must be a finite set of individuals available to mate with, and so on. In practice, our limited resources requirement is almost always met.

To better understand natural selection, let's follow this process with respect to a specific behavioral trait: how quickly an animal will approach a novel object in its environment, which is a behavior that has been well-studied in birds (Drent et al., 2003; van Oers et al., 2004a, 2000b, 2005). "Object" here is used in the broadest sense—for example, a novel object might be an individual from a species that has not been encountered before or a trap put out by humans or a new type of food in the environment. Approaching novel objects can be dangerous (if they turn out to be predators), but it might also yield benefits (if the novel object is a new type of prey). For simplicity, let's designate the time it takes for an individual to approach a novel object in its environment as the "approach" score.

We will now examine approach behavior by stepping through the three prerequisites mentioned—namely, variation, fitness consequences, and mode of inheritance. We will focus on a hypothetical population in a simplified example designed to illustrate the process of natural selection in the clearest possible manner. Let me emphasize again, however, that the details of both novel object approach behavior in birds, and group hunting in wild dogs (discussed earlier), have been well-studied by ethologists in more complicated experiments. Once we finish with our analysis of natural selection and approach behavior in our hypothetical population of birds, in the remainder of this chapter we will focus on discussing published experimental work in animal behavior.

VARIATION. For natural selection to act, there must be variation in the trait under investigation (Mousseau et al., 1999). Such variation is necessary for natural selection to have something to select between. If every animal in our hypothetical population of birds displayed the same approach score, it would be a waste of time studying natural selection on the approach trait in that population because there would be nothing for natural selection to select between (Dingemanse et al., 2002). For selection to act, individuals in our population must differ from one another with respect to approach score—if, for example, average approach scores in our birds range from 30 seconds (approach quickly) to 60 seconds (approach moderately) to 120 seconds (approach slowly), we have behavioral variation in approach score (Figure 2.6).

Variation in a trait can be caused by either environmental or genetic factors. We shall return to these two different forms of variation a bit later, but here we shall focus on **genetic variation**—in our case, behavioral variation in approach score that correlates with genetic differences between birds in our population. Genetic variation in a population can be generated in a number of ways. For

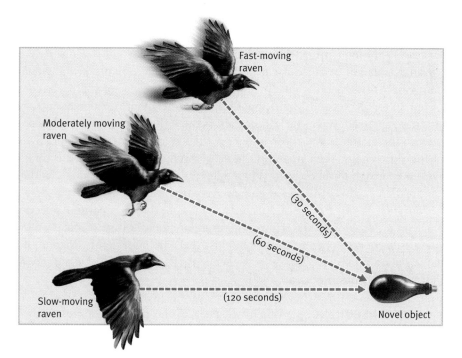

FIGURE 2.6. Natural selection and variation. For natural selection to act on a behavior, behavioral variation must be present in the population under study. In the case of novel object approach behavior, different birds may approach an object they have not previously encountered (for example, a new food source or a brightly colored glass vial, as shown here) slowly (taking 120 seconds to reach the object), moderately slowly (taking 60 seconds to reach the object), or quickly (taking 30 seconds to reach the object).

example, **mutation**—which is defined as any change in genetic structure—automatically creates new variation in a population.

Mutations can manifest themselves in many different ways, and can be caused by such factors as excessive exposure to X-rays, cosmic rays, radioactive decay, ultraviolet light, and various mutagenic chemicals. Genes are made up of DNA, which consists of strands of nucleotides composed of bases, a sugar, and a phosphate group. Addition and deletion mutations occur when a single nucleotide is either added or deleted from a stretch of DNA. Genes code for the production of enzymes and other kinds of proteins (which are made up of amino acids). So this type of mutation typically causes the production of an inactive enzyme, which may, in turn, affect an animal's behavior. Base mutations occur when one base in a nucleotide replaces another. Many base mutations can potentially affect protein function, and hence they may have an impact on an individual's reproductive success often, but certainly not always, by affecting behavior. Some base mutations do not cause changes in which amino acids are produced. These mutations are known as silent mutations. Transposition is a type of genetic mutation in which a section of DNA has its physical location changed from one part of a chromosome to a new location on that same chromosome, or even to a completely different chromosome. Rates of mutation, though fairly low per gene, are sufficiently high across an animal's genome to create significant amounts of new variation over evolutionary time.

In addition to mutation, another factor that affects variation in a population is **genetic recombination**. In sexually reproducing organisms—and the vast majority of animals reproduce sexually, as opposed to asexually—when pairs of chromosomes (one of which comes from the mother and one from the father) line up during cell division, sections of one chromosome may "cross over" and swap positions with sections of the other chromosome. This swapping creates new genetic variation. Crossing-over points are essentially random, and so virtually every possible crossover between a pair of chromosomes is possible in principle. As such, crossing over creates huge amounts of new genetic variation—including genetic variation in behavioral traits—in sexually reproducing organisms.

Although it may sound paradoxical, new genetic variants of a trait can enter a population via nongenetic pathways. The most common way for this to occur is through **migration**. Migration can increase genetic diversity in a given population because it can introduce new trait variants in individuals coming from other populations. In our population, the range of approach scores is from 30 to 120 seconds, but suppose that in a neighboring population some birds have approach scores of 150 seconds. If the differences in approach scores between the migrants and those in our population are a function of underlying genetic differences, then migration increases genetic variation in the time it takes to approach novel objects. When migrants mate with individuals in their new population, this generates even more genetic variation.

Variation is the first prerequisite that must be met for natural selection to act on a behavioral trait. However, variation alone is insufficient to allow natural selection to operate. Not only must there be behavioral variation, but that variation must have fitness consequences (Darwin, 1859; Dejong, 1994; Endler, 1986; Kingsolver et al., 2001).

FITNESS CONSEQUENCES. When we speak of the **fitness** consequences of a trait, we are referring to the change in an individual's reproductive success associated with what behavior that individual displays—for example, slow versus fast approach (Fisher, 1958; Grafen, 1988; Reeve and Sherman, 1993; Williams, 1966). In later chapters, we shall broaden this definition, but for now, "reproductive success" will refer to the mean number of reproductively viable offspring an individual produces.

In our case, variation in approach score must map on to changes in reproductive success, even if only weakly. Without this translation from variation in a trait to fitness differences associated with such variation, natural selection cannot act on approach behavior (or any behavior). To understand why, think about it like this: If we have behavioral variation, but all variants have the same effect on reproductive success, there is nothing for natural selection to select between. Suppose we have 100 birds, and to make things simple, let's imagine that 50 of them show approach scores of 30 seconds, and 50 display approach scores of 120 seconds—in this population, we clearly have variation in approach score. Let's assume that individuals with approach scores of 30 seconds produce an average of 4 offspring, and birds with approach scores of 120 seconds also produce an average of 4 offspring. Since individuals with different approach scores produce the same average number of offspring, variation in approach score (30 versus 120 seconds) does not translate into variation in fitness, and natural selection cannot act on approach score. On the other hand, if all individuals with lower approach scores of 30 had greater reproductive success than all individuals with higher approach scores, then behavioral variation does translate into fitness differences (Figure 2.7). The second prerequisite for natural selection has now been met, and the individuals with lower approach scores will be favored by natural selection.

Conventional wisdom in ethology is that fitness differences are almost always present if the investigator searches hard enough, and experimental work suggests that this is often the case (Endler, 1999; Gould and Lewontin, 1979; Mayr, 1983). In a sense, this is not surprising. The odds that two behavioral variants would have the exact same effect on reproductive success is very low, and we have already seen that over evolutionary time even small differences in reproductive success can have important consequences on the evolution of behavior.

FIGURE 2.7. Natural selection and fitness consequences. If approaching novel objects quickly enables a bird to be the first to reach a new food source, this may contribute to its survival, as it may get more of that food than birds with slower approach times. This variation in approach time will have fitness consequences if it leads to those approaching quickly having more eggs and hence more offspring.

The last prerequisite that needs to be in place before natural selection can operate is a mode of inheritance.

MODE OF INHERITANCE. In order for natural selection to act on a trait, that trait must be passed down from one generation to the next. That is, in addition to variation and fitness consequences, there must be some mode of inheritance in place for natural selection to act on a trait. Without a mode of inheritance, any fitness differences that exist with one generation are washed away, and natural selection cannot move our population of animals toward longer or shorter approach scores. To understand why, imagine that birds with approach scores of 30 seconds have (on average) 5 offspring, and that birds with approach scores of 120 seconds have (on average) 3 offspring. In this case, we have both variation and fitness consequences associated with behavioral variation. If there is no mode of inheritance in place, however, offspring will not resemble their parents with respect to approach score. That is, without a mode of inheritance, individuals who have low approach scores are no more likely to produce offspring with low approach scores than are individuals who have high approach scores, and vice versa. Any fitness associated with approach score would be lost in the next generation and natural selection would not be able to operate on this behavior.

Because genes are passed down from generation to generation, they are the most obvious candidate for a method of transmission. We shall focus on genetic transmission here, holding off our discussion of other modes of transmission until an in-depth discussion of cultural transmission in Chapter 5.

One way to study genes as a mode of transmission is through a population-wide **heritability** analysis, which measures the proportion of variance in a trait attributable to genetic variance (Hartl and Clark, 2006; Mousseau and

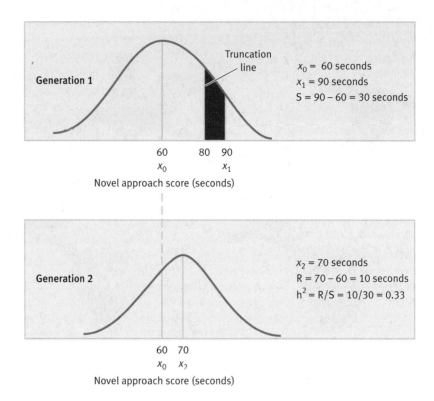

FIGURE 2.8. Heritability of novel object approach. Hypothetical results from our heritability experiment on novel object approach. The mean of *all* Generation 1 individuals (60 seconds) is labeled x_0, and the mean of those Generation 1 individuals that were allowed to breed (90 seconds) is labeled x_1. The mean of *all* Generation 2 individuals (70 seconds) is labeled x_2. $S = x_1 - x_0 = 30$ seconds, $R = x_2 - x_0 = 10$ seconds, $h^2 = R/S = 0.33$.

Roff, 1987). Recall that for natural selection to operate on a trait, there must be variation in that trait—in our case, variation in approach scores. But these *differences* in approach scores—indeed, in any behavior—can come about in many ways. Individuals displaying different approach scores may have been raised on different diets, been exposed to different learning opportunities, and so on. Behavioral differences can also be the result of genetic differences. It is these genetic differences that we use to measure heritability, and, in particular, that portion of genetic variance that is accessible to natural selection.

One means for measuring heritability is by designing a **truncation selection experiment**. In step 1 of an experiment examining heritability in approach scores, we measure the approach score of every bird in our population when it reaches 12 months of age. Suppose this gives us a mean approach score of 60 seconds for generation 1. Let's label this mean value x_0. Step 2 of our experiment is to *truncate*, or cut off, the population variation in approach scores by allowing only those individuals with approach scores greater than some value—for example, 80 seconds—to breed. We then calculate the mean approach score of those individuals that we have allowed to breed. Let us label that mean as x_1, and say that x_1 equals an approach score of 90 seconds in our population (Figure 2.8).

The difference between x_1 and x_0 is referred to as the selection differential, or S. In our case, S = 30 seconds. One way to think about S is as the maximal amount we could expect natural selection to change approach scores—the amount of change that we might expect if all the variation in approach score was variation upon which natural selection could act.

In step 3 of our truncation selection protocol, we raise the offspring produced by generation 1 birds, under identical conditions, until they have reached 12 months of age, and then we measure their approach scores. Let's label the mean approach score of these generation 2 individuals as x_2, and imagine this value to be 70 seconds. The difference between this mean (x_2) and the mean of the entire population in the first generation (x_0) is referred to as the response to selection, or R. It is a measure of how much natural selection has changed approach scores across generations 1 and 2. In our case, R = 10 seconds. Heritability is defined as R/S, and so in our population of birds, the heritability of approach is 10/30 or about 0.33. Another way to say this is that one-third of all the variance in approach is due to genetic variance—variation upon which natural selection can act.

Work in evolutionary biology, population genetics, and animal behavior all suggest that many traits—ranging from morphological to behavioral—show low (0.0 to 0.1) to moderate (0.1 to 0.4) heritability (Hoffmann, 1999; Mousseau and Roff, 1987; Price and Schulter, 1991; Weigensberg and Roff, 1996). As such, the heritability of approach behavior in our hypothetical population of animals falls within the typical range seen for behavioral traits.

The same protocol we have employed for measuring variability, fitness, and heritability of approach scores can be used for any number of different behaviors. This is not to say that obtaining concrete experimental evidence that natural selection operates on animal behavior *in the wild* is an easy task—it isn't, and it often takes years and years of effort to do so (Endler, 1986; Mousseau et al., 1999). There are many studies that *infer* how natural selection has operated on behavior in the wild, but experimental studies that measure natural selection in the field are very difficult to design and implement.

Behavioral Genetics

The sort of heritability analysis we just discussed is often undertaken by **behavioral geneticists** (Plomin et al., 2000, 2002). Behavioral geneticists are involved in many other activities that are linked to ethology, including:

▸ Using Mendel's laws of genetics to predict the distribution of behavioral phenotypes.
▸ Mapping genes for behavioral traits.
▸ Using other measures of heritability to determine what percentage of the variation in a behavioral trait is genetic and what percentage is environmental.

Let us take a look at each of these in turn.

MENDEL'S LAWS

Behavioral geneticists often use Mendel's laws to better understand the underlying genetics of behavioral traits. Mendel's first law—the principle of segregation—essentially states that individuals have two copies of each gene, that such genes remain distinct entities, and that these genes segregate (that is, distribute themselves) fairly during the formation of eggs or sperm. Gene

A

B

FIGURE 2.9. Satellite and independent ruff males. Some of the differences in the mating behavior of **(A)** satellite males and **(B)** independent males are controlled by a single gene with two alleles labeled S and s. The S allele is dominant and codes for satellite male behavior, while the s allele is recessive, and as such two copies of this allele are needed for the behavioral development of independent males. *(Photo credits: BS Thurner Hof).*

variants—alleles—can be **dominant**, meaning that at the genetic level, a single copy of the allele is all that is necessary for a trait to be expressed, or **recessive**, in which case two copies of an allele are necessary for the expression of a trait. To understand behavioral genetics and dominant and recessive alleles as they apply to animal behavior, let's consider the mating behavior of male ruff birds (*Philomachus pugnax*).

In ruffs, males display one of two behavioral strategies during the mating season (we shall return to these mating strategies in later chapters). "Independent males," which make up about 84 percent of the individuals in a population, guard small mating territories (technically referred to as lek arenas). "Satellite males," on the other hand, do not defend their own territories, but instead temporarily share an independent male's mating arena, and form a kind of alliance with independents, in which both individuals court simultaneously to attract the attention of females. Independent and satellite males differ not only in mating strategies, but in coloration and body mass, with satellites being generally smaller and in possession of lighter plumage (Bachman and Widemo, 1999; Hogan-Warburg, 1966; Lank et al., 1995; Figure 2.9). David Lank found that these two alternative mating types—independent and satellite—are primarily controlled by a single gene with two alleles labeled S and s. The S allele is dominant and codes for satellite male behavior, while the s allele is recessive and two copies of this allele are necessary for the development of an independent male. As such, SS and Ss males are satellites, and ss males are independents. It is remarkable that a single gene with two alleles codes for such a complex set of traits—mating strategy, size, and body mass. If we take the knowledge that our behaviors are coded by one gene with two alleles, and we combine that with a natural history–based understanding of mating preferences (which males with which genotypes are preferred as mates), we can make predictions about the distribution of SS, Ss, and ss genotypes over time.

As we shall see in a moment, the relationship between genotype and behavioral phenotype is often not nearly as simple as that seen in the case of ruff mating behavior. Many, if not most, behaviors have a much more complex underlying genetic structure.

LOCATING GENES FOR POLYGENIC TRAITS

In many cases, variation in more than a single gene is responsible for the expression of behavior. Using a number of experimental and quantitative techniques, behavioral geneticists are able to delineate the number of genes underlying such **polygenic** behavioral traits, and they sometimes can even pinpoint the location of such genes. Such findings can provide ethologists with a better understanding of the nature of variation in populations. This is somewhat different from the molecular genetic approach to behavior that we will discuss in Chapter 3, in which genes are often sequenced (the ordered arrangement of nucleotides is delineated) in order to understand the molecular genetic underpinnings of behavior (Kendziorski and Wang, 2006).

For polygenic behavioral traits, behavioral geneticists often search for a *set* of genes, each of which contributes a small amount to the expression of the trait of interest. Such a search is said to be looking for quantitative trait loci (QTLs). Sometimes behavioral geneticists actually locate QTLs, in the sense of delineating the exact region on a chromosome where QTLs lie; at other times, behavioral geneticists can place QTLs underlying a behavior on a specific chromosome, but they can be no more specific. To see how this works, let's examine the work of Jonathan Flint and his colleagues on QTLs and fear/fearlessness in mice (Flint et al., 1995; Solberg et al., 2006; Talbot et al., 1999; Yalcin et al., 2004).

Flint's group first examined fear by recording "open-field behavior" in mice. Open-field behavior measures fear expression when animals are placed in large, open, well-lit environments. Flint's group used two lines of mice that had been bred under artificial selection for many generations: one line of mice had been selected for high open-field activity, and the other for low open-field activity. The behavior of mice from both lines was measured in open-field tests, and, in addition, their fear response was measured when they were placed in two different types of mazes. Fear was measured in a number of different ways, including measuring the rats' activity level and the rates at which they defecate (low activity and high defecation rates are associated with fear in rodents).

After all the behavioral tests were complete and the more fearful mice were identified, the mice were dissected, and Flint and his colleagues collected DNA from the animals' spleens. By comparing variations in the sequencing of nucleotides on the DNA of these tissue samples, Flint and his colleagues were able to identify QTLs for fear on six different mouse chromosomes (1, 4, 12, 15, 17, and 18). More specifically, QTLs for fear during open-field trials were found on these six chromosomes, while QTLs for fear displayed in mazes were found on only a subset of these chromosomes (1, 12, and 15). That is, early work on QTLs and fear in mice found that different types of fear responses were controlled by different subsets of genes, and the researchers described the location of those genes.

Flint's group continued its work on mice, QTLs, and fear/fearlessness behavior, publishing follow-up papers in 1999, and then again in 2004 (Talbot et al., 1999; Turri et al., 2004). In each case, the technological advances in QTL analysis that had occurred since they did their first study in 1995 allowed Flint and his colleagues to provide us with an even more detailed picture of QTLs associated with fear. For example, the 2004 study involved 1,636 laboratory-bred mice, and examined the fear response shown by mice in five different laboratory environments (open field, mazes, mirrored chambers, and so on).

Across these five measures, researchers found evidence of QTLs associated with fear on fourteen different chromosomes (Turri et al., 2004). In other words, behaviors such as fear are often controlled by a large number of different genes, often located on many different chromosomes. If this were the case in natural populations of mice—that is, if many different genes were influencing fear/fearlessness—we would be likely to see a high degree of behavioral variability in this trait in our populations.

With the breakneck speed at which molecular genetics is progressing, and with collaborations on the rise between ethologists and behavioral geneticists, it is only a matter of time before our understanding of the genetics of behavioral traits becomes much more sophisticated and comprehensive.

DISSECTING BEHAVIORAL VARIATION

In addition to identifying and locating QTLs, behavioral geneticists are interested in better understanding the nature of the variation underlying behavioral traits. We have already touched on this point in our earlier discussion of heritability, but let's look at how behavioral variation occurs in a bit more detail, using some ethological data gathered in the field. In order to do so, we must first discuss another technique to measure the heritability of a trait.

In addition to the truncation selection method we outlined earlier, heritability can also be measured through **parent-offspring regression**. The idea here is simple. Parents pass on genes to their offspring, and so, when heritability is high, the behavioral variation one sees in offspring should map onto the behavioral variation observed in parents. The greater the role environmental variance—differences between the environments experienced by parents and offspring in relation to diet, location, and so forth—plays in determining variance in behavior, the lower the heritability of that behavior. To see how parent-offspring analysis can help us understand behavioral variance, we will look at Charles and Mary Brown's work on behavior in cliff swallows (*Petrochelidon pyrrhonota*; Figure 2.10). In particular, we will focus on using parent-offspring regression in dissecting the behavioral variance in an individual's preference for living in larger or smaller groups.

A **B**

FIGURE 2.10. Cliff swallows in their nests. Charles and Mary Brown have studied these birds for twenty years. In cliff swallows, preference for group size is a heritable trait. **(A)** Cliff swallow nests are often clustered together. **(B)** A closeup of one nest with chicks, and the mother standing next to the nest. *(Photo credits: Charles Brown)*

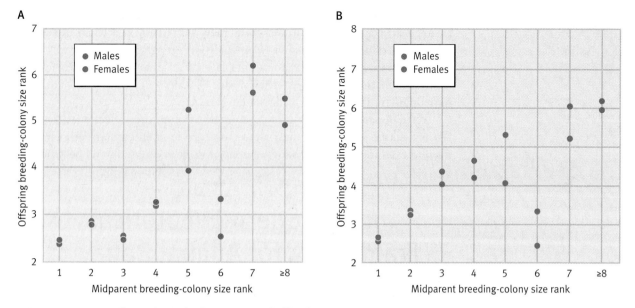

FIGURE 2.11. Breeding colony size in parents and offspring. There is a correlation between breeding colony size in parents and offspring in cliff swallows. Charles and Mary Brown sampled thousands of birds in their native habitat and found a strong correlation between parent and offspring colony size. This held true for all offspring **(A),** as well as for offspring who bred away from their natal site **(B).** *(From Brown and Brown, 2000)*

For the past twenty-five years, the Browns have conducted field studies of cliff swallow birds—a species in which group size affects survival, for example by affecting rates at which parasites move from bird to bird and the mortality resulting from parasitic infection (Brown and Brown, 2004a, 2004b). They tackled the question of how to dissect behavioral variation in group size preferences in two related experiments (Brown and Brown, 2000). In experiment 1, using five clusters of cliff swallow colonies, and an incredible 2,581 birds, Brown and Brown found that the group size in which individual swallows lived was statistically similar to the group size in which their parents lived. This was true for birds that bred at the same site as their parents, as well as for offspring that emigrated elsewhere, suggesting that the correlation between parent and offspring was not a function of living in the same place per se (Figure 2.11). If the correlation in group-size preference was due to parents and their offspring living in the same environment—that is, if this variance in group size was due to environmental variation—we would expect that correlation to disappear when offspring emigrated and lived in different environments from their parents. But that isn't what Brown and Brown found, suggesting that preference for group size is a heritable trait.

In their second experiment, Brown and Brown used nestlings from two *large* and five *small* colonies. Half the young from the nests in the large colonies were removed (the other half remained in the nest), and the young from small colonies were placed in their stead. Likewise, half the young in small colonies were replaced by young from large colonies. As such, in all their manipulated nests, Brown and Brown had offspring from both large and small colonies. This is referred to as a **cross-fostering experiment**, and of the almost 2,000 birds in this experiment, 721 were recaptured and used for a parent-offspring regression on preference for group size.

When examining the preference for group size in cross-fostered offspring, the Browns found a positive correlation with the group-size preferences of their genetic parents; a negative correlation was uncovered when group-size preferences of offspring and foster parents were compared. In other words, even after the cross-fostering, the young displayed the same group-size preference as their genetic parents (not their foster parents), suggesting a significant heritability for this complex behavioral trait.

To understand how the three prerequisites of natural selection, as well as the behavioral genetics studies, all tie together in contemporary ethology, we need to examine the modern foundations of work in evolution and behavior.

The Modern Theoretical Framework for Animal Behavior

The modern theoretical framework for natural selection as it applies to animal behavior can be traced to George C. Williams's book, *Adaptation and Natural Selection*, William D. Hamilton's pathbreaking papers on kinship and social behavior (see Chapter 8), Jerram Brown's book, *The Evolution of Behavior*, and Richard Dawkins's conceptually based book, *The Selfish Gene* (Brown, 1975; Dawkins, 1976, 1982, 1987; Hamilton, 1964; Williams, 1966). But perhaps the most important single contribution to both the theoretical and empirical framework underlying natural selection and animal behavior is E. O. Wilson's masterful synthesis, *Sociobiology* (Wilson, 1975). In *Sociobiology*, Wilson demonstrates the power of natural selection to shape behavior in everything from social insects to humans (Alcock, 2001). While there was an early social science backlash against Wilson's claim that sociobiological thinking can shed light on humans, ethologists and behavioral ecologists grabbed onto Wilson's compelling arguments on the power of natural selection to shape behavior, particularly social behavior (hence the term sociobiology; see the interview with Wilson at the end of Chapter 1).

SOCIOBIOLOGY AND SELFISH GENES

The sociobiological notion that genes—in our case, genes associated with behavior—are the units upon which natural selection acts, is often referred to as the "selfish gene" approach to ethology. The phrase "selfish genes" was first coined by Richard Dawkins in 1976. As Dawkins himself makes crystal clear, genes aren't "selfish" in any emotional or moral sense. In fact, genes aren't anything but a series of tiny bits of DNA put together in a particular sequence and orientation, and somehow distinct from other such tiny tidbits of DNA. Yet, genes can sometimes be treated as though they were selfish in that the process of natural selection favors those genes that increase the expected relative reproductive success of their bearers. From the gene's-eye perspective, that is all that matters (Dawkins, 2006; Grafen and Ridley, 2006).

Any gene that codes for a trait that increases the fitness of its bearer above and beyond that of others in the population will increase in frequency. So natural selection often, but not always, produces genes that *appear* to be selfish. Apply this approach to animal behavior, particularly animal social behavior, and you have one of the main ways in which ethologists think about genes and animal behavior (Alexander and Tinkle, 1981; J. L. Brown, 1975; Grafen and Ridley, 2006; E. O. Wilson, 1975). But it is worth emphasizing again that genes have no inherent qualities such as selfishness. Thinking of a gene as "selfish" just provides a convenient means to conceptualize some problems in animal behavior.

Since the sociobiological approach underlies many of the examples found throughout this book, it is useful here to examine a case study of how this approach works.

ANTIPREDATOR BEHAVIOR IN GUPPIES

The guppy has often been used by ethologists and behavioral ecologists to study aspects of natural selection, with dozens of papers a year published on some aspect of guppy ethology (Houde, 1997; Magurran, 2005). One reason for this interest in guppies is not only that they breed quickly, facilitating multigenerational studies, but that their population structure is ideal for studies of natural selection and behavior. Most guppy studies use fish from the Northern Mountains of Trinidad and Tobago. In many of these streams, guppies can be found both upstream and downstream of a series of waterfalls (Houde, 1997; Magurran, 2005; Seghers, 1973; Figure 2.12). These waterfalls act as a barrier to many of the guppy's predators. Upstream of such waterfalls, guppies are typically under only slight predation pressure from one small species of fish; in contrast, downstream of the waterfalls, populations of guppies are often under severe predation pressure from numerous piscine (that is, fish) predators.

High-predation and low-predation sites in the same streams are often kilometers apart, and as such, we might expect natural selection to operate differently in these populations. If the type of predators differ dramatically based on site, then natural selection should favor different traits in upstream and downstream guppy populations. Indeed, this turns out to be the case, and between-population comparisons in guppies have found differences with respect to many traits, including antipredator behavior, color, number of offspring in

A   **B**

FIGURE 2.12. Different guppy environments. (A) An upstream, low-predation stream in Trinidad, and **(B)** a downstream, high-predation stream. Guppies in these streams have been subject to different selection pressures. *(Photo credits: Lee Dugatkin)*

FIGURE 2.13. Colorful guppies. Guppies can differ on traits like color when between-population comparisons of guppies are made. Here we see a colorful male (right) and a female (left) from the Paria River in Trinidad. *(Photo credit: Anne Magurran)*

each clutch, size of offspring, aging patterns, and age at reproduction (Endler, 1995; Houde, 1997; Magurran, 2005; Reznick, 1996; Figure 2.13).

Using a combination of field and laboratory experiments, David Reznick and his colleagues have found that guppies from high-predation sites mature faster, produce more broods of smaller offspring, and tend to channel their resources to reproduction when compared to guppies from low-predation sites (Figure 2.14). Why? At high-predation sites, guppy predators tend to be much larger (Figure 2.15A) and can eat a guppy no matter how large it gets. At such sites, producing many smaller fish would seem to be favored, as this is akin to buying lots of lottery tickets and hoping that one is a winner. At low-predation sites, only a single small fish predator (*Rivulus hartii*) of guppies exists (Figure 2.15B). If guppies can get past a certain size threshold, they are safe from *R. hartii*. As such, natural selection favors females producing fewer, but larger, offspring that can quickly grow large enough to be out of the zone of the danger associated with *R. hartii*, and this is precisely what we see (Reznick, 1996).

Natural selection has also operated on various aspects of guppy *behavior* (Endler, 1995; Houde, 1997; Magurran, 2005; Reznick, 1996). One suite of behaviors that has been studied extensively in natural populations of guppies is their antipredator activities (Magurran, 2005; Magurran et al., 1995; Seghers, 1973). Depending upon whether they evolved in populations with heavy or

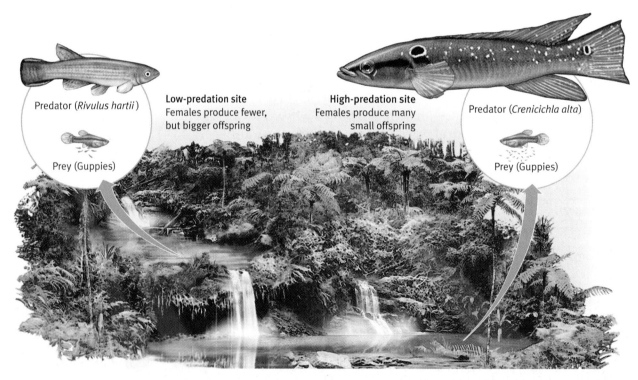

FIGURE 2.14. Natural selection and predation. Natural selection acts differently on guppy populations from high-predation sites (with *Crenicichla alta*) and low-predation sites (with *Rivulus hartii*). At high-predation sites, selection favors guppies producing many small young, but at low-predation sites, selection pressure is flip-flopped, favoring fewer, but larger, offspring. Offspring are pictured below female guppies in left and right circles above.

A **B**

FIGURE 2.15. Guppy predators. (A) A pike cichlid, *Crenicichla alta*. These predators are common in downstream sites native to guppies. **(B)** A killifish, *Rivulus hartii*. These small, fairly innocuous predators can eat only tiny guppies and are found in upstream (low-predation) sites in the rivers of Trinidad. *(Photo credis: Siegfried Baesler; © Jesús Salas y Carlos Garrido)*

light predation pressure, guppies, as well as sticklebacks and minnows, have a different suite of antipredator behaviors (Table 2.2).

Two components of antipredator behavior—called shoaling and predator inspection—have come under close scrutiny in guppies. Shoaling—swimming together in a group; also referred to as schooling—is a measure of group cohesiveness (Keenleyside, 1955; Pitcher, 1986), whereas **predator inspection** behavior refers to the tendency for individuals to move toward a predator to gain various types of information (Dugatkin and Godin, 1992; George, 1960; Pitcher, 1992; Pitcher et al., 1986).

TABLE 2.2. The effects of predation. An abbreviated list of some behaviors that are affected by predation pressure in guppies (*P. reticulata*), sticklebacks (*G. aculeatus*), and minnows (*P. phoxinus*). *(Adapted from Magurran et al., 1993)*

BEHAVIOR	EFFECT OF INCREASED PREDATION PRESSURE	SPECIES
Schooling	Larger and more cohesive schools	*P. reticulata* *P. phoxinus*
Evasion tactics	More effectively integrated in high-risk populations	*P. reticulata* *G. aculeatus* *P. phoxinus*
Inspection and predator assessment	Increase in inspection frequency	*G. aculeatus* *P. phoxinus*
	Increase in inspection group size	*P. phoxinus*
Habitat selection	Remain near surface and seek cover at edge of river	*P. reticulata*
Foraging	Increased feeding tenacity	*P. reticulata*
Female mating choice	Preference for less brightly colored males	*P. reticulata*
	Avoidance of sneaky mating attempts	*P. reticulata*
	Compromised by predator avoidance	*P. reticulata*
Male mating tactics	Increased use of sneaky mating tactics in high-risk populations	*P. reticulata*

From a sociobiological perspective, we might expect that guppies from high-predation sites would shoal (school) more tightly, and in greater numbers, than guppies from low-predation sites (Houde, 1997; Magurran, 2005; Magurran et al., 1995). Swimming in large groups provides more protection from predators than swimming in small groups, and should be more strongly favored at high-predation sites. The data from the field are in line with this prediction (Figure 2.16). Furthermore, guppies from high-predation sites inspect a predator more cautiously, but more often, than their low-predation counterparts. This too is in line with a sociobiological view of the guppy system, as cautiously, but frequently, examining any potential threat should be more strongly favored in areas of high versus low predation.

In the early 1990s, Anne Magurran and her colleagues learned of a unique

FIGURE 2.16. Natural selection affects group size. As a result of different selection pressures, preferred group size differs across guppy populations. **(A)** Group size where there is low-predation pressure leads to a preference for small groups. **(B)** Group size where there is medium- to high-predation pressure leads to a variety of group sizes. **(C)** Group size where there is very-high-predation pressure leads to a preference for larger group sizes. *(From Magurran and Seghers, 1991)*

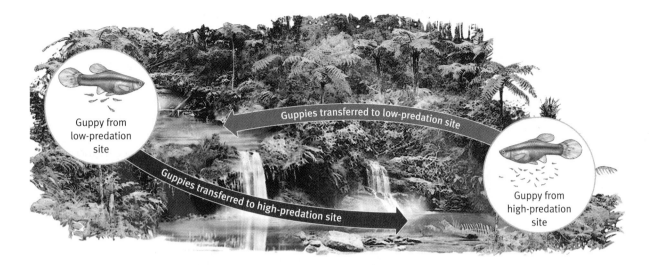

Guppy from low-predation site

Guppies transferred to low-predation site

Guppies transferred to high-predation site

Guppy from high-predation site

opportunity to examine a "natural experiment" on the evolution of antipredator behavior in guppies. It seems that back in 1957, one of the original researchers on guppy population biology, C. P. Haskins, transferred 200 guppies from a high-predation site (in the Arima River) to a low-predation site (in the Turure River) that had been unoccupied to that point by guppies. Magurran realized that this was a golden opportunity to examine natural selection on antipredator behavior. For if natural selection, via predation, shapes antipredator responses, then the lack of predation pressure in the Turure should have led to selection for weakened antipredator behavior in guppy descendants studied in the 1990s.

Magurran and her colleagues sampled numerous sites in the Turure (Magurran et al., 1992; Shaw et al., 1992). Genetic analysis suggested that the high-predation fish transferred from the Arima River back in 1957 had indeed spread all around the previously guppy-free site in the Turure River. More to the point, because of strong natural selection pressures, the descendants of the Arima River fish evolved shoaling and predator inspection behaviors that were more similar to those of guppies at low-predation sites than they were to the behaviors of their ancestors from the dangerous sites in the Arima River. This is precisely the sort of thing that had been found in other transplant experiments that had examined shifts in morphology and life history (Reznick, 1996; Reznick et al., 1990; Figure 2.17).

Magurran's group uncovered another curious finding. In addition to colonizing the low-predation areas of the Turure River (located upstream, where there are few predators), over the course of time the descendants of the Arima River fish moved downstream in the Turure River, back into areas of greater predation pressure. When tested, these fish showed antipredator behavior similar to that of their ancestors from the original high-predation site in the Arima River. One possible explanation is that the original colonizers spread fast, and since their antipredator behavior was beneficial when they reached high-predation sites in the Turure River, selection simply maintained such behavior. A more tantalizing, but to date untested hypothesis, is that the Arima River fish and their descendants colonized their new habitat at a much slower rate. If this were the case, natural selection may have shifted the colonizers and early descendants one way—toward the norm for low-predation sites—and then, later on, shifted the late descendants back in the opposite direction—toward the norm for fish from high-predation sites.

FIGURE 2.17. Transplants and natural selection. One way to examine the force of natural selection is to do reciprocal transplant experiments, which in effect switch selection pressures. Here, some guppies from high-predation sites (with *C. alta*) are transplanted to low-predation sites, and vice versa. Over the course of several years, transplanted populations converge on the characteristics of the fish in the populations into which they were transplanted.

In addition to nicely illustrating how one studies the evolution of behavior, the guppy example illustrates that while natural selection may take millions of years to shape some traits, this need not be the case—natural selection can act much more quickly. Upstream and downstream guppy populations have been separated from one another for less than 10,000 years, yet as a result largely of differences in predation pressure, natural selection has produced significant differences in behavior in guppy populations over this fairly brief evolutionary time period (Endler, 1995). Indeed, both Magurran and Reznick's work on transfer experiments demonstrates that natural selection can act on antipredator behavior in wild populations on the time scale of years to decades.

Adaptation

Now that we have a feel for how natural selection operates in shaping behavior, what shall we call the traits—behavioral or otherwise—that are almost always the result of this process? Such traits are typically referred to as **adaptations**, a term that is defined in many ways in the literature (Mayr, 1982; Mitchell and Valone, 1990; Reeve and Sherman, 1993; Sober, 1987). For our purposes, we shall simply note that natural selection produces adaptations—traits associated with the highest relative fitness in a given environment (Reeve and Sherman, 1993). For the guppies mentioned above, tight schooling and vigilant predator inspection are adaptations to life in high-predation streams.

Kern Reeve and Paul Sherman argue that a trait is an adaptation when that trait results in its bearers having the highest fitness among a *specified set of behaviors in a specified environment* (Reeve and Sherman, 1993). One critical aspect of this definition is that it shows that while natural selection produces adaptations, it is not necessarily true that adaptations are only the product of natural selection. If adaptations are traits that provide their bearers with the highest relative fitness in an environment, then any number of forces, including chance, could produce an adaptation. As long as the environment we are studying is the same environment in which natural selection operated, it's likely that most adaptations *are* the product of natural selection; nonetheless, under Reeve and Sherman's definition, adaptations *don't have to be* the product of natural selection (Gould and Lewontin, 1979). To see this, let us examine the question of behavioral adaptation and the egg-dumping behavior found in some populations of wood ducks (*Aix sponsa*; Figure 2.18).

In more than 100 different species of birds, females engage in **brood parasitism**, in which they place ("dump") their eggs into the nests of other individuals (Eadie et al., 1998; Payne, 1977; Rohwer and Freeman, 1989). If the eggs they dump in the nests of other birds hatch and are then raised by foster parents, the biological parents receive a huge benefit (new chicks), but they avoid the normal costs of parenting. Such brood parasitism is particularly common in waterfowl (Beauchamp, 1997). While waterfowl make up only about 2 percent of bird species, they account for more than 25 percent of the cases of parasitic egg dumping. In particular, brood parasitism is most prevalent in waterfowl that nest in tree cavities and man-made nest boxes.

Wood ducks typically nest in tree cavities created by woodpeckers or by limb breakage (Hauber et al., 2001). During the breeding season, females lay one egg per day and spend the remainder of their waking hours foraging. Males

FIGURE 2.18. Egg dumping by wood ducks. (A) A male and female wood duck at a man-made nesting box. **(B)** Many different wood ducks lay their eggs in the same nest, which may be adaptive in a native setting, but is maladaptive in man-made nests where many nests are clumped together. *(Photo credits: Paul Sherman)*

stay by their mates during the egg-laying period and then abandon the nest when females begin to incubate. A full clutch of ten to twelve eggs makes up more than 75 percent of a female's body mass (Bellrose and Holm, 1994).

Brad Semel and Paul Sherman studied one population of wood ducks that nest in man-made boxes in Missouri, and they found that a remarkable 95 percent of active nests were parasitized, despite many empty nest boxes that could be used to raise young. This produced the odd situation of nests having thirty to forty eggs, as opposed to the normal clutch of ten to twelve (Semel and Sherman, 1986; Figure 2.19). Many heavily parasitized nests were simply abandoned by the wood ducks, and no eggs in such nests hatched. Could this all possibly be adaptive?

Given the ecology and breeding biology of the wood duck, Semel and Sherman were interested in how such a system could lead to 95 percent of the active nests being parasitized when empty nest boxes were present. Were there some benefits accrued by females for egg dumping in an environment with nest boxes? Being good "adaptationists," Semel and Sherman laid out five potentially adaptive reasons for why females might dump their eggs. They hypothesized that females might do the following:

▸ Dump eggs to reduce the risk of predation on all their eggs at once, thereby engaging in what is called "bet hedging."
▸ Be forced to parasitize the nests of others for lack of suitable, hidden nests.
▸ Parasitize when their own nest is destroyed (by predation or storms).
▸ Gain some benefit by placing eggs in the nests of genetic relatives.
▸ Enhance their reproductive success in general by simply laying eggs in any available nest they come across.

FIGURE 2.19. Maladaptive behavior in wood ducks. Wood ducks typically nest in tree cavities (*left*). In such cavities, females generally lay ten eggs. When females nest in densely packed man-made boxes (*right*), a great deal of "egg dumping" occurs, where many females lay eggs in one box. This causes a decrease in reproductive success for all females and is not adaptive.

A

B
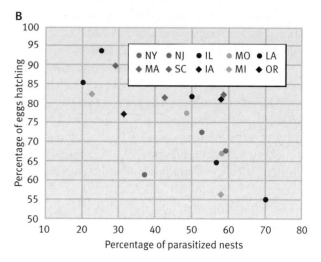

FIGURE 2.20. **Egg dumping and rearing young.** In wood ducks, the level of nest parasitism affects both the number of eggs laid **(A)** and the proportion of eggs that hatch **(B)**. NY = New York, NJ = New Jersey, IL = Illinois, LA = Louisiana, MA = Massachusetts, SC = South Carolina, IA = Iowa, MI = Mississippi, OR = Oregon. *(From Sherman, 2001, p. 138)*

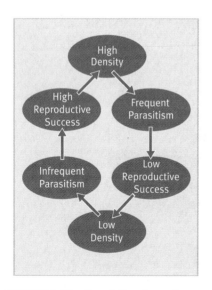

FIGURE 2.21. **Population dynamics and nest parasitism.** Sherman and Semel argue that both nest parasitism and population density cycle together. *(From Sherman, 2001)*

Using a brilliant combination of observation, experiment, and inference, Semel and Sherman were able to systematically discount each of the above five hypotheses, although some recent evidence suggests that kinship may play a small, indirect role in egg parasitism in wood ducks (Nielsen et al., 2006). Semel and Sherman found that the nests that were parasitized had *dramatically reduced reproductive success* (Semel et al., 1988, 1990; Figure 2.20). With such information in hand, we can ask whether the egg-dumping behavior that Semel and Sherman saw is adaptive. According to Reeve and Sherman (1993): "In applying our definition, the behavioral set includes parasitizing versus nonparasitizing conspecifics, the measure of fitness is hatchability of eggs, and the environmental context being examined is grouped, visible nest boxes. Under these conditions extreme brood parasitism lowers individual success. . . . Thus dump nesting is nonadaptive." In other words, the prevalence of brood parasitism in the population Semel and Sherman studied must be due to processes other than natural selection operating on parasitism and egg dumping *in that population.*

Sherman hypothesized that when nest boxes were not present (as was the case for most of the wood duck's history) and good territories were dispersed throughout the environment, there was likely a very high premium placed on finding good cavities in which to nest (Sherman, 2001). Thus, females may have egg dumped in such cavities, and they may have benefited from such parasitism (Figure 2.21). But when nest boxes were present and clumped, as in Semel and Sherman's population, such egg dumping was no longer adaptive under Reeve and Sherman's definition. Natural selection may very well have favored brood parasitism in the wood duck's past, but the nest boxes radically changed the population ecology of this species, such that egg dumping was no longer adaptive in Semel and Sherman's population. Indeed, today more and more ethological research is examining "maladaptive" behavior in changed environments (Neff and Sherman, 2004; Sih et al., 2004a, 2004b).

While most behaviors that we see in animals are likely adaptations and the product of natural selection, the wood duck example shows that this need not be the case. Maladaptations are likely to occur when man-made changes cause an unnatural scenario to suddenly be common, as in the case of brood parasitism in ducks.

Sherman and Semel's work nicely illustrates how animal behaviorists can test for behavioral adaptations and behavioral maladaptations. But these studies are also important because they highlight the testing of multiple alternative hypotheses (Chamberlin, 1897). That is, rather than focus on one possible explanation for egg dumping, Sherman and Semel constructed a list of alternative hypotheses, and they systematically tested each hypothesis to see which best explained egg dumping. This is a very powerful approach for studying behavior.

Genetic Techniques to Test Hypotheses in Animal Behavior

In addition to genes playing a fundamental role in the process of natural selection per se, animal behaviorists also employ genes as tools to test specific hypotheses that often center on the notion of genetic relatedness. Two examples of this approach are presented below.

KINSHIP AND NAKED MOLE RAT BEHAVIOR

By definition, genetic relatives (siblings, parents, offspring, and so on) share many of the same genes. Because of this genetic similarity between kin, we expect more cooperative and altruistic behavior among kin than among unrelated individuals. In fact, as we shall see in Chapter 8, according to basic kinship theory, the more related individuals are, the more we expect to see cooperative and altruistic behaviors (Hamilton, 1964). To see how we can use genes as a tool to test this idea, we shall look into the fascinating, but bizarre life of naked mole rats (*Heterocephalus glaber*; Figure 2.22).

Few mammals have captured the fancy of both scientists and laymen to the extent of the naked mole rat (Jarvis, 1981; Sherman et al., 1991). These

FIGURE 2.22. Naked mole rats. Naked mole rats show very high within-colony relatedness. This maps nicely onto numerous cooperative and altruistic behaviors common to this species, such as digging tunnels, sweeping dirt or debris out of the tunnels, grooming the queen, or defending against predators. Here, we see workers in the process of digging a tunnel. Naked mole rats use their sharp teeth to break up the dirt and then move it back through the tunnel to a worker who throws it out of the tunnel. *(Photo credit: Gregory G. Dimijian/Photo Researchers, Inc.)*

TABLE 2.3. The relationship between social behavior in naked mole rats and social insects. Comparisons between naked mole rats and eusocial insects indicate basic similarities in such characteristics as reproductive division of labor, overlapping generations, and communal care of young. *(From Lacey and Sherman, 1991)*

SPECIES	SIMILARITIES TO NAKED MOLE RATS	DIFFERENCES FROM NAKED MOLE RATS
Paper wasp (*Polistes fuscatus*)	Single breeding female per colony Aggressive domination of other colony members by reproductive female No permanent sterility in subordinate foundresses Size-based subdivision of nonbreeding caste Similar colony sizes (20–100 workers) Slightly larger size in queens than in workers	All female workers Haplodiploid genetics New nests each spring Outcrossing promoted by dispersal of reproductives from nest site Carnivore
Honeybee (*Apis mellifera*)	Single breeding female per colony Colony reproduction by fissioning (swarming) Age polyethism among nonreproductives Slightly larger size in queens than in workers	All female workers Haplodiploid genetics Primarily chemical, not behavioral, reproductive suppression of workers Permanently "sterile" nonreproductive females Vastly larger colonies in honeybees Outcrossing promoted by aerial mating aggregations Nectarivore
Wood termite (*Kalotermes flavicollis*)	Single breeding female per colony Diploid genetics Male and female workers Delayed caste fixation Division of labor among nonbreeders Extremely long life of reproductives Diet of plant material; breakdown of cellulose by gut endosymbionts Allo- and autocoprophagy Opportunity for workers to become reproductives if they escape the breeder's influence Working behavior begins before adulthood	Chemical, not behavioral, reproductive suppression Vastly larger colonies in termites Queens many times larger than workers Outcrossing promoted by aerial mating aggregations

small, hairless rodents of tropical Africa display **eusociality**, an extreme form of sociality that is present in many social insect groups (Table 2.3). Naked mole rats were the first vertebrates to display the three characteristics associated with this extreme form of sociality, namely:

▸ A reproductive division of labor, wherein individuals in certain castes reproduce and individuals in other castes do not.
▸ Overlapping generations, such that individuals of different generations are alive at the same time.
▸ Communal care of young.

Naked mole rats live in large groups, in which a *single queen* and one to three males are the only individuals that mate and reproduce in the entire colony. Although intra-colony aggression certainly exists in this species, cooperation is the first thing that jumps out at anyone studying naked mole rats (Reeve, 1992; Reeve and Sherman, 1991; Stankowich and Sherman, 2002). Nonreproductive male and female naked mole rats, who live much shorter lives than reproductive naked mole rats, undertake a wide variety of cooperative behaviors, such as digging new tunnels for the colony, sweeping debris, grooming the queen, and defending against predators (Lacey and Sherman, 1991; Pepper et al., 1991). But why? Why do individuals yield exclusive reproduction to a single queen and a few males, as well as work for the colony? The answer in part centers on the high genetic relatedness between individuals within naked mole rat colonies.

As mentioned above, basic kinship theory suggests that the more genetically related individuals are, the more cooperation they will show with each other. Using this as their theoretical framework, Kern Reeve and his colleagues hypothesized that naked mole rats are very cooperative with others in their colony because they are close genetic relatives (Reeve et al., 1990).

To test this idea, Reeve's group sampled the DNA of fifty naked mole rats and then employed a molecular technique called "DNA fingerprinting" to examine the genetic relatedness among colony members (DeSalle and Schierwater, 1998; Jeffreys et al., 1985). Using DNA from liver, muscle, and brain samples, they created three DNA "probes" to separate out three distinct DNA fragments for each mole rat. These probes produced a series of prominent black bands, which consisted of between 1.6 and 1.8 kilobytes of DNA. Individuals had an average of about twenty-nine such distinct bands, and these bands together represented the **DNA fingerprint** of that mole rat. DNA fingerprints of different individuals could then be compared—the better the bands matched up, the more closely related were the individuals (Reeve et al., 1992).

Reeve and his colleagues found that because of very high levels of inbreeding—a result of mating between relatives—the average genetic relatedness in these colonies of cooperative naked mole rats was extremely high, as predicted by kinship theory (see Braude, 2000, for an alternative view). The exact value they came up with was an average relatedness of 0.81 within naked mole rat colonies. To put this in some perspective, unrelated individuals have a value of 0 for this indicator, brothers score (on average) 0.5, and the most related of all individuals, identical twins, score 1.0 (Figure 2.23). Thus, naked mole rat individuals, on average, fall

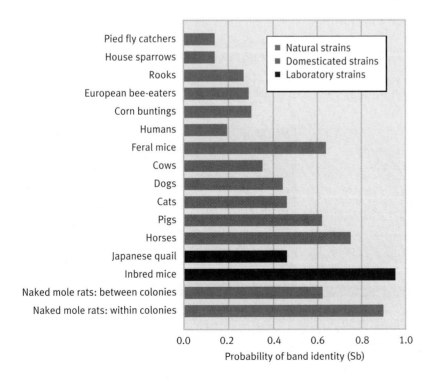

FIGURE 2.23. Naked mole rats show high levels of genetic relatedness. Reeve and his colleagues used what is known as Jeffrey's molecular genetic probe to ascertain relatedness among individuals. They found that naked mole rats in a colony were more genetically related to one another than any non-inbred strain of animal known. *(From Reeve et al., 1990)*

between normal siblings and identical twins on a relatedness scale, and they even lean toward the identical twins' side of the equation. In the case of the naked mole rats, then, genetic techniques were used to test a theory about kinship and social behavior that is derived from sociobiological and selfish gene thinking.

COALITION FORMATION

Another context in which genetic relatedness is important, and where molecular genetic techniques have been used to assess such relatedness, is **coalition** formation in animals (Harcourt and de Waal, 1992). In coalitions, the result of an interaction between a pair of animals is affected by a third individual, who aids one of the other interactants. The recipient of such aid is then more likely to obtain the resource for which it is vying (for example, food, mates, shelter). Coalitions have been examined most extensively in primate species, but they have also been the subject of study in many other animals, including hyenas, wolves, lions, cheetahs, coatis, eiders, and dolphins (Chapais, 1992; Harcourt and de Waal, 1992; Figure 2.24).

Aiding another individual against a third party is often a dangerous activity, and injuries to coalition members are common (Harcourt and de Waal, 1992). As such, animal behaviorists have hypothesized that coalitions should often be formed among genetic relatives, who stand to gain the most by aiding each other, as this would increase the probability that copies of their genes would make it into the next generation (Harcourt and de Waal, 1992; Mesterton-Gibbons and Sherratt, 2007; Noe and Hammerstein, 1995; see Chapter 8). That being said, determining which animals in natural populations are genetically related can be very difficult, unless a thorough genealogy is available; hence ethologists often rely on molecular genetic techniques to measure relatedness.

Male lions form cooperative coalitions in patrolling their group's territorial borders (Packer et al., 1988; Packer and Pusey, 1982). Although such territorial defense is dangerous, larger coalitions are particularly adept at defending their territories against intrusions from other lion groups (Bygott et al., 1979; Packer et al., 1988; Whitehead and Connor, 2005). As part of their long-term study of lion behavior, one of the questions that Craig Packer, Anne Pusey, and their

A

B

FIGURE 2.24. Coalitions. Males, often brothers, form long-lasting coalitions that have significant fitness effects on all members. **(A)** Two cheetahs in a coalition survey the area, looking in different directions for the appearance of prey. **(B)** The two cheetahs in the coalition both flush out and capture prey. *(Photo credits: Tim Caro)*

FIGURE 2.25. A pride of lions. In lions, males form coalitions and patrol and guard their territories. *(Photo credit: Craig Packer)*

colleagues addressed was whether such large male coalitions were typically made up of genetic relatives (Packer et al., 1991; Figure 2.25).

To tackle this question, they turned to DNA fingerprinting and examined the number of DNA bands shared by coalition members. What they found was that while small coalitions were sometimes made up of relatives and sometimes not, larger coalitions were always composed of relatives (Packer et al., 1991). It seems that when coalitions are small, each male in the coalition has about equal reproductive success. On the other hand, when coalitions are large, some individuals have very low reproductive success, while others have very high reproductive success. The only way then to promote the formation of large groups, given that individuals risk low reproductive success by joining such groups, is to have some added benefit (Figure 2.26). Kinship provides that benefit, as even when individuals themselves have low reproductive success in large coalitions, they are in fact helping raise the fitness of their higher-ranking genetic relatives. Since their relatives share many of the genes they themselves have, those on the low end of the coalition totem pole still get some indirect fitness benefits by joining such coalitions. This adaptationist perspective on coalition formation became clear only as a result of the now readily available molecular genetics techniques that ethologists have at their disposal.

FIGURE 2.26. Coalition size and kinship. The variance in reproductive success increases as coalition size goes up in lions. In large groups, one or two individuals produce most of the young, with other coalition members fathering far fewer offspring. Larger coalitions are more likely to be made up of kin, providing an indirect benefit to those males that do not father many cubs. The numbers by each point indicate the number of cubs fathered by each male in that coalition, and a box around the number indicates that the males are close relatives. *(From Packer et al., 1991)*

Phylogeny and the Study
of Animal Behavior

In *On the Origin of Species*, Darwin summarized his ideas on evolution in "two great laws" that centered on (1) conditions of existence, and (2) common ancestry. When Darwin spoke of the "conditions of existence," he was describing the living (biotic) and nonliving (abiotic) environment that sets the stage on which natural selection operates. In other words, the effect that a given variant of a trait has on reproductive success is not absolute, but depends on the environment in which an organism finds itself—that is, it depends on the conditions of existence. The first part of this chapter has been devoted to examining animal behavior and natural selection, and so here we shall focus on Darwin's other great law— common ancestry—as it applies to the study of ethology.

Species that share a recent common ancestor tend to resemble one another in many respects for the very reason that they share a common ancestor. For Darwin, common ancestry was important because it helped explain "that fundamental agreement in structure which we see in organic beings in the same class, and which is quite independent of their habits of life" (Darwin, 1859). For example, from an ethological perspective, suppose that Species 1 and Species 2 —let's say two species of squirrels—evolved from a common ancestor, labeled Species 3. If Species 1 and 2 display the same set of antipredator behaviors, one possible reason for this similarity is that both Species 1 and 2 possess this suite of traits because their common ancestor, Species 3, possessed it.

In a moment, we shall look at some case studies that elaborate on the ways that ethologists incorporate **phylogeny**—that is, evolutionary history through common descent—into their studies of animal behavior. Before that, however, let us walk through a brief primer on phylogeny, so that we have a solid conceptual basis for applying phylogeny to questions of animal behavior.

PHYLOGENETIC TREES

To study common ancestry, evolutionary biologists construct **phylogenetic trees**, which depict the evolutionary history of a group of species, genera, families, and so forth. These trees graphically depict the phylogeny of the groups of organisms in question. The term "phylogeny" was first introduced by a German contemporary of Darwin, Ernst Haeckel, who was deeply involved in disseminating ideas on evolution throughout Europe. Although Darwin himself did not use the word phylogeny until the fifth edition of *On the Origin of Species*, he was clearly thinking about phylogenetic trees as early as 1837, twenty-two years before the publication of the first edition (Dayrat, 2005). Indeed, Figure 2.27A depicts a hypothetical tree that Darwin included as the only figure in the first edition of *On the Origin of Species*, whereas Figure 2.27B shows the first sketch of a phylogenetic tree from Darwin's early notebooks.

The first step in the process of building phylogenetic trees is to measure some set of traits, often referred to as characters, in the organisms under study. Traits can, for example, be structural, developmental (embryological), molecular, or most relevant to us, behavioral. Until the molecular revolution of the 1970s, almost all trait measurements were morphological or anatomical—for example,

A

B

FIGURE 2.27. Darwin and phylogenetic trees. **(A)** Hypothetical phylogenetic tree from *On the Origin of Species*. Ancestral species A–L are on the bottom and time is along the y axis *(From Darwin, 1859)*. **(B)** First known sketch of an evolutionary tree by Charles Darwin, who drew it in an early Notebook in 1837. Notice the "I think" in the top left corner. In both A and B, we see divergence over time. *(Reproduced by permission of Syndics of Cambridge University Library)*

bone length, tooth shape, and so on—and much of that was gathered from fossil evidence. In this context, a trait need not correspond to a single structural measurement, such as bone length. It can instead be a measure of a number of related structures, such as jaw shape, the relative position of a group of bones, and so forth. With the advent of molecular genetics, many so-called "traits" measured today are DNA sequences, and these molecular genetic maps can be used to help build phylogenies by comparing and contrasting sequences across different species.

Not all traits are equally valuable in constructing phylogenies. To understand why, we need to distinguish between two basic types of traits—homologies and homoplasies. A **homology** is a trait shared by two or more species because those species shared a common ancestor. For example, all female mammals produce milk for their young, and they all possess this homologous trait because mammals share a common ancestor that produced milk.

A **homoplasy** is a trait that is not due to descent from a common ancestor shared by two or more species, but instead is almost always the result of natural selection acting independently on each species. A classic example of a homoplasy is shown by the wings of birds, mammals (for example, bats), and insects (Figure 2.28). Superficially, the wings found in these different groups are constructed in a similar manner, but this is not because wings were present in a common ancestor of birds, mammals, and insects. In the case of wings, natural selection pressures in the three taxa were similar enough that an appendage associated with flight would have some of the same basic characteristics. Such homoplasies—the result of shared natural selection pressure—are referred to as **analogies**, and the process leading to the production of analogous traits is called **convergent evolution**.

Homologous traits are used in phylogeny building because they reflect shared evolutionary histories. Homoplasies, on the other hand, while they do shed light on natural selection, do not reflect the historical relationships between species and, in fact, distort and misrepresent these relationships when used in

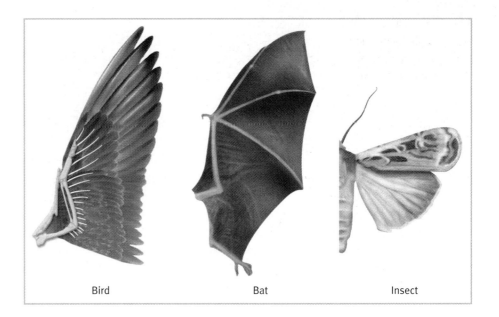

FIGURE 2.28. Convergent evolution in wing structure. Similarities and differences in the wings of birds, bats, and insects.

Bird   Bat   Insect

phylogenetic tree building. Ideally, we would like to be able to build phylogenetic trees by including homologies, but eliminating homoplasies. In practice, however, this is very difficult to do, as it is often hard to distinguish between homologies and homoplasies (Delsuc et al., 2005).

When attempting to construct phylogenetic trees, we need a method to ascertain which varieties of a trait appeared first—that is, which are ancestral—and which varieties are derived from these ancestral states. When we study the historic order in which different varieties of a trait appear, we are examining what is referred to as **polarity**, or the direction of historical change in a trait.

Evolutionary biologists have many ways for determining polarity, including using the fossil record in conjunction with techniques for dating fossils. Indeed, for most of the history of evolutionary biology, the fossil record was the primary source for adding a temporal component to phylogenetic trees. With this sort of information in hand, evolutionary biologists could then use morphological and anatomical data to try to group together species (families, genera, and so on) based on similarities and differences. For example, species sharing many anatomical similarities would be grouped together more closely than those sharing fewer anatomical similarities, and researchers could then build a phylogeny based on this (and the data from the fossil record).

Today, molecular genetic data are also being used to group species together. To do so, DNA sequences from different species are compared against one another at the nucleotide level. Statistical comparisons of DNA sequences are made, and phylogenetic groupings are established based on nucleotide similarities and differences across species. In addition, complex mathematical models that include an estimate of the rate of molecular genetic change can be used to calculate the amount of time that would be required to produce the nucleotide differences we have measured. In essence, even in the absence of information from the fossil record, these molecular genetic data allow us to work backward from extant (present-day) species, and calculate the most likely phylogenetic history that would produce the molecular genetic similarities and differences we see today.

When evolutionary biologists use the techniques described above, they often end up with many possible phylogenetic trees, each of which *might* represent the true phylogenetic history of the taxa they are studying. But, of course, there is only one actual phylogenetic history for any taxa, so we need a method for distinguishing between candidate trees. Researchers have developed a number of techniques—many of which are mathematically complex—to handle the problem of distinguishing between possible phylogenetic trees (Felsenstein, 2004; Hillis et al., 1992). The most common of these techniques is **parsimony analysis**. The concept of parsimony is most often associated with the ideas of a fourteenth-century philosopher named William of Ockam (sometimes spelled Occam), who argued that "entities are not to be multiplied beyond necessity." This concept is now referred to as Ockam's razor, and within evolutionary biology it has been taken to mean that the phylogenetic tree that requires the least number of evolutionary changes is the most likely to be correct.

When our morphological and molecular genetic analyses produce similar phylogenetic trees, our confidence increases that our phylogenetic tree is correct. In addition, as more morphological, molecular genetic, and fossil evidence is uncovered in the future, we can examine whether the new data are consistent with our phylogenetic tree. If they are, we gain confidence that our tree accurately reflects the evolutionary history of the taxa we are studying.

Ethologists use phylogenetic trees in many ways. One typical approach would be for animal behaviorists to begin the process by using an already established phylogenetic tree for the taxa they are studying (for example, a tree based on the methods discussed above). Then, ethologists could take the behavioral data they have—let's say data on mating systems—and superimpose them onto a phylogenetic tree to examine the evolutionary history of mating systems. That is, they take the mating systems data they have collected on each species and place them on a phylogenetic tree, so that mating systems can be viewed in the context of evolutionary history. Once this is done, animal behaviorists can ask questions such as: Which of the mating systems seen today are derived? Which are ancestral? In addition, they can make inferences about the mating systems of species that predated those they are studying, even if they are extinct. This is done by using statistical techniques to calculate which ancestral state (of mating system) would require the fewest number of evolutionary changes to produce the mating systems that we see in our extant species.

Ethologists can also use existing phylogenetic trees to make inferences about natural selection and convergent evolution. Once we know something about the phylogenetic history of the group we are studying, we can ask whether certain selection pressures consistently favor one behavioral variant or another *independent of phylogenetic history*. For example, do males in species with intense male-male competition for mates have larger testes than males from species that have less male-male competition? Is this trend independent of the phylogenetic history of the species we are studying? If, for example, we see that all species that have male-male competition and males with large testes are descended from a common ancestor with both these traits, we can explain this relationship by common ancestry. If all species that have male-male competition and males with large testes are not descended from a recent common ancestor with both these traits, we can infer that natural selection has independently favored large testes size over and over again in species with male-male competition.

Now that we have walked through a brief primer on phylogeny, let's look at a few more detailed examples in which ethologists have used phylogenetic analyses to shed light on animal behavior.

PHYLOGENY AND PARENTAL CARE

Ethologists often use phylogenetic analysis to try to reconstruct the order in which a suite of behaviors has appeared over evolutionary time. We shall use this approach here to focus on the evolution of parental care behavior. At the most basic level, there are four "states" that capture parental care systems in animals: no parental care, maternal care, paternal care, and biparental (maternal and paternal) care. We can then ask: In what historical order, if any, do these forms of parental care most often appear? For example, if we assume that no parental care is the primitive, or original, state in the taxa we are studying, do we most often see maternal care appear next? Paternal care? Biparental care? And once we establish the answer to that question, what parental care system typically follows the one that followed no parental care? In addition, we can ask any number of questions about what other traits—for example, nest-building behavior—are most associated with a particular form of parental care.

Early theories on the order in which various parental care systems evolve focused on fish and anuran frogs (Gross and Sargent, 1985). These analyses suggested a "stepping-stone" model in which parental care appeared in the following order: no parental care, paternal care, biparental care, and finally maternal care (as a result of male desertion). The sample size for these analyses, however, was relatively small, and subsequent studies in the same groups produced contradictory results (Goodwin et al., 1998; Summers et al., 1999).

To better address the order in which parental care systems typically evolve—if such an order even exists—we need to work with a large group of species. Ideally we would use a group in which we see each variety of parental care (many times), and one in which we have good information on the phylogenetic relationship between species. One such group consists of ray-finned fish (the *Actinopterygii*), which contain on the order of 400 families of fish, which in turn are made up of over 20,000 species (Figure 2.29). Indeed, ray-finned fish make up more than one-half of all known vertebrate species, and include the group most often studied by ethologists—namely, the bony fish, or teleosts.

FIGURE 2.29. Parental care in fish.
Various forms of parental care (maternal care, paternal care, both maternal and paternal care, and so on) have been uncovered in ray-finned fish. Here we see a male clown anemonefish tending the eggs laid by its mate. This fish shows the bright coloration and paternal care often found in species with external fertilization. *(Photo credit: Fred Bavendam/Minden Pictures/Getty Images)*

To begin their phylogenetic study of parental care in ray-finned fish, Judith Mank and her colleagues first used morphological data (including data from fossils) and molecular genetic data, and then employed various techniques for assessing trait polarity. They used this information to build a phylogenetic tree of 224 families of ray-finned fish and then examined the evidence for parental care in these various families (Mank et al., 2005). That is, their phylogenetic tree was not built using data on parental care behavior—instead, inferences about the evolution of parental care were made based on the tree Mank and her colleagues built using morphological and molecular genetic data. To do this, they began by categorizing the species in their established phylogenetic tree by using already published data on parental care—no parental care, maternal care, paternal care, or biparental care—and then they examined the order in which these systems appeared over evolutionary time. Second, because ray-finned fish have two fairly distinct ways of reproducing—external or internal fertilization—they asked whether particular parental care systems were associated with either external or internal fertilization. Finally, because male color pattern and nest-building behavior have been found to play an important role in fish mating systems, they examined whether the presence or absence of male coloration and/or the presence or absence of nest-building behavior was associated with specific parental care systems.

First, let us look at some baseline findings. Parental care was found in approximately 30 percent of the families of ray-finned fish analyzed by Mank and her colleagues. In external breeders, parental care was found in 25 percent of the families studied. For internally fertilizing fish, parental care was found in 90 percent of the families analyzed.

Mank and her colleagues found that in ray-finned fish paternal care evolved on twenty-two independent occasions—in other words, there were twenty-two independent occurrences of a shift from "no parental care" in an ancestral species to paternal care in a descendant species. Maternal care and biparental care also evolved independently numerous times within the ray-finned fish (Figure 2.30). No evidence, however, was found for the stepping-stone model

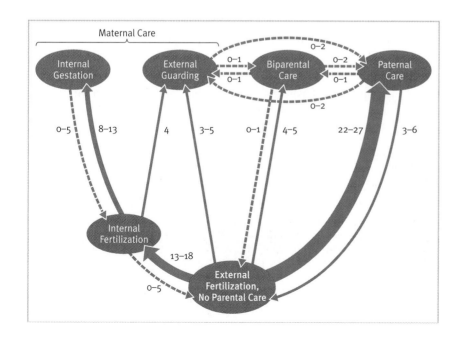

FIGURE 2.30. The phylogenetic history of parental care in ray-finned fish. Thickness of the arrows reflects relative numbers of evolutionary transitions (numerals near arrows indicate the estimated range of the number of transitions). Dashed arrows indicate cases in which transitions are unclear. *(From Mank et al., 2005)*

described earlier. Indeed, aside from the fact that paternal care was the most likely evolutionary state to emerge from no parental care, no clear ordering of parental care systems was found.

Other findings from Mank and her colleagues included:

1. Maternal care tended to evolve after species had moved from external to internal fertilization.
2. In species with external fertilization, paternal care was often found alongside intense male coloration and nest construction.
3. Male coloration was also associated with systems in which females fertilized their eggs internally.

Overall, then, Mank and her colleagues' ambitious phylogenetic analysis did not find evidence for a sequential stepping-stone model of the development of parental care. Instead, what they found was evidence for multiple origins of all parental care systems (particularly paternal care), as well as some fascinating evolutionary relationships between parental care, nesting behavior, mode of fertilization (external or internal), and male coloration pattern.

PHYLOGENY, MATING SYSTEMS, AND MALE AGGRESSION

Ethologists have long argued that males may benefit from being aggressive when sexually receptive females are present, and less aggressive otherwise (Emlen and Oring, 1977; Orians, 1969). That is, if males can assess female sexual receptivity, natural selection may favor males fighting one another for access to females, since the payoff for such aggression, when receptive females are around, may be very high. If sexually receptive females are not present (or if males cannot assess sexual receptivity), the costs of males fighting one another may outweigh the benefits, and hence selection may favor less aggression on the part of males. To test these ideas, we would ideally like to examine male aggression in closely related species that differ as to the availability of sexually receptive females. *Nasonia* wasps fit that description well.

Wasps of the genus *Nasonia* lay their eggs inside a host species, and their larvae feed on the host as they develop. *Nasonia* females lay between 20 and 140 eggs in the pupae of flesh flies and blow flies, and once males emerge from their eggs, they remain on the surface of the pupae and await the emergence of females and subsequent mating opportunities (Whiting, 1967). This group provides a model system for examining the relationship between the evolution of male aggression and female sexual receptivity in a phylogenetic context, because the phylogeny of three closely related species of *Nasonia* wasps is well established, and male aggression and female sexual receptivity can be observed, recorded, and mapped onto this phylogeny.

Jason Leonard and Chris Boake systematically measured the amount of male-male aggression in three species of *Nasonia*—*Nasonia vitripennis*, *Nasonia giraulti*, and *Nasonia longicornis* (Leonard and Boake, 2006). To do this, they observed the wasps on a fly pupae for periods of thirty minutes, and quantified aggressive behaviors such as "wings up," "charge," lunge," "grab," and "pursue," as well as responses to aggression such as "back up," "flee," and "kick." They

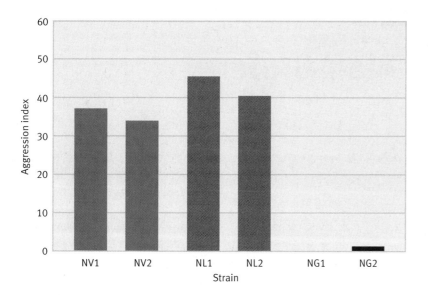

FIGURE 2.31. **Aggression and wasps.** The mean level of aggression for three different species of wasps, including two strains of *Nasonia vitripennis* (NV), two strains of *N. longicornis* (NL), and two strains of *N. giraulti* (NG). *(From Leonard and Boake, 2006)*

found that *N. vitripennis* and *N. longicornis* displayed high levels of male-male aggression, while this aggression was rare in *N. giraulti* (Figure 2.31).

What accounts for the species-level differences in male-male aggression? The answer is tied to the number of receptive females available in the three *Nasonia* species. In a separate experiment from the one described above, every tenth female to emerge from a pupae was captured and then dissected by Leonard and Boake. The researchers then examined whether a female was *already* pregnant when she emerged from the pupae—such within-host mating is not uncommon in some insects. What Leonard and Boake found was that virtually *all N. giraulti* females were already pregnant when they emerged from the pupae; in other words, no emerging females were receptive to male courtship (Figure 2.32). On the other hand, very few *N. vitripennis* females were pregnant when they emerged, and hence most emerging females were receptive to courting males. The data on *N. longicornis* were intermediate between that of the other two species (but leaned toward little within-host mating). Male

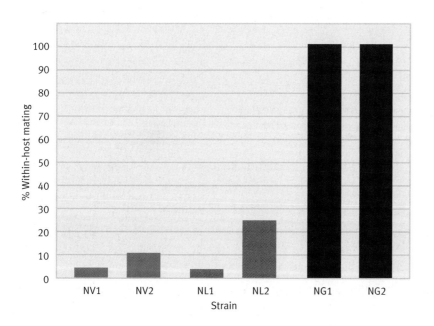

FIGURE 2.32. **Mating in wasps.** The mean level of within-host mating for three different species of wasps, including two strains of *Nasonia vitripennis* (NV), two strains of *N. longicornis* (NL), and two strains of *N. giraulti* (NG). *(From Leonard and Boake, 2006)*

INTERVIEW WITH

Dr. Alan Grafen

If you had to explain natural selection to an alien who knew nothing of life on earth, how would you do it?

Richard Dawkins has convincingly argued that all adaptive complexity must arise through natural selection. It follows that an alien capable of communicating with me would themselves be the product of natural selection, and furthermore would be likely to come from a civilization that had understood how adaptive complexity arose. Thus, I would look forward to hearing what the alien had to tell me about natural selection.

Some have argued that the process of natural selection is a tautology—something that is circular, and true by definition. Where have they gone wrong?

They've almost certainly read the wrong explanation. You can't read Darwin's *Origin of Species*, or Dawkins's *The Selfish Gene*, and pay attention, and come away thinking natural selection is a tautology. It is one of the features of natural selection that nearly everyone thinks they intuit the idea without being exposed to it! Indeed, Darwin's correspondence suggests he suspected that even Thomas Henry Huxley, who came to be known as "Darwin's bulldog," did not understand natural selection very well.

There are surely people who claim that special relativity is a tautology, or that Newtonian mechanics is fatally flawed, but they are a tiny green-inkish minority. The anti-intellectuals' assault on natural selection is conducted on a broader front and,

more worryingly, seems to be much more acceptable in respectable company.

The idea of natural selection needs to be treated with respect, so don't waste your time arguing with someone who thinks he's worked it all out for himself and claims to have

discovered a mistake in it! Insist that he should have a proper explanation in front of him, make him point to the line where he doesn't follow the argument, and do your honest best to help him over his obstacle.

Can it really be true that the same process—natural selection—operates on everything from viruses to humans?

That is what science is like. Gravity too operates on everything from viruses to humans and, just like natural selection, it operates in

some ways just the same, and in other ways very differently, because of the different context.

Why is there such reluctance in the social science community to accept that natural selection has shaped much of our own behavior?

This is an interesting question, but there is another foot that may have a boot on. Might a social scientist not ask "Why is there such reluctance in the biological community to accept that human behavior has unique aspects and essentially cultural aspects for which biology provides no framework?"

It is a primary duty of an academic to respect other subjects, and the seriousness of their intellectual work, so we should not try to maneuver social scientists into giving up their lines of enquiry or their conceptual frameworks.

It is actually quite hard to understand another subject's basic ideas, and this leads to trouble whenever subjects grow into new areas and acquire new neighbors. To have a dialog with people absolutely requires mutual respect and a serious attempt at understanding each others' positions.

One of my own papers, "Fertility and Labour Supply in *Femina economica*" was a consciously constructed attempt to build a model in which the same behavior could be understood biologically and economically. The resolution of the conflict between the points of view is all done formally and mathematically in that paper. There is no simple "one side is right, the other is wrong"—rather the explanatory forces are partly overlapping and partly intertwined.

It seems uncontroversial that at some level, biology will have something important to say about human behavior, and equally, that many of the patterns of behavior and explanations already discovered by social scientists will remain unaffected by biology. But in between these two easily accepted propositions lie many areas in which only detailed study and analysis can determine the role, if any, biology should play. Useful study of those areas can be done only by people with a good understanding both of the social sciences and of biology.

In what way has our fundamental understanding of the process of natural selection been changed by the revolution in molecular genetics?

Molecular biology has revolutionized the detailed facts we can discover about the organisms we're studying. Do female birds have offspring by more than one male in the same nest? How long ago did humans and chimps diverge? The range of useful facts will no doubt grow and grow.

There is one, terribly important, aspect of natural selection that is completely unaffected by molecular biology, and it is in many ways the very core of Darwin's argument: that

the only known process capable of producing complex adaptations is natural selection. This argument was developed mathematically by the great biologist (and statistician and geneticist) R. A. Fisher, and Bill Hamilton wrote in his encomium on the variorum edition of Fisher's *Genetical Theory of Natural Selection*: "And little modified even by molecular genetics, Fisher's logic and ideas still underpin most of the ever broadening paths by which Darwinism continues its invasion of human thought."

The only known process capable of producing complex adaptations is natural selection.

There is a tendency, particularly prevalent for obvious reasons among some practitioners, to believe that new technologies require a revisiting of all old knowledge. As if the discovery of the telescope might revise our view of how frequently the moon circles the earth. Read the *Origin of Species*, and be persuaded of the reality and biological significance of natural selection. Read G. C. Williams's *Natural Selection and Adaptation* (1966) and understand how to reason about natural selection. Read Dawkins's *The Selfish Gene* and see how Darwin's logic, rendered logically explicit, unifies the range

of evolutionary theories biologists apply today. Biologists know a lot about natural selection, and molecular genetics will not make any substantial difference to their arguments.

Molecular genetics is nevertheless a hugely important scientific enterprise, both medically and intellectually. What *does* it have to offer to students of natural selection? For one thing, many more examples of Darwinian adaptations. To learn about the workings of the ribosomes, or DNA topoisomerases, or hundreds of other fabulous molecules, is to be filled with wonder at the achievements of natural selection, just as much as the sonar of bats or the workings of the vertebrate eye. In some ways the molecular examples are more impressive, because they reveal how life itself is possible at a very fundamental level.

The problem Darwin solved in 1859 has remained solved. While nothing in molecular genetics is likely to require the re-opening of that case, molecular genetics *will* continue to supply further examples of adaptations and fuel further sophistications of our understanding of natural selection.

Dr. Alan Grafen is a professor at Oxford University, where he is member of the Animal Behavior Research Group. He is the coauthor of Modern Statistics for the Life Sciences (Oxford University Press, 2002) and is one of the leading theoretical biologists in the area of evolution by natural selection.

TABLE 2.4. Aggression, within-host mating, and sexual receptivity in *Nasonia* wasps. Leonard and Boake examined the relationship between male aggression, within-host mating, and female sexual receptivity in *Nasonia vitripennis*, *N. giraulti*, and *N. longicornis*.

SPECIES	MALE-MALE AGGRESSION	WITHIN-HOST MATING	SEXUAL RECEPTIVITY OF EMERGING FEMALES
N. vitripennis	high	almost none	high
N. giraulti	low	almost always	low
N. longicornis	high	some, but intermediate between the two other species	moderate

aggression and female receptivity indeed seem to be linked (Table 2.4). It is only when receptive females emerge from the pupae that we see male-male aggression, which makes good sense from an adaptationist perspective, as it is only then, and not when females emerge pregnant, that male aggression may lead to mating opportunities.

With this data in hand, Leonard and Boake could then map their behavioral results onto the phylogeny of these three *Nasonia* species and make some inferences about whether high male-male aggression and no within-host mating were the original state in *Nasonia*, or whether these were the derived states (those that appeared subsequent to the original state). Fortunately, a molecular phylogeny was available for *Nasonia* (Campbell et al., 1993). This phylogeny indicates that *N. vitripennis* is the oldest of the three species examined by Leonard and Boake, dating back somewhere between 200,000 and 1 million years. *N. giraulti* and *N. longicornis* evolved more recently (Figure 2.33). The phylogenetic information suggests that the high levels of male-male aggression

FIGURE 2.33. Phylogeny of *Nasonia* wasps. A phylogenetic tree of *Nasonia* wasps. *N. vitripennis* is the oldest of the three species examined by Leonard and Boake, dating back somewhere between 200,000 and 1 million years (as shown by the length of the horizontal line on the tree). *N. giraulti* and *N. longicornis* evolved more recently. The tree shows two strains (LBII and R5 11) of *Nasonia vitripennis* (NV), two strains (IV7 and IV 14) of *N. longicornis* (NL), and two strains (R2 and RVRV) of *N. giraulti* (NG), as well as another species of wasp (*Trichomalopsis dubius*) from a separate genus that is somewhat older than *N. vitripennis*. *(From Campbell et al., 1993)*

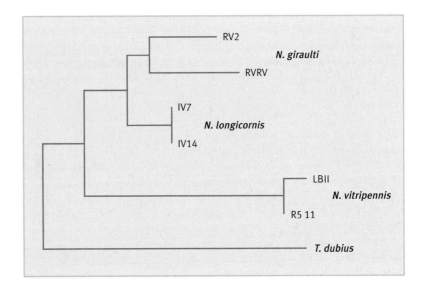

RV2
N. giraulti
RVRV
IV7
N. longicornis
IV14
LBII
N. vitripennis
R5 11
T. dubius

and high female receptivity seen in *N. vitripennis* make up the ancestral state in the genus *Nasonia*, as they are present in the oldest of the *Nasonia* species studied. The low levels of male-male aggression and female receptivity in *N. giraulti* is then the derived, or more recent, state of these behaviors. *N. longicornis*, which shows high levels of male-male aggression, but mixed levels of female receptivity, appears to be in the early stages of divergence from *N. vitripennis*, and moving toward the derived states seen in *N. giraulti*.

Leonard and Boake's work on *Nasonia* wasps is a nice example of the way that the phylogenetic approach and the adaptationist approach can complement one another in the study of animal behavior.

In this chapter, we have focused entirely on ultimate or "why" questions in animal behavior. This entailed understanding the process of natural selection, and how selection pressures shape animal behavior, as well as examining how evolutionary history—phylogeny—can help shed light on questions in ethology. It is important to recognize that just because we have discussed natural selection and phylogeny in different sections does not imply that they are unconnected to one another. This is not the case. Along with mutation, recombination, and the other sources of new genetic variation, the phylogenetic history of a species impacts the variation available for natural selection to act upon at any given time. Conversely, when natural selection shapes traits in Species 1 it is, to some extent, affecting the way that *descendants* from Species 1 will look, act, and so on.

Ultimate questions are often contrasted with proximate questions, which focus on immediate causes of behavior (release of a hormone, firing of a neuron, and so on). If we think of this chapter as a primer on ultimate questions, then Chapter 3 will be such a primer for proximate questions. But, once these two chapters are complete, we will be integrating both proximate and ultimate perspectives into each and every chapter for the remainder of the book.

SUMMARY

1. Artificial selection is the process of humans choosing certain trait varieties over others through implementing breeding programs that cause one or more selected varieties to increase in frequency. We have been shaping animals and plants by the process of artificial selection for the better part of 10,000 years.

2. Much of animal behavior work revolves around the notion that behavior, just as any trait, has evolved by the process of natural selection. The process of natural selection requires limited resources, variation, fitness differences, and heritability. For example, if we have a number of different foraging variants displayed by individuals in a population, and these variants translate into fitness differences and are heritable, then natural selection will act to increase the frequency of the foraging variant associated with the greatest relative fitness.

3. Even a small selective advantage—on the order of 1 percent per generation—is sufficient for natural selection to dramatically change gene frequencies over evolutionary time.

4. Among other things, behavioral geneticists use Mendel's laws of genetics to predict the distribution of behavioral phenotypes, to search for QTLs, and to determine what percentage of the variation in a behavioral trait is genetic and what percentage is environmental.

5. In addition to viewing the gene as one of the fundamental units by which behavioral traits are transmitted, ethologists also employ molecular genetics as a tool to allow them to test basic models of behavioral evolution. For example, molecular genetic techniques are often employed to test detailed predictions regarding kinship and the evolution of cooperation.

6. Natural selection produces adaptations—traits with the highest relative fitness in a given environment—but, not all adaptations are necessarily produced by natural selection.

7. To study common ancestry, evolutionary biologists construct phylogenetic trees, which depict the evolutionary history of various species, genera, families, and so forth. These trees graphically depict the phylogeny, or history of common descent, between the groups of organisms in question.

8. A homology is a trait shared by two or more species because those species shared a common ancestor. A homoplasy is usually the result of natural selection acting independently on each species.

DISCUSSION QUESTIONS

1. How was it possible for Darwin to come up with his theory of natural selection in the complete absence of a science of genetics? Many modern studies in ethology rely on genetics, particularly molecular genetics, as a critical tool. How did Darwin manage without this tool?

2. Jacques Monod once referred to natural selection as a tinkerer. Why is this a particularly appropriate analogy for how the process of natural selection operates?

3. Read Reeve and Sherman's (1993) paper, "Adaptation and the goals of evolutionary research," in volume 68 (pp. 1–32) of the *Quarterly Review of Biology*. After reviewing all the definitions of "adaptation," do you agree with Reeve and Sherman's approach to this subject? If you do not agree, explain why not by listing your reasons.

4. When considering how much variation in a behavioral trait is genetic and how much is environmental, how does the "uterine environment," in which a fetus matures, complicate matters?

5. Secure a copy of Gould and Lewontin's (1979) paper, "The spandrels of San Marcos and the Paglossian paradigm: A critique of the adaptationist programme" in volume 205 (pp. 581–598) of the *Proceedings of the Royal Society of London, Series B*. List both the merits and flaws in Gould and Lewontin's approach. Overall, do you think their critique is a fair one?

6. Maternal care behavior has been documented in such diverse groups as insects, fish, and mammals. Why would it probably be a mistake to use maternal care as a character in any analysis that examined the phylogenetic relationship between these very different groups? Cast your answer in terms of convergent evolution.

SUGGESTED READING

Darwin, C. (1859). *On the origin of species*. London: J. Murray. The starting point for modern ethology and a joy to read.

Dawkins, R. (1976). *The selfish gene*. Oxford: Oxford University Press. The book that introduced the term "selfish gene" and all its implications.

Reeve, H. K., Westneat, D. F., Noon, W. A., Sherman, P. W., & Aquadro, C. F. (1990). DNA "fingerprinting" reveals high levels of inbreeding in colonies of the eusocial naked mole rat. *Proceedings of the National Academy of Sciences, U.S.A., 87,* 2496–2500. A nice overview of the manner in which molecular genetics can shed light on behavioral adaptations.

Weiner, J. (1995). *The beak of the finch: A story of evolution in our time*. New York: Vintage Books. A Pulitzer Prize–winning book on Peter and Rosemary Grant's work on evolution in the Galápagos finches.

Williams, G. (1966). *Adaptation and natural selection*. Princeton: Princeton University Press. A critical approach to adopting the adaptationist perspective. Regarded by many as a must-read for those studying animal behavior.

3

Proximate Factors

uppose that I am attending a roundtable discussion on visual acuity in birds. Sitting in the room with me are four scientists. The speaker on the podium is discussing visual acuity in robins (Figure 3.1), and on the screen in front of us is information on the anatomy of a robin's eye, the neuronal underpinnings of robin vision, and even information about the molecular genetics underlying visual acuity in robins.

When she has finished her presentation, the speaker asks everyone in the room to briefly explain visual acuity in robins from the perspective of their particular discipline. Our first scientist proceeds to explain how natural selection produced an increase in visual acuity over time. She outlines the process of natural selection on vision, and describes how better vision produces a robin that is a superior forager and more adept at avoiding predators. Our next speaker stands up and explains how the curvature of the eye leads to better understanding of why modern-day robins have better visual acuity than some other birds. The third scientist then describes the neural circuitry underlying vision and how that will shed light on increased visual acuity in robins. Finally, our fourth scientist proceeds to detail the changes associated with robin vision at the molecular genetic level, and how these changes are critical to understanding vision in robins.

Who's right? They all are, but their explanations are at different levels of analysis. The first speaker has provided an ultimate explanation—one based on evolutionary processes—while the last three scientists have provided answers, all of which may be correct, at the proximate level. Ever since Tinbergen discussed the four sorts of questions ethologists ask (regarding immediate stimuli, development, survival function, and phylogeny; see Chapter 1), animal behaviorists have understood the importance of studying behavior both from an ultimate and a proximate perspective. That is, various subdisciplines in ethology look at all the issues raised at our roundtable. Indeed, in the long run, one goal of animal behaviorists is to integrate these different perspectives, to the greatest extent possible, into a comprehensive view of animal behavior.

FIGURE 3.1. Different perspectives on a trait. Four different scientists studying a robin's eye could come up with different, but mutually compatible, explanations for the bird's visual acuity.

Ultimate and Proximate
Perspectives

When faced with questions about the nature of behavior, the most common error made by those not trained in the field of ethology is to confuse the level at which a behavior is being analyzed. For example, we can answer the question "Why do songbirds sing?" in terms of physiology, neurobiology, survival value, relationship to other species of birds, and so on (Sherman, 1988). Confusion arises when you ask a question about behavior at one level of analysis, and I answer your question at a different level. I might give you an answer to why songbirds sing based on the bird's voice box (syrinx), its musculature, and the nervous system connecting the syrinx to the brain, when in fact you were looking for a reply that explains birdsong in terms of why natural selection seems to have favored this trait in many different species, or perhaps the role that phylogeny plays in explaining birdsong. When we talk past each other this way, it is because we are approaching the question from different conceptual pathways—one dealing with immediate causation (proximate) and one centering on forces that have shaped a trait over evolutionary time (ultimate). In order to solve what Paul Sherman refers to as the "levels of analysis" problem in behavior, we need to understand both ultimate and proximate causation, so as not to confuse them (Alcock and Sherman, 1994; Mayr, 1961; Reeve and Sherman, 1993; Sherman, 1988).

We have examined ultimate causation in Chapter 2, so Chapter 3 shall serve as a primer on proximate causation. Once we have completed our primers on ultimate and proximate causation, we shall integrate both approaches into all of the remaining chapters of this book

One way to think of the distinction between proximate and ultimate perspectives is to recognize that proximate questions include "How is it that . . . ?" and "What is it that . . . ?" sorts of questions, while ultimate questions are typically of the form "Why is it that . . . ?" (Alcock, 2001, 2003; Figure 3.2). In that sense, proximate and ultimate explanations complement one another. Sometimes proximate causes are defined as those that are not evolutionary in nature. But this is probably not the most productive definition for two reasons. First, as we shall see, it can often be very useful to understand evolutionary (ultimate) forces when asking "how" and "what" questions, and that utility can get lost if we define proximate causation as everything that isn't evolutionary. Second, this definition makes it seem as if the proximate level of analysis is less important than analysis at the ultimate level, and that is not the case.

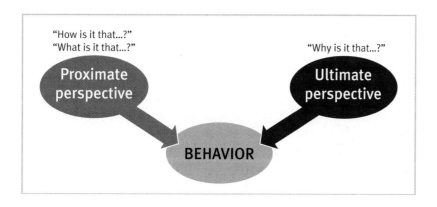

FIGURE 3.2. Causes of behavior. One can study behavior from both a proximate and an ultimate perspective.

Conceptually, we need to think in different ways when we undertake proximate and ultimate analyses. In a proximate analysis, we are working with factors that operate within the lifetime of an organism, in the here and now, rather than inferring (or testing) historical arguments as we do in an ultimate analysis about what evolutionary forces have operated in the past or how such evolutionary forces might operate in the future. At the same time, it is important to recognize that there are fundamental links between proximate and ultimate analyses. Suppose we are undertaking a proximate analysis of some behavior—let's say male aggressiveness. If we understand something about the natural selection pressures that have acted on male aggression, that can help us design a better way to do our proximate analysis. For example, if we know that male aggression is directed toward other males to gain access to food, we might focus on different proximate factors than if we know that male aggression is directed toward other males during the breeding season in order to secure access to females. As we shall see later in the chapter, many times, although certainly not always, the proximate underpinnings of foraging and mating behaviors are different, and in that sense our understanding of natural selection might help provide focus for our proximate analysis. Conversely, our proximate analysis might provide information that will help us better understand how natural selection has shaped male aggression. We might find that the hormones involved in male aggression also lower a male's resistance to disease, suggesting that we need to incorporate this disease effect into our natural selection model of male aggression. What's more, and just as importantly, our proximate analysis, by shedding light on neurobiology, endocrinology, molecular genetics, and so on, will help us to better understand the raw material that natural selection may operate on in the future. That is, our proximate analysis will shed light on the variation available for natural selection to act on in the future.

Before we focus our attention on proximate causation alone, an example of how animal behaviorists employ both proximate and ultimate perspectives to address a single trait may help elucidate the relationship between these two approaches, and will serve as a nice starting point for an in-depth look at the proximate level of analysis. To do this, we shall consider Geoff Hill's thorough and ingenious work on plumage (that is, feather) coloration in the house finch (*Carpodacus mexicanus*).

In the house finch, males are more brightly colored than females. The question that Hill addressed was the nature of differential plumage coloration in male and female house finches. Conceptually, the question of differential plumage coloration in finches is a problem that can be examined from both a proximate and an ultimate perspective (Figure 3.3). That is, we can ask *what* causes males and females to differ in plumage coloration and also examine *why* such color differences persist over evolutionary time. In addressing these questions, we will venture into a discussion that involves foraging behavior, mate choice, and parental care, all of which play a part in understanding the proximate and ultimate underpinnings of plumage coloration in male and female house finches. We will begin by examining Hill's work on proximate causation, and then move on to his work on ultimate causation. But it should be noted that it is not necessarily the case that proximate studies precede ultimate studies—just as often the converse is true.

To examine the proximate basis for plumage, Hill employed within- and between-population comparisons and controlled feeding experiments. We must recognize that, from the start, Hill knew that plumage coloration in the male

FIGURE 3.3. Natural variation. Significant natural variation exists in house finch coloration. This set the stage for Hill's work on the proximate and ultimate questions on plumage coloration. *(Photo credit: Geoff Hill)*

house finch was a result of carotenoid—primarily red—color pigments that were ingested by the birds, and that this finding has been corroborated many times over the years (Brush and Power, 1976; Hill, 1992, 1993a; Hill et al., 2002; Inouye et al., 2001). What is particularly interesting in this light is that birds are unable to synthesize their own carotenoid pigments, and they rely completely on diet for this substance (Brush, 1990; Brush and Power, 1976; Goodwin, 1950). Hill's work, and that of others, demonstrated that at the proximate level, differences in *male* plumage within and between populations of finches were correlated with the amount of carotenoids in their diet—that is, differences in plumage were due to *developmental differences* in what carotenoid-based foods males ate as they matured, as well as which of these foods males added to their diets as adults. Differences in plumage had yet to be addressed in females, and it is to such differences that we now turn (Brush and Power, 1976; Butcher and Rohwer, 1989; Hill, 1993c).

Hill undertook a series of controlled feeding experiments on two groups of females who were fed a fixed diet while housed in aviaries at the University of Michigan. Both groups were fed a commercially made finch food, and both groups had their diets supplemented with water and apples. In one of these groups, however, the water and apples were treated with canthaxanthin—a red carotenoid pigment. Females in the canthaxanthin treatment developed much brighter plumage after their diet was supplemented, but females fed just normal apples and water maintained a drab plumage pattern.

From a proximate perspective, we can now address two issues: (1) what causes between-population differences in female coloration, and (2) what causes differences in plumage coloration between males and females. These sorts of "what causes" questions are often where a proximate analysis begins. With respect to differences between females across populations, it appears that the *differential availability* of carotenoid (primarily red) pigments in food across populations is critical. For example, Hill found differences in female plumage coloration between individuals from Michigan, New York, and Hawaii (Hill, 1993a, 1993c). These differences appear to be a function of the amount of carotenoid-based food sources in these localities: the more such food is present in the foraging environment, the brighter the average female is in a population.

From a proximate perspective, the answer to the question "What causes differences in plumage coloration between females?" centers on how much carotenoid-based food is present in the physical environment. Differences in the developmental environment, in this case the amount of carotenoid-based food available to females as they matured, as well as during their adulthood, help explain differences in female plumage coloration.

Differences in plumage color between males and females within a population appear to be due to differences in the way in which males and females forage, rather than to the availability of carotenoid-based foods for males and females. At the behavioral level, males actively search for carotenoid-based foods. While females don't avoid carotenoid foods, they are much more passive in terms of searching for such items. Here, the proximate analysis focuses our attention not solely on the amount of carotenoid-based food present in the environment, but also on differences in foraging strategies in males and females.

This proximate explanation for differences in male and female coloration leads us nicely to our discussion of ultimate questions. Hill argued that the reason that females don't actively search for carotenoid-based foods is that, whereas colorful males receive significant benefits for having colorful plumage

FIGURE 3.4. Plumage manipulation.
As part of Hill's study on plumage coloration, he artificially brightened (top left photo to top right photo) or lightened (bottom left photo to bottom right photo) the plumage coloration of male house finches. *(Photo credit: Geoff Hill)*

(see below), females do not. As such, females focus on maximizing the calories they get per unit time, not the amount of carotenoids that they ingest.

In conjunction with his work at the proximate level, Hill conducted numerous experiments to examine the ultimate cause of differences in male and female plumage coloration (Hill, 1990, 1991, 1993b). Once Hill knew that foraging behavior was correlated with plumage color and that males actively searched for carotenoid-rich foods, he could ask why—that is, why do males actively search for carotenoids that increase their plumage coloration? What's in it, fitness-wise, for males to do this? We have now shifted our conceptual framework from the proximate to the ultimate. With that in mind, also remember that this shift to an ultimate analysis was a result of findings that arose from our proximate analysis.

To examine the ultimate reason that males are more colorful than females, Hill used hair dyes to either brighten or lighten the plumage coloration of a group of wild eastern male finches (Figure 3.4). Then he examined how such manipulations affected female mate choice (Table 3.1). Males that had their color

TABLE 3.1. Plumage manipulation. Hill examined how brightening and lightening plumage coloration affected a suite of variables in male house finches. There were 40 males in the brightened condition, 20 males in the sham control, and 40 males in the lightened condition. (From Hill, 1991)

MALE CHARACTERISTICS	BRIGHTENED	SHAM CONTROL	LIGHTENED	STATISTICAL SIGNIFICANCE (P)
Original plumage score	140.7	139.9	141.00	0.95
Manipulated plumage score	161.6	139.9	129.40	0.0001
Proportion paired	1.0	0.6	0.27	0.0001
Time to pair (days)	12.1	20.2	27.80	0.07

experimentally enhanced were much more likely to get a mate than males whose colors had been experimentally lightened. This result alone provided powerful evidence that one of the ultimate reasons that males search for carotenoid-rich food is that females are attracted to males with bright plumage. Hill went on to examine precisely *why* females prefer males with bright plumage. This is an ultimate question regarding mate choice in females—namely, are there fitness benefits for females who make good choices with respect to male plumage coloration?

Recent work from the Hill lab suggests that one benefit to mating with redder-colored males is that such males appear to be better able to fight off pathogens. When Hill and Farmer inoculated twenty-four male house finches with *Mycoplasma gallicepticum*, a bacterial pathogen, they found that males with more elaborate plumage coloration were able to rid themselves of this disease more quickly than drabber-colored males (Figure 3.5). As such, females may expose themselves to fewer pathogens by selecting males that are more resistant to disease over males that are less resistant (we explore this in more depth in Chapters 6 and 16). In addition, if such disease resistance is inherited, by choosing the more disease-resistant males as mates, a female's offspring will be better able to stave off disease (Duckworth et al., 2001; Hill and Farmer, 2005).

A second fitness-related benefit that females may receive by choosing brighter-colored males over drabber-colored males centers on parental care and food provisioning. When examining the relationship between male color and male parental care in eastern populations of house finches, Hill found that the mean number of times a male fed a chick at his nest was positively correlated with the intensity of his plumage coloration, with brighter males feeding chicks more than twice as often as drabber males (Hill, 1991; Figure 3.6A). Females may then prefer redder males because such males make good fathers, at least with respect to feeding. Yet, this cannot be the only fitness-related explanation for why females prefer redder males, as recent work from western populations of house finches has found that, in these populations, more colorful males provide less parental care than drabber males, but females still prefer the more colorful males as mates (Badyaev and Hill, 2002; Duckworth et al., 2004; McGraw et al., 2001).

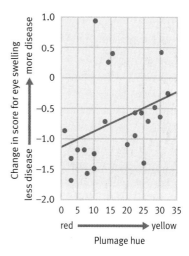

FIGURE 3.5. Plumage coloration and recovery from infection. Birds were infected with *Mycoplasma gallicepticum*, which caused eye swelling, and the rate at which they recovered from this infection was linked with their plumage coloration. Birds with more red coloration (who had eaten food with more carotenoid pigments) recovered more quickly (in later phases of the experiment) than birds with more yellow coloration (who had eaten food with fewer carotenoid pigments). *(From Hill and Farmer, 2005)*

A

B

FIGURE 3.6. Plumage, feeding, and heritability. (A) Brighter male house finches feed their young at higher rates than drabber male finches. **(B)** A significant positive relationship exists between father and son plumage brightness scores in house finches. *(From Hill, 1991)*

There is a third benefit that females may receive by choosing more colorful over less colorful males as mates. In eastern populations, female house finches may obtain indirect fitness-related benefits by mating with brightly colored males, as such males appear to be better foragers, and hence they may survive with a relatively high probability. If the traits responsible for this increased survival are passed on to offspring, then mating with colorful males may produce very fit offspring. Hill found that males with lots of red plumage produced sons with colorful plumage (Figure 3.6B). Given that red plumage coloration can't be inherited—as such coloration is diet dependent—this suggests that males that are good foragers, and thus have the carotenoids needed to produce colorful plumage, produce sons that are also good foragers.

Hill's work is an excellent example of how ultimate and proximate (particularly developmental) perspectives can provide an in-depth picture of animal behavior. Among other things, it showed how proximate explanations of what causes differences in coloration can also point the way to ultimate reasons for why there are such differences.

In the remainder of this chapter, we will examine the following proximate factors affecting behavior:

- hormones,
- neurobiology,
- molecular genetics,
- development.

Before proceeding to the next section, it is important to place the remainder of this chapter within the larger scope of the entire book. Once we complete the "primer chapters" (Chapters 2–5), Chapters 6–17 will deal with a series of eleven major behavioral venues (foraging, predation, cooperation, aggression, and so on). It would clearly be impractical, indeed impossible, to discuss a hormonal, neurobiological, molecular genetic, and developmental example of each of the areas covered by Chapters 6–17 within this primer chapter, and so I am forced to choose. What I have attempted to do is combine the four proximate approaches with examples of the behaviors covered in the later chapters of the book in a way that demonstrates how broadly these four approaches can be applied. At the very least, I hope that this presentation provides a sense of the interdisciplinary nature of work in animal behavior.

There is a sense in which dividing proximate causation into four components—hormonal, neurobiological, molecular genetic, and developmental—is artificial. For example, neurobiological differences often underlie hormonal changes in behavior (and vice versa), and one could argue that all hormonal and neurobiological differences associated with behavior can be understood at the molecular genetic level. As another example, hormonal differences can lead to behavioral differences that translate into animals having very different experiences during development. Conversely, developmental differences can lead to different hormonal responses to some stressor in the environment, as well as affect various properties of neurons associated with behavioral responses. All of this is to say that the relation between hormonal, neurobiological, molecular genetic, and developmental causation is complex, and that boundaries between them can be difficult to define. My justification for separating them here is that before we can understand the complicated *interaction* between these four types of causation, we need a basic understanding of how each one works. Once that is accomplished, toward the end of the chapter, we will integrate molecular genetic, developmental, hormonal, and neurobiological approaches in discussing studies of a single species—the honeybee.

Hormones and Proximate Causation

A bit of background will help set the stage for our discussion of proximate causation, hormones, and behavior. The **endocrine system**, a powerful communication network that strongly influences many aspects of animal behavior, is composed of a group of ductless glands that secrete hormones (derived from the Greek word for "excite") directly into the bloodstream (in vertebrates), or into fluid surrounding tissue (in invertebrates). In vertebrates, the glands producing hormones include the adrenal gland, the pituitary gland, the thyroid gland, the pancreas, the gonads, and the hypothalamus. Within these glands are endocrine cells, which synthesize and then secrete hormones into the bloodstream (Figure 3.7). Hormones act as molecular messengers that affect target cells that reside some (relatively long) distance from the gland secreting the hormone. Many glands can secrete more than one hormone, and the same hormone can have different effects on different target cells. Hormones affect many traits, including behavior, both directly and indirectly through changes in cell metabolism or DNA expression. Correct functioning of the endocrine system is of fundamental importance to behavioral functions and to the modification of rates and directions of various cellular functions. Malfunctioning of hormones, either through diminished secretion (hyposecretion) or excessive secretion (hypersecretion), affects functions such as growth, metabolism, reactions to stress, aggression, and reproduction.

It is important to keep in mind that the endocrine system is not a disconnected amalgam of ductless glands. Oftentimes, hormones secreted by

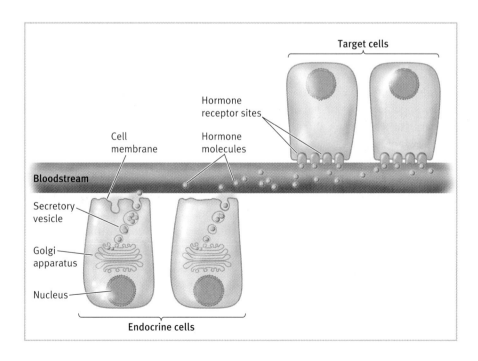

FIGURE 3.7. Endocrine cells and target cells. A schematic of how endocrine cells work and how hormones eventually affect target cells. Enzymes in the Golgi apparatus process proteins into hormone molecules and package them inside secretory vesicles. These vesicles fuse with the cell membrane and release the hormone molecules into the bloodstream. The hormone molecules travel through the bloodstream until they reach the receptor sites of the target cell, where they bond and initiate a series of interactions. (Adapted from Nelson, 2005)

one endocrine gland stimulate the production and secretion of hormones from another gland. This chain has important behavioral consequences. For example, in response to the production and secretion of CRH (corticotropin-releasing hormone) from the hypothalamus, the anterior pituitary gland secretes ACTH (adrenocorticotropic hormone), which in turn stimulates the adrenal glands to produce glucocorticoid hormones like cortisol. These glucocorticoids play a critical role in the production of stress-related behaviors—for example, reduced aggression in the presence of dominant individuals. Conversely, the secretion of some hormones *inhibit* the production of hormones in other ductless glands, rather than *promoting* such production. As such, we need to think of the endocrine system as an interconnected and complex communication network that has both direct and indirect effects on animal behavior.

In a moment, we will examine the basic structure of the endocrine system, and in particular, how hormones indirectly and directly affect animal behavior. Before we do, it is worth noting that there is an important exception to the rule that hormones are produced by ductless glands. Some hormones, called **neurohormones**, can be released into the blood via neurons (almost always located in the brain) that secrete these hormones directly into the bloodstream (Nelson, 2005). For example, as we will see later on, the neurohormone octopamine plays an important role in the changes in foraging behavior in animals such as honeybees.

Hormones are almost always transported through the bloodstream, and with one exception (the cells in the lens of the eye), all cells in the body have a direct blood supply. This means that hormones can reach virtually every cell in the body (Nelson, 2005), but that does not necessarily mean that they have an effect on every cell in the body. A hormone will only have an effect on a cell if the cell has the correct receptor site for that hormone. Cells with the receptor site for a particular hormone are referred to as target cells for that hormone. The receptor site (often on the surface of a cell) and the hormone act as a lock-and-key system that is known as the hormone receptor complex. A receptor (lock) is not activated until the correct hormone (key) reaches it, and a hormone has no effect on a cell unless the cell has the correct receptor. For our purposes, what this means is that the relationship between animal behavior and endocrinology is only put into play when hormones reach target cells.

In this lock-and-key system, once a hormone reaches a cell and bonds with the receptor site, a series of interactions occur that affect the expression of genes and the synthesis of proteins. Precisely how these changes occur depends on the specific hormone we are studying, but changes in gene expression and protein synthesis either directly or indirectly affect an animal's behavior. For example, increased gene expression or protein synthesis could, through a series of intermediary steps, lead to an increase in foraging behavior or an increase in aggressive behavior, or perhaps both.

Of course, the lock-and-key system we just described is only put into operation when a hormone is released into the bloodstream. What causes the release in the first place? The answer to this question often lies in the complex ways that animals respond to stimuli in their environment. To see this, let's look at one component of the endocrinology of reproductive behavior in birds.

Many bird species breed during the spring and summer, when temperatures are warmer and food is more plentiful. Changes in day length are an excellent cue for seasonal change, and in many birds, levels of the hormones gonadotropin (which stimulates sperm production) and testosterone increase in males as day

FIGURE 3.8. Day length, hormones, and behavior. Many bird species breed during the spring and summer, and changes in day length are an excellent cue for seasonal change. As day length changes, it affects circulating levels of testosterone (T). Increases in T increase the probability that males are aggressive toward one another (to gain access to females), guard their mates, build nests, and defend their brood.

length increases. Testosterone binds to receptor cells in the brain, and is associated with various behaviors related to mating and paternal care—for example, males are more likely to be aggressive toward one another to gain access to females, guard their mates, build nests, and defend their brood when testosterone is high. Thus, environment change (day length) is associated with increased levels of testosterone, and increased levels of testosterone affect how animals respond to environmental stimuli like the presence of other males and the appearance of nest predators (Ball, 1993; Dawson, 2002; Wingfield et al., 2001; Figure 3.8). When ethologists experimentally manipulated day length in the laboratory, they discovered that delaying the onset of increased day length can have profound effects on male testosterone levels (which remain low) and all of the testosterone-mediated behaviors we have just described.

If we think of animals as an engineer might, we realize that they possess three interactive systems (Figure 3.9): (1) an input system made up of all the sensory systems (smell, sight, and so on), (2) a central processor made up of

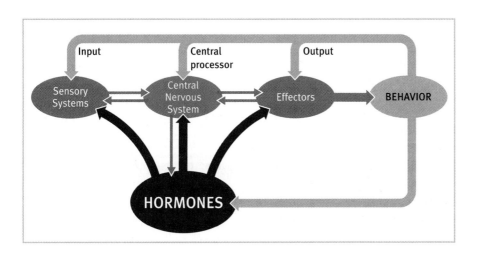

FIGURE 3.9. Complex effects of hormones. Hormones can affect input systems (sensory systems like those for smell, sight, or hearing), central nervous system functions (processing), and output systems (for example, effectors like muscles controlling movement). (Adapted from Nelson, 2005)

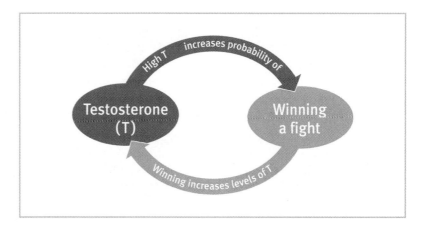

FIGURE 3.10. Testosterone (T) and aggression. A positive feedback loop exists between levels of T and probability of winning a fight. High levels of T increase the probability of winning, while winning further increases circulating levels of T.

integrators that process and integrate the sensory information received, and (3) output systems—effectors such as muscles that move when stimulated (Nelson, 2005). What hormones do is change the probability that a specific sensory input leads to a specific output.

Hormones can affect the probability that a specific sensory input leads to a specific behavioral response in many ways. Hormonal changes might *modify* some ongoing behavior, or they might *trigger* the onset of a behavior. In addition, hormones might *prime* animals so that they would be more or less likely to behave in a specific way in a specific environment. For example, when testosterone is at a high level, males are more likely to engage in aggressive behavior than when testosterone levels are low. That is, when baseline levels of testosterone are high, males are primed for aggressive behavior, in the sense that they are more likely to display aggression when encountering another male than they are otherwise. With testosterone, as with many hormones, there is a hormonal-behavioral feedback loop in play. If an animal wins a fight, partly as a result of behaviors resulting from high baseline levels of testosterone, this may increase the probability of winning future fights by further increasing testosterone levels or by lowering the level of stress hormones such as cortisol (Figure 3.10).

Hormones also affect the *organization* of behavior systems during early development. To see this, let's examine the effect of hormones on behavior in mice. Female mice, like many female mammals, gestate many fetuses at the same time. If a developing male mouse fetus is surrounded by female fetuses, it is often exposed to lower levels of circulating testosterone (Figure 3.11). When such males mature they tend to be less aggressive and less sexually active than males who were surrounded by male fetuses when in utero. Here we see a case in which the entire behavioral repertoire associated with aggressive interactions could be fundamentally altered by hormonal effects early on in development.

While the specific relationship between behavior and the endocrine system in various species is different, early work by Hans Selye found that the behavioral/endocrinological response to danger—sometimes called the "fight or flight" response—is very similar across different types of stress. Subsequent work found that this fight or flight response was similar across many vertebrate species, including humans (Nelson, 2005; Selye, 1936; Stratakis and Chrousos, 1955). To understand the complex interaction between the endocrine system and behavior in a bit more detail, let's examine some of the specifics of the fight or flight response.

When a stressor—a predator, for example—is sensed by an individual, the hypothalamus initiates a response, which works along two pathways. In the

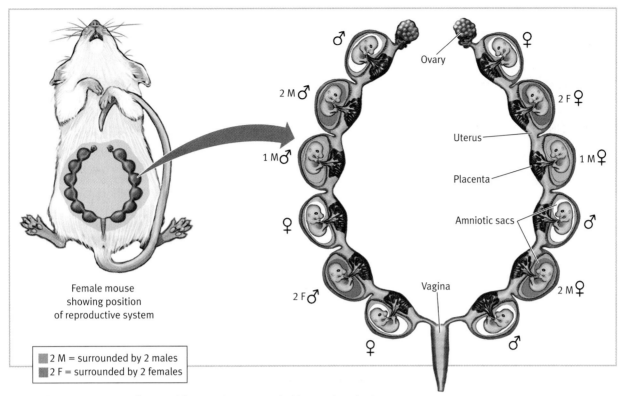

FIGURE 3.11. Intrauterine position. Males surrounded by two females in utero act relatively "feminized," while females surrounded by two males act relatively "masculinized." These behavioral differences are typically a result of differential exposure to hormones while in utero. 1M = surrounded by one male; 2M = surrounded by two males; 2F = surrounded by two females. *(From vom Saal, 1989)*

first pathway, the adrenal glands begin to secrete epinephrine (also known as adrenaline), and norepinephrine is secreted by both the adrenal glands and certain nerves in the central nervous system. This burst of epinephrine and norepinephrine leads to a quick and very large increase in blood sugar, which, along with oxygen, is delivered quickly to vital organs. In particular, the brain, skeletal muscles, and heart are recipients of both increased blood sugar and oxygen. As a result of the increased sugar and oxygen, circulation increases and "nonessential" systems—for example, the digestive and reproductive systems—are shut down. All of this allows for an appropriate behavioral response to whatever the stressor—in our case, a predator—may be. The increase in sugar might enable the animal to quickly flee from a predator or perhaps to fight off this danger.

In a second pathway, another "responsive reaction" chain is also put into motion when a stressor is sensed. Here corticotropin-releasing hormone (CRH), growth hormone-releasing hormone (GHRH), and thyrotropin-releasing hormone (TRH) are secreted by the hypothalamus. CRH in turn stimulates the anterior pituitary gland to increase the production of ACTH, which then stimulates the adrenal gland to secrete cortisol, which converts noncarbohydrates into sugars—energy that can be used to handle the stressor in question, by, for example, fleeing quickly from danger or standing put and fighting. The adrenal gland also increases its production of aldosterone, which increases water retention and hence reduces bleeding if the stressor causes injury. These two parallel hormonal/behavioral responses to stressors nicely illustrate the intricate and

FIGURE 3.12. Helping in male Mongolian gerbils. Male helping behavior as a function of prior intrauterine position has been examined in Mongolian gerbils. *(Photo credit: Julian Barker)*

FIGURE 3.13. Testosterone measurements. Circulating testosterone levels for males that were surrounded by zero (2F), one (1M), or two (2M) other males while in utero. *(Adapted from Clark et al., 1991)*

complex ways that organisms respond to dangers in their environment. It is only when stress is chronic that the endocrine system fails to respond in the appropriate manner.

With our brief overview of the endocrine system and behavior complete, let's move on to examine a few case studies from the animal behavior literature.

THE LONG-TERM EFFECTS OF IN-UTERO EXPOSURE TO HORMONES

Let us return to the case of in-utero exposure to testosterone that we mentioned earlier. In a number of rodent species, the sex of the two siblings surrounding an individual in utero can have dramatic effects on testosterone level and an individual's behavior after birth (Ryan and Vandenbergh, 2002; vom Saal, 1989). Behaviorally, males that were surrounded by two other males in utero (labeled 2M males) are more aggressive than males that were surrounded by two females (labeled 2F males). In addition, 2M males mark their territories by scent and mount more females than 2F males, both in the laboratory and the field (Drickamer, 1996; Ryan and Vandenbergh, 2002; vom Saal and Bronson, 1978). To better understand the behavioral endocrinology of testosterone and intrauterine position, let's examine mating and parental care in male gerbils (*Meriones unguiculatus*). Male Mongolian gerbils are known to huddle over their young and groom them (Figure 3.12). Researchers examined whether such behavior was affected by in-utero testosterone effects.

In gerbils, the position of males while in utero affects the level of testosterone to which they are exposed. In 1991, Mertice Clark and her colleagues used a technique called radioimmunoassay to measure in-utero testosterone levels of 2M and 2F males (Clark et al., 1991). What they found was that testosterone levels in 2M males were significantly higher than in 2F males (Figure 3.13). It is still not clear exactly what causes this difference, but it is likely, in part, a result of 2M males being exposed to higher levels of testosterone in their amniotic sacs as a result of being surrounded by two other males (Clemens et al., 1978). These in-utero differences between 2M and 2F males have long-term consequences—adult 2M males have twice the level of circulating testosterone levels as adult 2F males (Clark et al., 1991, 1992a; Even et al., 1992; vom Saal, 1989). With this in mind, Clark and her colleagues examined whether testosterone differences that had been initiated in utero, and continued through life, affected male reproductive behavior, both in terms of obtaining mates and providing parental care (Clark and Galef, 2000; Clark et al., 1992b, 1998).

Clark and her team began their comparison of the mating behavior of 2M and 2F males by housing a single male (either 2M or 2F) and a single female together in a cage. They then measured how long it took before the male sexually mounted the female, and the time it took between mounting the female and ejaculation. Results were clear—2M males not only mounted females more quickly, but they ejaculated sooner (similar results have been uncovered in comparisons of 2M and 2F mice) (vom Saal, 1989; vom Saal et al., 1983). Given these differences in mating behavior, it was not surprising when follow-up experiments indicated that 2M males also sired more offspring after being paired with a female than did 2F males.

The long-term consequences of intrauterine position on testosterone are not limited to mating behavior. Theory suggests that testosterone level plays an

FIGURE 3.14. In-utero position and subsequent parental behavior. Males that were surrounded by two males while they were in utero (2M males) provided less parental care when they matured than did males that were surrounded by two females when in utero (2F males). *(From Clark et al., 1998)*

important role in explaining the negative correlation between mating success and parental care often found in male birds and mammals (Feder et al., 2000; Ketterson and Nolan, 1999). Researchers have found that males with high levels of testosterone tend to spend more time and effort searching for mates, but devote less effort to parental care.

The work described above demonstrates increased mating effort on the part of 2M males, and so Clark and her team examined whether 2M males also dispensed less parental care (Clark and Galef, 1999; Clark et al., 1998). To test this, twenty-three 2F males and twenty-one 2M males were each housed individually with a female, until the female was pregnant and gave birth. Once a female had given birth, the behavior of males toward pups was examined. Both when their mates were present, and when their mates were absent, 2M males spent significantly less time in contact with pups than 2F males (Figure 3.14). To be more confident that the differences between 2M and 2F males were linked to relatively higher testosterone levels in 2M males, Clark and Galef undertook a follow-up experiment in which they castrated adolescent males to experimentally reduce testosterone level. Such castrated males increased the time they spent caring for pups. When castrated males had their testosterone levels brought back to normal, through silicon implants, their parental behavior decreased, suggesting a causal link between testosterone and parental care (Clark and Galef, 1999; Clark et al., 2004; Figure 3.15).

It appears, then, that intrauterine position affected circulating levels of testosterone, which in turn affected both males' mating behavior and their parental care, nicely illustrating the complex, long-term, and often indirect, effects of hormones on animal behavior.

STRESS HORMONES AND SPATIAL MEMORY IN RATS

Ethologists and behavioral endocrinologists are very interested in the way in which hormones affect memory (de Quervain et al., 1998, 2000; Sapolsky, 2003). This is in part because of the implications such work might have on understanding learning disabilities in humans (Alderson and Novack, 2002; Sauro et al., 2003), and in part because learning and memory play such a

FIGURE 3.15. Testosterone and male parental care. When male Mongolian gerbils were castrated, they spent more time with pups than did "sham" castrated males that had undergone a similar operation but were not actually castrated. *(From Clark et al., 2004)*

fundamental role in shaping animal behavior across a wide variety of taxa (Chapter 4). While not always the case, high levels of glucocorticoid hormones—often called "stress hormones"—interfere with spatial memory skills in many animals (McEwen and Sapolsky, 1995; Sapolsky, 1999; Sapolsky et al., 2000). In this section, we will examine Dominique de Quervain and his colleagues' work on how one such glucocorticoid hormone—corticosterone—affects spatial memory in rats (de Quervain et al., 1998).

To examine spatial memory in rats, de Quervain and his team used a device called a water maze. Rats are put into a large tank of dark and murky water, and some distance from where the rat enters the water, there is a single small platform that is underwater (but close enough to the surface to serve as a resting place for the rat). When first put into the tank, rats swim around randomly, but eventually they come across the hidden platform, and when they do, they use it as a refuge. That is, after a rat finds the platform, which was hidden by the murky water, it tends to remain there, and it avoids expending more energy swimming around the water maze tank. As they are put through more and more trials in the water maze, rats become better and better at finding the platform.

Based on prior work on rodents, de Quervain and his colleagues hypothesized that a stress-induced increase in corticosterone would impair a rat's spatial memory regarding the position of the platform. To test this hypothesis, the researchers gave rats eight trials in the water maze, and then they divided the rats into four groups (Figure 3.16). In Group 1, rats received a shock thirty

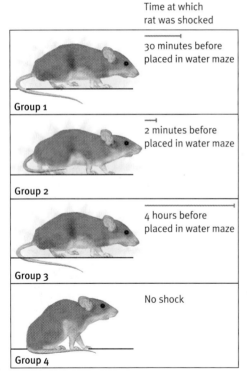

Time at which rat was shocked

Group 1 — 30 minutes before placed in water maze

Group 2 — 2 minutes before placed in water maze

Group 3 — 4 hours before placed in water maze

Group 4 — No shock

Underwater platform

Swimming rat

Water maze

FIGURE 3.16. Water maze apparatus and learning trials. De Quervain and his colleagues examined stress and learning in rats by using a water maze in murky water that had a platform that the rats could not see but could learn to find. In Group 1, rats received a shock thirty minutes before their ninth trial. The shock was administered two minutes before the ninth trial in Group 2 rats, and four hours before the ninth trial in Group 3 rats. Rats in Group 4, the control group, received no shock before their ninth trial.

A

B

FIGURE 3.17. **Shock and spatial memory in rats.** **(A)** In the experiment by de Quervain and his colleagues, rats that received a shock thirty minutes before their trial in the water maze spent less time near the platform (target) than did rats in the other three groups (control, shock at two minutes before trial, and shock at four hours before trial). **(B)** The swimming path of the control rat was consistently near the target (T), indicating that its memory for the location of the platform was not impaired, while the swimming path of the rat that was shocked thirty minutes before being put in the water maze was random, indicating that its memory for the location of the platform was impaired by the shock. *(From de Quervain et al., 1998)*

minutes before they were next placed in the water—that is, rats were shocked thirty minutes before their ninth trial in the water maze. In Group 2, the shock was administered two minutes before the ninth trial; and in Group 3 it was administered four hours before the ninth trial. A fourth group—the control group—received no shock before their ninth trial. The researchers found that rats in Groups 2 and 3 spent about as much time near the platform as did rats in the control group. That is, shocks that were administered two minutes or four hours before a trial did not impede spatial memory for the location of the platform. Rats in Group 1—those that experienced the shock thirty minutes before the trial—did show impaired memory for the location of the platform (Figure 3.17).

These behavioral results provided de Quervain and his team with critical information about what hormonal changes may have been associated with impaired spatial memory. Unlike other hormones affecting memory, corticosterone's effects on spatial memory are often displayed about thirty minutes after stress is induced, and then these effects dissipate over the next few hours. Corticosterone's effects on spatial memory would then only be predicted for Group 1, where shock was administered thirty minutes before the water maze trial. This is because the time between shock and testing in the water maze was too short for corticosterone effects to be manifest in Group 2 (two minutes), and too long for such effects to occur in Group 3 (four hours). De Quervain and his team measured corticosterone levels in rats in all four groups. As predicted, they found that, compared to the control group, only rats in Group 1—the group with decreased ability to find the area of the platform—had higher levels of corticosterone, suggesting an important memory-inhibiting role for this hormone.

De Quervain and his team examined the role of corticosterone on spatial memory in two follow-up experiments. In one of these, they injected rats with a drug called metyrapone, which inhibits the production of corticosterone by blocking certain chemical reactions in the adrenal glands, where corticosterone is produced. When rats were injected with metyrapone, individuals that were shocked before their trial in the water tank did not show impaired memory compared to control animals. That is, when corticosterone production was blocked, the inability of rats to find the platform in the maze was reversed, again suggesting that corticosterone was associated with spatial memory tasks in rats.

In their second follow-up experiment, instead of shocking rats thirty minutes before their last trial in the water maze, de Quervain and his colleagues injected rats with corticosterone thirty minutes before a trial. If corticosterone changes in response to stress were behind the impairment of spatial memory, then rats that have their corticosterone levels experimentally increased should also show impaired spatial memory in the water maze. Results suggest that this was the case, as rats injected with corticosterone (but not shocked) thirty minutes before being placed in the water maze tank also showed impaired memory when it came to finding the platform.

Taken together, the work by de Quervain and his team is a beautiful example of how the behavioral endocrinology of spatial memory can be studied in a controlled environment. The combination of behavioral experiments with measurements of corticosterone, experimental manipulations of corticosterone, as well as manipulation of chemicals that block the production of corticosterone allows us a much deeper understanding of the role that endocrinology plays in impaired spatial memory.

Neurobiological Underpinnings of Behavior

Because of its function with respect to chemical communication, we have seen what an important role the endocrine system plays in the proximate analysis of behavior. But the endocrine system, which relies strictly on chemical communication, has its limitations, particularly with respect to speed of response, which is usually on the order of minutes to hours. A second communication network—the nervous system—involves an electrical impulse system that is constructed for much quicker responses. This section of the chapter will serve as a sort of primer on the nervous system and behavior, giving an overview of the neurobiological underpinnings of behavior.

Animals possess specialized nerve cells, called neurons, which share certain similarities regardless of what message they conduct. Before we trace an impulse along the nervous system and see how it affects an animal's behavior, let us examine the basic structure of a neuron. Each neuron has a cell body that contains a nucleus and one or more nerve fibers. Fibers that transmit electrical information from one cell to another are called **axons**. Axons can range in size from less than a millimeter to over a meter long. Axons also differ in terms of diameter. This is important because the speed of the nervous impulse affects the speed at which animals respond behaviorally, and the thicker the diameter of an axon, the faster the nervous impulse travels along it.

Each neuron has only a single axon. The first section is called the axon hillock, and the last section consists of the axon terminals (sometimes called

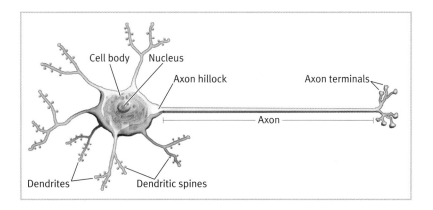

FIGURE 3.18. Nerve cell. Information is collected by dendrites (which often have dendritic spines projecting off their surface), conducted along an axon, and transmitted to neighboring cells from the axon terminals across the synaptic gap to their dendrites.

synaptic terminals). There may be many branches of axon terminals, and it is from these branches that information leaves a neuron as it passes along the nervous system (Figure 3.18).

Neurons receive impulses from other cells via fibers called **dendrites**. A neuron may have thousands of dendrites, forming what is called a dendritic tree. In addition, in certain types of neurons, each "branch" on this dendritic tree may have many "dendritic spines" that receive input from other cells. Later in the chapter, we shall see that the number of these dendritic spines can increase as a function of behaviors associated with spatial navigation, but for now, what is important is that because of dendritic trees and spines, each neuron can receive information from many other neurons.

THE NERVOUS IMPULSE

Let's now trace what happens from the point at which the nervous system of an animal responds to something in the environment to the point at which we observe some sort of behavioral response. Suppose the external stimuli is tactile—that is, the animal is touched by something. In response to this stimulus, a wave of electrical activity sweeps down along the axons of sensory nerve cells that are in contact with the skin. Not all stimuli produce such a response. For this process to begin, the stimulus—the external touch—must exceed the nerve cell's "threshold." Technically, the threshold is a function of the amount of change in the voltage across a neuron's membrane, but for our purposes, what is most important is that stimuli that don't meet this threshold fail to cause the nerve cell to fire, and stimuli above the threshold always cause the nerve cell to fire.

To use an analogy from electrical engineering, nerve cell thresholds are the equivalent of on-off switches, rather than a dimmer switch. Any stimulus greater than the threshold, regardless of how much greater, causes the nerve cell to fire. In other words, the nerve cell fires in exactly the same manner whether the stimulus is 1 percent greater than the threshold or 1,000 percent greater. Such a system is not without its problems. For instance, if a nerve cell fired differently as a function of the degree to which a stimulus overshot the threshold, this might provide an organism with a better ability to gauge the intensity of a stimulus. But even though the nerve cell fires the same way each time its threshold is reached, organisms are still able to use their nervous systems to gauge the strength of a stimulus in at least two ways: (1) the number of times that a neuron fires increases with the strength of the stimulus, and (2) the number of neurons that fire in response to a stimulus also increases as a function of stimulus strength.

Once an impulse has reached the end of an axon, it must be transmitted to other neurons. This can be accomplished by an electrical impulse jumping across the synaptic gap between neurons or, more commonly, by the release of a neurotransmitter—for example, acetylcholine—from thousands of synaptic vesicles located on the tips of the branches at the end of the axon terminals. Neurotransmitters migrate across the synaptic gap and are absorbed by the membrane of the next neuron. If the next neuron is sufficiently stimulated— that is, if its threshold has been met—it will fire. This process continues over and over as the nerve impulse migrates along its neural path. Although they travel very short distances (20 to 30 nanometers), the existence of neuro- transmitters adds a chemical component to the nervous system—that is, a nervous impulse requires both electrical and chemical transmission.

The neural pathway that was initiated by an animal being touched may end when the terminal neurons in the pathway *innervate* (stimulate) some *effector*, such as a muscle, to take action; in this case, terminal neurons might stimulate foraging behavior by opening or closing the jaw muscle (if the animal has encountered potential prey) or initiate flight behavior by innervating muscles associated with such flight (if the touch was that of an aggressive, dominant group member). In other instances, depending upon the stimulus, nerve pathways might end with the secretion of a chemical that causes an endocrine gland to secrete a hormone. This idea that terminal neurons cause secretion of hormones that affect behavior reminds us that the neural and endocrinological communication systems are not independent of one another, but part of a communication "web" that provides an organism with infor- mation about its external and internal environments.

This communication web can work in many ways. Our example in- volving the neuroethological response to touch focused on a stimulus that causes an excitatory response along the nervous system, eventually trans- lating into an animal taking some behavioral action (for example, foraging, fleeing). But we should note that some stimuli cause inhibitory effects, whereby a neuron sends a signal that does not meet the threshold of the cell that receives the signal, eventually resulting in the inhibition of behavior. Such inhibitory responses might be lifesaving—as a result of this process an animal might, for example, freeze in the presence of predators that hone in on the motion of prey.

At a very general level, nervous systems across many animals show some consistent evolutionary trends:

▸ Nerve cells that served specific functions—including functions linked to behavior—became clustered.
▸ Over evolutionary time, nervous systems became centralized, with longitudinal nerve cords becoming the major highway across which nervous impulses travel. The front end of the longitudinal nerve cord became dominant, leading to the evolution of the brain.

With this brief review of the animal nervous system in hand, we can now move on to examine how ethologists might address proximate questions using a neurobiological, or more specifically, a neuroethological approach.

NEUROBIOLOGY AND LEARNING IN VOLES

Here we shall examine spatial learning in voles from a neuroethological perspective, beginning with some basics about vole behavior. Male meadow voles (*Microtus pennsylvanicus*) are polygamous (see Chapter 7), meaning that they mate with more than one female during a breeding season (Figure 3.19). In addition, male meadow voles have very large home ranges—home ranges that are sometimes ten times the size of that of a female, and that often encompass the home ranges of many females (Gaulin and Fitzgerald, 1986, 1989). Given that males have larger home ranges than females, and that they must keep track of females within those home ranges, animal behaviorists predicted that males would have better navigational skills than females.

When Steve Gaulin and Randall FitzGerald ran male and female meadow voles through a series of mazes in the laboratory, they found that indeed males showed superior spatial learning abilities. Gaulin and FitzGerald also examined spatial learning skills in a second species, the prairie vole (*Microtus ochrogaster*). Prairie voles are monogamous, and males and females have home ranges that are approximately equal in size. Because males do not have larger home ranges, and do not have to navigate across many female home ranges, ethologists hypothesized that the difference in spatial learning in males and females that was seen in the polygamous meadow vole would be absent in the monogamous prairie vole. When Gaulin and FitzGerald tested prairie voles in mazes, they found no difference between the spatial abilities of males and females of this species (Figure 3.20).

From a neuroethological perspective, we can (1) examine the neural substrate underlying the differences in male and female spatial learning abilities in voles, and (2) examine how components of the nervous system change as a function of a spatial learning experience. First, let us compare males and females in both polygamous and monogamous species of voles. In so doing, we shall focus on the hippocampus, an area of the cerebral cortex of the brain that is known to be important in spatial navigation (Eichenbaum et al., 1990; Morris et al., 1982; O'Keefe and Nadel, 1978).

FIGURE 3.19. Meadow voles.
Meadow voles (*Microtus pennsylvanicus*) have been the subject of much work on behavior, neurobiology, and endocrinology. *(Photo credit: Phil Myers, Museum of Zoology, University of Michigan)*

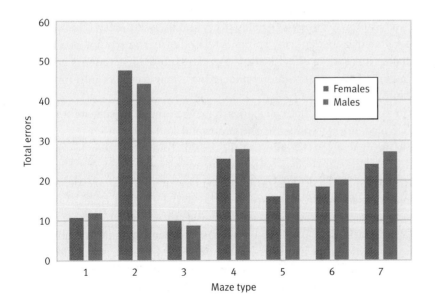

FIGURE 3.20. Learning in voles. No significant differences in learning mazes (as shown here by the number of errors on seven maze types) were found in monogamous prairie voles, indicating no differences in spatial learning between male and female prairie voles. In contrast, male meadow voles made significantly fewer errors on the seven mazes than did female meadow voles (not shown here), indicating that male meadow voles had superior spatial learning abilities than did female meadow voles. *(Adapted from Gaulin and FitzGerald, 1989)*

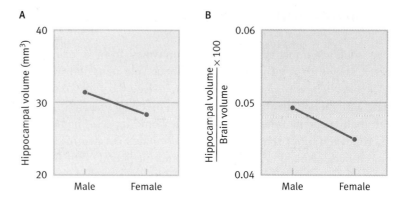

FIGURE 3.21. Sex difference in size of hippocampus. In meadow voles, males have a larger hippocampus, both in **(A)** absolute size and in **(B)** relative size, than do females. *(From Jacobs et al., 1990)*

Based on the spatial learning results described above, Lucia Jacobs and her colleagues hypothesized that males in polygamous species would have larger hippocampuses than females, but that no such sex difference in hippocampal size would be seen in monogamous species of voles. For their experiments, the researchers used meadow voles as the polygamous species (as above), but they chose the pine vole (*Microtus pinetorum*), rather than the prairie vole tested by Gaulin and Fitzgerald, as their monogamous species.

When Jacobs and her team compared the size of the hippocampus in relation to overall brain size, they found sex differences in meadow voles, but they did not find sex differences in pine voles (Jacobs et al., 1990; Figure 3.21). This sort of comparative approach is a powerful neuroethological tool. Behavioral differences between species can lead to predictions about neurobiological differences regarding the hippocampus, and these predictions can then be tested under controlled conditions.

Work on spatial learning and neurobiology in rodents is not restricted to between-species comparisons, nor is it restricted to studies on the hippocampus. Researchers have found that the parietal and prefrontal cortex areas of the brain also play an important role in the spatial learning process, and in particular that the number of dendritic spines is correlated with learning. For example, in rats, the parietal and prefrontal cortex areas of the brain show a greater density of dendritic spines in males versus females (Kolb and Stewart, 1996). Exactly how the number or density of dendritic spines is related to learning is not clear, but it is likely that an increase in either leads to a greater interconnectedness between neurons, and that this greater interconnectedness may translate into improved learning abilities.

FIGURE 3.22. Sex differences in water maze trials. Male meadow voles spent more time near the platform in water maze trials than did female meadow voles. *(Adapted from Kavaliers et al., 1998)*

Martin Kavaliers and his colleagues have examined spatial abilities and the number of dendritic spines in the prefrontal and parietal cortex of male and female meadow voles (Kavaliers et al., 1998). To do this, they tested both male and female meadow voles in the water maze we discussed earlier, and they determined spatial learning by measuring how quickly the voles learned to find the hidden platform in the maze over the course of eight trials. As in the Gaulin and FitzGerald study, males were consistently superior to females at the spatial learning task, both in terms of the speed of learning and the ability to retain the information they had learned (Figure 3.22). Once the spatial learning trials were completed, a subset of the brains of males and females was dissected and the number of dendritic spines in their prefrontal and parietal cortex was measured. Kavaliers and his team found that males had more dendritic spines than females in both areas of the cortex (Figure 3.23).

The Kavaliers study demonstrates that learning and neuronal density are correlated, but it does not tell us about causation. It might be that male meadow voles had more dendritic spines than females before the water maze trials, and hence had superior spatial learning abilities. Or it could have been that males and females had the same number of dendritic spines before the water maze test, but that learning during the water maze trials might have increased spine density in males, but not in females. Or perhaps both are true. No studies to date on voles allow us to distinguish between such possibilities, but May-Britt Moser and her colleagues have provided evidence from rats suggesting that dendritic spine number can be changed by spatial learning experience (Moser et al., 1994).

Moser and her team measured spatial learning skills in rats using both the water maze test and a second spatial learning task that involved finding food that was hidden in a cage. After the spatial learning trials, the researchers dissected the brains of a subset of these animals to measure dendritic spine number and density. A group of control animals was not exposed to either type of spatial learning task, and the researchers also dissected their brains. Given that rats were randomly assigned to the control and spatial learning groups and hypothesizing that the number of dendritic spines changed as a result of spatial learning, we would expect that the rats that went through the spatial learning trials would have more dendritic spines than the control animals. Moser and her team found just such a relationship in rats (further studies with voles will have to determine if this relationship also exists in voles).

This work by Moser and her colleagues is a good example of what is called **neural plasticity**—defined as the ability of neurons to undergo change as a function of experience (Huttenlocher, 2002; Jenkins et al., 1990). Work on neural plasticity is a very active area of research in neuroethology, and will no doubt grow in scope in the coming years.

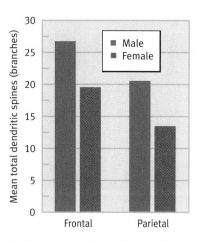

FIGURE 3.23. Sex difference in number of dendritic spines. In meadow voles, males have more dendritic spines (branches) in both the frontal and the parietal cortex of the brain than do females. *(From Kavaliers et al., 1998)*

VOCALIZATIONS IN PLAINFIN MIDSHIPMAN FISH

In their long-term work on the plainfin midshipman fish (*Porichthys notatus*), Andrew Bass and his colleagues have uncovered what they refer to as type I and type II males (Bass, 1998; Bass and Zakon, 2005; Figure 3.24). Behaviorally, type I and type II males act very differently. Type I males build nests, are four times larger than type II males, have a very high gonad-body size ratio, and produce sounds in a number of different behavioral contexts (Table 3.2). Type I males generate short duration grunts when engaged in aggressive contests with other males, or longer duration "hums" when courting females (Bass and McKibben, 2003; Bass and Zakon, 2005; Brantley and Bass, 1994). If females choose a type I male, they remain on the nest and lay eggs there.

Type II males are small, with low gonad-body ratios. They are often referred to as "sneakers" because they do not build nests, but rather lurk around the nests of type I males, where they dart in and shed sperm in an attempt to fertilize the nesting female (see Chapter 6 for more on this behavioral strategy). In addition, unlike type I males, type II males do not hum to attract females, and they only occasionally produce grunt sounds.

FIGURE 3.24. Vocal fish. In plainfin midshipman, some male types produce vocalizations while others do not. **(A)** The two smaller fish on the ends are type II sneaker males (who do not sing), while the fish that is second from the left is a "singing" type I parental male. **(B)** A type I male in his nest with his brood attached to the rocks. *(Photo credits: Andrew Bass)*

TABLE 3.2. Traits of type I and type II males. A summary of the differences between type I and type II plainfin midshipman, and a comparison with plainfin midshipman females.

SEXUALLY POLYMORPHIC TRAITS	TYPE I MALE	TYPE II MALE	FEMALE
nest building	yes	no	no
egg guarding	yes	no	no
body size	large	small	intermediate
gonad-size/body-size ratio	small	large	large (gravid), small (spent)*
ventral coloration	olive-gray	mottled yellow	bronze (gravid), mottled (spent)*
circulating steroids	testosterone, 11-ketotestosterone	testosterone	testosterone, estradiol
vocal behavior	hums, grunt trains	isolated grunts	isolated grunts
vocal muscle	large	small	small
vocal neurons	large	small	small
vocal discharge frequency	high	low	low

Gravid connotes pregnant: spent connotes post-pregnant

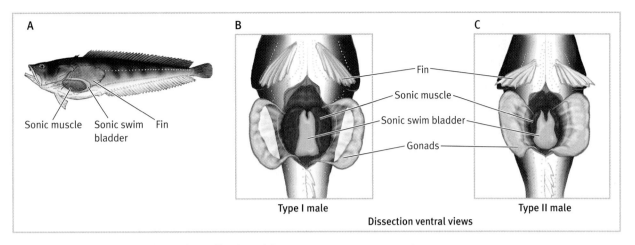

FIGURE 3.25. Sonic muscles and vocalization. (A) The vocal organ of the plainfin midshipman is made up of a pair of sonic muscles attached to the walls of the swim bladder. **(B)** Sonic muscles of type I males are well developed in comparison with muscles from type II males **(C)**. *(From Bass, 1996, p. 357)*

Because type I and II males have different vocalization patterns, there has been a good deal of work done on the neurobiological underpinnings of sound production in this species. The vocal organ of the midshipman is a set of paired sonic muscles attached to its swim bladders (Figure 3.25). Since all males—both type I and type II—have such sonic muscles, what causes the differences in sound production between the two types of males? Part of the answer lies in the fact that type I males have larger sonic muscles (with more muscle fibers), and this difference in size affects sound production (Bass, 1992; Bass and Marchaterre, 1989). But the difference in size of the sonic muscles is only part of the reason that type I and type II males produce such different vocalizations. To understand why, we need to realize that each of the sonic muscles is innervated by what is called a sonic motor nucleus that runs from the hindbrain of the fish down along the spine to the sonic muscles. The two sonic motor nuclei themselves are innervated by "pacemaker" neurons that generate impulses in a regular cyclic, rhythmic pattern. Indeed, Bass and his colleagues have mapped out much of what they call a "vocal pattern generator," and have found differences in the rate at which pacemaker neurons generate impulses. The pacemaker neurons in type I males fire at a rate that is 15 to 20 percent higher than that of type II males, helping to explain differences in the vocalizations of type I and II males, and hence differences relating to reproductive behavior and aggression.

Using the plainfin midshipman as a case study, Bass and his colleagues have demonstrated a tight linkage between neurobiological and endocrinological approaches to sound production in type I and II males (Bass and Zakon, 2005; Remage-Healey and Bass, 2007). For example, a hormone called arginine vasotocin (AVT) inhibits activity in neurobiological circuitry associated with the production of sounds in type I males, but AVT does not affect vocal motor activity and sound production in type II males. On the other hand, the hormone isotocin (IT) has the exact opposite effect, inhibiting activity in the neurobiological circuitry associated with sound production in type II males, but having no effect on sound production in type I males (Bass and Baker, 1990, 1991). The linkage between hormones, neurobiology, and sound production in the midshipman may have some important general applications for other vertebrate groups. This is because the areas of the brain involved in sound production in the midshipman—more specifically, the preoptic and anterior hypothalamus—are similar to brain sections involved in sound production in numerous other species. In that sense, midshipman are a "model species" for examining the interplay of the neuronal and endocrinological systems involved in the production of sound. Another way to think about this is that the plainfin midshipman show how *internal* communication systems—endocrinological and neuronal—help us understand an *external* communication system, namely sound production (Goodson and Bass, 2001).

SLEEP AND PREDATION IN MALLARD DUCKS

While it is clear that sleep is necessary for normal functioning in animals, sleep nonetheless poses a difficult problem—sleeping individuals are more susceptible to being attacked by predators. Here we shall explore the proximate underpinnings of an incredible antipredator behavior seen in a number of creatures—sleeping with one eye open and one eye shut. This type of sleep was first recorded in chickens (Spooner, 1964), and is best examined in John Rattenborg and Steve Lima's studies of sleep and antipredator behavior in mallard ducks (*Anas platyrhynchos*) (Rattenborg et al., 1999a, 1999b, 2000).

Mallards, it seems, have the ability to sleep with one eye open and one hemisphere of the brain awake (Ball et al., 1988). In essence, these birds sleep with half their brain awake and half their brain asleep, in what is referred to as unihemispheric sleep. Rattenberg and Lima examined unihemispheric sleep in mallards and found that not only could they sleep with one eye open, but mallards on the periphery of the group, where they are more susceptible to predation, relied on unihemispheric sleep more than birds in the center of a group. Indeed, birds on the periphery of the group slept with the eye outward, away from their group and toward areas of potential predation (Figures 3.26 and 3.27).

How do mallards manage this split-brained sleep? It seems that these birds are capable of putting one hemisphere of the brain—the hemisphere active

FIGURE 3.26. Unihemispheric sleep. (A) Percent of time ducks spent with one eye closed or both eyes closed as a function of position in the group (at the group's center or on its edge). (B) When ducks were at the edge of a group and had one eye open, they spent much more time looking away from the group's center than when they had one eye open and were at the center of the group. *(From Rattenborg et al., 1999a)*

Infrared cameras

FIGURE 3.27. Sleeping apparatus. This experimental housing unit was employed to record eye state and electrophysiology of four mallard ducks. Eight infrared cameras were used to allow the movement of each eye of each mallard to be recorded. Birds on the extreme left and right were considered to be on the edges of the group. *(From Rattenborg et al., 1999a)*

during sleep—into what is called slow-wave sleep (Rattenborg et al., 1999a, 1999b). "Slow-wave" here simply refers to the frequency of the brain waves that investigators record using a device called an electroencephalogram (EEG). Slow-wave sleep in birds has a signature (in terms of wave frequency and amplitude) that is quite different from other states of sleep or wakefulness. This slow-wave state allows quick responses to predators, but it does not interfere with the sleeping half of the bird's brain until danger is present. EEG recordings indicate that the part of the brain controlling the open eye during unihemispheric sleep showed the low frequency range characteristic of slow-wave sleep, while the other half of the mallard's brain showed EEG patterns that were similar to those of true sleep.

Much of the work on unihemispheric sleep has been undertaken in birds, but they are not the only group in which this form of sleep has been documented. Although most mammals sleep with both halves of the brain asleep (bihemispherically), aquatic mammals are an exception. In aquatic mammals like dolphins, whales, fur seals, and sea lions, unihemispheric sleep is thought to allow individuals to swim to the surface and breathe during sleep (Lyamin and Chetyrbok, 1992; Mukhametov et al., 1988; Figure 3.28). Various techniques have been used across these studies to measure activity in the two sides of the brain, including brain temperature measurements, in which temperature was found to be higher in the "awake" side of an animal's brain than in the "sleeping" side (Berger and Phillips, 1995; Kovalzan and Mukhametov, 1982).

Using such tools as electroencephalograms and brain temperature measurements, animal behaviorists have been able to study brain dynamics during sleep—an activity that often lasts eight hours/day. These analyses shed light not only on animal behavior per se, but they have also revealed completely new brain activities that are of general interest to neurobiologists, one such activity being unihemispheric sleep.

FIGURE 3.28. Sleep in aquatic mammals. In some aquatic mammals, like the fur seal, unihemispheric sleep is thought to allow individuals to swim to the surface and breathe during sleep. Here the fur seal is shown sleeping on its left side as its left hemisphere sleeps. The right hemisphere remains awake, controlling paddling of the left flipper and keeping its nostrils above water. When the right hemisphere sleeps, the left hemisphere controls paddling of the right flipper and breathing. *(From Rattenborg et al., 2000)*

Molecular Genetics and Animal Behavior

We will now move on to a proximate analysis of animal behavior that centers on the burgeoning field of molecular genetics. It may seem strange to think of studies on molecular genetics as somehow being proximate analyses. After all, most of the primer chapter on natural selection (Chapter 2) was written in an evolutionary light and typically focused on how selection favors one behavioral genetic variant over another. In Chapter 2, we also examined how molecular genetics can be used to test various ethological hypotheses. Genes, however, can also be used in the proximate explanation of a trait in a very straightforward manner. If, rather than expounding on what *selective* forces are involved in gene frequency change, a study is instead designed to address which specific gene or set of genes code for a trait, then we are using genes as a proximate causative factor. If a study finds that some variant of gene X is associated with a variant of behavior Y, we are casting genes in a proximate, rather than an ultimate, light. Identifying the genes behind behavior traits is a large-scale endeavor going on in hundreds of labs around the world today. Researchers involved in this area have examined the molecular genetic underpinnings of traits such as foraging, mate choice, aggression, division of labor, and so on (Table 3.3). Below we examine two case studies involving proximate explanations at the molecular genetic level: (1) ultraviolet vision in birds, and (2) song acquisition in birds.

ULTRAVIOLET VISION IN BIRDS

The effect that a single change at the molecular genetic level can have on traits that are important to animals (as well as ethologists) is remarkable. Consider the case of ultraviolet (UV) vision, which is found in a wide array of animals, including fish, amphibians, reptiles, birds, insects, and mammals (Jacobs, 1992; Salcedo et al., 2003; Shi et al., 2001; Yokoyama, 2002). UV vision in vertebrates

TABLE 3.3. Molecular genetics and animal behavior. Examples of social behavior and the specific genes that have been linked to such behaviors in a suite of different organisms. (From Robinson et al., 2005)

BEHAVIOR	ORGANISM	GENE
Foraging		
Rover versus sitter phenotype	*Drosophila melanogaster*	*foraging*
Roamer versus dweller phenotype	*Caenorhabditis elegans*	*egl-4 (egg-laying defective 4)*
Division of labor: onset age of foraging	*Apis melllifera*	*foraging*
Division of labor: onset age of foraging	*A. mellifera*	*malvolio*
Division of labor: foraging related?	*A. mellifera*	*period*
Division of labor: foraging related?	*A. mellifera*	*ace (acetylcholine esterase)*
Division of labor: foraging related?	*A. mellifera*	*IP(3)K (inositol 1,3,5 triphosphate kinase)*
Division of labor: exocrine gland function	*A. mellifera*	*Royal jelly protein*
Foraging specialization: nectar versus pollen	*A. mellifera*	*Protein kinase C*
Social feeding	*D. melanogaster*	*npf (neuropeptide F)*
Social feeding (aggregation)	*C. elegans*	*npr-1 (neuropeptide receptor family 1)*
Mate recognition and courtship		
Vocal learning, vocalization	*Taeniopygia guttata; Homo sapiens*	*FOXP2 (winged helix/forkhead protein)*
Vocal learning, song recognition	*T. guttata*	*zenk (Zif269/Egr1/ NGFIA/Krox24); others*
Pheromone-mediated communication	*Mus musculus domesticus*	*V1R, V2R (vomeronasal receptor, families 1 and 2)*
Pheromone-mediated communication	*D. melanogaster*	*Gr68a (Gustatory receptor 68a)*
Pheromone-mediated communication	*Bombyx mori*	*BmOR1 (olfactory receptor 1)*
Male courtship	*D. melanogaster*	*fruitless; others*
Male courtship; timing of mating	*D. melanogaster*	*period*
Female receptiveness (lordosis)	Rodents	Estrogen responsive genes
Post-mating behavior		
Refractoriness to mate, ovipositioning, decreased longevity	*D. melanogaster*	Genes for seminal proteins
Monogamy, parental care	Rodents	*V1aR, OTR (vasopressin receptor 1A; oxytocin receptor)*
Maternal care	*Rattus norvegicus*	*GR (glucocorticoid receptor)*
Attachment to mother	*M. m. domesticus*	*Orpm (opioid receptor-μ)*
Maternal care, pup retrieval	*M. m. domesticus*	*Dbh (dopamine β-hydroxylase)*
Social hierarchies		
Territorial versus nonterritorial males	*Haplochromis burtoni*	*GnRH1 (gonadotropin releasing hormone 1)*
Dominant versus subordinate males	*Procambarus clarkii*	*5HTR1, -2 (serotonin receptor type 1 and 2)*
Dominance interactions		
Aggression	*M. m. domesticus*	*Maoa (monoamine oxidase A)*
Aggression	*Macaca mulatta*	*5HTT (serotonin transporter)*
Subordinate behavior	*M. m. domesticus*	*Dvl1 (disheveled)*

FIGURE 3.29. A small change goes a long way. A single amino acid change is all that separates the coding for ultraviolet versus violet perception in the zebra finch. *(Photo credit: Ann and Rob Simpson)*

is determined by retinal visual pigments and is used in the context of mating, foraging, hunting, and social signaling (Bennett et al., 1996; Church et al., 1998; Fleishman et al., 1993; Viitala et al., 1995). For example, female zebra finches use ultraviolet wavelength in determining which males they select as their mates (Church et al., 1998). Yet, until recently, little was known about UV vision's proximate underpinnings. What allows some organisms, but not others, to hunt, signal, and attract mates in this wavelength?

Using molecular genetic cloning techniques, Yokoyama and his colleagues examined UV vision in zebra finches (*Taeniopygia guttata*; Yokoyama et al., 2000; Figure 3.29). Zebra finches are able to see in UV, and via *a single amino acid change* (C84S), the researchers were able to transform the ultraviolet pigment—the substance that allows the birds to see in UV—into a violet pigment that doesn't allow for UV vision. Thus, with the change of a single amino acid, ultraviolet light perception was gone and violet perception was present.

Even more remarkably, Yokoyama and his colleagues performed the reverse experiment using chickens and pigeons, neither of which possess ultraviolet pigments (Kawamura et al., 1999). Using sections of DNA that were very similar to those found in the finch, Yokoyama and his colleagues were able to generate ultraviolet pigments from violet pigments, again by changing a single amino acid. One change in amino acid, and pigeons and chickens were able to see in UV wavelength via ultraviolet pigments.

Following the work of Yokoyama and his associates, a number of studies have further elucidated the molecular genetic, proximate underpinnings of ultraviolet vision in animals. For example: (1) evidence now suggests that the molecular genetic underpinnings of ultraviolet vision in invertebrates such as fruit flies can also be tied to changes in a single amino acid (Salcedo et al., 2003), (2) evidence that in some birds in which the ancestral species had lost the UV pigment, some descendant bird lineages, like the canary and the budgerigar, regained UV pigment by a single amino acid change (Shi and Yokoyama, 2003), and (3) molecular genetic analysis has led to the reconstruction of ancestral green visual pigments in the zebra finch (Chinen et al., 2005).

As a whole, this set of work demonstrates not only the power of molecular genetics to help unravel proximate questions in animal behavior, but it also illustrates that what appears to be a complex trait like ultraviolet vision—a trait that functions in the context of mating, foraging, and so on—can originate from simple changes at the molecular level.

SONG ACQUISITION IN BIRDS

As we will see in numerous places throughout this book, songbirds use their songs in many different contexts, including attracting potential mates and fending off intruders from their territory. A molecular genetic approach to birdsong highlights the role of **gene expression**—that is, the expression of a gene as a result of environmental or behavioral triggers. For example, at a very general level, researchers have found that the expression of the *FOXP2* gene in brain regions is associated with both song perception in birds and language acquisition in humans (Enard et al., 2002; Haesler et al., 2004; Teramitsu et al., 2004).

The zebra finch has become a model system to illustrate the relationship between gene expression and birdsong. Early work in this species by David Clayton, Claudio Mello, and their colleagues involved exposing zebra finches to birdsong, and then measuring messenger RNA (mRNA) levels in the brain of these birds (Mello et al., 1992). Messenger RNA is a single-stranded RNA that is critical for protein synthesis, and Clayton and his colleagues focused on mRNA levels in a section of the forebrain called the neostriatum, because this section of the brain is associated with song pattern recognition, song discrimination, and the processing of auditory cues in birds. These researchers found that mRNA levels associated with a gene called *zenk* increased after the birds heard zebra finch songs, and that was associated with an increase in the number of neurons in the neostriatum (Figure 3.30). It is still not clear precisely how the increased mRNA levels and neuron development associated with *zenk* expression are tied to song learning. The protein produced by the mRNA may affect the auditory neurons, which are connected to song recognition. More generally, there is some evidence that *zenk* may be part of a complex genetic pathway leading to the neural plasticity we discussed earlier in the chapter—this neural plasticity is critical to song learning in birds (Mello et al., 2004).

Other research also supports the role of *zenk* in zebra finch birdsong: (1) zebra finches exposed to the song of another species (the canary) showed a much reduced mRNA response to the other species' birdsong, and (2) no

A   **B**

FIGURE 3.30. *Zenk* **and exposure to song. (A)** Induction of *zenk* mRNA in the forebrain of a male zebra finch that has been exposed to zebra finch song for forty-five minutes. **(B)** Same area in male who was not exposed to song. *(From Mello et al., 1992, p. 6819; courtesy Claudio Mello)*

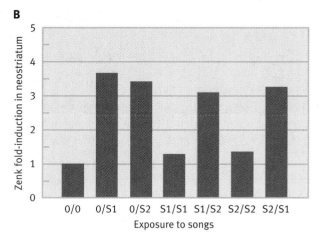

FIGURE 3.31. *Zenk* **levels and habituation. (A)** Induced *zenk* mRNA levels decreased with increased exposure to the same song in male zebra finches. **(B)** Induced *zenk* mRNA levels increased when a male zebra finch was exposed to a new song. The researchers exposed each group to one song for two and a half hours (training), followed by another song for thirty minutes (testing); the two songs were designated as stimulus 1/stimulus 2 (0 = no song, S1 = exposure to song 1, S2 = exposure to song 2). Note that the S1/S2 and S2/S1 bars, which represent the case of exposure to new songs, are higher than the S1/S1 and S2/S2 bars. *(Adapted from Mello et al., 1995)*

increase in *zenk* expression was uncovered after the birds were placed in either a "no song" experimental treatment, or when they heard "tone bursts" that did not correspond with the song of any bird species.

If a zebra finch is played the same conspecific song repeatedly, all of the strong responses described above begin to decrease, and slowly return to their baseline levels—that is, to the levels seen before exposure to the song for the first time (Figure 3.31A). This sort of **habituation** is often seen when an animal is exposed to the same stimulus over and over. In a series of fascinating experiments, Clayton and his team examined the interaction between expression of the *zenk* gene and habituation of zebra finches to familiar song. That is, the researchers wanted to understand not just how gene expression was affected by hearing song, but also they wanted to know how gene expression was affected by *repeated exposure* to birdsong.

To examine habituation and the expression of *zenk*, Mello, Fernando Nottebohm, and Clayton first exposed a zebra finch to the song of a conspecific and found the same increase in mRNA and neural recruitment to the forebrain discussed earlier (Mello et al., 1995). Once a bird had habituated to a familiar song, the song of a new zebra finch was played, and an increase in mRNA and neural recruitment to the forebrain was once again recorded. These results suggest that after repeated exposure, a song is categorized by a bird as "familiar," and it no longer elicits the molecular genetic and neural changes associated with increased *zenk* expression (Figure 3.31B).

The idea that animal behaviorists, in collaboration with researchers in other fields, are beginning to understand the bird's initial response to song, and its eventual habituation to song at the molecular genetic level, highlights the new and growing power of molecular genetic tools in ethology.

Development and Animal Behavior

In his classic paper, "On the Aims and Methods of Ethology," Niko Tinbergen emphasized the importance of developmental factors in shaping an animal's behavior (Tinbergen, 1963). Tinbergen and those who followed in his footsteps were using development in a broad sense meant to encompass everything from the in-utero effects we discussed in rodents to the specific effects that environmental factors might have after birth on the behavior of a developing organism (Stamps, 2003; West et al., 2003). Environmental factors relevant to development and behavior include abiotic (nonliving) components of the environment. For example, exposure to navigating cliff faces during development might help a ram cope better with life on cliffs when it is an adult. Developmental factors also include biotic (living) components of the environment. During its development, our ram might learn about the behavior of its predators, and how best to avoid danger from such predators. In such a case, we might ask the proximate question: How does experience with biotic factors such as predators affect the subsequent behavior of an organism? We could then cast our answer in terms of learning. In addition, developmental factors might involve learning to escape predators by watching others in one's social group solve the same problem—that is, developmental factors might include aspects of social learning.

Throughout this book, we will explore a myriad of ways that development affects behavior. Here, we focus on two case studies, examining: (1) early development and its effect on parental behavior in the oldfield mouse, and (2) development, temperature, and ovipositing behavior in wasps.

EARLY DEVELOPMENT AND ITS EFFECT ON PARENTAL BEHAVIOR IN THE OLDFIELD MOUSE

Mammals and birds tend to become better parents as they produce more and more offspring. Direct experience as a parent, however, is only one way to learn how to become a successful mother or father. Developmental factors early in life can also potentially affect future parental behavior. For example, in many species of birds and mammals, some individuals remain in their natal group, even after they themselves are capable of reproduction, and they often help their parents raise additional broods of offspring (that is, the younger siblings of the helpers). Is it possible that such developmental experience may affect subsequent parenting success in helpers who eventually leave their natal territory? Susan Margulis and her colleagues examined this possibility in oldfield mice (*Peromyscus polionotus*).

Data on helping behavior among oldfield mice in natural settings are extremely difficult to gather, but a significant body of indirect evidence suggests that some females remain at the nest and help their mothers raise the next clutch of young. For example, natural history data suggest that a mother can be both pregnant and nursing a brood of mice, while an older brood still remains at the nest, providing ample opportunity for potential helpers to aid in rearing their younger siblings (Foltz, 1981). Margulis tested whether "experienced" females—

that is, females that remained at their parents' nest during the rearing of a litter of their younger siblings—were subsequently better mothers to their own offspring than "inexperienced" females who did not remain at the nest while younger broods of siblings were being reared (Margulis et al., 2005). Thus, they examined whether a developmental trajectory involving helping one's mother affected the helper's own parenting behavior.

In order to avoid cause-and-effect problems, Margulis and her colleagues experimentally created inexperienced and experienced females by removing (or not removing) females from their natal nests. They began their work using a large colony of mice housed at the Brookfield (Illinois) Zoo, and they used mice that were ten to fifteen generations removed from wild-caught individuals. Margulis and her team formed a series of male-female pairs. Quickly thereafter, mating occurred, and pups were born. In the "inexperienced female" (IF) treatment, IF females were removed from the nest at twenty days of age and they were raised in all-female groups until the experiment began. In the "experienced female" (EF) treatment, when EF females were twenty days old they were *not* removed from the nest but rather remained at the nest with their pregnant mother until she gave birth again and weaned a second brood. At that point, EF females were removed from the nest and reared in an all-female group until the experiment began.

At the start of the experiment, IF and EF females were paired with inexperienced males, with whom they mated and produced offspring, and the females' parental activities and offspring survival were recorded. Results suggest that all females—both EF and IF—became better parents as they produced more and more broods over time, but the key comparison was between inexperienced and experienced females at any given point in time. Here, Margulis and her colleagues found that the broods of experienced females survived with a higher probability than those of inexperienced females, in part due to the superior nest-building behavior displayed by experienced females (Figure 3.32). The results indicate that the developmental experience of being present when one's mother raises a subsequent clutch of offspring has long-term consequences for parenting abilities.

FIGURE 3.32. Nest building and experience. The proportion of females that did not start building nests was lower in experienced females (green) versus inexperienced females (orange). Experienced females began to build nests sooner and built superior nests than inexperienced females because they learned to do so when exposed to their pregnant mother. *(From Margulis et al., 2005)*

DEVELOPMENT, TEMPERATURE, AND OVIPOSITING BEHAVIOR IN WASPS

One abiotic factor that often has profound developmental consequences in animals is temperature. Animals that are native to colder climates often show developmental differences when raised in warmer environments, and vice versa. Temperature, for example, is known to have strong effects on olfactory senses in insects (Herard et al., 1988), and since olfaction is a primary way in which insects interact with both abiotic and biotic factors in their environment, developmental differences caused by temperature have become an area of interest in ethology.

Joan van Baaren and her colleagues examined temperature-related developmental changes that occur in *Anaphes victus*, a parasitoid wasp species. Parasitoids usually lay their eggs inside a host species, and adult females learn how to avoid hosts that have already been parasitized (Papaj and Lewis, 1993; Papaj et al., 1989). Van Baaren and her colleagues tested whether the temperature that female larvae were exposed to during development would affect their ability to learn how to find suitable hosts when they themselves were ready to lay eggs (van Baaren et al., 2005). Conceptually, here we are considering the manner in which the environment interacts with an animal's ability to learn, which then affects how parasitoids infect their hosts.

To examine the effect of temperature on learning and host choice behavior, van Baaren's team raised larvae at 4°C in two experimental treatments, one of which lasted three weeks, and one of which lasted twelve weeks. In addition, they ran a control treatment in which larvae were not exposed at all to a temperature of 4°C. After this, female larvae were raised at a more typical temperature for this species (24°C). Their ability to find suitable hosts was later examined when these females were ovipositing (laying) their own eggs (Figure 3.33). When

FIGURE 3.33. Temperature, learning, and egg laying. Exposure to cold temperature (4°C for three weeks for larvae in Group 1, 4°C for twelve weeks for larvae in Group 2) during development had significant effects on a female wasp's ability as an adult to discriminate between hosts of different quality. Larvae in Group 3, who were continuously raised at normal temperatures of 24°C, did not experience these effects. Exposure to cold temperature also had a strong negative effect on the speed at which females learned to avoid already parasitized hosts, as they had to choose to lay their eggs in patches in which none of the hosts had been parasitized (left), half had been parasitized (center), or all had been parasitized (right). Orange circles indicate a parasitized host. *(Based on van Baaren et al., 2005)*

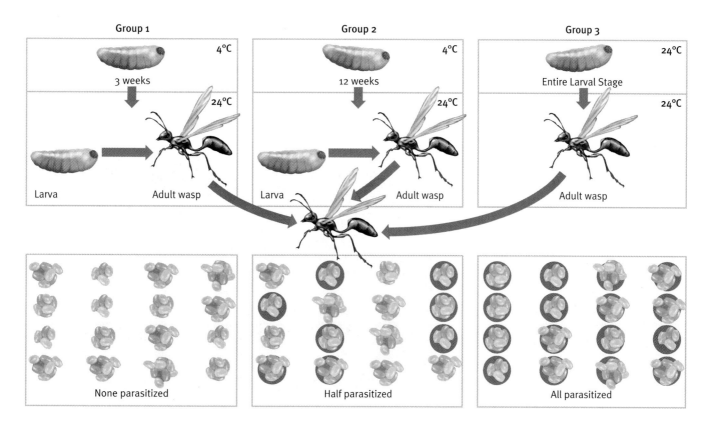

tested, females were presented with three different patches, which differed in the number of good hosts (unparasitized) and "bad" hosts (already parasitized). Van Baaren and her colleagues then measured the number of eggs the females laid, and the ability of the females to learn to avoid already parasitized hosts.

The results indicate that exposure to cold temperature during development had significant effects on: (1) the number of eggs a female laid inside a host, and (2) the female's ability to discriminate between hosts of different quality. Although it is not clear exactly why, the longer a female had been exposed to cold temperatures during development, the fewer eggs she laid in hosts. Equally interesting is the finding that exposure to cold temperature had a strong negative effect on the speed at which females *learned* to avoid already parasitized hosts. Although von Baaren and her colleagues do not know exactly how this occurs, exposure to cold may have affected a female's ability to use visual cues to distinguish between hosts that had already been parasitized and nonparasitized hosts. This is an incredibly important decision in the life of a parasitoid, and our proximate analysis has allowed us to understand it at a deeper level.

Foraging in Honeybees: An Integrated Proximate Analysis

We will now look at a series of different types of proximate analyses, all undertaken in a single species—the honeybee (*Apis mellifera*; Figure 3.34). Ethologists have had a long-standing fascination with honeybees. When Niko Tinbergen, Konrad Lorenz, and Karl von Frisch won the 1973 Nobel Prize for their seminal work in ethology, it was based in part on von Frisch's work on foraging in honeybees (Hinde, 1973; Marler and Griffin, 1973). But this fascination with honeybee behavior can be traced further back, to Darwin himself, who wrote a great deal about the behavior of these social insects. Indeed, by Victorian times, the British public had fallen in love with bees, particularly when they discovered that worker bees who were fed "royal jelly" developed into queens. What's more, they were spellbound by the idea that the same bee egg develops into a male

FIGURE 3.34. Honeybee foraging. The proximate underpinnings of foraging behavior in honeybees have been studied in depth by Gene Robinson and his colleagues. *(Photo credit: George D. Lepp/Corbis)*

if it remains unfertilized, but develops into a female if it unites with a drone's sperm (Prete, 1990, 1991; Richards, 1987). This fascination with bees, by both scientists and nonscientists, meant that Darwin could not (and did not) ignore these creatures and their curious behaviors in *On the Origin of Species*.

Here we shall use honeybee foraging behavior as a case study of an integrated proximate approach toward animal behavior, primarily focusing on the work coming out of Gene Robinson's laboratory. We shall in turn examine the effects of neural structures, genes, development, and hormones on honeybee foraging behavior.

MUSHROOM BODIES AND HONEYBEE FORAGING

We begin our integrated proximate analysis with a discussion of neuroethology and foraging behavior in bees. Because many organisms, including honeybees, must navigate around in search of food outside of their hives or nests, the ability to remember and retrieve information from the environment is critical. As we have seen, in vertebrates this spatial navigation is often associated with the hippocampus. In invertebrates, however, it is most often linked with a cluster of small neurons located at the front of their brain. This cluster, known technically as the *corpora pedunculata*, is often referred to as the **mushroom bodies** (Capaldi et al., 1999; Fahrbach, 2006; Figure 3.35). Both the mushroom bodies and the hippocampus are often associated with spatial navigation, suggesting that a proximate analysis of spatial navigation and neuroethology in invertebrates may lead to results that are also of interest to researchers working on similar questions in vertebrates (Davis, 1993; Kandel and Abel, 1995).

Mushroom bodies play a central role in spatial navigation and foraging behavior in honeybees—a species that often travels many kilometers in search of food (Visscher and Seeley, 1982). Whereas younger bees generally reside within the hive, an age-based task allocation system exists such that older bees primarily give up in-hive tasks, such as cleaning the hive and feeding the larvae, and switch to foraging outside of the hive (Robinson, 1992). Such foragers use both visual and olfactory cues in their search for food.

When they first leave their home hive, rather than immediately commencing a search for food in the nearby environment, would-be foragers often turn back toward the nest and hover up and down for several minutes, in what is referred to as an "orientation flight" (Willmer and Stone, 2004). This behavior apparently orients the foragers to the relative position of their nest in the environment. Bees often start undertaking orientation flights when they are about one week old and begin actually foraging when they are about three weeks of age. Ginger Withers, Susan Fahrbach, and Gene Robinson examined bees of different ages and bees that undertake different tasks within a colony (foraging versus caring for the larvae in the hive) to see whether the size of their mushroom bodies differed as a function of age or task allocation. The researchers found that the mushroom bodies of foragers were 14.8 percent larger than those of the other groups (one-day-old bees and nurses) that they measured, suggesting a strong proximate role for mushroom bodies and foraging (Withers et al., 1993; Figure 3.36). This is a particularly striking finding because the relative volume of other nerve clusters in the honeybee brains remained relatively unchanged as a function of age and task allocation, and only the mushroom bodies increased in relative size.

FIGURE 3.35. Mushroom bodies. The mushroom bodies—shown in light blue—are clusters of neurons located at the front of the bee brain and are involved in spatial learning. The yellow denotes the optic lobes of the bee brain. *(Photo credit: Birgit)*

FIGURE 3.36. Mushroom bodies and foraging. Mushroom bodies were larger in foragers than in bees that remained in a colony (1-day-old bees and nurses who care for the larvae in the hive). *(From Withers et al., 1993)*

To further examine whether foraging-related experience per se affected growth in mushroom body volume, Withers and her team induced early foraging behavior in a colony of bees. Whereas normal bees begin this task at about twenty days of age, bees in the experimental treatment began foraging at seven days of age. The configuration of the mushroom bodies in these precocious foragers resembled that of normal-aged foragers, suggesting that activities surrounding foraging may also directly trigger a series of neural-based changes in mushroom body volume, illustrating yet another instance of neural plasticity (Sigg et al., 1997; Withers et al., 1993).

GENES, mRNA, AND HONEYBEE FORAGING

To examine the possible molecular biological underpinnings of the developmental shift from working in the hive by younger bees to foraging outside the hive by older bees, Alberto Toma and his colleagues capitalized on prior findings that suggested that the *period* (*per*) gene influences circadian rhythms and development time in fruit flies (Konopka and Benzer, 1971; Kyriacou et al., 1990). As such, they focused on the *per* gene as a "candidate" gene involved in control of the developmental changes in foraging that occur in honeybees (Fitzpatrick et al., 2005; Robinson et al., 2005). More specifically, they examined how *per* messenger RNA (mRNA) levels might influence the developmental changes associated with becoming foragers (Toma et al., 2000).

Toma and his colleagues measured mRNA levels in the brains of three sets of laboratory-raised bees. The three groups of bees were composed of individuals that were four to six, seven to nine, and twenty to twenty-two days old. In addition, individuals in a group of one-day-old bees were marked and added to a natural colony of bees in the field. Researchers recaptured marked individuals at day 7 and day 24 of their experiment, and they measured their *per* mRNA levels. Results demonstrate a clear relationship between *per* mRNA level, age, and foraging in honeybees. In both laboratory and natural populations, *per* mRNA was significantly greater in older individuals that foraged for food and brought such food to their colony, when compared to younger bees that remained at the hive (Figure 3.37).

It is possible that increased *per* mRNA levels could be due to age differences alone, rather than to the age-related shift to foraging behavior. Toma examined whether *per* mRNA increases were strictly associated with age, or whether *per* mRNA and foraging were correlated even if age could be removed as a factor. As in the Withers experiment described above, Toma studied "precocious" foragers— that is, foragers that begin searching for food outside of the nest at about seven days old. These precocious foragers provided Toma and his colleagues with the chance to remove age effects from the *per* mRNA/foraging connection, as they now had a sample of bees that foraged but were much younger than typical food gatherers. Precocious foragers had *per* mRNA levels that did not differ from those of typical (older) foragers, suggesting a fundamental link between *per* mRNA and foraging, as opposed to a more general connection between *per* mRNA and development. We still do not know the direction of the causality here—is increased *per* mRNA level a cause or a result of increased foraging?— but the correlational link is well-established (Bloch et al., 2001).

Over the last few years, with the explosion of molecular genetic technology, a much more detailed picture of genes, mRNA abundance in the brain, and

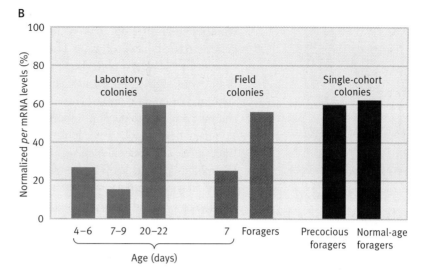

FIGURE 3.37. Foraging, age, and mRNA. (A) Foraging bees have significantly higher levels of *per* mRNA than younger, nonforaging bees. This difference could be due to age, behavior caste (forager versus nonforager), or both. **(B)** Some individual bees developed into precocious foragers who began searching for food much earlier than usual. When ten-day-old precocious foragers were compared to normal foragers (twenty-two-day-old foragers), Toma and his colleagues found no statistical differences in *per* mRNA levels. *(From Toma et al., 2000)*

foraging in honeybees has emerged. For example, in a large-scale study of 5,500 genes, Charles Whitfield, Anne-Maire Cziko, and Gene Robinson found that changes in mRNA levels associated with 39 percent of these genes (that is, about 2,145 of the 5,500 genes examined) were involved in the transition from hive work to foraging behavior in honeybees (Whitfield et al., 2003).

These sorts of large-scale genomic approaches to animal behavior will become more and more common as the genomes of more species are sequenced (Robinson et al., 2005; Sumner, 2006). The challenge will be figuring out how to go from the massive amount of data gathered when a genome is sequenced to understanding any specific animal behavior. For example, although the field of genomics and behavior is growing quickly, at the present time we can't examine each of these 2,000 plus genes and mRNA products associated with the transition to forager, nor would we want to, as little is known about exactly how these genes and their mRNA products operate in the transition to honeybee forager.

We can, however, examine one more well-studied gene associated with the transition to foraging in honeybees to give us a finer understanding of the proximate underpinnings of social insect foraging. Here we will discuss the work of Yehuda Ben-Shahar, Nichole Dudek, and Gene Robinson, who examined the effect of the gene *malvolio (mvl)* on manganese transport to the honeybee brain, and its subsequent implications for foraging in this species (Ben-Shahar et al., 2004). The gene *mvl* is an excellent candidate for this sort of work, as earlier experiments have shown that it affected the way in which fruit flies responded to sucrose (an important component of honeybee food and drink).

In honeybees, foragers who specialize in collecting pollen have a higher responsiveness to sucrose than those that specialize in nectar foraging, and both types of foragers have a stronger response to sucrose than younger "nurse"

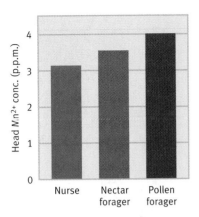

Figure 3.38. Pollen foragers, nectar foragers, and manganese. Pollen foragers have more manganese in their heads than both nectar foragers and nurses. *(From Ben-Shahar et al., 2004)*

bees (who feed the larvae) in the hive. Ben-Shahar and his colleagues examined whether such differences were linked to differences in *mvl* transport of manganese to the honeybee brain. They discovered that both the amount of manganese in the head of a honeybee and the amount of *mvl* mRNA in the honeybee brain were high in pollen foragers and nectar foragers, and low in nurses. As such, if we compare nurses with all foragers (pollen and nectar foragers), we see that *mvl* appears to play an important role in foraging behavior.

At a finer scale, if we look at pollen foragers versus nectar foragers, we uncover even more evidence suggesting a link between *mvl* and foraging. Recall that pollen foragers show a stronger response to sucrose than do nectar foragers. If *mvl* plays an important role in foraging, then we would expect to see more manganese in the heads of pollen foragers versus nectar foragers, and the evidence suggests that this is the case (Figure 3.38). Further evidence for the proximate link between *mvl* and foraging can be found in the fact that when bees were experimentally treated with manganese, their response to sucrose increased, and they made the transition from nurse to forager at an early age.

HORMONES AND HONEYBEE FORAGING

The last part of our proximate analysis of honeybee foraging behavior focuses on endocrinological effects. As bees mature into foragers that leave the nest, they experience an associated increase in levels of juvenile hormone (JH), particularly a form of juvenile hormone called JH III (Hagenguth and Rembold, 1978; Wyatt and Davey, 1996). To better understand the relationship between juvenile hormone and foraging behavior, Joseph Sullivan, Gene Robinson, and their colleagues removed (allatectomized) the corpus allatum—the gland that produces JH—in experimental groups of bees in four colonies (Sullivan et al., 2000, 2003; Figure 3.39). This group of allatectomized bees was then compared to two control groups, one in which the bees went through a similar surgical procedure but did not have their corpus allatum removed, and the other in which the bees were anesthetized only. By experimentally removing the source of JH, this procedure allowed the

FIGURE 3.39. Bee surgery. To examine the effect of juvenile hormone (JH) in honeybee foraging, Sullivan removed the corpus allatum—the gland that produces the hormone. The inset shows a view through the incision. *(Adapted from Sullivan et al., 2000)*

researchers to examine whether changes in JH *caused* foraging-related changes, as other work from the same laboratory had found that changes in foraging behavior do not cause changes in JH level (Elekonich et al., 2001).

Sullivan and his team found that although both allatectomized bees and control bees eventually commenced foraging in three of the four colonies observed, bees that had been allatectomized (and thus had no JH) began foraging significantly later than did bees in the control groups. When allatectomized bees did commence foraging, they returned to the nest much less often than did bees in the control treatments, suggesting a causal link of JH in foraging-related development in honeybees. Sullivan and his team uncovered additional support for this link between JH and foraging when they found that no other major behavior shifts resulted from removing the corpus allata—just changes related to foraging (Sullivan et al., 2000, 2003).

If increased JH levels were causing increased foraging behavior, then the researchers hypothesized that experimentally increasing the JH levels in allatectomized bees would result in a return to normal foraging behavior by the bees. Experiments designed to test this idea have found that when allatectomized bees were given a dose of a chemical called methoprene—a chemical that is similar to JH—they showed no differences in age-related foraging when compared to controls, providing even stronger evidence for the role of JH in foraging behavior in honeybees (Robinson, 1985, 1987; Robinson et al., 1989).

Let us examine a second case in which a neurohormone, called octopamine, has been linked to increased foraging activity in honeybees. Early work had shown that octopamine modulates learning and memory in honeybees, and also affects their visual, olfactory, and gustatory senses (Erber et al., 1993; Hammer and Menzel, 1998; Scheiner et al., 2002). Foraging bees have more octopamine in their brains than do nurse bees that stay at the hive, and this hormone reaches its highest concentration when a bee switches from nest-bound activities to foraging activities for the hive (Schulz et al., 2003; Wagener-Hulme et al., 1999). With this information in hand, Andrew Barron and Gene Robinson asked the following question: Did an increase in octopamine affect other activities in newly foraging bees, or just flight activities related to foraging?

Barron and Robinson found two lines of evidence that the effects of octopamine were specific to foraging activities (Barron and Robinson, 2005): (1) while experimental treatment with octopamine increased flight activity related to foraging, it did not increase a second flight-related behavior—the removal of corpses from the colony, and (2) when bees treated with octopamine were exposed to other hormones associated with the production of a new brood of offspring, they increased their foraging behavior (to feed a now larger hive), but they did not increase other activities associated with caring for the new brood.

Controlled experimental work on octopamine, along with juvenile hormone, illustrates the ways in which a proximate perspective of the honeybee endocrine system can shed light on a fundamentally important behavior in the life of a bee—foraging.

Honeybee foraging, then, allows us to employ many of the approaches we have outlined in this chapter in a single case, providing us with a comprehensive proximate understanding of a behavior that has been of interest to ethologists since the time of Darwin.

INTERVIEW WITH

Dr. Geoffrey Hill

Why do you think so few ethologists design experiments to test both proximate and ultimate questions? Why do researchers tend to specialize in one or the other?

Increasing specialization has been a trend in Western culture for hundreds of years, and specialization in all endeavors is accelerating in the twenty-first century. Science is a reflection of society at large, and in modern science all researchers are specialists. Consider a scientist during the time of Darwin or Newton. Scientific meetings in the nineteenth century included researchers from all branches of science and every scientist was conversant and up to date on the latest discoveries in all fields of science. Part of the inspiration for Darwin's theory of natural selection was a book that he read that presented a new theory for geological processes. Today scientists cannot realistically stay abreast of discoveries even within a single discipline like biology or chemistry. With the explosion of knowledge in past decades, a scientist has to spend all of his or her time just keeping up with the latest research in a very narrow subdiscipline like behavioral ecology. So, it is not surprising that many researchers who are focused on ultimate questions related to the function and evolution of behaviors do not engage in parallel lines of research investigating the proximate neural or hormonal mechanisms underlying the behaviors that they study. The techniques for one scientific approach are essentially unknown to individuals trained in another scientific approach.

A trend in modern science that helps to counteract the move toward increasing specialization is collaboration. Collaborative, multi-disciplinary studies, are drawing in more top scientists, and many funding agencies are actively encouraging multidisciplinary studies by providing

special funding for such projects. Collaborative projects allow a topic to be studied from both ultimate and proximate perspectives by combining the skills and knowledge of scientists with different training. Such collaborative efforts can lead to breakthroughs in our understanding of behavioral processes.

What drew you to focus your research program on bird behavior?

Since I was a pre-teen I've been a bird nut. I got my first pair of binoculars when I was eleven and I've been chasing birds ever since. I'm very fortunate in being able to

turn my hobby into my profession. I never seriously considered studying anything but bird behavior. As much as I enjoyed finding and identifying different species of birds as a young birdwatcher, my greatest exhilaration came when I captured birds, put bands on their legs, and followed and chronicled their individual successes and failures. There is really nothing like walking onto a university campus where every individual house finch is wearing colored bands that I placed on their legs and slowly gaining an understanding of why the birds behave as they do.

Early on in my career, I made the conscious decision to give up some travel opportunities and focus on common local bird species that are logistically easy to study. At times I envy my colleagues who get to travel to exotic locations for their studies of bird behavior, but the exhilaration of having a tractable population of birds where I can conduct convincing tests of key behavioral hypotheses is more than compensation for travel opportunities lost.

Generally speaking, how do you think proximate and ultimate perspectives interact in helping us to better understand animal behavior?

I think we clearly need both ultimate and proximate explanations of all behavioral phenomena if we want to really understand them. The two levels of explanation do not work in opposition to each other—they reinforce one another. Evolution of behaviors can only proceed within the constraints of the underlying proximate mechanisms. Proximate mechanisms are shaped by evolution. An understanding of proximate control of behavioral traits inevitably leads to new insights about how they function and why they evolved. Conversely, an evolutionary prospective can guide studies about proximate mechanisms and make such mechanisms more comprehensible.

As an example of how ultimate and proximate studies reinforce each other, consider studies of red coloration in fish and birds. Explaining such red coloration was a focus of both physiologists and ethologists in the mid-twentieth century, but through several decades these two groups of scientists paid little attention to each other's work. During this period, ethologists showed that red coloration often functioned in mate attraction, and physiologists determined that red coloration of both birds and fish was commonly created by deposition of carotenoid pigments. Moreover, physiologists discovered that carotenoid pigments could not be synthesized by birds or fish but had to be ingested as macromolecules. Coming out of this era, scientists had both a proximate and ultimate understanding of red coloration, but a comprehensive understanding of red coloration eluded both groups.

A breakthrough in the understanding of red coloration (and ornamental traits in general) occurred when pigment physiology was united with observations of mating preferences and sexual selection theory. Observations and bits of information that seemed disconnected and inexplicable suddenly made perfect sense. Carotenoid pigmentation was a useful criterion in mate choice because carotenoid pigments cannot be synthesized. These pigments have to be ingested, and acquisition and utilization of carotenoid pigments

could be interrupted by environmental conditions. Red pigmentation was a signal of success in dealing with environmental challenges. This conclusion could only have been reached by working from and uniting the foundations laid by initial proximate and ultimate studies.

Suppose, for the sake of argument, that a hypothetical "house finch genome project" was now complete. How would this sort of information affect the way you studied behavior in this species?

A finch genome would lead to breakthroughs in our understanding of many aspects of the behavioral ecology of house finches, such as the genetic basis for behaviors, the co-evolution of display traits and preferences for such traits, and the link between genetically based immunity and ornamentation. There is no house finch genome project in the works, but the genome of the domestic chicken has already been sequenced, and the first songbird genome—from the zebra finch—is currently in the works. The chicken genome is already very useful for interpreting genetic data from house finches, and a zebra finch genome will be even more useful, even though zebra finches are in a different songbird family than house finches.

Even without a house finch genome, my colleagues and I have seen great opportunities for testing behavioral hypotheses with new genetic tools, and I've been increasingly involved in genetic work with house finches. I do not ever actually get into the lab and do DNA work. My genetic studies are a great example of the sort of collaborative research that I mention above. I provide data sets on behavior and reproductive history and blood samples as a source of DNA from my field studies, and my collaborators

sequence the DNA and interpret the genetic information.

Over the next five years, what sort of advances in the proximate study of behavior do you envision?

We live in an exciting age of discovery. Breakthroughs in DNA sequencing and gene expression will revolutionize our understanding of the genetic control of many traits, including behavioral traits. In addition, equipment for all sorts of analytical analyses—from hormone assays to action potentials along individual neurons—will allow behaviorists to gain a firmer understanding of the mechanistic basis of behaviors. Truly exciting, but perhaps more than five years away, is the delivery of specific doses of hormones or neurotransmitters to specific tissues of the body or the instantaneous measurement of circulating hormones or the release of neurotransmitters. Such ability to manipulate the chemistry of the body or to measure short-term changes in body chemistry will rapidly advance our understanding of the proximate bases for behaviors.

As great a tool as these new analytical methods present, it will always be the creative application of technology by insightful researchers that leads to breakthroughs in our understanding of how nature works.

Dr. Geoffrey Hill is a professor at Auburn University. His work on the house finch is a classic example of employing both proximate and ultimate perspectives when studying animal behavior. This work is summarized in his wonderful book, A Red Bird in a Brown Bag: The Function and Evolution of Colorful Plumage in the House Finch *(Oxford University Press, 2002).*

SUMMARY

1. One way to distinguish between proximate and ultimate perspectives is to remember that the former tends to address "How is it that . . . ?" and "What is it that . . . ?" questions, while the latter addresses "Why is it that . . . ?" questions. If we were, for example, examining vision in birds, a proximate perspective might lead us to ask how the visual system is set up or what the neurobiological and molecular underpinnings of vision are. An ultimate, or evolutionary, approach would focus on why the visual system is designed as it is. One of the most frequent errors made by those who are not trained in the field of animal behavior is to confuse proximate and ultimate perspectives.

2. Proximate and ultimate approaches complement one another and together provide a comprehensive picture of the ethological trait under study. In order to understand why a trait is designed as it is (an ultimate question), an understanding of exactly how it is built (a proximate question) is often essential. Similarly, if we are interested in understanding how a trait is designed (a proximate question), our analysis can only be aided by knowing what the trait was designed to do (an ultimate question).

3. In this chapter, we have seen how endocrinology, neurobiology, molecular genetics, and development can be construed as important factors in the proximate analysis of behavior.

4. The endocrine system, a powerful communication system that strongly influences many aspects of animal behavior, is composed of a group of ductless glands that secrete hormones—molecular messengers—directly into an animal's bloodstream. Correct functioning of the endocrine system is of fundamental importance to behavioral functions and to the modification of rates and directions of various cellular functions.

5. The nervous system provides an electrical impulse ideally designed for instantaneous communication. Animals possess specialized nerve cells called neurons that share certain similarities, regardless of what message(s) they conduct. Understanding how neurobiology affects behavior is an important component to proximate analyses of behavior.

6. Molecular genetics can be a powerful tool in proximate analyses of behavior. Genes can be used in the proximate explanation of a trait by studying which specific gene or set of genes code for a trait. Studies of animal behavior and molecular genetics, and identifying (and sometimes sequencing) the genes behind behavioral traits, are large-scale endeavors going on in many labs around the world today.

7. Development in a broad sense encompasses everything from the in-utero effects to the specific effects that environmental factors might have after birth on the behavior of a developing organism. Environmental factors relevant to development and behavior include both abiotic (nonliving) and biotic (living) components of the environment.

8. The example of honeybee foraging behavior allows us to bring together numerous different approaches to the proximate study of behavior—molecular genetic, hormonal, developmental, and neuronal approaches—in a single system, and in so doing, provides us with a comprehensive understanding of the proximate underpinnings of a behavior that has fascinated ethologists since the time of Darwin.

DISCUSSION QUESTIONS

1. Go back and reexamine one of the behaviors we discussed in Chapter 2 (ultimate causation). Suggest how one would go about studying this behavior from a proximate perspective, and how the ultimate and proximate perspectives together provide a richer understanding of whatever behavior you have chosen.

2. Find the 1998 special issue of *American Zoologist* (vol. 38), which was devoted to proximate and ultimate causation. Choose two different papers in this issue, and compare and contrast how they try to integrate proximate and ultimate causation.

3. If you could design some behavioral endocrinology experiments to add to the integrative work we discussed on plumage and carotenoid food in finches, what sort of experiments would you design? How would these experiments complement what is already known?

4. How does the work on the neuroethology of learning in voles illustrate the way that proximate studies can use between-population and between-sex comparisons to help us better understand animal behavior?

5. The entire genome of the honeybee has recently been sequenced. How might this affect work on molecular genetics and behavior in this species? Are there any pitfalls you can imagine to having such a large genetic database available to behavioral researchers?

SUGGESTED READING

Adkins-Regan, E. (1998). Hormonal control of mate choice. *American Zoologist, 38,* 166–178. A review of the endocrinology of mate choice.

Alcock, J., & Sherman, P. (1994). The utility of the proximate-ultimate dichotomy in ethology. *Ethology, 96,* 58–62. A short defense of the proximate/ultimate classification.

Bass, A. H., & McKibben, J. R. (2003). Neural mechanisms and behaviors for acoustic communication in teleost fish. *Progress in Neurobiology, 69,* 1–26. A nice illustration of how animal nervous systems play a critical role in behavioral decision making.

Capaldi, E., Robinson, G., & Fahrbach, S. (1999). Neuroethology of spatial learning: The birds and the bees. *Annual Review of Psychology, 50,* 651–682. A review of the neural underpinnings of spatial learning.

Robinson, G. E., Grozinger, C. M., & Whitfield, C. W. (2005). Sociogenomics: Social life in molecular terms. *Nature Reviews Genetics, 6,* 257–271. An updated review of molecular genetic approaches to behavior.

West, M. J., King, A. P., & White, D. J. (2003). The case for developmental ecology. *Animal Behaviour, 66,* 617–622. Also Stamps, J. (2003). Behavioural processes affecting development: Tinbergen's fourth question comes of age. *Animal Behaviour, 66,* 1–13. Two reviews of developmental approaches to animal behavior.

Learning

FIGURE 4.1. Damselflies. Damselflies learn about predation threat through chemical cues. *(Photo credit: Kim Taylor/ natureplace.com)*

earning about biotic and abiotic components of an environment may provide animals with any number of benefits. For example, prey species often live in areas that contain both predatory and nonpredatory species, and learning to distinguish between them clearly has fitness consequences. Even encounters with predators are not always the same, as at any given time some predators are in hunting mode while others are not actively hunting prey (Chivers et al., 1996). If prey can learn to distinguish between dangerous and benign encounters with potential predators, they may free up time for other activities such as foraging or mating—in other words, learning about possible predation pressure may allow animals to more optimally handle the trade-offs they face in everyday life.

In aquatic systems, recognition of predators often involves processing chemical stimuli (Ferrari et al., 2005; Ferrari et al., 2006a, 2006b; Ferrari and Chivers, 2006). If the food that a potential predator eats produces a chemical cue that is recognizable to its prey, then this chemical cue acts as "the scent of a predator" and may provide an opportunity for such prey to learn what is dangerous and what isn't (Crowl and Covich, 1990; Gelowitz et al., 1993; Howe and Harris, 1978; Keefe, 1992; Mathis and Smith, 1993a,1993b; Wilson and Lefcort, 1993). Douglas Chivers and his colleagues examined this possibility by studying learning and antipredator behavior in the damselfly (*Enallagma spp*; Chivers et al., 1996; Figure 4.1). What makes Chivers's study especially interesting is that it nicely shows how to distinguish *learning* about predators from *innate behavioral responses* that prey may display toward predators.

Damselfly larvae are found in ponds with minnows, and both species are often attacked and consumed by pike (*Esox lucius*). Chivers and his colleagues hypothesized that damselfly larvae might learn about the potential dangers associated with pike encounters by using chemical cues. To test this hypothesis, the researchers fed pike predators either minnows, damselflies, or mealworms. Minnows and damselflies are prey for pike, whereas mealworms are not and thus served as a control. After four days on one of these three diets, a pike was removed from its tank, and damselflies that had never before had any contact with a pike were exposed to the water from the pike's tank.

When damselfly larvae were exposed to the water containing chemical cues from a pike that had eaten damselflies or a pike that had eaten minnows, Chivers and his colleagues found that the damselfly larvae significantly curtailed their foraging behavior. They did not reduce their foraging behavior, however, when they were exposed to the water treated with pike that consumed mealworms (Figure 4.2). Because damselflies are found in the same ponds as minnows, but the damselflies tested by Chivers had never before experienced a pike, these results strongly suggest that damselflies innately associate the scent of pike plus damselfly or pike plus minnow with danger, but they make no such association between pike, mealworm, and danger. That is, the damselflies here hadn't learned anything; they simply were predisposed to respond to the smell of pike and prey (minnows and damselflies) as dangerous.

Chivers's team followed up their initial experiment by examining the role of learning and antipredator behavior in damselflies. Here they took the damselflies that had been exposed to the three treatments above (water from pike plus damselfly, water from pike plus minnow, and water from pike plus mealworm) and isolated them for two days. Then each and every damselfly was exposed to water from a pike that had been fed mealworms. With respect to learning and antipredator behavior, we now have two particularly interesting

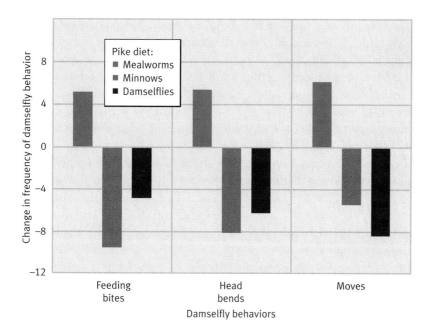

FIGURE 4.2. Chemically mediated changes. Numerous aspects of damselfly behavior, including the frequency of feeding bites, head bends, and moves, were changed as a function of whether the damselflies were exposed to chemical stimuli from a pike predator that had eaten mealworms, minnows, or damselflies. *(From Chivers et al., 1996)*

groups of damselflies: (1) damselflies that were initially exposed to water from pike plus damselfly, but that were subsequently exposed to pike plus mealworm water, and (2) damselflies that were initially exposed to water from pike plus minnow, but that were subsequently exposed to pike plus mealworm water.

Damselflies in these two treatments responded to the scent of pike plus mealworm by decreasing their foraging activities. Recall that in the first experiment, damselflies did *not* curtail feeding when they encountered the smell of pike plus mealworm for the first time, but they did curtail feeding in this second experiment. This suggests that, based on their earlier experience in the first experiment, damselflies in the second experiment had learned to associate pike plus *the scent of any potential prey* with danger, and this translated into a reduced foraging rate even when they encountered the scent of pike and mealworm.

What Is Individual Learning?

In this chapter, we shall examine the role that **individual learning** plays in animal behavior. The role of social learning—that is, learning from other individuals—will be the subject of the next chapter. In our analysis of individual learning—henceforth referred to as learning in the rest of this chapter—we will start by addressing three interrelated questions: How do animals learn? Why do animals learn? What do animals learn?

Before tackling these overarching questions, it is important to address a few baseline issues, first and foremost among them being: What do we mean when we speak of learning? This is a complicated question, but the definition of learning we will adopt here is simple, straightforward, and fairly widely accepted within psychology. When we speak of learning, we are referring to a relatively permanent change in behavior as a result of experience (Shettleworth, 1998). This definition does have a downside, in that it is not clear how long a time period is encompassed by the words "relatively permanent." That being said, this is a working definition, already adopted implicitly by most ethologists, and it will serve our purposes here well.

It is interesting to note that the phrase "relatively permanent" was added to an older definition of learning, which was something akin to "a change in behavior as a result of experience." The insertion of "relatively permanent" was meant to address a particularly difficult problem regarding what constitutes learning. Sara Shettleworth describes the problem as follows: A rat that experiences no food for twenty-four hours is more likely to eat than a rat that has just been fed. Most people would say that hunger per se, not any learning by the rat, explains its increased proclivity to forage, even though the experience of *not being fed* did affect the rat's behavior when it was presented with food (Shettleworth, 1998). Insertion of the phrase "relatively permanent" into our description of learning eliminates this problem.

Adopting "a relatively permanent change in behavior as a result of experience" as our definition of learning, we see an interesting relationship between learning and what evolutionary ecologists refer to as "phenotypic plasticity" (Harvell, 1994; Levins, 1968; Stearns, 1989; Tollrian and Harvell, 1998; Via and Lande, 1985; West-Eberhard, 1989, 2003). A **phenotype** is typically defined as the observable characteristics of an organism (Walker, 1989), and **phenotypic plasticity** is broadly defined as the ability of an organism to *produce different phenotypes* depending on environmental conditions. For example, many invertebrates such as the bryozoan *Membranipora membranacea* live in colonies (Harvell, 1998). When living in such colonies, individuals typically lack the spines that are often used as an antipredator defense in related species. These spines are simply not grown when *Membranipora membranacea* develops in the absence of predators. Yet, individuals will grow spines relatively quickly when exposed to predatory cues (Harvell, 1991, 1994; Tollrian and Harvell, 1998; Figure 4.3). The resultant change, from spineless to spined, constitutes a case of phenotypic plasticity. The phenotype of this bryozoan shifts dramatically as a result of environmental changes—in our case, the addition of a predator—and hence is thought of as "plastic" (Figure 4.4).

A

B

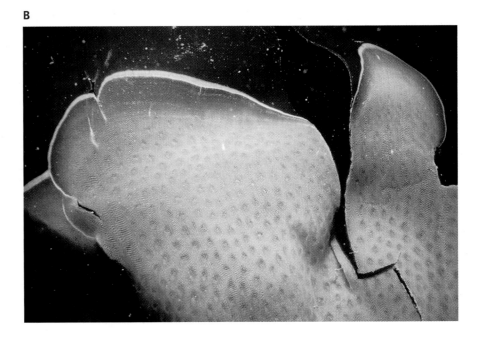

FIGURE 4.3. Inducible defenses. In some bryozoans, like *Membranipora membranacea*, colonies produce spines when predators are present. **(A)** Spines are shown protruding from a colony as a defense against predators, and **(B)** an overview of a colony of *Membranipora membranacea*. *(Photo credits: Ken Lucas/ Visuals Unlimited; © Sue Daly/naturepl. com)*

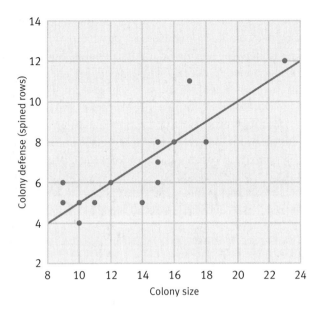

FIGURE 4.4. Phenotypic plasticity. When colonies of the bryozoan *Membranipora membranacea* are exposed to chemical stimuli from a predator, individuals in these colonies grow defense spines. Here we see the response to a single "dose" of water conditioned with bryozoan predators. Large colonies produce more spines. *(From Harvell, 1991, p. 4)*

If learning is "a relatively permanent change in behavior as a result of experience," it then becomes one type of phenotypic plasticity if we think of behavior as part of a phenotype (Dukas, 1998a). That is, if we replace "behavior" with "phenotype" in our definition of learning, phenotypic plasticity becomes the broader category under which learning is subsumed. So all learning is a type of phenotypic plasticity, but not all phenotypic plasticity involves learning. To better see this, consider the "flushing" behavior often seen in foraging birds.

While searching for food, birds may move their tails and wings in a way that flushes insects out from cover—insects that the bird then eats. In the painted redstart (*Myioborus pictus*), for example, when individuals are under branches, they increase their wing and feather motion and flush insects from the overhanging branches. One hypothesis to explain this flushing behavior is that the birds learn that when they are under branches and flap their wings, they will get food. On the other hand, this response could be innate rather than learned.

Piotr Jablonski and his colleagues tried to distinguish between the two hypotheses. What the researchers found is that, while it is true that birds in nature increase their wing-flapping behavior when they are under branches, the same increase in wing flapping also occurs in the laboratory, even when the birds are not rewarded for such behavior. That is, when Jablonski's team put naive birds under branches, they started flapping more as well, even when they got no food for doing so (Jablonski et al., 2006). As such, flushing insects under branches does represent a case of phenotypic plasticity—the ability of an organism to *produce different phenotypes* depending on environmental conditions—but is not a case of learning.

How Animals Learn

In this section, we shall delve into *how* animals learn what they learn. There is a huge psychological literature on this, both theoretical and empirical, and I am making no pretensions of covering this issue in any detail. Rather, I hope to review some basic ideas on how animals learn, or what psychologists often refer to as the processes underlying learning. Our discussion of how animals learn will follow an outline developed by Cecilia Heyes, both because of its conciseness and its attempt to tie *how* animals learn to *why* they learn (Heyes, 1994). Heyes notes that there are three commonly recognized types of experience that can lead to learning. We will touch on these three types of experience—namely, single stimulus, stimulus-stimulus, and response-reinforcer—and, in the process, look at the various categories and subcategories of learning that they facilitate.

LEARNING FROM A SINGLE-STIMULUS EXPERIENCE

In many ways, the simplest experience that can lead to learning involves a single stimulus—a stimulus that can take almost any form. For example, let's imagine that we are interested in studying learning in rats. Let's further imagine that numerous times throughout the day a researcher simply places an arbitrary cue in a rat's cage. We will make the cue a blue-colored stick, which is considered an arbitrary cue because it had no relevance to the rat before we began our experiment (Figure 4.5). Rats will often take note of such a disturbance and turn their heads in the direction of the blue stick. If, *over time*, the rats become more likely to turn their heads in the direction of the blue stick—that is, if they become more sensitive to the stimuli with time, **sensitization** has occurred. Conversely, if, over time, the animals become less likely to turn their heads, **habituation** is said to have taken place. Sensitization and habituation are two simple single-stimulus forms of learning.

The process of habituation is of great concern to experimental ethologists, particularly to those who work in the laboratory. It can become quite difficult to examine certain types of behaviors if animals habituate quickly to stimuli. For example, in many ethology experiments involving antipredator behavior, predators may be housed such that visual interactions between predator and prey are possible, but the predator can't actually harm the prey (Figure 4.6). This ethical compromise spares the life of the potential prey, but it creates a scenario in which the prey may now habituate to the predator, having learned that the predator cannot in fact move close enough to present any real danger (Huntingford, 1984). Because of these sorts of issues, ethologists often need to

FIGURE 4.5. Habituation and sensitization. Numerous times each day a blue stick is placed in a rat's cage. If the rat takes less and less notice of the stick, habituation has occurred. If the rat pays more attention to the blue stick over time, sensitization has taken place.

Predator fish   Prey fish

FIGURE 4.6. Habituation as a problem. Suppose the antipredator behavior of the smaller fish on the right is the subject of investigation. If the experimental protocol involves keeping the prey species in one tank (right) and the putative predator in another tank (left), the prey may learn that the predator is not dangerous and habituate to its presence.

go to great lengths to be certain that habituation has *not* occurred in their study system (Rowland and Sevenster, 1985).

Conservation biologists also worry about habituation in animals that may be trained in captivity and then released into the wild. In the safety of the lab, such animals may have habituated to certain stimuli that might prove very dangerous upon the animals' release into the wild (Bauer, 2005). Nonetheless, animal trainers, particularly those working with economically valuable animals such as horses, often try to habituate the animals they work with to various stimuli, so that the animals become less frightened by stimuli that often elicit innate fear responses (Christensen et al., 2006).

A single stimulus that results in habituation or sensitization may have many consequences for learning processes. If an animal habituates to a stimulus, this may interfere with later attempts to get the animal to associate that stimulus with some other cue. For example, if rats habituate to the blue stick, it might prove more difficult for them to subsequently learn that the blue stick signals the arrival of food. On the other hand, if sensitization to a single cue has occurred, it may facilitate the association of the sensitized stimulus with other cues.

PAVLOVIAN (CLASSICAL) CONDITIONING

Suppose that rather than giving a rat a single stimulus like the blue stick, from the start we *pair* this stimulus with a second stimulus, let's say the odor of a cat—an odor that rats have an inherent fear of. Now, five seconds after the blue stick is in place, we spray the odor of a cat into one corner of the cage (Figure 4.7). If the rat subsequently learns to associate stimulus 1 (blue stick) with stimulus 2 (cat odor) and responds to stimulus 1 by climbing under the chip shavings in its cage as soon as the blue stick appears, but *before* the odor is sprayed in, we have designed an experiment in **Pavlovian** *or* **classical conditioning** (Kim and Jung, 2006).

Stimulus 2
Unconditioned
Stimulus (US)

Stimulus 1
If paired with Stimulus 2 may
become Conditioned Stimulus (CS)

FIGURE 4.7. Paired stimuli. Five seconds after a blue stick (Stimulus 1) is placed in a rat's cage, the odor of a cat (Stimulus 2) is sprayed in as well. The question then becomes: Will the rat pair the blue stick with danger (cat odor)?

This form of conditioned learning was first developed by Ivan Pavlov in the late 1800s (Pavlov, 1927; Figure 4.8). At the most basic level, Pavlovian conditioning experiments involve two stimuli—the conditioned stimulus and the unconditioned stimulus (Domjan, 2005, 2006). A **conditioned stimulus (CS)** is often defined as a stimulus that initially fails to elicit a particular response, but comes to do so when it becomes associated with a second (unconditioned) stimulus. In our rat case, the blue stick is the conditioned stimulus, as initially the rat will probably have no fear of this object. The **unconditioned stimulus (US)** is a stimulus that elicits a vigorous response in the absence of training. In our rat case, the US would be the cat odor, which inherently causes a fear response in rats. Once the rat has learned to hide after the blue stick (CS) alone is in place, we can speak of its hiding as being a **conditioned response (CR)** to the presence of the blue stick (Figure 4.9).

Before examining Pavlovian conditioning in a bit more detail, we must define a few more terms. In the learning literature, any stimulus that is considered positive, pleasant, or rewarding is referred to as an **appetitive stimulus.** Appetitive stimuli include food, the presence of a potential mate, a safe haven,

FIGURE 4.8. Ivan Pavlov and classical conditioning. Pavlov is watching a classical conditioning experiment as it is being conducted in his laboratory. In the experiment, a device to measure salivation has been attached to the dog's cheek, the unconditioned stimulus is a dish containing meat powder, and the conditioned stimulus is a light. *(Photo credit: Sovfoto)*

CS

Conditioned Response
(CR) = hiding

FIGURE 4.9. Conditioned response. If the rat pairs the blue stick (CS) and the cat odor (US), then it will hide under the chips when the blue stick alone is presented. Such hiding represents a conditioned response (CR).

and so on. Conversely, any stimulus that is unpleasant—shock, noxious odors, and so forth—is labeled an **aversive stimulus**. Another important distinction made in the learning literature is between positive and negative relationships. When the first event (placement of the blue stick) in a conditioning experiment predicts the occurrence of the second event (cat odor), we have a positive relation between events. Conversely, if the first event predicts that the second event will *not* occur—imagine that a blue stick is always followed by *not* feeding an animal at its normal feeding time—we have a negative relationship. Positive relations—for example, blue stick predicts cat odor—produce **excitatory conditioning**, while negative relations—for example, blue stick leads to no food at a time when food is usually presented—produce **inhibitory conditioning**.

Pavlovian conditioning experiments can become very complicated by adding in second-order conditioning to the experimental equation (Figure 4.10). In second-order conditioning, once a conditioned response (CR) has been learned by pairing US and CS1, a new stimulus is presented before CS1, and if the

CS2   CS1   CS2

CS1   Panel 1   CR   Panel 2   Panel 3   CR

FIGURE 4.10. Second-order conditioning. In panel 1, a rat has *already been conditioned to associate the blue stick with a cat odor.* In panel 2, a red light is flashed on before the blue stick is placed in its cage. In panel 3, the rat displays a conditioned response when just the red light is turned on. In such a case, second-order conditioning to the red light has taken place.

new stimulus itself eventually elicits the conditioned response then the new stimulus has become a conditioned stimulus (CS2). In our case, any rats that learned to hide when the blue stick was present might now see a red light (the second-order stimulus, CS2) preceding the appearance of the blue stick. Once the rat has learned to pair the red light with the danger associated with cat odor, we can speak of second-order Pavlovian conditioning.

BLOCKING, OVERSHADOWING, AND LATENT INHIBITION. The effects of Pavlovian conditioning impact not only behavior per se, but also what is referred to as *learnability*. We will explore three types of learnability: overshadowing, blocking, and latent inhibition. To see how these operate, let's consider an experiment with four groups of rats. Suppose that Group 1 individuals undergo a standard Pavlovian paradigm with two stimuli: the blue stick (CS1) and a cat odor (US). In Group 2, a second conditioned stimulus (CS2), a red light, is always presented s*imultaneously* with the blue stick, just prior to the presence of the cat odor (Figure 4.11). Subjects from both groups are then tested in response to the blue stick alone. If the red light is **overshadowing** the blue stick, rats in Group 2 will respond less strongly to the blue stick than will rats in Group 1. The CS2 has made it more difficult for the rats to pair the blue stick and the cat odor—it has retarded the rats' ability to learn.

Now let us add a third group to our experiment. In Group 3, individuals are first trained to associate the blue stick with the cat odor, but after this, the red light is presented at the same time as the blue stick, and this compound stimulus is paired with the cat odor. Recall that in Group 2, the blue stick and the red light were always presented together. Rats in Group 3 differ from

FIGURE 4.11. Overshadowing. Group 1 rats have learned to associate just a blue stick and a cat odor, whereas Group 2 rats have learned to associate both a red light and a blue stick (together) with the cat odor. In the test arena, Group 1 and Group 2 rats are examined when just the blue stick is present. If Group 2 rats respond less strongly to the blue stick than Group 1 rats, overshadowing of the blue stick by the red light has taken place in the Group 2 rats.

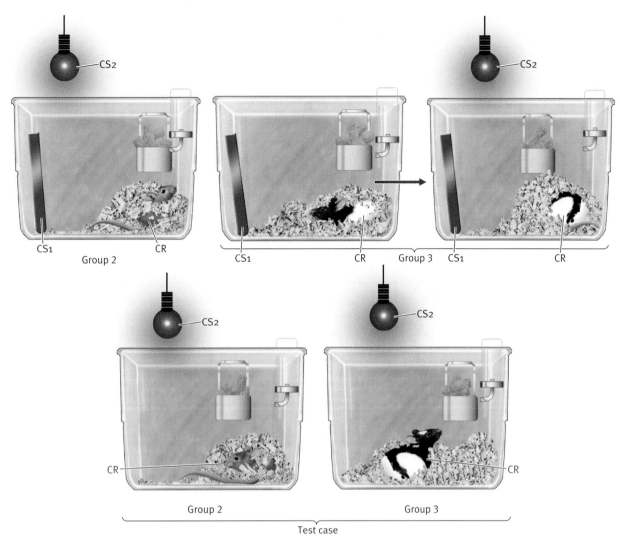

FIGURE 4.12. Blocking. Group 2 rats are trained to associate the red light and the blue stick (together) with the cat odor. Group 3 rats are initially trained to associate just the blue stick with the cat odor, but then they are trained to associate the joint presence of the stick and the light with the cat odor. Individuals from both groups are then tested in the presence of just the red light. If Group 3 individuals react less strongly than Group 2 rats to the light, blocking of the ability to pair the red light alone with the cat odor has occurred in the Group 3 individuals.

those in Group 2 in that they first learned to associate the blue stick and cat odor before any red light was added to the protocol. Now, after the animals are trained, let us compare the reaction of rats in Groups 2 and 3 when they are presented with the stimulus of a red light. **Blocking** occurs when those in Group 3 respond less strongly to the red light than individuals in Group 2 (Kamin, 1968, 1969). It is as if initially learning to associate the blue stick alone with the cat smell *blocked* Group 3 subjects' ability to pair the red light with the cat odor (Figure 4.12).

Finally, let's consider a fourth group of rats that is initially exposed to a blue stick, but no cat order, for a long period of time. If we find that when we then try to pair up the blue stick with cat odor at some subsequent point in time, the rats in this group have more difficulty learning than the rats in Group 1 (where we have standard Pavlovian pairing), then we say that **latent inhibition** is responsible for this learning deficit in Group 4.

INSTRUMENTAL (OPERANT) CONDITIONING

Instrumental conditioning, also known as **operant** or **goal-directed learning**, occurs when a response made by an animal is reinforced by reward or punishment. One of the most fundamental differences between Pavlovian and instrumental learning centers on the fact that, in the latter, the animal must undertake some action or response in order for the conditioning process to produce learning. The classic example of instrumental learning is a rat pressing some sort of lever (that is, taking an action) to get food to drop into his cage. Rats associate pressing on the lever (response) with food (outcome) and quickly learn this task.

Not all instrumental learning, however, is as easy to quantify as in the rat case. Michael Domjan illustrates this nicely by considering a dog that barks at intruders until the intruders go away (Domjan, 1998). Clearly, the dog has to bark (undertake an action) to make the intruder go away (produce an outcome), but does this illustrate instrumental *learning* in nature? Did the dog learn that barking (the response) made the intruder leave (the outcome)? It is certainly possible. But it is equally plausible that a novel intruder induced the barking, and that this barking simply continued until the intruder disappeared. In this case, the dog may have learned nothing. The difficulties inherent in these sorts of cases are why operant conditioning experiments are most often undertaken in the laboratory.

The earliest work on instrumental learning was that of Edward Thorndike and involved testing how quickly cats could escape from "puzzle boxes" that Thorndike had constructed (Thorndike, 1898, 1911). When Thorndike placed a cat in a locked box, the cat initially tried all sorts of things to get out of its confined space. Some of these behaviors, by chance, led to a successful escape from the box. Thorndike postulated that the cat began to pair certain behaviors that it undertook in the box with a positive effect—escape—and it was then more likely to use such behaviors when confined, and his data supported this contention. Combining the findings from his puzzle box experiment with other results he had obtained, Thorndike postulated the **law of effect**. This law states that if a response in the presence of a stimulus is followed by a satisfying event, the association between the stimulus and the response will be strengthened. Conversely, if the response is followed by an aversive event, the association will be weakened.

Thinking on the subject of instrumental learning was revolutionized by the work of B. F. Skinner, who argued that much work in this area ignored the fact that behavior was a continuous, free-flowing variable (Skinner, 1938). To remedy this problem, Skinner devised what is now known as a Skinner box. His idea was to create a continuous measure of behavior that could somehow be divided into meaningful units. When a rat pushes down on a lever, it is making an **operant response** because the action changes the rat's environment by adding food to it (Figure 4.13). The fact that "lever pushing" is a relatively unambiguous event that is easily measurable, and that it occurs in an environment over which the rat has control, has greatly facilitated the work of psychologists doing research within the instrumental learning paradigm.

FIGURE 4.13. Skinnerian rats. To test various theories of animal learning, rats are often placed in "Skinner boxes," where they have to take an action (here, pressing a button) to get a reward of food or water. *(Photo credit: Walter Dawn/Science Photo Library/Photo Researchers, Inc.)*

There is still some debate among psychologists over the relative merits of Pavlovian and instrumental learning techniques. From our perspective, however, much of this debate, though interesting in its details, is not relevant, in that over the years both instrumental and Pavlovian conditioning techniques have become very fine-tuned and have provided much in the way of understanding how animals learn what they learn.

Why Animals Learn

With an understanding of *how* animals learn, we can now take a definitively more evolutionary perspective and ask *why* animals learn. In so doing, we will need to recall how adaptationists think. If we imagine that the ability to learn is under some sort of complex genetic control, we can ask whether this ability is favored by natural selection, and if so, under what circumstances. In so doing, we will be addressing three related questions: (1) How can within-species studies help us understand natural selection and learning? (2) How can population comparisons be used to shed light on the evolution of learning? (3) What theories examine how learning evolves in different environments?

WITHIN-SPECIES STUDIES AND THE EVOLUTION OF LEARNING

Psychologists have done thousands, perhaps tens of thousands, of studies of learning in animals, particularly in rodents and pigeons. For the most part, until recently, these experiments have not been designed to take into consideration the natural environment of the organism, nor the evolutionary forces acting on the organism. This is due, at least in part, to a history that includes work both by Edward Thorndike and Ivan Pavlov in which they argued that, aside from the details, the qualitative features of learning are the same in all animals, including man—that is, all animals learn in a fundamentally similar fashion (Bitterman, 1975; Pavlov, 1927; Thorndike, 1911). This view became widely accepted, with such psychologists as B. F. Skinner and Harry Harlow promoting it (Harlow, 1959; Skinner, 1959). M. E. (Jeff) Bitterman, a leader in the field of comparative animal learning, notes that "work on learning has been dominated from the outset by a powerful theory which denies that learning has undergone any fundamental evolutionary change" (Bitterman, 1975, p. 699). If Thorndike and Pavlov were right that the particular environment an organism evolved in has no effect on learning, the same sort of learning should be seen in all creatures that learn, regardless of the sort of learning tasks with which they are presented.

In adopting the adaptationist approach, the above claim seems hard to imagine. Could it really be true that natural selection has not acted on the ability to learn? Rather, it seems that the ability to learn should be under strong selection pressure, with individuals who learn appropriate cues that are useful in their particular environment being strongly favored by natural selection. Those who adopt this view are said to be in the "ecological learning" school, and their influence is getting stronger as our knowledge about evolution and learning increases (Dukas, 1998a; Johnston, 1985; Shettleworth, 1998). Such ecological learning first emerged in the psychological literature with the work of John Garcia and his colleagues.

GARCIA'S RATS. In the mid-1960s, Garcia and his team ran a series of learning experiments using rats. Experiments on rat learning were hardly news in either the psychological or biological community, but Garcia's results made both groups rethink their approach to studies of learning (Garcia et al., 1972; Seligman and Hager, 1972). What is particularly amazing about Garcia's work is that in many ways the protocol he used was very similar to that already being used in psychology experiments centered on learning. In essence, Garcia simply attempted to have rats form an association between a series of cues (Garcia and Koelling, 1966). One of those cues was either "bright-noisy" water (that is, water associated with a noise and an incandescent light) or "tasty" water (that is, water with a particular taste). The researchers then paired bright-noisy water or the tasty water with one of the following negative stimuli: radiation, a toxin, immediate shock, or delayed shock. For example, in the bright-noisy water/radiation treatment, bright-noisy water would be presented and the rats who had been trained to this cue would drink the water and then be exposed to radiation that would make them ill.

Garcia and Koelling found a fascinating interaction between the type of punishment a rat received for drinking water and the type of water that the rat consumed. X-ray and toxin treatments, each of which made the rat physically ill, were easily associated with the tasty water (gustatory) cues, but not with the bright-noisy (audiovisual) cues. That is, the rats quickly learned that tasty water was to be avoided after this cue was paired with X-rays or toxins, but they did not learn to avoid bright-noisy water after it was paired with X-rays or toxins. In contrast, when Garcia and Koelling examined the rats that were given shock treatments, they found that shock was easily paired with the bright-tasty water (audiovisual cue), but not with tasty water (gustatory cue).

Garcia and Koelling explained their views by adopting an adaptationist stance (see Chapter 2)—something quite unusual for psychologists of the 1960s. They argued that natural selection would favor the ability to pair gustatory cues (tasty water) with internal discomfort (getting ill). After all, many instances of internal discomfort in nature are likely to be caused by what an animal has consumed, and rarely are food cues associated with audiovisual cues (as in the bright-noisy water treatment). On the other hand, peripheral pain, like that caused by a shock, might be more commonly associated with some audiovisual cue like hearing or seeing a conspecific or a predator, and so again natural selection should favor the ability to pair these cues together.

In another apparent blow to orthodoxy in psychological learning circles of the period, Garcia found that learning in rats will occur without immediate reinforcement (Garcia et al., 1966). Most psychologists believed that delays in reinforcement on the order of seconds can cripple animal learning, yet Garcia found that learning occurred, even after delays of seventy-five minutes, when injections of noxious substances were paired with drinking saccharin-flavored water. From an evolutionary perspective, the work of Garcia and his colleagues makes perfect sense. In nature, one would expect a delay between the time that a rat consumed a substance and any subsequent negative effect of such consumption. As such, natural selection would have favored rats that were able to associate what they ate with becoming ill, even if separated by significant time intervals.

OPTIMAL FORGETTING IN STOMATOPODS. The ability to remember events plays an obvious role in animal learning. In fact, depending on your precise definition of memory, learning is impossible without some form of memory. Psychologists have long studied memory and learning by, for example, looking at **extinction curves** (graphical representations of the weakening and then ending of paired associations) in learning experiments. Such experiments typically test how long an animal will remember some paired association once the pairing itself has stopped. Such tests are critical to numerous aspects of psychological learning theory, but they fail to ask a question that jumps to the surface when an adaptationist approach to the subject of memory is invoked. Namely, given the ecology of the species, might natural selection shape an optimal memory span? That is, while psychologists tend to focus on how long associations last, an evolutionary animal behaviorist would ask why we see variation in the length of time that stimuli stay paired, and how natural selection may have favored certain extinction curves over others.

It may be that certain events in an animal's life are timed such that it would be beneficial to remember them for X days, but after this time period, remembering and acting on such memories would be either of no benefit or perhaps even detrimental. For example, imagine a forager who is able to remember the location and amount of food in patches. If patches are renewable, then while it may pay to remember the location of a food patch, it doesn't necessarily pay to remember how much food was there the last time you visited, as this might lead to erroneous decisions that are based on outdated information (Figure 4.14).

Before proceeding to examine an example of how behavioral ecologists and ethologists might test the idea of optimal memory, it is important to realize that no natural selection model of any behavior predicts that an animal will reach some global optimum. Rather, natural selection models predict that, given the constraints that an animal faces, selection will favor moving as close to an optimum as possible (Alcock, 1998; Mayr, 1982). In other words, ethologists don't search for the best of all possible solutions to a problem and assume that selection will take us there, but rather they recognize that many constraints prevent selection from ever reaching such a global optimum.

With respect to learning there are, in all likelihood, neurobiological constraints on memory and other cognitive functions, and these serve as guideposts for the limits of natural selection's ability to shape memory capacity (Dukas, 1998a, 1998b;

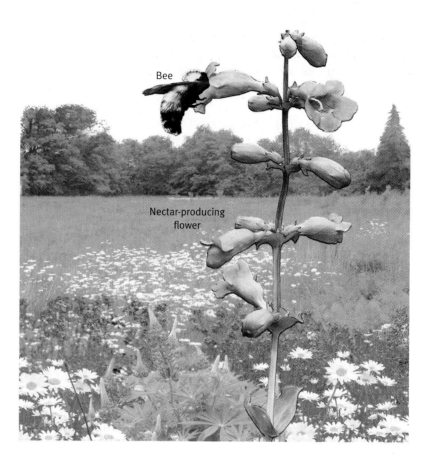

Bee

Nectar-producing
flower

FIGURE 4.14. How long to remember? Imagine a bee foraging at a nectar-producing flower. While it might pay for the bee to remember the flower's location, it might not be beneficial to remember specific nectar content, as that shifts within and between days.

Shettleworth, 1998). That being said, it is interesting to note that neurobiologists have found that a relatively small number of neurons seem needed to store a relatively large amount of memory-related pieces of information (Morton and Chiel, 1994; Singer, 1994).

To see how ethologists might tackle the question of natural selection and memory, we will consider Roy Caldwell's 1992 study of aggressive behavior in the stomatopod crustacean *Gonodactylus bredini* (Caldwell, 1992; Healey, 1992). Male and female *G. bredini* share a nest cavity for a few days before they breed, and they actively repel all intruders from this area (Caldwell, 1986; Dingle and Caldwell, 1972; Shuster and Caldwell, 1989). Very shortly after mating, however, the male leaves the breeding cavity and goes out in search of a new mate. Caldwell set up an experimental design that allowed him to examine whether the males who left the brood cavity and the females they left behind recognize one another after the male's desertion, and if so, for how long and why (Caldwell, 1992).

It turns out that both male and female *Gonodactylus bredini* remember one another after the male has left. Males are less likely to be aggressive toward their former mates, while females put up a weaker resistance to such males. With respect to memory, males and females recognize one another for at least two weeks—the duration of the experiment, and relatively speaking, a long time (Caldwell, 1992). What makes this study fascinating is that, based on his understanding of stomatopod biology, Caldwell hypothesized that individuals might actually be able to recognize each other for up to four weeks. But why four weeks?

It turns out that the females guard their brood for four weeks, after which the brood leaves its cavity for good. At the four-week point, then, males need not worry about being aggressive toward former mates, as such aggression will not harm their own brood (Figure 4.15). In other words, Caldwell predicted that there is an optimal time to recognize former mates, and that this optimum is set by the self-interest of the interacting parties. For *Gonodactylus bredini*, this optimum is set at four weeks, and Caldwell predicted that male and female stomatopods will either forget each other after this time period, or at the very least, they will act as if they had forgotten each other.

Unfortunately, Caldwell's experiment did not run for four weeks. But suppose it had, and suppose he had found that, up to four weeks, males behaved less aggressively toward former mates, but no longer did so after this time. It would be difficult, if not impossible, to determine whether the stomatopods actually forgot information or simply ignored information that they still retained. This is a general problem in animal learning studies, however, and is beyond the scope of what we are addressing here. That is, since we measure learning by what an animal does, in the absence of language, it is hard to be specific about what is going on cognitively when an animal doesn't do something. Did it forget? Did it not act on the information it possessed? There are some ways around this, but they are often circuitous (Roper et al., 1995). For example, if an animal is placed in an obvious life-and-death situation and fails to perform a learned behavior that would save its life, we can, in all likelihood, infer that it simply forgot the appropriate life-saving behavior, rather than that it recalled such behavior but ignored it. In any case, the stomatopod study raises some fascinating questions about how natural selection might be acting on some aspect of learning and memory in animals.

FIGURE 4.15. Stomatopod threat. Male and female stomatopod crustaceans share a cavity for a few days before they breed. Although the males leave the breeding cavity soon after mating, they tend to remember their former mates and to be less aggressive toward them during the weeks that their brood remains in the cavity. This is a photo of a male *Gonodactylus smithii* in a threat position. *(Photo credit: Roy Caldwell)*

POPULATION COMPARISONS AND THE EVOLUTION OF LEARNING

In Chapter 2, we learned that one technique that ethologists employ to understand the evolution of behavior is to compare behavior across different populations of the same species. Oftentimes such studies compare two or more populations to one another and make predictions about behavioral similarities and differences between these populations, based both on a knowledge of their ecology and some hypotheses about how natural selection has operated in each (Balda et al., 1998; Bitterman, 1975; Dukas, 1998a; Johnston, 1985; Macphail, 1987; Marler and Terrace, 1984; Rozin, 1988; Shettleworth, 1998). Here we will adopt this approach with respect to how natural selection has shaped learning in doves and sticklebacks.

LEARNING, FORAGING, AND GROUP LIVING IN DOVES. Animals in groups often find food faster and have more time available for foraging (Krebs and Davies, 1993). With respect to learning, Pascal Carlier and Louis Lefebvre predicted that individuals who live in groups should learn more quickly than territorial (and hence more isolated) individuals (Carlier and Lefebvre, 1996). Ideally, one would like to test this hypothesis in a single species, where natural selection has favored group living in some populations, but solitary living in others. Zenaida dove populations from Barbados (*Zenaida aurita*; Figure 4.16) fit the bill perfectly, as solitary living (via territoriality) is the norm in one dove population studied by Carlier and Lefebvre, while in another population

FIGURE 4.16. Zenaida doves. Zenaida doves from populations where individuals live in groups appear to be better at learning foraging tasks than individuals from populations where doves are territorial. *(Photo credit: Jean-Philippe Paris)*

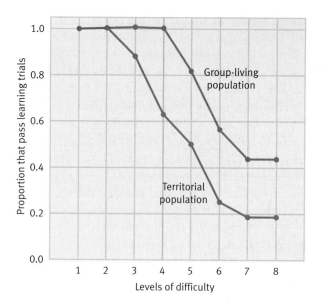

FIGURE 4.17. Group living and learning. More birds from the group-living population surpassed the "learning criteria" for foraging tasks than did birds that had lived alone (territorial population). As the learning task became more difficult, fewer birds passed, but birds from the group-living population consistently did better than those from the territorial population. *(From Carlier and Lefebvre, 1996, p. 1203)*

only nine miles away, group living is the norm. Because these populations are geographically close to one another, differences in other environmental variables, above and beyond those associated with territoriality, were likely to be fairly minimal.

Sixteen doves from each of the group-living and territorial populations were captured and brought into the laboratory. All subjects were then individually presented with the challenge of learning how to operate an experimental apparatus that required the birds to pull on a metal ring, which then opened a drawer containing food. Carlier and Lefebvre found clear evidence that group-living doves learned this task more quickly than did birds from the territorial population (Figure 4.17; see also Sasvari, 1985). Furthermore, they found that the more difficult the learning task the birds had to solve, the more pronounced the between-population differences.

Let's examine two possible explanations for these differences (Carlier and Lefebvre, 1996). First, the animals may have already differed in foraging experience before the experiment, and hence some of the differences the researchers uncovered may have been due to what individuals had experienced, and potentially learned, prior to being brought into the laboratory. Second, above and beyond what experiences any given set of birds took into Carlier and Lefebvre's experiment, natural selection may have operated on learning ability across these populations. The verdict is still out as to which of the possibilities best explains differences between dove populations. But in principle, one could obtain a much clearer idea of which of these explanations is more powerful by raising both territorial and group-living doves in the laboratory under controlled conditions, and testing whether differences in learning still remained. If they did, this would suggest that natural selection had favored learning more strongly in the group-living population of doves.

LEARNING AND ANTIPREDATOR BEHAVIOR IN STICKLEBACKS. As just discussed, one way to partially circumvent the confounding effects of personal experience per se and natural selection acting on learning abilities in interpopulational studies of learning is through the use of controlled laboratory experiments. In the lab, it becomes possible to raise individuals from two very different populations in a similar environment, and hence minimize experience differences across populations. This is just what Huntingford and Wright did in their study of avoidance conditioning in two populations of three-spined stickleback fish (*Gasterosteus aculeatus*; Huntingford and Wright, 1992).

Along with guppies, sticklebacks have become a favorite species for testing ethologically based hypotheses regarding interpopulation differences (Godin, 1997; Wooton, 1976). The reason for the interest in using sticklebacks in such a context stems from the fact that many stickleback populations are very similar, with often only a single critical variable—predation pressure—differing across populations. Some sticklebacks live in locales that contain a variety of different predators, and some populations live in lakes with virtually no predators.

Huntingford and Wright raised individuals derived from predator-rich and predator-free streams in the laboratory, and during their development none of the individuals had any interaction with predators. An adaptationist approach to population differences would suggest that natural selection should have acted more strongly on antipredator strategies—including learning about danger—in the sticklebacks from the predator-rich population.

Huntingford and Wright started by training eight sticklebacks from each of their population groups to associate one side of their home tank with food. They found no differences in learning across populations in the context of foraging alone—individuals from both populations were equally adept at learning that food would come to one side of their tank. Then, after a stickleback had learned that one side of its tank was associated with food, fish were subject to a simulated attack from a heron predator. Huntingford and Wright then examined whether between-population differences emerged in terms of how long it took to learn to avoid the side of the tank associated with heron predation (and food) (Figure 4.18).

While all but one fish from both populations learned to avoid the dangerous end of their tank, fish from high-predation areas learned this task more quickly

FIGURE 4.18. Learning in sticklebacks. The number of stickleback fish from **(A)** low-predation and **(B)** high-predation sites that failed to reach the avoidance learning criteria (orange bars) and the number of sticklebacks swimming into the dangerous compartment (green bars). As the number of fish remaining decreases, the number of fish that have met the learning criteria increases. *(From Huntingford and Wright, 1992)*

than did fish from predator-free populations. Two lines of reasoning support the hypothesis that natural selection has operated on learning and antipredator behavior in these populations of sticklebacks. First, Huntingford and Wright's laboratory protocol minimized the probability that individual experiences differed significantly across the populations they examined. Second, and equally important, Huntingford and Wright did not find between-population differences in all learning contexts; when the task was a simple association of food and place, no population differences in learning emerged. The researchers only discovered interpopulational differences with respect to learning and antipredator behaviors in the behavioral scenario in which they hypothesized natural selection was operating—in learning to avoid areas associated with predators.

A MODEL OF THE EVOLUTION OF LEARNING

In addition to empirical examinations on the evolution of individual learning, a number of mathematical models have been developed to examine when natural selection might favor the ability to learn (Bergman and Feldman, 1995; Boyd and Richerson, 1985; Dopazo et al., 2003; Hinton and Nowlan, 1987; Irwin and Price, 1999; Odling-Smee et al., 2003; Stephens, 1991, 1993). Theoreticians typically begin the process of modeling the evolution of learning by taking a cost-benefit perspective. Imagine a behavioral scenario in which the options are to respond to some stimuli with a fixed genetically programmed response, or to respond to stimuli based on prior experience in the same situation—that is, by learning. Are the net benefits associated with learning greater or less than the net benefits that might be associated with a fixed genetic response to some stimuli?

Ethologists, behavioral ecologists, and psychologists have argued that natural selection should favor the ability to learn over the genetic transmission of a fixed trait when the environment an animal lives in changes often, but not too often. To see why, we must recognize two assumptions that underlie many of these models: (1) most models assume that there is some cost to learning, even if it is only a very small cost, and (2) when we speak of learning in such models we are referring to the ability to learn being a trait that has an underlying genetic basis. Both of these assumptions appear to be met in fruit flies, in whom both genetic variation in the ability to learn, as well as a fitness cost of learning have been documented (Mery and Kawecki, 2002, 2003). With the model's assumptions now made clear, we can ask why environments that change often (but not too often) favor the evolution of learning.

When the environment *rarely changes*—and hence the environment that offspring encounter is similar to that of their parents—information is best passed on by genetic transmission of inflexible traits, since such a means of transmission avoids the costs of learning. On the other end of the spectrum, if the environment is *constantly changing*, there is nothing worth learning because what is learned is completely irrelevant in the next situation. When the environment is constantly changing, acting on past experience is worthless, as past experience is of no predictive value. Hence, genetic transmission of a fixed response, rather than a costly learned response, is again favored. Somewhere in the middle, in between an environment that never changes and one that always changes, learning is favored over the genetic transmission of a fixed response.

In this zone, it is worth paying the cost of learning. The environment is stable enough to favor learning, but not so stable as to favor genetic transmission.

David Stephens agrees that the starting point in modeling genetic transmission of fixed traits versus the ability to learn should indeed be the stability of an animal's environment (Stephens, 1991, 1993). But Stephens challenges the assumption about environmental stability as it is represented in these models, saying that many models conflate two types of stability that need to be separated.

The model that Stephens himself developed breaks environmental predictability into two sections: (1) predictability within the lifetime of an individual, and (2) predictability between the environment of parents and offspring. These two types of predictability can be very different, and conflating them may hinder our understanding of the evolution of learning (Table 4.1). For example, consider a case in which early in life the offspring of species A move to environments that are far removed from those of their parents, and that the environment to which they migrate is stable over the course of their lifetime. In such a case, between-generation environmental variability in species A is quite high, while within-lifetime environmental variability is much lower. This potentially important distinction is lost when models lump together within- and between-generation environmental variation.

Learning is favored in Stephens's model when predictability within the lifetime of an individual is high, but environmental predictability between generations is low. To see why, let's walk through each of the possible scenarios in Table 4.1. In boxes 1 and 2, predictability within generations is low, and so neither strategy does particularly well. But since learning has a cost associated with it, genetic transmission of a fixed response is favored. Fixed genetic transmission is again favored in box 4, because with high predictability at all levels, the cost of learning is never worth the investment. Only in box 3, with high within-generation predictability but low between-generation predictability, is learning favored. Learning is favored here because, once an organism learns what to do, it can repeat the appropriate behaviors during its lifetime. But isn't this the sort of predictability that usually favors a fixed genetic transmission? It is indeed, but now the environment changes so much between generations that genetic codes for fixed traits would fail at that level despite working within the lifetime of an individual.

TABLE 4.1. Stephens's model for the evolution of learning. The key variables in this model are within-lifetime environmental predictability and between-generation environmental predictability.

		WITHIN-LIFETIME PREDICTABILITY	
		Low	High
BETWEEN-GENERATION PREDICTABILITY	Low	Ignore experience (1)	Learn (3)
	High	Ignore experience (2)	Ignore experience (4)

What Animals Learn

As we have already seen, we don't necessarily expect to observe learning in every conceivable behavioral scenario, nor in every species. That being said, if the ability to change behavior based on prior experience is a significant force in shaping animal behavior, then we should generally expect to see learning in a wide variety of contexts. In order to provide a broad (but brief) overview of animal learning, in this section we shall examine evidence for learning with respect to habitat selection, mating, familial relationships, and aggression. One prominent omission from this list is "learning about food sources"—a topic that we discussed earlier in the chapter and that we will discuss in depth in Chapter 10.

Some researchers have sought to go beyond studying learning per se, and are examining animal intelligence. There has been research on apes learning sign language, parrots learning expanded vocabularies, sea lions learning object discrimination, among other studies. Yet, this work remains controversial, both because it is difficult to define intelligence, and because some believe that the results produced to date can be explained by conditioning rather than cognitive thought on the part of the animal. Much more work remains to be undertaken to better understand the evolution of intelligence in animals.

LEARNING WHERE HOME IS LOCATED

Learning plays a fundamental role in habitat selection in many animal species. For example, while some aspects of bird migration are known to be instinctual, learning also plays a critical role in the long journeys often involved in migration (Able, 1999; Alerstam et al., 2003; Dingle, 1996; Dyer, 1998; Gauthreaux, 1997; Mettke-Hofmann and Gwinner, 2003). More generally, learning likely plays an important role in habitat selection (see Chapter 13), including learning territory boundaries, the identity (and possibly the personality) of neighboring individuals, and the nature and value of resources in a given area (Beecher et al., 1998; Eason et al., 1999; Fisher, 1954; Getty, 1987; Godard, 1991). Here we will focus on the role of learning in the orientation and migratory behavior of fish (Braithwaite and de Perera, 2006; Dodson, 1988; Giske et al., 1998; Odling-Smee and Braithwaite, 2003).

There are numerous theories on how fish make the often very long migration back to their natal stream as adults. For example, there is some evidence that fish use celestial and magnetic compasses (Quinn, 1984), while other studies find that fish may use drifting currents (Miller et al., 1985) or some physiological change (for example, a change in temperature or oxygen intake) in response to their current position to guide them back home (Barkley et al., 1978). At the same time, however, more and more evidence demonstrates that learning may play a role in fish migration (Dodson, 1988).

Juvenile salmon appear to learn the odors associated with their natal streams, and they subsequently use such information to guide their way home (Dittman and Quinn, 1996; Dittman et al., 1997; Nevitt et al., 1994; Quinn and Dittman, 1990; Figure 4.19). Dittman and his colleagues examined the age at which young salmon learn about their home streams, and whether such

FIGURE 4.19. Pink salmon migration. In some species of fish, learning plays a role in orientation and migration. *(Photo credit: Tom Walker/ Photri)*

learning is age-dependent in hatchery-reared coho salmon (*Oncorhynchus kisutch*). At different stages during development, young salmon were exposed to either natural odors or an artificial odor (beta-phenylethyl alcohol) and then tested in the presence of such odors when they matured into adults. Results from the beta-phenylethyl alcohol treatment show clearly that learning the odor of the natal stream was taking place when the young matured from the parr stage—a post-larval stage when fish have dark "parr bars" on their sides—to the smolt stage—a stage that follows the parr style and at which salmon are first ready to migrate—but not earlier. Only salmon that had been exposed to this artificial odor as young smolts were attracted to this smell when they matured into adults. This age-dependent learning effect is particularly interesting, as learning occurs at the same time as a surge in plasma thyroxin levels, suggesting a possible hormonal underpinning to migratory learning (Kudo et al., 1994).

Lema and Nevitt followed up the lead that thyroxin may play an important role in learning during salmon migration (Lema and Nevitt, 2004). They hypothesized that an increase in thyroid hormone in the parr-smolt transition might increase the production of cells associated with the salmon's olfactory system, as this olfactory system also undergoes dramatic change during the transition to the smolt stage (Dittman et al., 1997; Jarrard, 1997; Nevitt et al., 1994).

To test their ideas, Lema and Nevitt surgically implanted pellets containing thyroid hormone in one group of parr, and they surgically implanted a placebo pellet in a second group of parr. When they compared groups, they found that the experimental group had higher levels of circulating thyroid hormones (as would be expected because of the implanted pellets), but they also found that the experimental group showed an increase in cells associated with the development of the olfactory system. More specifically, Lema and Nevitt saw a rise in what are called "multipotent" progenitor cells. These cells typically differentiate into olfactory receptor nerves, indicating a clear link between thyroid hormone and olfactory-based learning in migratory salmon (Dukes et al., 2004; Lema and Nevitt, 2004).

LEARNING ABOUT YOUR MATE

Given the fundamental importance of finding a willing and able mate, one might expect that animals would use any possible information available to them to help in the process of searching for potential mates (Pfaus et al., 2001). If an individual could learn to associate certain cues with mating opportunities, this ability would surely reap long-term fitness benefits (Graham and Desjardins, 1980; West et al., 1992; Zamble et al., 1985, 1986). Michael Domjan and his colleagues have been examining Pavlovian learning and mate choice in a number of different species, but here we will touch on their work with the Mongolian gerbil (*Meriones unguiculatus*) (Domjan et al., 2000).

Mongolian gerbils are burrowing desert rodents that rely on chemical communication during many forms of social exchange, including the formation of pair bonds (Thiessen and Yahr, 1977; Ågren, 1984). Given this, Ron Villarreal and Domjan ran an experiment that first allowed pair bonds to form between a male and a female. The researchers presented one group of males with an olfactory cue (mint or lemon) and then gave them access to their partners. They presented males in another (control) group with the odor, but they did not provide them with access to females following this presentation. Males that experienced the pairing of an odor and subsequent access to a pairmate learned relatively quickly to approach an area where access to the female was signaled by an odor, while males in the control group made no such association (Villarreal and Domjan, 1998).

Villarreal and Domjan took their work a step further and went on to examine whether females learned to associate an odor with the presence of their pairmates, and whether any male/female differences emerged. Females did learn to pair odor and access to their pairmates—conditioned females responded to odor cues by approaching the area associated with this cue, and any differences between males and females disappeared over time, suggesting that discrepancies between male and female gerbils in learning to pair a cue with the presence of a mate may not be great in nature.

Domjan and Karen Hollis have hypothesized that differences between males and females in their learning abilities should be positively correlated with differences in male and female parental investment (Domjan and Hollis, 1988). The more that parental investment is shared equally, the more the sexes should be similar in terms of learning ability, particularly with respect to learning the location of partners. One way to think about Domjan and Hollis's hypothesis is in terms of how much each sex is willing to invest in future offspring (Trivers, 1974). In the case in which both males and females provide resources for offspring, selection pressure for learning ability should be strong on both sexes. Assuming the appropriate cognitive infrastructure, in such a case we expect males and females to have the ability to learn where their mate—the co-provider of resources for their offspring—is at any given time. This "learning the location of mates" ability may also be demonstrated during courtship.

In many mating systems, only a single sex provides resources for offspring, and that sex is predominately the female sex. There are many reasons for this (see Chapters 6 and 7), but for the purposes of Domjan and Hollis's hypothesis, what this translates into is that males in such systems should be better at learning about the location of mates than females. To see why, think about it like this: In terms of parental care for subsequent offspring, females are a valuable resource for males, as they alone provide food for offspring. From a

A **B**

FIGURE 4.20. **Parental investment and learning ability.** **(A)** Parental investment is shared in blue gourami, and differences in learning between the sexes is small. **(B)** In Japanese quail, the females care for the young, as shown by this female at the nest with her eggs, and there is no parental investment by males, but males show greater learning abilities than females. *(Photo credits: © Wil Meinderts/FotoNatura/Minden Pictures; public domain)*

parental care perspective, males are much less valuable a resource to females. Males then are under strong selection pressure to find receptive females, while females can almost always find males that are willing to mate. Hence, in such mating systems, selection for learning locations associated with potential mates is stronger in males than in females. More experimental work needs to be done in this area, but some support for this hypothesis has been found. First, in both Mongolian gerbils and gourami fish, parental investment is shared and learning differences between the sexes are small. Second, in contrast to Mongolian gerbils and gourami fish, in Japanese quail, where there is no parental investment on the part of males, males show significantly greater learning abilities than do females (Gutierrez and Domjan, 1996; Hollis et al., 1989; Villarreal and Domjan, 1998; Figure 4.20).

LEARNING ABOUT FAMILIAL RELATIONSHIPS

How animals recognize each other as kin or nonkin is still a subject of contention, but in some species learning may play a role in such recognition (Fletcher and Michener, 1987; Hepper, 1991). If animals can learn how they themselves are related to others, as well as how different individuals in their group are related to one another, natural selection might favor altruistic and cooperative behavior being preferentially allocated to close genetic kin. Here we shall examine learning and kin recognition in the context of helpers-at-the-nest.

As we discussed in Chapters 2 and 3, in some species of birds and mammals, individuals forego direct reproduction and instead help their relatives raise their offspring (Brown, 1987; Solomon and French, 1996; Stacey and Koenig, 1990). Oftentimes, this simply involves offspring remaining at their natal nest and helping their parents raise a subsequent brood (the helper's siblings). But this is only one way in which helping may emerge. For example, young, reproductively active long-tailed tits (*Aegithalos caudatus*) breed independently as soon as they

FIGURE 4.21. Learning who is kin. Young, long-tailed tits (*Aegithalos caudatus*) often become helpers at the nests of their close genetic relatives, helping to build nests and to forage for food to feed the chicks. As helpers, they accrue indirect fitness benefits by contributing to the survival of their close genetic kin. *(Photo credit: Andrew MacColl)*

FIGURE 4.22. Playback calls and kin. Individual birds showed a strong preference for the calls given by their close genetic kin, staying for a longer time near the speakers that gave off the calls of their kin. *(From Sharp and Hatchwell, 2005)*

can (Figure 4.21). In this species, however, most nests fall victim to predation on the young. At that point, breeders often become helpers at the nests of their close genetic relatives, and such helpers accrue indirect fitness benefits by helping to raise their kin (Hatchwell et al., 2004). This brings up a number of fascinating questions, including: How do the birds know who are kin? Do they learn who is kin, and who isn't, and if so, how?

To address these questions, Stuart Sharp and his colleagues ran a series of experiments that focused on a specific call—the "churr" call—made by long-tailed tits. This call develops before young birds fledge and leave the nest, and it remains very consistent throughout the lifetime of an individual (Sharp and Hatchwell, 2005). "Churrs" are given by males and females in the context of short-range communications, such as those regarding nest-building and aggression (Gaston, 1973; Hatchwell et al., 2001; Sharp and Hatchwell, 2005).

Sharp and his team began by employing a "playback" experiment, in which an individual would hear the taped call of either a close genetic relative or a nonrelative. Individual birds showed a strong preference for the calls given by their kin (Figure 4.22). Following the playback experiment, Sharp and his colleagues designed an experimental protocol to assess whether the birds learned the churr calls of their relatives, or whether their preference was based on genetic predispositions for certain types of churr calls. They ran a cross-fostering experiment (see Chapter 2), in which chicks were either raised with their biological parents, or were switched to another nest and raised by foster parents.

A number of lines of evidence suggest that the churr call is in fact learned: (1) The calls of foster siblings raised together were about as similar as the calls of biological siblings raised together; (2) the calls of biological siblings raised apart were as dissimilar as the calls of unrelated individuals in nature; (3) the songs of foster parents and their foster offspring were very similar, whereas the songs of biological parents and their offspring were different when those offspring were raised by foster parents. These results all suggest an important role for learning in the development of churr calls.

The typical scenario for kinship and learning in long-tailed tits would then unfold like this: Young fledglings would almost universally be raised in the nests of their biological parents. As they matured, they would develop a churr call that was similar to that of their parents, and they could use their parents' call as a template for determining relatedness. Once the young fledglings left their nest, if they failed at independent breeding, they could distinguish between kin and nonkin based on their learned churr call, and they could preferentially dispense aid to kin.

LEARNING ABOUT AGGRESSION

Ethologists and behavioral ecologists have had a long-standing interest in aggressive behavior (see Chapter 14; Archer, 1988; Dugatkin, 1997a; Gadagkar, 1997; Huntingford and Turner, 1987). In the animal behavior literature, aggression is often partitioned into two components—intrinsic and extrinsic factors (Landau, 1951a, 1951b). Intrinsic factors usually refer to traits that correlate with an animal's fighting ability (Parker, 1974a), with the most common of these factors being some measure of size (Archer, 1988; Huntingford and Turner, 1987; Hurd, 2006).

Extrinsic factors include what have come to be known as "winner" and "loser" effects (see Chapter 14). Winner and loser effects are usually defined as an increased probability of winning an aggressive interaction based on past victories, and an increased probability of losing an aggressive interaction based on past losses, respectively. Our question here will be whether learning is involved with either winner or loser effects. To address this question experimentally, ideally we would work with a species in which aggression per se was well understood, so that we could have a strong baseline from which to launch into studying learning and winner and loser effects in the context of such aggression. It is for this reason that Karen Hollis and her colleagues worked on learning and winner and loser effects in blue gourami fish (*Trichogaster trichopterus*), a species in which males are territorial and aggression has been studied in numerous contexts (Hollis et al., 1995).

Hollis and her team had previously demonstrated that male blue gouramis could be trained to associate a light with either the presence (+) or absence (−) of an intruder male in their territory. They found that after the presentation of the light cue, two individuals that had both learned that a light meant the presence of another fish were much more aggressive than two fish that associated a light with the absence of another individual, presumably because the former were prepared for a fight (Figure 4.23). This work, in and of itself, does not touch on the issue of winner and loser effects per se, but rather sets the stage for experimental work that does.

Hollis used a similar protocol to that described above to examine the effect of conditioned learning on winner and loser effects (Hollis et al., 1995). The essential idea was to examine whether conditioning (Pavlovian learning) could have long-term effects on territorial males by creating the start of a series of encounters that would produce a winner or loser effect. Half the gouramis in the study were trained to associate a red light with the presence of a territorial intruder. The other half were control males who were presented with the red light six hours before they saw a territorial intruder, and as a result of the time delay, did not associate the red light with an intruder. Hollis's experiment involved two contests. In the first contest, after a red light was turned on, trained males and controls were pitted against each other until a clear winner and loser emerged. As expected from the earlier work, trained males were much more likely to win such encounters.

FIGURE 4.23. Pavlovian fish. Males that had learned to associate a light with the presence of another male were more aggressive when the light cue was present than were males that did not associate the light with the presence of another male. *(From Hollis, 1984)*

FIGURE 4.24. Winners and losers.
(A) Males that won in contest 1 were more likely to win in contest 2 (WW) than were males that had lost in contest 1 (LW).
(B) Males that lost in contest 1 were more likely to lose in contest 2 (LL). *(From Hollis et al., 1995, p. 129)*

In the second contest, winners and losers from the first contest were paired up with new intruders three days later. In these pairings, no red light was shown to either fish. All individuals that won their fights in the second contest turned out to have been winners in the first contest as well, and these individuals were the very trained males that had seen the signal light before their first encounter (Figure 4.24). That is, males trained through conditioning were not only more likely to win initial encounters, but they also won subsequent encounters in which the stimulus they had been trained with was now absent. A similar effect was found with respect to losing. Those males that were trained to associate the red light and an intruder, but lost their fight in the first contest, were likely to lose to new intruders even in the absence of the stimulus. These results suggest that learning may be a powerful force in shaping aggressive interactions.

Molecular Genetics and Endocrinology of Learning

In this section, we will examine the way in which modern techniques in both molecular genetic analysis and endocrinology are shedding light on some proximate aspects of learning. Both studies focus on fear avoidance learning in rats, but the lessons drawn from these studies may apply to learning in a wide variety of contexts.

MOLECULAR GENETICS OF LEARNING IN RATS

Psychologists have been using rats as a model system for studying learning for the better part of a century. Recent work on learning has attempted to tie together long-term "breeding" experiments in rats with the molecular underpinnings of various types of learning. As a case in point, Shumin Zhang and his colleagues recently examined the molecular genetics of avoidance learning in two genetically selected lines of rats that have been selectively bred for over forty years (Brush, 2003; Brush et al., 1999; Zhang et al., 2005).

The two lines of rats—known as the Syracuse High Avoidance (SHA) line and the Syracuse Low Avoidance (SLA) line—were bred from a single, large population of rats in 1965. Each generation of rats was tested on its tendency to avoid auditory and visual cues associated with a foot shock. Although the protocol varied slightly over time, the basic scenario was that a rat was placed in a cage with two compartments, and could freely move between these compartments. Just before a series of foot shocks was to be delivered to the compartment that the rat was in, a light and a tone were set off. The rat underwent ten training sessions in such a protocol. Rats were then tested in sixty "avoidance" trials to see how often they would move to the other compartment once the sound and tone were presented—that is, the rats were tested as to whether they paired these signals with shock and would attempt to avoid such shock. In each generation, those rats that were best at avoiding shock (SHA) were bred with one another, and those that were poorest at such an avoidance task (SLA) were bred with one another.

Over the course of more than forty years of breeding, SHA animals eventually avoided shocks in forty of sixty trials (on average), while the SLA typically displayed such avoidance learning in none of the sixty trials. Other work had shown that the SHA and SLA rats were equally active in their normal daily routines and that they did not differ in their ability to detect shock or the visual and auditory cues used during the experiments. But these two strains of rats did differ in "fearlessness," with the SLA rats showing much higher levels of anxiety in a series of experiments that were separate from the avoidance learning trials described above. It seems that SLA rats were both anxious and poor at learning to avoid unpleasant cues (shocks), while the converse held true for SHA rats. Further support for this association comes from studies that demonstrate that rats that were administered drugs that are known to reduce anxiety became better at avoidance learning (Fernandez-Teruel et al., 2002; Pereira et al., 1989; Sansone, 1975).

To better understand the molecular underpinnings of the learning differences between the SHA and SLA lines of rats, Zhang and his colleagues ran a series of sophisticated molecular genetic tests to determine whether these lines showed differences in gene expression in the hypothalamus—an area of the brain known to be important in avoidance learning as well as anxiety (Zhang et al., 2005). To begin their work, Zhang's team ran rats from both lines through ten training sessions and then through sixty avoidance learning trials. Then they selected SHA rats that showed avoidance learning in 70 percent (or more) of their trials and SLA rats that displayed such avoidance learning in less than 10 percent of their trials.

After the learning trials, SLA and SHA rats were allowed to rest and then were killed and dissected. The researchers removed and measured the hippocampus of each rat for gene expression. Initially sifting through gene expression in 7,500 genes, Zhang and his team were able to distill their system down to eight candidate genes that were differentially expressed in the SLA and SHA rat lines. Four of these genes—*Veli1, SLC3a1, Ptpro,* and *Ykt6p*—showed greater expression in the hippocampus of SHA rats, while four others—*SLC6A4/ 5HTT, Aldh1a4, Id3a, and Cd74*—were expressed in greater quantities in the brains of SLA rats. Zhang and his colleagues argue that such a finding supports the claim that complex traits like avoidance learning may be controlled by many genes, each of which contributes only a small amount to phenotypic expression.

The list of genes mentioned above may seem like "alphabet soup" to someone without advanced training in molecular genetics, but these genes may have very important practical implications for humans. For example, the *SLC6A4/5HTT* gene is integrally involved in the reuptake of the neurotransmitter serotonin in rodents. Similar work in humans has demonstrated that differences in serotonin use correlate with anxiety, depression, and suicidal thoughts (Gross et al., 2002; Hariri et al., 2002; Munafo et al., 2003). Thus, experimental work in rats may also shed important light on the genetics of anxiety and depression in humans.

ENDOCRINOLOGY OF LEARNING IN RATS

The molecular genetic studies we have just discussed elucidate one proximate factor underlying learning in rats. Let us continue along these lines and now review a case study in which another proximate factor associated with learning in rats—hormones, and in particular stress hormones—has been examined.

Glucocorticoids—for example, corticosterone—are hormones that play a large role in the stress responses and learning of many animals (de Kloet et al., 1999). In fact, experimental work shows that not only do glucocorticoids have an effect on learning and memory in adult animals, but that when pregnant female rats are stressed, and glucocorticoid levels rise, the offspring of such females show high levels of anxiety and perform suboptimally in learning tests (Lemaire et al., 2000; Weinstock, 1997). In both mature individuals and juveniles, glucocorticoids easily cross the "blood-brain" boundary and enter the brain, where they can affect emotional state and cognitive abilities. This may explain why stressing pregnant mothers affects anxiety in their offspring.

The hippocampal section of the brain contains receptors to which glucocorticoids bind, including the mineralocorticoid receptor (MR) (de Kloet et al., 1998). In order to better understand the relationship between glucocorticoids, stress, and learning, Ana Herrero and her colleagues administered a series of behavioral tests to a group of rats and then measured various hormones in the animals after they were exposed to the tests. Their results are correlational rather than causal, but they shed new light on learning and stress (Herrero et al., 2006). Herrero and her team first exposed a group of rats to tests designed to examine the fear response (one test involved rats moving through a maze, and the second involved measuring how rats respond to large open fields). Rats appear to fear open environments—that is, environments lacking cover—and both of these tests involve placing a rat in an open environment and examining its stress response to that environment. The researchers assessed the rat's stress by measuring such variables as the amount of time the rat spent frozen (unmoving) and the rate at which the rat defecated (see Chapter 2). The higher these values, the greater the stress and anxiety attributed to the animal. Some rats were only exposed to one fear test, and others were exposed to both fear tests. Rats exposed to both tests were consistent in that they were either anxious in both, or not anxious in either.

Once Herrero and her colleagues had established that rats are consistent in their response to open environments, they ran 140 rats through one fear test, and they classified the rats as "high-anxiety" or "low-anxiety" animals. Subsequent to this, rats were tested on their spatial learning skills. This involved placing the rats in a water maze and measuring their abilities to find and remember the location of a submerged escape platform on which they could rest. At various points in their experiments, Herrero's team killed and dissected the rats, and measured either their plasma corticosterone levels—a rough measure of the amount of corticosterone circulating in their blood—or the number of mineralocorticoid receptors in their hippocampus.

Although all animals—those classified as high and low anxiety—eventually learned to swim to the submerged platforms, high-anxiety individuals took significantly longer than low-anxiety animals to learn to do so, mostly because high-anxiety animals spent more time swimming close to the edge of the water tank (Figure 4.25). In other words, low-anxiety rats were better at this spatial learning task. When blood corticosteroid levels were measured in rats that had been run through the water maze, Herrero found that high-anxiety animals had higher corticosterone levels than did low-anxiety animals (see Chapter 3). In addition, high-anxiety animals had *fewer* mineralocorticoid receptors in their hypothalamus. This makes some sense, as having fewer mineralocorticoid receptors results in a reduced ability to bind corticosterone, and hence to an increase in circulating stress hormones—which we know is true for the high-anxiety rats.

FIGURE 4.25. Anxiety and learning in a water maze. (A) High-anxiety (HA) individuals took significantly longer than low-anxiety (LA) animals to learn to swim to the submerged platform, mostly because high-anxiety animals spent more time swimming close to the edge of the water tank, as shown in **(B)** diagrams of the rats' swimming paths in their first three training trials. *(From Herrero et al., 2006)*

It is not clear what the cause-and-effect relationship is in Herrero's studies. It may be, for example, that rats with few mineralocorticoid receptors and high circulating corticosterone became anxious in the open environment tests, and then scored poorly in the water maze test. Or it could be that the open environment tests caused a change in the levels of mineralocorticoid receptors and circulating corticosterone, and that animals with increased circulating corticosterone and decreased mineralocorticoid receptors then did poorly on the water maze test. Further experiments are needed to decipher a cause-and-effect relationship, but the work of Herrero and her colleagues clearly demonstrates that there is a link between stress hormones, stress hormone receptors, anxiety, and learning.

Phylogeny and the Neurobiology of Learning

Phylogenetic work on learning is still in its infancy. While psychologists and ethologists have a long-standing interest in many aspects of learning, it is only recently that evolutionary biologists have been mapping learning onto phylogenetic trees. This is in part a result of evolutionary biologists focusing on "innate" versus learned behavior, and in part due to insufficient data on learning across a broad spectrum of organisms. In any event, more phylogenetic work on learning is beginning to appear, and here we shall focus on William Wright's studies that tie together neurobiology, learning, and phylogenetic analysis (Marinesco et al., 2003; Wright, 1998, 2000; Wright et al., 1996).

Learning has been documented in many species of mollusks. In particular, snails in the family *Aplysiidae* have become a model system for studying the neurobiology of learning, in large part because the nervous system of these

INTERVIEW WITH

Dr. Sara Shettleworth

How did you become interested in studying learning? Were you trained as a psychologist or a biologist?

As an undergraduate, I was drawn to psychology by the introductory course taught by Henry Gleitman. He is a wonderful lecturer who went on to write a popular introductory textbook and win awards for his teaching. Much of the course dealt with the then-current controversies in learning theory, and I found the interplay of theory and experiments fascinating.

In graduate school I was exposed to biological approaches to behavior, which piqued my interest in what role learning played in the natural lives of animals. As it happened, it was at about that time that conditioned taste aversion was discovered by Garcia and his colleagues, and not long afterwards Brown and Jenkins first described autoshaping in pigeons. These discoveries were absolutely mind-blowing at the time because they seemed to show that learning was not a completely general process. Animals learned some things with very minimal input and others not at all. To understand these patterns, we might need to take into account the role that learning might play in the animal's natural life. Although I have worked on quite a number of different species and learning problems since then, it has always been with a commitment to this point of view. As for biological training, I have been fortunate to collaborate or otherwise be associated with biologists who are interested in psychological questions, and I think we have learned a lot from one another.

Do we know of any species of animal that can't learn something?

I don't know of any. Considering that even the single-celled organism *Stentor* can modify its behavior in simple ways, as shown by Jennings 100 years ago, it might be hard to find one that did not at least show habituation or sensitization.

Is there any reluctance in mainstream psychology to study learning from an evolutionary perspective? If so, why?

Historically, learning and memory have been studied pretty much in isolation from anything about the biology of the species doing the learning. People have suggested that the prominence of learning in American psychology and its abiological emphasis are attributable to the American faith in the importance of the environment as opposed to hereditary factors in individual development and adult achievement. In Henry Plotkin's excellent book about evolutionary psychology, *Evolution in Mind*

(Penguin, 1997), there is a nice little history of the relationship between psychology and evolutionary thinking. This is definitely changing, partly due to discoveries within psychology like those I mentioned in answering question 1. The increasingly important role of neuroscience and genetic manipulations of the nervous system in psychology probably also play a role in making people think more and more of psychology as, in effect, part of biology. At the same time, behavioral ecologists have brought the evolutionarily based study of behavior full circle, back to an interest in causal mechanisms and development, which tended to be neglected in the early days of that field. Indeed, the term *cognitive ecology* has been invented to refer to the study of the role of cognitive mechanisms—perception, learning, memory, and the like—in solving ecological problems. This can only lead to more cross-disciplinary communication, collaboration, and training, which in the long run may have an impact on thinking in psychology.

How much of a quagmire is the terminology used in the study of learning? To the outside reader it seems as if there are endless definitions and subdefinitions. Is that a fair statement?

No, I don't think it's fair. Fields of science all have their own specialized terminologies, which are necessary to convey specialized ideas and distinctions that can't be expressed concisely in ordinary language.

When I ask psychology students to read literature from behavioral ecology, they find terms like ESS, MVT, conspecific, homology versus analogy, phylogeny, and the like, pretty baffling.

What do you think ethologists can glean from work on human learning?

In his famous paper "On Aims and Methods of Ethology," Tinbergen pointed out that a complete understanding of behavior includes answers to four questions. Two of them are "What is the current (or proximate) cause of this behavior?" and "How does it develop in the individual?" (The others are "How did it evolve?" and "How does it function?" or "What is its survival value?") Causation and development are essentially what psychologists study, even if the species and behaviors are somewhat limited. So it seems obvious that ethologists and psychologists (whether they study humans or other animals) should have a lot to learn from each other.

Could you weigh in on the "modular mind" debate? Do you think learning is better viewed as one all-purpose algorithm, or as a series of smaller programs, each designed by selection to allow animals to cope with particular sorts of problems (foraging, mating, etc.)?

I am definitely of the "modular mind" school because I think it makes more functional sense and because it also makes better sense of some data. It is also a more sensible way to approach a broad comparative psychology than the old idea that species differ in some single dimension like "intelligence." I have written about this in a couple of recent chapters (Shettleworth, 2000, 2002). However, along with other psychologists of this persuasion, I tend to think of modules more as cognitive subunits that perform distinct information-processing operations rather than as mechanisms for separate biological functions like mating and food-finding. For example, learning and using information from landmarks might be identified as a distinct (modular) part of spatial cognition, but it could be employed in finding food or mates or a nest. Of course, there have been rather few tests of whether this is really correct. At least in rats in laboratory tests, spatial learning seems to proceed

> The term *cognitive ecology* has been invented to refer to the study of the role of cognitive mechanisms— perception, learning, memory, and the like—in solving ecological problems.

similarly whether the animal is rewarded with food (i.e., foraging) or escaping from a water tank or some other aversive situation. There may also be some differences in the details, but it is not clear whether or not this is due to the different motivational systems in play or for some other reason like sheer strength of motivation.

What's the next breakthrough to look for in the study of animal learning?

Although there are still many unanswered questions about animal learning and cognition that need to be studied entirely at the level of behavior, at present there is probably more research on learning being done by behavioral neuroscientists and geneticists than by people like me who focus on behavior of normal intact animals. Thus, statistically it is most likely that the biggest breakthroughs will be made in studies of the neural and molecular basis of learning. However, while much work of this kind simply uses traditional behavioral tests like maze learning or Pavlovian conditioning, some behaviorally sophisticated researchers in this area are making novel observations about how animals learn and remember. For example, in a quest to develop simple tests for rats in which the animals would remember many items of information, Howard Eichenbaum and his colleagues discovered that—not surprisingly given their nocturnal way of life— rats are extraordinarily good at olfactory learning. A rat can learn and remember the significance of many different odors and at the same time. As well, when odors are used, rats can easily learn kinds of tasks that they would learn only with great difficulty, if at all, with visual stimuli, which have traditionally been used. This example illustrates how an integrated approach to learning can lead to new findings: by using ethologically relevant stimuli the researchers have revealed new facts about animal learning and memory, as well as making possible investigations of the neural basis of learning that would not be possible otherwise.

Dr. Sara Shettleworth is a professor at the University of Toronto, Canada. Her work integrating biological and psychological approaches to the study of animal cognition and learning ranks her as a leader in that field.

snails contains only about 20,000 large and individually recognizable neurons that are grouped into about ten clusters (called ganglia). Compared to the number of neurons in other animals typically used in learning experiments, this is a remarkably small number. Moreover, the fact that the neurons are physically large makes these animals especially promising for work on the neurobiology of learning (Hawkins et al., 2006; Kandel, 2001).

Wright and his colleagues used six species of snails—including four species in the family *Aplysiidae*—to examine the neurobiology of learning from a phylogenetic perspective (Wright et al., 1996). They studied learning in the context of "defensive withdrawal" behavior in snails, which typically involves a snail withdrawing its soft body parts from outside of its shell and moving them under the shell in response to danger. They chose defensive behavior because a significant body of literature already existed on this antipredator adaptation, providing Wright and his team with some important background information about the behavior they were going to analyze.

The sea hare, *Aplysia californica*, is the best studied of the snail species in which learning has been examined. When Wright undertook his study, it was already clear from work on *A. californica* that one critical neurobiological component of learning in snails was the neurotransmitter serotonin (Mercer et al., 1991). For example, in the case of learning and defensive withdrawals, serotonin modulates the neurons that initiate withdrawal responses and how they change over time. In particular, serotonin appears to affect sensory neurons in two ways: (1) Serotonin causes an increase in the duration of the electrical signal that travels along the axon, and (2) serotonin increases the number of action potentials that are fired (Baxter and Byrne, 1990; Mercer et al., 1991; Sugita et al., 1994). These changes then appear to allow the animal to learn about whatever stimulus facilitated the increase in serotonin in the first place.

Wright and his colleagues examined how neurons associated with defensive withdrawals responded to exposure to serotonin in four *Aplysiidaen* species—*Aplysia californica*, *Dolabella auricularia*, *Bursatella leachii*, and *Dolabrifera dolabrifera*—as well as in two more distantly related snail species. Their protocol involved bathing neurons in serotonin and measuring whether this affected the number and strength of action potentials associated with neurons involved in withdrawal responses. A response in action potential was seen in three of the four *Aplysiidaen* species. The one exception was *D. dolabrifera*, in which neither the number nor the duration of action potentials increased.

A phylogenetic analysis of the species in Wright's study shows that *D. dolabrifera* is a fairly recently derived species, and that it evolved from a lineage that had shown a response to serotonin. That is, the response to serotonin and its cascading effects on withdrawal response were lost in *D. dolabrifera*. Perhaps more importantly for our discussion of a phylogenetic approach to learning and neurobiology, Wright's findings suggest that since *D. dolabrifera* did not show a response to serotonin, but other *Aplysiidaen* species did show such a response, *D. dolabrifera* might fare worse on learning tasks associated with defensive withdrawals.

To examine whether the neurobiological differences that emerged from his phylogenetic analysis translate to differences in learning, Wright ran a series of experiments on learning and defensive behaviors in both *A. californica* and *D. dolabrifera* (Wright, 1998). Because *D. dolabrifera* lacks the serotonin-induced changes in sensory-neuron firing, Wright and his colleagues hypothesized that they would not fare as well on learning tasks as *A. californica*.

A

B

FIGURE 4.26. Learning in snails. *Aplysia californica* but not *Dolabrifera dolabrifera* snails learn to withdraw for longer periods of time after being shocked. *(From Wright, 1998, p. 331)*

Wright measured learning in the context of a "defensive withdrawal" of the tail and mantle in both species of mollusk. A snail would receive a series of electrical shocks in the tail area, and Wright would then measure how long it took an animal to move its tail and mantle back into its shell, and how such a withdrawal from outside of the shell changed over time. Wright employed four different learning protocols. What he found was that, in most instances, learning was seen in *Aplysia*, but not in *Dolabrifera* (Figure 4.26). In other words, the neurobiological differences in the serotonin systems that were revealed based on a phylogenetic analysis of mollusks were associated with major differences in the ability to learn in *Aplysia* and *Dolabrifera*.

In this chapter, we have examined both proximate and ultimate perspectives of individual learning, including work on Pavlovian conditioning and operant conditioning. We have examined how, why, and what individuals learned in a suite of behavioral venues (predator-prey interactions, migration, the search for mates, aggression, and so on). In the next chapter, we will examine similar issues in the context of social learning and cultural transmission.

SUMMARY

1. Psychologists have defined learning in many ways. When we speak of learning here, we are referring to "a relatively permanent change in behavior as a result of experience." This definition does, however, have a downside, in that it is often difficult to determine how long a time period constitutes "relatively permanent."
2. The ability of organisms to learn provides them with the opportunity to respond in a very flexible fashion to environmental change. Learning, in the most general sense, is considered a form of phenotypic plasticity.
3. The simplest form of learning involves a single stimulus. Sensitization and habituation are two simple, single-stimulus forms of learning. Habituation in particular is often of concern to experimental ethologists, whose interpretation of results can be confounded if animals habituate too quickly to stimuli.

4. Pavlovian, or classical, conditioning experiments involve two stimuli—the conditioned stimulus and the unconditioned stimulus. A conditioned stimulus (CS) is defined as a stimulus that fails initially to elicit a particular response, but comes to do so when it becomes associated with a second (unconditioned) stimulus. Second-order conditioning, excitatory conditioning, inhibitory conditioning, learnability, blocking, overshadowing, and latent inhibition are issues often addressed in Pavlovian conditioning experiments.

5. Instrumental conditioning, also known as operant or goal-directed learning, occurs when a response made by an animal is somehow reinforced. One fundamental difference between Pavlovian and instrumental learning centers on the fact that, in the latter, the animal must undertake some "action" or "response" in order for the conditioning process to produce learning.

6. Interpopulation comparisons in learning, as in studies of sticklebacks and doves, are a powerful tool employed by ethologists interested in learning. By making comparisons across populations that differ in their abilities to learn, ethologists can address both proximate questions (what are the differences?) and ultimate questions (why do such differences occur?).

7. Ethologists, behavioral ecologists, and psychologists have long argued that learning is favored over the genetic transmission of a fixed trait when the environment in which an animal lives changes often, but not too often. David Stephens has expanded on this idea by investigating within- and between-generation variability, and he finds that learning is favored when predictability within the lifetime of an individual is high but predictability between generations is low.

8. Animals learn in many different contexts, including, but not limited to, foraging (what to eat?), habitat selection (where to live?), predators (what's dangerous?), mates (what constitutes a mate, and what constitutes a good mate?), and familial relationships (who is genetic kin?).

9. Modern techniques in both molecular genetic analysis and endocrinology are shedding light on learning. Researchers, for example, have studied the molecular genetics of avoidance learning in two genetically selected lines of rats. Evidence suggests that, at the proximate level, differences in avoidance learning are associated with eight candidate genes that were differentially expressed in these two lines of rats.

10. Phylogenetic work on learning is still in its infancy, as it is only recently that evolutionary biologists have been mapping learning onto phylogenetic trees. This is in part a result of evolutionary biologists' focus on "innate" versus learned behavior, and in part due to insufficient data on learning across a broad spectrum of organisms. That said, work tying together neurobiology, learning, and phylogenetic analysis is becoming more and more common.

DISCUSSION QUESTIONS

1. Following up on the "optimal forgetting" study in stomatopods that we discussed in this chapter, can you think of other situations in which it might pay for animals to forget, or at least not act on, information they have obtained? Try and come up with three cases, and write a paragraph on each case justifying its selection.

2. Obtain a copy of parts I and II of Tooby and Cosmides's 1989 article "Evolutionary psychology and the generation of culture," in volume 10 (pp. 29–97) of the journal *Ethology and Sociobiology*. After reading this article, explain how "Darwinian algorithms" work and how they relate to our discussion of animal learning.

3. Read Domjan and Hollis's 1988 chapter "Reproductive behavior: A potential model system for adaptive specializations in learning," which appeared in Bolles and Beecher's book, *Evolution and learning* (pp. 213–237). Then outline how classic psychological models of learning can be productively merged with evolutionary approaches to learning.

4. Design an experiment that can distinguish between the two alternative explanations for interpopulational differences in dove foraging, as described in Carlier and Lefebvre's 1996 "Differences in individual learning between group-foraging and territorial Zenaida doves," which appeared in volume 133 (pp. 1197–1207) of the journal *Behaviour*.

5. Why do you suppose phylogenetic work on learning was slower to emerge than phylogenetic studies on morphological, anatomical, or even "fixed" behavioral traits?

SUGGESTED READING

Domjan, M. (2005). *The principles of learning and behavior*, 5th ed. Belmont, CA: Wadsworth Publishing. An excellent primer on the psychology and biology of learning.

Johnston, T. (1985). Introduction: Conceptual issues in the ecological study of learning. In T. D. Johnston & A. T. Pietrewicz (Eds.), *Issues in the ecological study of learning* (pp. 1–26). Hillsdale, NJ: Lawrence Erlbaum Associates. The "ecological" approach to learning is outlined in this edited volume.

Kim, J. J., & Jung, M. W. (2006). Neural circuits and mechanisms involved in Pavlovian fear conditioning: A critical review. *Neuroscience and Biobehavioral Reviews, 30*, 188–202. A review of Pavlovian conditioning and the role that neurobiology plays in this form of learning.

Krebs J. R., & Inman, A. J. (1992). Learning and foraging: Individuals, groups, and populations. *American Naturalist, 140*, S63–S84. A review of learning and its role in foraging studies.

Shettleworth, S. (1998). *Cognition, evolution and behavior*. New York: Oxford University Press. A very detailed treatment of behavior and evolution, with much on learning.

5

Cultural Transmission

FIGURE 5.1. Imo the monkey. Imo, a Japanese macaque monkey, introduced a number of new behaviors (for example, potato washing) that spread through her population via cultural transmission. *(Photo credit: Umeyo Mori)*

In our discussion of genetics and heritability in Chapter 2, we noted that for natural selection to act on a behavior, a mechanism for transmitting that behavior across generations is required. When Mendel's work on genetics was rediscovered in the early 1900s, it became obvious that genes are a means of transmitting traits across generations, enabling natural selection to act on genetically encoded traits. In fact, until recently, evolutionary biologists and ethologists operated under the assumption that genes were not only *one* way to transmit information across generations, they were the *only* way. Slowly, this view is beginning to change. Recall, for example, our discussion in Chapter 1 of Jeff Galef's fascinating work on foraging and information transfer across generations of rats. More generally, there is a growing recognition of the importance of the **cultural transmission** of behavior—often defined as the transfer of information from individual to individual through social learning or teaching—both within and between generations of animals (see below for more on the definition of cultural transmission; Bonner, 1980; Boyd and Richerson, 1985; Danchin et al., 2004; Heyes and Galef, 1996; Laland and Janik, 2006; Odling-Smee et al., 2003; Reader and Laland, 2003; Zentall and Galef, 1988).

To get a glimpse of how cultural transmission operates in nonhumans, let's consider the case of Imo, a Japanese macaque monkey that lived on Koshima Islet, Japan, in the 1950s (Kawai, 1965; Kawamura, 1959; Figure 5.1). Imo's story begins when ethologists studying her troop of macaques threw sweet potatoes on the sandy beach for the monkeys to gather and eat. When Imo was a year old, she began to wash the sweet potatoes in water before she ate them. This novel and creative behavior, which was never before seen in Imo's population, allowed her to remove all the sand from the sweet potatoes before she ingested them. But what made this new behavior remarkable is not that Imo found a novel solution to cleaning her food; rather, the key feature of this system is that many of Imo's peers and relatives learned the skill of potato washing from Imo via **social learning**, which is usually defined as the process of learning by watching others. By 1959, most infant macaques in Imo's troop intently watched their mothers, many of whom had acquired Imo's habit, and they learned to wash their own sweet potatoes at early ages. Because a novel behavior—potato washing—had spread through Imo's troop by social learning, we can speak of potato washing in terms of cultural transmission (Figure 5.2).

FIGURE 5.2. Potato washing in monkeys. In Japanese macaques living on Koshima Islet, Japan, the skill of potato washing appears to be transmitted culturally. *(Photo credits: Frans de Waal)*

When Imo was four, she introduced an even more complicated new behavior into her group. In addition to the sweet potatoes that researchers gave the moneys on Koshima Islet, they also occasionally treated the monkeys to a food item to which the macaques were partial—wheat. The introduction of this new source, however, caused a problem, which was that the wheat was provisioned to the monkeys on a sandy beach, and wheat and sand mixed together are not nearly as appealing a meal as wheat alone. So, Imo came up with a novel solution—she tossed her wheat and sand mixture into the water, where the sand sank and the wheat floated. As with the sweet potatoes, it was only a matter of time before her groupmates also learned this handy trick from her. It took a bit longer for this trait to spread through the population, however, as monkeys aren't used to letting go of food once they get it, so it was hard to learn to throw the sand-covered wheat into the water. But eventually this new behavioral trait spread to many group members via cultural transmission.

Imo's actions were not the only ones to attract attention about the cultural transmission of behavioral traits, as many similar cases are now on record. Michael Huffman, for example, found another case of cultural transmission in macaques (Huffman, 1996; Nahallage and Huffman, 2006). Huffman's study revolved around twenty years of work on the Japanese macaques of the Iwatayama National Park in Kyoto, Japan. Early in his work, Huffman began to observe a behavior never before noted in macaques—individuals would play with stones, particularly right after eating (Hiraiwa, 1975; Figure 5.3).

In the Iwatayama National Park where Huffman studied macaques, stone play behavior was first observed in 1979 when Glance-6476, a three-year-old female macaque, brought rocks in from the forest and started stacking them up and knocking them down. Not only that, Glance-6476 was very territorial about her stones and took them away when approached by other monkeys. When Huffman returned to study Glance's troop four years later, stone play (also referred to as to stone handling) "had already become a daily occurrence and was already being transmitted from older to younger individuals." Interestingly, cultural transmission in this system seems to work down the age ladder, but not up. While many individuals younger than Glance-6476 acquired her stone

FIGURE 5.3. Stone play in monkeys. Michael Huffman has found that one population of Japanese macaques in the Iwatayama National Park in Kyoto has created a tradition of "stone play" in which individuals stack up stones and then knock them down. *(Photo credit: Michael Huffman)*

FIGURE 5.4. Stone play tradition spreads. Orange bars represent verified stone handlers, and green bars represent individuals not verified as stone handlers. Note the increase in the frequency of the tradition with time. *(From Huffman, 1996, p. 276)*

play habit, no one over her age added stone play to their behavioral repertoire (Figure 5.4).

Charmalie Nahallage and Huffman later examined stone play in a captive troop of macaques in the Primate Research Institute in Kyoto, Japan (Nahallage and Huffman, 2006). When they did a detailed study of the use of stone play in juvenile and adult macaques, they uncovered age-specific differences in the use of culturally acquired behavior. Juveniles tended to engage in many short bouts of stone play that involved vigorous body actions (for example, shaking, running, and jumping). This pattern of behavior is consistent with what is called the "motor training" hypothesis of play behavior (see Chapter 15), which suggests that stone play may facilitate the development of perceptual skills, as well as neural and cognitive development (Bekoff and Byers, 1981). Adults, on the other hand, engaged in fewer, but longer bouts of stone play, which may slow down the deterioration of cognitive processes often seen in aging primates (Figure 5.5).

Stone play has now been uncovered in other captive troops of macaques like the monkeys that Nahallage and Huffman study. But this behavior has never been documented in wild populations that are not provisioned by humans. As such, stone play appears to occur only in populations that have significant

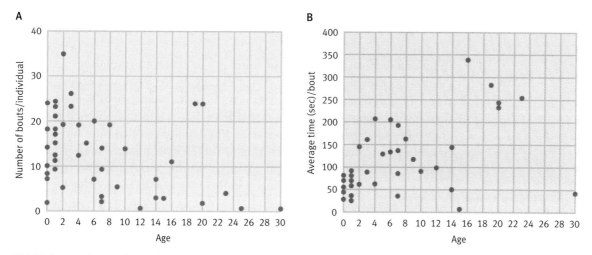

FIGURE 5.5. Stone play and age. (A) The number of stone play sessions decreases with age. **(B)** The average time per stone play session increases with age. *(From Nahallage and Huffman, 2007)*

"leisure time"—that is, in populations that are freed up because their food is provided for them (Nahallage and Huffman, 2007).

Cultural transmission has also been extensively documented in other primates, including our closest living relatives, the chimpanzees (Whiten, 2005; Whiten and Boesch, 2001; Whiten et al., 1999, 2005). Over the course of the last thirty years, six long-term studies of natural populations of chimpanzees have documented an incredible array of culturally transmitted traits, ranging from "swatting flies" and opening nuts with stones, to squashing parasites with leaves. In some cases, researchers have clear evidence of young chimps watching and learning these behaviors from adults; in other cases, the evidence is more indirect (see Chapter 15).

When looking across these chimpanzee populations, we see a hallmark signature of cultural transmission: numerous traits are culturally transmitted in each and every population, but populations differ from one another in terms of *which* traits are transmitted culturally. For example, hammering open nuts with stones is seen in two chimp populations, but it is absent in four. If this behavior were genetic, we might expect it to be seen in all the chimp populations or none of them. If it were culturally transmitted, however, we might expect that it would arise by individual trial-and-error learning in some populations, but not in others. For example, hammering nuts, once it arose by such trial-and-error learning, could quickly spread by cultural transmission, but only in the populations that were lucky enough to have one of their members stumble on the solution in the first place.

The reason for opening a discussion of cultural transmission with primate examples is not because they provide the most convincing experimental evidence of cultural transmission recorded in animals. Rather, these studies are observational, and they lack the controlled experimental manipulations that underlie other work on nonhuman cultural transmission (Galef, 2004). Nonetheless, we opened our discussion of cultural transmission with these examples of food washing, stone handling, hammering open nuts, and swatting away flies because they dramatically illustrate that cultural transmission in animals can be a powerful force and that it occurs in nonhuman animals, as well as in humans.

What Is Cultural Transmission?

In order to understand the role of cultural transmission in animal societies, we need to begin with a definition. What exactly do we mean when we speak of cultural transmission in animals? This turns out to be a more difficult question than it might appear at first glance (Figure 5.6). In fact, even back in 1952, anthropologists already had more than 150 definitions of culture and cultural transmission (Kroeber and Kluckhohn, 1952). Evolutionary and behavioral biologists, however, have tended to focus on one general definition that is summed up nicely by Robert Boyd and Peter Richerson in their book *Culture and the Evolutionary Process* (1985).

Slightly modifying Boyd and Richerson's definition, we will speak of cultural transmission as a system of information transfer that affects an individual's phenotype by means of either teaching or some form of social learning (Boyd and Richerson, 1985). Again, recall the Norway rats we discussed in Chapter 1. As scavengers, rats often encounter potential new foods. The downside of scavenging is that many novel foods may in fact be dangerous to eat. Scavenging is an ideal behavior in which to examine the cultural transmission of information, as new items are always being encountered, and information on their potential danger constantly needs to be updated. Obtaining some sort of information about food from other rats is one way to update knowledge about the suitability of novel foods. In fact, Norway rats learn what new foods to try by smelling their nestmates and subsequently trying the new food items that such nestmates have recently ingested (Galef and Wigmore, 1983; Galef, 1996). Returning to our definition of what constitutes cultural transmission, one aspect of a rat's phenotype—in this case, what sorts of food it eats—is modified by information that it has learned from other individuals.

FIGURE 5.6. What constitutes cultural transmission? Clearly the child is learning to use utensils by watching others (that is, through cultural transmission). The chimp on the right, however, also has learned his nut-cracking skills from watching others. Should this also count as a culturally transmitted behavior?

FIGURE 5.7. Imitation in infants. Imitation is a form of social learning that begins early in humans. Here the infant claps his hands in imitation of his mother clapping her hands. *(Photo credit: Jerry Tobias/Corbis)*

WHAT'S SO IMPORTANT ABOUT CULTURAL TRANSMISSION?

Before moving on to what exactly constitutes social learning and teaching in animals, let us briefly touch on an issue that ethologists, psychologists, and anthropologists often raise when discussing cultural transmission in animals. "Why," the question goes, "is there so much focus on cultural transmission?" After all, we spent a great deal of time on the topic of learning in Chapter 4, and if cultural transmission is just one form of learning—that is, learning from other individuals—why not simply consider it a special kind of learning and move on? In other words, as Boyd and Richerson ask, "Why not simply treat culture as a . . . response to environmental variation in which the 'environment' is the behavior of conspecifics?" (Boyd and Richerson, 1985). Why not think of cultural transmission as just another means by which organisms adapt to the environment, and leave it at that?

The answer to these questions is that learning from other individuals in a group differs dramatically from individual trial-and-error learning in two important ways. To begin with, cultural transmission involves the spread of information *from individual to individual* (Figures 5.7 and 5.8). That is, if you learn from others and they learn from you, information can be spread through a population in a very efficient manner. This potentially translates into the behavior of a single individual in a population dramatically shifting the behavior patterns seen in an entire group—recall how Imo's novel food-washing techniques spread via cultural transmission. This is simply not the case for other types of learning. What an individual learns via individual learning—the sort of learning we discussed in Chapter 4—disappears when that individual dies (and perhaps before). When cultural transmission is in play, however, what is learned by one individual may be passed down through endless generations. If Imo had learned to clean her sweet potatoes by washing them in water in a population in which social learning was absent, this foraging innovation would have vanished when she died. Instead, some fifty years later, one can still go to Koshima Islet and see these monkeys washing their sweet potatoes.

FIGURE 5.8. Cultural transmission via teaching. Teaching is a form of cultural transmission in which the teacher imparts some information to a student faster than the student could learn it on her own. This piano teacher is teaching her young student how to place her hands to produce particular chords on the piano. *(Photo credit: fotosearch)*

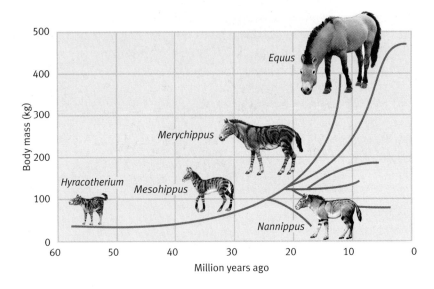

FIGURE 5.9. Speed of change. In some cases, natural selection may take millions of years to produce major changes, as in horse evolution. Cultural evolution works on a much faster time scale. Natural selection can work much quicker than in the horse case, but it is generally much slower than cultural evolution. *(From Ridley, 1996)*

Cultural transmission can occur within a population very quickly, which makes it a particularly potent form of information transfer. When natural selection acts to change the frequency of genes that code for behavior, the time scale can range from a few dozen generations (as in the guppy case we explored in Chapter 2) to much longer time scales (thousands of generations). And when natural selection acts on major morphological change, the time scale may be millions of generations (Figure 5.9). Cultural transmission of information, on the other hand, operates much faster, and can easily cause important changes in the behavior seen in populations in just a handful of generations. In fact, cultural evolution can have a dramatic impact within a single generation (Boyd and Richerson, 1985, 2004, 2005; Henrich et al., 2005; Odling-Smee et al., 2003; Reader and Laland, 2003).

EFFECTS OF OTHERS ON BEHAVIOR

Cultural transmission relies in one sense or another on a "model" individual (also called a demonstrator or tutor) and an "observer," who learns a specific behavior or response from the model (Figure 5.10). Yet, it is important to recognize that there are situations that involve an interaction between observers and models, but that do *not* constitute social learning or teaching. In these cases—labeled

FIGURE 5.10. Cultural transmission in humans. Many of the behaviors we acquire as we develop are learned via a combination of individual and social learning. *(Photo credits: Damon Fourie/Stone; Jacques Copeau/FPG)*

local enhancement and social facilitation—the observer is drawn to an area by a model or by the action of a model, or is simply in the presence of others, but the observer does not learn a particular behavior or response from the model, and hence cultural transmission is not occurring. We will first examine local enhancement and social facilitation before moving on to instances of cultural transmission via social learning and teaching.

LOCAL ENHANCEMENT. William Thorpe coined the term **local enhancement** to describe the case in which individuals learn from others, not so much by doing what they observe, as by being drawn to a particular area because another individual—a model—was in that location (Heyes, 1994; Thorpe, 1956, 1963; Figure 5.11). In other words, when local enhancement is in play, a model simply draws attention to some aspect of the environment by the action she undertakes there (for example, digging for worms). Once the observer is drawn to the area, she learns on her own.

As an example of local enhancement, consider foraging behavior in colonially nesting cliff swallows, birds that feed in groups ranging in size from 2 to 1,000 individuals (see Chapter 2). Charles Brown has found that, in addition to the actual transfer of information between groupmates (Brown, 1986), local enhancement facilitates foraging, as some individuals are drawn to good foraging areas because others birds are foraging there.

Local enhancement can be a powerful force, as shown in Michael Webster and Paul Hart's experiment examining foraging behavior in sticklebacks (Webster and Hart, 2006). In this experiment, fish encountered two habitats that differed in the density of available food. After two weeks, sticklebacks

FIGURE 5.11. Local enhancement. If fish 1 is drawn to where fish 2 is foraging (near a stone), but then learns nothing else from fish 2, local enhancement is at work.

learned to associate one of these habitats with more food and the other with less. Once fish had established a preference based on what they had learned, Webster and Hart allowed these trained fish to see a model that was foraging in the habitat with less food. Individuals observing the model were more likely to choose the suboptimal foraging patch, even though that choice conflicted with their own foraging experiences. Thus, the role of local enhancement was stronger than that of personal experience.

SOCIAL FACILITATION. **Social facilitation** differs in a subtle, but important, way from local enhancement. During local enhancement, the *action* of a model draws attention to some aspect of the environment. But under social facilitation, the *mere presence* of a model, regardless of what he does, is thought to facilitate learning on the part of an observer (Zajonc, 1965). For example, there are many instances in the foraging literature in which increased group size caused increased foraging rates per individual, perhaps because individuals had learned that they were safer in the presence of conspecifics (Giraldeau and Caraco, 2000; Stephens and Krebs, 1986; Figure 5.12).

FIGURE 5.12. Social facilitation. In social facilitation, the mere presence of a model(s) draws in an observer. Here our lone starling is attracted to a group, not because of what group members are doing or where they are, but simply because it is drawn to the presence of others. "Safety in numbers" might be a benefit to such facilitation.

Social facilitation and local enhancement can be experimentally separated from one another. To see this, consider a series of experiments that Elisabetta Visalberghi and Elsa Addessi ran on foraging behavior in capuchin monkeys (Visalberghi and Addessi, 2000; Figure 5.13). These researchers examined what factors affected a capuchin monkey's probability of taking in a novel food. In one treatment, a *lone* capuchin was tested on its tendency to try a new food type (vegetables that had been color dyed). In a second treatment, a capuchin and the novel food type were on one side of a test cage, and a group of capuchins was on the other side of the cage. No food was placed on the side of the cage with the group. The third treatment was identical to the second, except that a familiar food type was placed on the side of the cage with the group, which made it likely that they would eat the food. Now the lone capuchin saw not only a group, but a group that was eating food, but not eating the novel food type (Figure 5.14).

When comparing across their treatments, Visalberghi and Addessi found evidence indicative of local enhancement, but not of social facilitation. Evidence for local enhancement was uncovered in that during any given observation period, capuchins in treatment 3 (lone capuchin + group with food) were more likely to be eating food than capuchins in treatment 1 (lone capuchin). Local enhancement was occurring as the lone capuchin's attention was drawn to the novel food when it saw the other capuchins eating the food and then proceeded to eat more itself. No definitive evidence for social facilitation, however, was uncovered. While a comparison of treatments 1 and 2 (lone capuchin versus lone capuchin + group without food) did uncover more foraging in treatment 2, this difference was not statistically significant—that is, the mere presence of others who were not eating did not lead the lone capuchin to eat significantly more of the novel food.

FIGURE 5.13. Capuchin foraging.
Foraging in capuchins (*Cebus paella*) has been examined with respect to both local enhancement and social facilitation. These capuchin monkeys are foraging on palm nuts. *(Photo credit: Tui De Roy/Minden Pictures/Getty Images)*

SOCIAL LEARNING

Examples of social learning—observers learning specific behaviors or responses from models—abound in the psychological literature on humans, as well as in the ethological literature on animals (Bandura, 1977, 1986; Dugatkin, 2000; Heyes and Galef, 1996; Rosenthal and Zimmerman, 1978; Zentall and Galef,

Alone | Group present | Group plus food

N = Novel food   **F** = Familiar food

FIGURE 5.14. Social facilitation and local enhancement in capuchin foraging. The experimental design for the three treatments used in the Visalberghi and Addessi study. *(From Visalberghi and Addessi, 2000)*

FIGURE 5.15. Watch, learn, and decide. Chimps learn how to "fish" for termites by watching others. Individual chimps are clearly capable of judging how effective a foraging technique this is, and choosing whether or not to add it to their behavioral repertoire.

1988; Figure 5.15). Social learning is sometimes referred to as "observational learning" in the psychology literature. A classic example of an experiment on social learning in humans is Albert Bandura's "bobo" doll study (Bandura et al., 1961; Giancola and Chermack, 1998). In this experiment, children were exposed to one of two treatments. In one treatment, children were working on an art project when an adult in the room began punching and kicking a "bobo" doll. This doll was inflatable and weighted at the bottom, so it snapped back up when knocked down. In the other treatment, children working on an art project saw a calm adult. In this treatment, the bobo doll was still in the room; it just wasn't being assaulted by an adult. Children from both groups were then given the choice of playing with aggressive toys or nonaggressive toys.

The children exposed to the "violent adult" treatment not only chose to play with aggressive toys, but they often beat up the doll and yelled the same things that the adult had yelled, while children in the other treatment played much more calmly (Figure 5.16). No doubt, some readers will look at the bobo doll experiment and think "Of course Bandura got the results he did; it's obvious to anyone that this is what would happen." But two things should be kept in mind when looking at these results: First, Bandura didn't "have to" obtain the results he did. The kids could have ignored the adult punching the bobo doll, or they could even have been particularly nice in response to the adult's aggressive behavior. In fact, some social psychology theories predicted that watching aggression would somehow reduce the observers' aggressive tendencies by providing an outlet. It could have worked that way in Bandura's experiment; it just didn't. Second, science is full of examples in which researchers actually did the experiment to test "something that was obviously true," and they found out that it wasn't. The only way to know for sure is to do the experiment. The same thing can be said of work on social learning in animals. In retrospect, it might seem obvious that rats learn what to eat and what not to eat by social learning. But it didn't have to turn out that way. Rats could have ignored any information they obtained from smelling their nestmates, but they didn't.

Social learning can take many different forms in both humans and non-humans. Below we examine two forms of social learning—imitation and copying.

FIGURE 5.16. The bobo doll experiment. In Bandura's classic bobo doll experiments, the power of social learning is frighteningly evident, as young children treated the bobo doll as aggressively as the adult they observed. *(Photo credits: Albert Bandura)*

IMITATION. George Romanes was one of the first scientists to actually raise the possibility that cultural transmission plays an important role in animal life. In a series of books, Romanes argued that imitation is integral to a wide variety of animal actions (Romanes, 1884, 1889, 1898). Since Romanes wrote his books more than a century ago, the term **imitation** has been used in many different ways in the psychological literature (Byrne, 2002; Heyes and Galef, 1996; Miklosi, 1999; Whiten, 1992). Cecilia Heyes argues that imitation involves the "acquisition of a topographically novel response through observation of a demonstrator making that response . . ." (Heyes, 1994). As such, to demonstrate imitation, there must be some *new* behavior learned from others, and that behavior must involve some sort of *new spatial (topographic) manipulation* as well as lead to the achievement of some goal (Figure 5.17). We have already touched on a good case of imitation at the start of this chapter. When Imo washed her sweet potatoes in water before she ate them, and others in her group

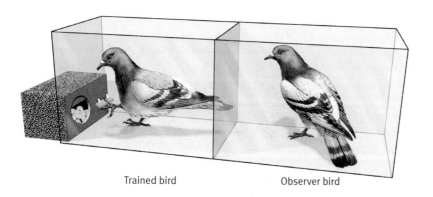

Trained bird   Observer bird

FIGURE 5.17. Imitation. Here an observer bird watches a trained pigeon who must lift its foot and push on a lever to open a small circular entrance to a food source. Imitation occurs when the observer learns this new task by watching the model lift its leg and push the lever down.

FIGURE 5.18. Blue tit birds learn to open milk bottles. Blue tit birds learned to peck open the top of milk jugs decades ago. This behavior may have spread via cultural transmission. *(Photo credit: Roger Wilmhurst/Foto Natura/Minden Pictures)*

observed and then learned this novel behavior, which requires a new sequence of spatial actions, imitation was taking place.

Another instance of imitation can be seen in the behavior of blue tit birds (*Parus caeruleus*) in Britain in the 1940s. At the time, glass milk bottles covered with foil caps were delivered to people's homes and left on their doorsteps by milkmen in the morning. Some customers found that the foil caps on the top of the milk bottles were being torn off before they could retrieve the freshly delivered bottles from their doorsteps (Figure 5.18). J. Fisher and Robert Hinde argued that this new behavior had been accidentally stumbled upon by a lucky blue tit and that others learned this nifty trick, at least in part, from watching the original milk thief (Fisher and Hinde, 1949). That is, birds observed a demonstrator taking action to manipulate the foil by pecking at it and tearing through to the milk. This was a novel response that was learned by the observers, who then also undertook the spatial actions necessary to achieve the goal of obtaining milk from the bottle.

Jeff Galef and his colleagues have also uncovered an interesting example of imitation in birds. In this study, budgerigars (parakeets) observed others lifting a flat cover off a dish, using either their beak or their foot (Galef et al., 1986). Those budgerigars that observed a model that used its beak to gain access to food were themselves likely to use their beaks when placed in the same situation, while those budgerigars observing a model that used its foot to unlock hidden food also used their feet. That is, the birds learned a topographically novel response from watching others.

Several interesting problems arise when we think critically about imitation. For example, when individual 1 attempts to imitate individual 2, it can only see individual 2's movements, but not the muscle activation underlying such movements. So how does individual 1 know what to do to make such movements itself? This is referred to as the correspondence problem (Brass and Heyes, 2005). Another problem associated with imitation is that of "perspective taking." Suppose, for example, that you and I are facing one another, and I raise my right hand and move it in circles. If you wish to imitate this action, you need to take into account our positions relative to one another. If you simply raise the hand that was on the same side as the hand I raised, you would be raising your left hand, and not imitating my action.

Behavioral neuroscience is beginning to shed light on both correspondence and perspective-taking problems (Rizzolatti et al., 2006). Studies on these questions in humans often involve subjects who are placed in a magnetic resonance imaging (MRI) device and given some problem to solve while activity in their brain is scanned by the MRI machine. Typically, the problem is very simple—for example, tapping a specific finger a set number of times, or repeating a particular musical chord on the guitar. These studies indicate that certain sections of the brain—the inferior frontal gyrus, the dorsal and ventral premotor cortex, as well as other areas—are consistently active during imitation (Decety et al., 2002; Grezes and Decety, 2001; Grezes et al., 2003; Iacoboni et al., 2001; Koski et al., 2002; Muhlau et al., 2005). Interestingly, our brains respond more strongly to opportunities to imitate an action when we see another human doing it than when we see the same action being performed by a robot (Kilner et al., 2003; Tai et al., 2004).

There is less behavioral neuroscience work on these issues in nonhumans, but that is beginning to change. For example, work on imitation in monkeys has found that a set of "mirror" neurons in what is referred to as the F5 area of the premotor area of the monkey brain is very active when a monkey observes an action—such as grasping a piece of food on a tray—and then repeats that action (Rizzolatti and Craighero, 2004; Rizzolatti et al., 2001). What makes the mirror neurons in the F5 area of the brain particularly relevant is that some of these neurons are motor neurons (neurons that are needed to repeat an act during imitation) and some are visual neurons (neurons that are necessary for watching a model). An action must first be observed before mirror neurons will fire, again suggesting a connection to imitation. Indeed, these neurons will fire if an individual sees a hand manipulating an object, but not if he sees the object alone nor if he sees the object being manipulated by a tool (Gallese et al., 1996; Rizzolatti et al., 1996). Some evidence suggests that mirror neurons in humans also reside in the equivalent of the F5 section of our brains, and that such neurons are involved in human imitation as well.

COPYING. When animals **copy** one another, an observer repeats what he has seen a model do. Oftentimes, the copier is then rewarded for whatever behavior it has copied. Imagine one animal observing another animal foraging in a certain way. If, after being rewarded—receiving food—the observer adopts the foraging technique of the model, copying has taken place. In the psychological literature, the rewards associated with copying can be extrinsic (the food items in the above case) or intrinsic (related to animal emotions and feelings). Copying differs from imitation in that what is copied need not be novel and need not involve learning some new topographical action. That is, an individual can copy the action of another, even if he already knows how to do what the model is doing, and even if it does not involve learning some new spatial orientation to do what the model does. As a case in point, animals generally know how to choose a mate, but they may still copy the mate *choice* of a model.

Some of the strongest evidence to date of copying comes from what is referred to as mate-choice copying, during which an individual—usually a female—copies the mate choice of those around her. Dugatkin examined female mate-choice copying in guppies (*Poecilia reticulata*) using a ten-gallon aquarium situated between two separate end chambers constructed of clear Plexiglas (Dugatkin, 1992a). A single male was put into each of these end chambers. The "observer" female—the individual that potentially copies the behavior of other females—was placed in a clear Plexiglas canister in the middle of the central aquarium. At the start of a trial, one male was put into

Male guppy — Observer female guppy — Model female guppy — Male guppy

FIGURE 5.19. Mate-choice copying. The experimental apparatus used in the guppy mate-choice copying experiments.

each end chamber (Figure 5.19). Removable glass partitions created left or right sections of the aquarium into which another female—the "model" female—was placed. A key component of this experiment was that the placement of the model—either near the male in the left end chamber or near the male in the right end chamber—was determined by the flip of a coin. This was done to rule out the possibility that one male may have been more attractive than the other and that the model and the observer independently each chose that male.

Once the model, the observer, and the two males were in place, fish were given ten minutes during which the observer female could watch the model female near one of the two males. The model female and the glass partitions were then removed, and the observer female was released from her canister and given ten minutes to swim freely and choose whichever male she preferred (as indicated by which end chamber she swam near). In these trials, the observer female chose the male that had been chosen by the model female seventeen out of twenty times.

While the results of this experiment are consistent with the hypothesis that females copy the mate choice of others, there are several alternative explanations. For example, since guppies live in social groups ("schools" of fish), the observer female might simply be choosing the area that had recently contained the largest number of fish (in this case, two) (Magurran and Seghers, 1990; Seghers, 1973). A control treatment was conducted to test this "schooling hypothesis." It was identical to the above protocol, except that females were placed in the end chambers. In this case, the observer female chose the female in the end chamber closest to the model in only ten out of twenty trials. As such, the tendency to school (stay near two fish rather than one fish) per se does not explain the results of the first experiment; if it had, observer females would have chosen the end chamber closest to where the model had been placed. Using a protocol similar to that of the guppy experiments, mate-choice copying has also been uncovered in a number of different species of fish, as we well as in some birds and mammals (see Chapter 6).

Another example of copying can be found in the fear response of mice to biting flies (also called stable flies, *Stomoxys calcitrans*; Kavaliers et al., 1999, 2001). After a mouse is bitten by stable flies, one of its defensive responses is to bury itself under whatever debris that it can find (Figure 5.20). When a naive mouse observes another mouse being bitten by flies and then burying itself, the observer quickly buries itself when it is exposed to flies—that is, the observer

Stable fly bites model mouse as observer mouse watches.

Stable fly

Observer   Model

Model mouse hides in debris (bedding, shredded paper) as observer mouse watches.

Observer   Model

Twenty-four hours later, when exposed to stable fly, observer mouse hides in debris.

Stable fly

Observer

FIGURE 5.20. Copying a defensive response. After a mouse is bitten by stable flies, one of its defensive responses is to bury itself under debris. A mouse that observes another mouse being bitten by a stable fly and then hiding will copy the hiding behavior of the model mouse as soon as it is exposed to a fly.

does not wait until it is bitten to adopt a defensive position, but does so as soon as it is exposed to the flies. Thus, it copies the defensive action of the model.

In order to understand something about the molecular genetics of copying in these mice, Martin Kavaliers and his colleagues focused on what is known as the NMDA receptor (Kavaliers et al., 2001). At the cellular level, this receptor plays an important role in neural plasticity—that is, neural flexibility—which itself is an important component of learning and memory (see Chapter 3). When Kavaliers and his colleagues blocked the NMDA receptor of an observer mouse, using what is called an NMDA antagonist chemical, they found that the observer did not learn to bury itself as soon as it was exposed to flies. That is, the NMDA antagonist blocked copying in these mice. A similar experiment used rats that could copy a model's foraging behavior and also found that blocking the NMDA receptor impeded social learning by means of copying (Roberts and Shapiro, 2002).

TEACHING IN ANIMALS

Given the complexity that we associate with teaching, the notion that animals teach each other is one of the more contentious aspects of the literature on animal cultural transmission (Caro and Hauser, 1992; Franks and Richardson, 2006; Hauser, 1997, 2000; Hauser and Konishi, 1999; Leadbeater et al., 2006; Thornton and McAuliffe, 2006). While there are many definitions of **teaching**, the concept usually implies that one individual serves as an instructor or teacher, and at least one other individual acts as a student who learns from the teacher (Caro and Hauser, 1992; Ewer, 1969; Fragasy and Perry, 2003; Galef et al., 2005; Maestripieri, 1995).

Teachers have a much more active, not to mention complicated, role than just being a model that another individual mimics, as in social learning. In a review on teaching in animals, Tim Caro and Marc Hauser suggest that for a behavior to be labeled as "teaching," a teacher must provide an immediate benefit to students but not to herself, she must teach only naive "students," and she must impart some new information to students faster than they would otherwise receive it. This definition is interesting, not only because of the emphasis on what must take place for teaching to occur, but also for what kinds of behaviors are excluded from the realm of teaching. For example, in the case of the blue tits opening the foil caps of milk bottles in Britain in the 1940s, imitation rather than teaching was taking place. While blue tits learned how to open foil caps by observing others, those who opened the caps did so regardless of who watched them. According to Caro and Hauser's definition, they weren't teaching other birds anything since they opened the milk bottles in the same way even if they were alone and thus they weren't modifying their behavior only in the presence of naive observers. They were indeed obtaining immediate benefits for themselves in that they obtained the milk after they opened the bottles.

What sort of examples might fall under the Caro and Hauser definition of teaching? Consider a female cat who captures live prey and allows her young to interact with this prey, making sure that such prey doesn't escape along the way. If mother cats only engage in this behavior when in the presence of young cats, we may have a true case of teaching. Anecdotal examples of this genre of teaching have been documented to some extent in domestic cats (Baerends-van Roon and Baerends, 1979; Caro, 1980; Ewer, 1969), lions (Schenkel, 1966), tigers (Schaller, 1967), and otters (Liers, 1951). Teaching has been examined in more detail in both cheetahs (Caro, 1994a) and meerkats (Thornton and McAuliffe, 2006). Consider Caro's description of three ways that mother cheetahs used "maternal encouragement" to facilitate hunting skills in their offspring (Figure 5.21):

> Firstly, they pursued and knocked down the quarry but instead of suffocating the victim allowed it to stand and run off. By the time the prey had risen, the cubs had normally arrived. Second, mothers carried live animals back to their cubs before releasing them, repeatedly calling (churring) to their cubs. Third, and less often, mothers ran slowly during their initial chase of a prey and allowed their cubs to overtake them and thus be the first to knock down the prey themselves. (Caro, 1994a, pp. 136–137)

While this sort of behavior is consistent with teaching, it is not sufficient to demonstrate teaching, as it is unclear whether young cheetahs accelerated their

A

B
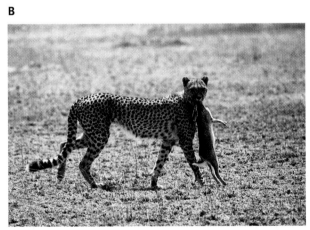

FIGURE 5.21. Cheetah teaching? (A) A mother cheetah brings a Thomson's gazelle to her cubs, and allows them to "kill it," even though it was already dead. **(B)** Until the young cheetah is taught how to hunt, it can only kill small items like the hare shown here. *(Photo credits: Tim Caro)*

hunting skills as a result of these interactions with their mother or for other reasons (Caro and Hauser, 1992; Galef et al., 2005).

A more recent example of teaching has been documented in meerkats, a species in which young pups are incapable of catching their own prey. At about a month old, these pups begin following groups of foragers, and the pups are assisted in their own foraging attempts by older groupmates called "helpers" (Figure 5.22). Many of the prey that meerkats ingest are difficult to catch and, in the case of scorpions, are also quite dangerous. Helpers will often incapacitate scorpions by removing their stingers and presenting them to pups as food. Alex Thornton and Katherine McAuliffe observed that very young pups were either fed dead or incapacitated scorpions, but as the pups got older, the helpers presented them more and more often with live scorpions (Thornton and McAuliffe, 2006).

To experimentally examine whether helpers were teaching pups how to forage on dangerous prey, the researchers took advantage of the fact that helpers respond to the begging calls of pups even when pups cannot be seen, and that such begging calls change in predictable ways as pups age. When Thornton and McAuliffe had a group of young pups, but played the calls of older pups, helpers were more likely to bring live prey over to the pups. When the group contained older pups, but the researchers broadcast the begging calls of younger pups, helpers were more likely to bring over dead or incapacitated scorpions. Thus, helpers were clearly changing what type of prey they delivered in a manner that would both help and teach the pups.

Thornton and McAuliffe found additional evidence for teaching by helpers in that such helpers: (1) spent significant time monitoring pups after presenting them with food, (2) retrieved prey when pups lost their food, (3) on occasion, further modified a scorpion (removing the stinger, killing the scorpion, and so on) after it was lost but later retrieved by the pups, and (4) nudged pups who were reluctant to eat scorpions. This nudging often increased the probability that the pups would eat the scorpion that they had initially rejected. All in all, the evidence that helpers modified their behavior in costly ways—spending time that they could have used to forage for themselves but instead spent with pups—and that such modifications helped pups learn how to forage on dangerous prey suggests teaching on the part of meerkat helpers.

COMMON THEMES IN EXAMPLES OF ANIMAL TEACHING. Caro and Hauser searched for common themes that underlie cases of teaching, and they found two candidates. First, except for the meerkat case (which was undertaken after Caro and Hauser's analysis), almost all instances of animal teaching focus on the parent/offspring relationship. This may strike you as intuitive, but remember that in many animal societies, young can learn from others besides their parents. Furthermore, in principle, adult animals could presumably teach other adults. This certainly suggests something special about the costs and benefits of teaching in the parent/teacher, offspring/student relationship. The kinship that bonds teacher and student—that is, parent and offspring—may be one of the only benefits large enough to make up for the costs of teaching (Caro and Hauser, 1992; Galef et al., 2005).

Second, Caro and Hauser argue that cases of teaching tend to fall into one of two categories: "opportunity teaching" and "coaching." When opportunity teaching is taking place, teachers actively place students in a "situation conducive to learning a new skill or acquiring knowledge." In contrast, coaching has taken place when the teacher directly alters the behavior of students by

FIGURE 5.22. Meerkat foraging and teaching. Older groupmates assist younger pups in their foraging attempts and also teach the younger pups to catch prey, including dangerous scorpions, as shown here. (*Photo credit: Alex Thornton*)

Panel 1

Panel 2

Panel 3

FIGURE 5.23. Three types of cultural transmission. In vertical transmission systems (panel 1), information is passed from parent to child. When horizontal transmission (panel 2) is in operation, an individual learns from peers. In oblique transmission (panel 3), young individuals learn from adults who are not their parents.

encouragement or punishment. The majority of examples of animal teaching fall under opportunity teaching, presumably because this type of teaching is probably the simpler of the two. The meerkat example, however, shows nicely how both forms of teaching can be in play in the same system. Meerkats use opportunity teaching by manipulating prey for young pups, while at the same time coaching pups by nudging them and thereby encouraging them to try new, potentially dangerous, food items.

Modes of Cultural Transmission

With a better understanding of what constitutes teaching and social learning, we are now ready to delve into cultural transmission in a bit more detail. To begin this process, we shall examine three different modes of cultural transmission: vertical, horizontal, and oblique transmission (Cavalli-Sforza and Feldman, 1981; Figure 5.23).

VERTICAL CULTURAL TRANSMISSION

FIGURE 5.24. Cultural transmission in finches. Birdsong in some species of finches is learned culturally. *(Photo credit: Greg Lasley Nature Photography)*

Vertical cultural transmission occurs when information is transmitted across generations from parent(s) to offspring. This type of cultural transmission might take place through either teaching or social learning—offspring might simply learn from their parents by observation, or parents might teach a behavior to their offspring. For example, in some finch species, vertical transmission is taking place when males learn the song that they will sing from their fathers, and when females develop song preferences in potential mates based on the songs their father sang (Grant and Grant, 1996; Figure 5.24).

Vertical cultural transmission has been studied in bottlenose dolphins (*Tursiops truncatus*), who are known to imitate one another, both in the laboratory and in the wild, and who live in groups that are structured in a

FIGURE 5.25. Beaching behavior. Dolphins may trap fish by stranding them on a beach and then surging out of the water to catch them. The dolphins then quickly return to the water with their prey. *(Photo credit: Neil Lucas/Nature Picture Library)*

way that allows for transmission of behavioral traits from parents to offspring (Kuczaj et al., 1998; Xitco and Roitblat, 1996). In particular, researchers have focused on vertical transmission of bottlenose dolphin foraging skills, as this species displays a complex and rich assortment of different foraging strategies. For example, one fascinating, and quite surprising, foraging strategy called "beaching" or "beach hunting" involves a dolphin surging out of the water and onto a beach to catch a single fish, and then quickly returning to the water with its prey (Mann and Sargeant, 2003). This form of beaching of individual fish is a fairly rare behavior—in a long-term study of one bottlenose dolphin population in Shark Bay, Australia, only four adult females and their calves were observed beaching with any consistency (Sargeant et al., 2005). Another form of beaching among other dolphins, however, has been observed in salt marshes in the southeastern United States, where one to six dolphins isolate a school of fish and herd the fish toward land, creating a wave to send them onto the land and then surging out of the water to capture the stranded fish (Hoese, 1971; Figure 5.25). Yet, while beaching can be profitable when successful, it can also be quite dangerous, as beachers may get stranded.

Janet Mann and her colleagues found that only calves born to mothers that themselves were "beachers" displayed this specialized foraging strategy. They then undertook a detailed genetic analysis involving mitochondrial DNA and found that beaching was not a genetically transmitted trait. Rather, the behavioral evidence suggests that young calves learn beaching from their mothers, and that this is likely a result of the young calves spending a great deal of time with their mothers and learning this dangerous foraging tactic via vertical cultural transmission.

A second fascinating case of vertical transmission of foraging strategies has also been observed in the bottlenose dolphins of Shark Bay, and is the first known case of tool use in dolphins (Krutzen et al., 2005). Here the foraging behavior is called "sponging" and involves female bottlenose dolphins breaking a marine sponge off the seafloor and placing it over their mouth, and then using this tool to probe the seafloor for fish prey (Smolker et al., 1997; Figure 5.26). As with beaching behavior, sponging is seen almost exclusively in females, and a detailed molecular genetic analysis suggests that this trait is not transmitted genetically. Instead, young females in one particular Shark Bay lineage learn sponging from their mothers.

FIGURE 5.26. Sponging behavior in dolphins. Female bottlenose dolphins break a marine sponge off the seafloor and place it over their mouth. This tool is used to probe the seafloor for fish prey and to protect them from scrapes and stings as they forage. *(Photo credit: Janet Mann)*

HORIZONTAL CULTURAL TRANSMISSION

Cultural transmission is not limited to the transfer of information from parents to their offspring. In humans, for example, everyday experiences demonstrate that most information comes from peers—people who are of the same approximate age group. This type of transmission of information, called **horizontal cultural transmission**, operates not only for adults, but for children as well. In fact, in humans, horizontal transmission of information is so powerful that adults spend much of their time trying to subdue its effects on their offspring. We want our children to learn some things from their peers, but not everything.

Horizontal cultural transmission plays a role in animal as well as human behavior. Consider the case of horizontal transmission of foraging-related information in guppies, a species in which fish segregate into schools based on which members are about the same age and size as one another. Kevin Laland and Kerry Williams trained guppies of approximately the same age to learn different paths to a food source—a long path and a short path (Laland and Williams, 1998). Not surprisingly, it was more difficult to train fish to take the longer path when both paths were present, but Laland and Williams found a clever way (involving what amounts to trapdoors) to do so.

Once the "long-path" and "short-path" groups were trained, Laland and Williams slowly removed the original members of each group and replaced them with new "naive" individuals who didn't know either of the paths to the food source. Initially, groups contained five trained guppies, then four trained individuals and one untrained, then three trained individuals and two untrained, and so on, until none of the original trained group members remained. The question, then, was whether the fish remaining at the end of the experiment—none of which were trained to a particular path—maintained the "traditional" path taken by the original fish in their group.

Laland and Williams found that in both the short-path and long-path groups, guppies at the end of the experiment still followed the path to which the original fish had been trained. Horizontal transmission of information was clearly in operation, as the only "models" from which to learn were same-aged individuals. What makes this experiment particularly interesting is that it demonstrates that cultural transmission can produce "maladaptive" (long-path use), as well as adaptive (short-path use) behavior. In fact, horizontal transmission in the long-path groups not only resulted in guppies acquiring the "wrong" information, it actually made it more difficult for the fish in that treatment to subsequently learn to use the shorter path (Brown and Laland, 2002; Reader et al., 2003).

OBLIQUE CULTURAL TRANSMISSION

Oblique cultural transmission refers to the transfer of information across generations, but not via parent/offspring interactions. In this form of cultural transmission, young animals simply get their information from adults that are not their parents. This sort of transmission might be particularly common in animal species where there is no parental care, and hence where most young/old interactions would be between nonrelatives.

Oblique transmission has been uncovered in many scenarios, such as predator recognition in blackbirds (see Chapter 11), but let us just examine one for the moment—learned snake aversion in rhesus monkeys. Early work

FIGURE 5.27. Monkeys and fear of snakes. Rhesus monkeys in the field often fear snakes after watching others respond to such potential danger. Monkeys raised in the lab, who do not normally fear snakes, can be made to fear them through observing older monkeys reacting fearfully to snakes. Young monkeys were shown this video of an older monkey who fled to the back of the cage and cringed in fear at the sight of two snakes. *(Photo credit: Sue Mineka)*

comparing wild- and laboratory-raised primates found that the lab-raised animals who never saw a snake did not respond to snakes in the same manner as wild-raised individuals who had the chance to experience snakes in nature (Hall and Devore, 1965; Seyfarth et al., 1980; Struhsaker, 1967). Knowing this, Susan Mineka and her colleagues examined whether oblique cultural transmission played a role in the fear of snakes (Cook et al., 1985; Mineka and Cook, 1988; Mineka et al., 1984).

Mineka began her laboratory-based experiment with juvenile rhesus monkeys who were not afraid of snakes. Shortly after observing an adult model respond to snakes with typical fear gestures and actions (Figure 5.27), juveniles themselves adopted these same gestures (for at least three months). It made no difference whether the individuals observed were the subjects' parents (vertical transmission) or unrelated adult monkeys (oblique transmission)—exposure to adult models showing fear in the presence of snakes led to observers showing similar fear responses. Mineka also found that when observers saw a model who had been trained to display fear in the presence of a neutral object—a flower—the observers did not display fear when they were exposed to flowers, suggesting that a predisposition to fear snakes is interacting with oblique cultural transmission (Cook and Mineka, 1989). Further evidence of this interaction can be seen in the fact that monkeys who had first seen an adult model interact with a snake in a nonfearful manner, but then saw a second model respond with fear to snakes, displayed less fear than individuals exposed only to a model who had displayed fear. These monkeys were culturally "immunized" against associating snakes and fear (Mineka and Cook, 1986).

The Interaction of Genetic and Cultural Transmission

If, as it seems to be the case, cultural and genetic transmission both operate on animal behavior, then we can search for cases in which both forms of transmission are in play in the same system. To better achieve a fundamental

FIGURE 5.28. Finch songs across generations. If male songs are culturally transmitted from father to son, then the songs of the sons should resemble those of their father and their paternal grandfather, but not those of their maternal grandfather. *(From Grant and Grant, 1996)*

understanding of how such interactions work, let's consider two different case studies that examine the interaction of genes and culture in two dramatically different animal systems—birds and fish.

THE GRANTS' FINCHES

Peter and Rosemary Grant's work probably best simulates what Charles Darwin might be doing were he alive today (Weiner, 1995). Like Darwin, the Grants have been studying finches in the Galápagos Islands, and like Darwin's work, their studies are already considered classics. Among the many problems the Grants have tackled is the role of cultural transmission in the evolution of finch song. In Galápagos finches, cultural transmission not only facilitates birdsong, but it interacts in an unexpected manner with the genetics of reproductive isolation and speciation in these birds (Grant and Grant, 1994, 1997).

The medium ground finch (*Geospiza fortis*) and the cactus finch (*G. scandens*) both inhabit the Galápagos Island of Daphne Major. Although these are considered to be different species, some cases of interbreeding between these two finch species have been uncovered, and the hybrids do not appear to suffer a decrease in fitness as compared to the two pure species—that is, there is no fitness penalty for hybridization across ground and cactus finches. Yet, despite the fact that there seems to be no fitness cost for hybridization, medium ground finches and cactus finches rarely interbreed. Why? Without barriers blocking interbreeding, why don't the many species of finches just merge into one species? More specifically, does cultural transmission play a role in inhibiting such a merger (Freeberg, 2004; Lachlan and Servedio, 2004; Nelson et al., 2001; Slabbekoorn and Smith, 2002)?

In finches, male birdsong plays a prominent role in the mating process, and, as in all songbirds, male finches learn the songs they sing. When the Grants studied the songs sung by ground and cactus finches during the mating season, they found that these songs were transmitted across generations via cultural transmission (Grant and Grant, 1996). The evidence for the cultural transmission of birdsong comes from comparing the songs of sons, fathers, and grandfathers. To see why, consider the case in which fathers and sons have very similar songs. This could be due to the song being a genetic trait passed from father to son, or it could be due to the cultural transmission of the song from father to son. Now, compare the songs of sons to those of their paternal and maternal grandfathers. If songs are genetically controlled, we should see that the songs of sons are similar to the songs of both their paternal and maternal grandfathers, since they inherit genes from both grandfathers. But, if the songs are culturally transmitted from father to son, then the songs of the sons should resemble those of their paternal grandfather, but not those of their maternal grandfather. This is because the paternal grandfather would have transmitted the song to the father, who would then have transmitted the song to the son. The evidence suggests that the songs of sons resemble the songs of their paternal grandfathers, but not the songs of their maternal grandfathers (Figure 5.28). Thus, birdsong appears to be culturally transmitted.

The Grants also found that the songs of these two species were quite different from one another. For example, the song of the cactus finch has shorter components that are repeated more often than the components of the song of the ground finch. These differences in their songs—a culturally transmitted trait—have a dramatic impact on gene flow across species. Of 482 females sampled, the vast majority (over 95 percent) mated with males who sang the song appropriate to their own species. Thus, cultural transmission of song allows females to recognize individuals of their own species. In addition, females tend to avoid males who sing songs that are similar to the songs that their own fathers sang, which suggests that song also plays a role in preventing inbreeding. Thus, because song is culturally transmitted from father to son, females may decrease the probability of mating with blood relatives when they avoid mating with males who sing like their fathers.

In their long-term study, the Grants uncovered eleven cases in which the male of one species sang the song of another species. In most of these cases, cross-species breeding would then occur, resulting in hybrid offspring. In other words, remove the normal pattern of cultural transmission and the barrier to breeding across species disappears, suggesting a new and exciting avenue of research in the interaction of cultural transmission and genetics. In this example, then, we see how powerful cultural transmission of traits can be in that it can have significant effects on such evolutionary issues as cross-species hybridizations resulting from interbreeding.

GUPPY MATE CHOICE

As we have seen earlier in the chapter, female guppies copy the mate choice of other females (Dugatkin, 1992a). Observer females who viewed a model female choose one male over another were much more likely to choose that male themselves. In addition to this type of cultural transmission of information, genetic transmission of traits also plays an important role in guppy mate-choice behavior (Houde, 1997; Magurran, 2005).

Guppies from some populations—most notably, fish from the Paria River in Trinidad and Tobago—prefer to mate with males that have lots of orange body color. Interpopulational comparisons suggest that this preference of Paria River females for males with more orange body color is heritable (Houde, 1988; Houde and Endler, 1990). In addition, orange body color itself is a heritable trait in Paria River males (Houde, 1992; Houde, 1994).

To examine how genetic and cultural transmission interact in shaping mate choice in females from the Paria River, Dugatkin set up an experiment with four different treatments (Dugatkin, 1996b). In each treatment, a female was exposed to a pair of males. In treatment I, males were matched for orange body color (the mean difference in orange color between the males was less than 4 percent). In treatments II, III, and IV, males differed in total orange body color by an average of 12 percent (II), 24 percent (III), and 40 percent (IV). In each and every treatment, the experiment was designed such that observer females always saw a model female near the male with less orange body color. That is, the information being culturally transmitted to models was always in direct opposition to a female's genetic predisposition to choose males with more orange body color as mates.

Results of the experiment show that females in treatment I—in which males were matched for orange body color—copied each other's mate choice. When males differed in orange body color by an average of 12 or 24 percent (treatments II and III, respectively), females consistently preferred the less orange of the two males, again following the mate choice of the model female;

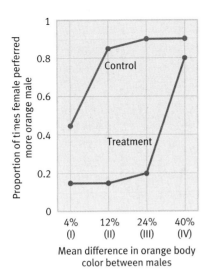

FIGURE 5.29. Mate-choice copying in guppies. Control trials demonstrate that when a female chooses between males that differ in orange body color, and no model female is present, she shows a strong preference for more orange males. In the treatment trials, a model female was always placed near the less orange male. When males differed by small (12%) or moderate (24%) amounts of orange, copying the other female's mate choice overrode the female's innate preference for more orange males. When males differed by large (40%) amounts of orange, copying opportunities didn't change the female's genetic predisposition to choose orange males. *(Based on Dugatkin, 1996b)*

in these treatments, culturally transmitted information overrode a female's genetic predisposition to mate with males with lots of orange body color. But when male orange body color differed by an average of 40 percent (treatment IV), females consistently preferred the more orange of the two males, thus overriding any effects of copying (Figure 5.29).

These results suggest that it may be possible to experimentally examine the relative strength of both cultural transmission and genetic predisposition. In the guppy system, it appears that whether or not females copy a model's mate choice is affected by a threshold difference in the amount of orange body color in the male. If the male's orange body color is beneath this threshold, the effects of copying are predominant. But if the orange body color is above this threshold, genetic preferences mask any cultural effects. This sort of finding reinforces the idea that both genetic and cultural transmission can shed light on important issues in the study of animal behavior, and it demonstrates that a comprehensive understanding of ethology will often, but certainly not always, require that both forms of transmission be taken into account.

Cultural Transmission and Brain Size

In this chapter, we have seen examples of cultural transmission in everything from fish to primates (B'shary et al., 2002). Clearly, at least some forms of cultural transmission are possible even in animals with very tiny brains. That being said, it may very well be that some sort of relationship between large brain size and cultural transmission exists. The key to finding such a relationship (if it does exist) is to search in the right places, and to ask precisely the right questions.

E. O. Wilson has suggested that in a population of large-brained animals, new innovations—the discovery of novel solutions to problems—might pop up and spread more often than would happen in a population of small-brained animals. The data on this question are mixed (Dunbar, 1992; Sawaguchi and Kudo, 1990). But Simon Reader and Kevin Laland, in the most comprehensive study to date, found that across more than 100 species of nonhuman primates, there was a significant positive correlation between brain size and both innovation and tool-use frequency, thus confirming the predicted trends (Dunbar, 1992; Reader and Laland, 2002; Sawaguchi and Kudo, 1990).

Reader and Laland defined innovations as "novel solutions to environmental or social problems." Using this definition, they uncovered 533 recorded instances of innovations, 445 observations of social learning, and 607 episodes of tool use that covered 116 of the 203 known species of primates. They then mapped out these behaviors against something called "executive brain" volume, a measure that includes both the neocortex and striatum sections of the brain (Jolicoeur et al., 1984; Keverne et al., 1996). Innovation, social learning, and tool use all had a positive correlation with absolute executive brain volume. That is, even when the large discrepancy in body size across the 166 species of primates included in the study is taken into account, it appears that it is the absolute size of the primate brain, not brain size in relation to body size, that correlates best with social learning, tool use, and innovation (Figure 5.30). Put simply, big brain size, per se, matters in primates.

FIGURE 5.30. Effects of increasing brain size in primates. Reader and Laland determined the executive brain ratio (the executive brain size divided by the brainstem size) to examine the relationship between innovations and social learning and brain size. They found: **(A)** As the executive brain ratio of primates increases so too does the occurrence of new innovations. This same relationship holds true when innovation is plotted against absolute executive brain size. **(B)** The occurrence of social learning also increases with an increase in primate brain size. This same relationship was found when social learning was plotted against absolute executive brain size. *(From Reader and Laland, 2002)*

A similar trend between large brain size and an increased propensity toward innovation was found for birds in North America, Britain, and Australia (Lefebvre et al., 1997a, 1997b, 2004; Sol et al., 2005b). This relationship has interesting implications for questions relating to the conservation and ecology of birds (Sol et al., 2005a, 2005b). For example, Daniel Sol and his team examined whether the relationship between brain size and innovation impacted bird species when they were moved to novel environments through large-scale, human "introduction" programs (where humans introduce a new species to a novel habitat). Using global data on more than 600 such introduction programs, Sol and his colleagues found that bird species in which individuals had a high brain size/body ratio were more likely to survive and thrive (that is, to have greater "invasion potential") after introduction to novel environments than were species with lower brain size/body ratios. In addition, the researchers found that when large-brained species were introduced to novel environments, they increased their rate of innovation—for example, by using a new foraging technique—which in turn increased their probability of success (their "invasion potential") in their new habitats.

In this chapter, we have seen that cultural transmission is different from individual learning in that it involves learning from others, and its effects last beyond the lifetime of the individual. Cultural transmission can lead to a quick shift to a new behavior or response throughout a population in ways that are not possible through individual learning. We have also seen that cultural transmission is not unique to humans, and that it has been observed in fish, birds, rats, and (other) primates.

Having worked our way through an introductory chapter and four primer chapters, we are now ready to explore specific animal behaviors in more depth, beginning with sexual selection.

Dr. Cecilia Heyes

Why study cultural transmission in animals? Isn't culture the sort of subject that sociologists examine?

There are many reasons why the study of culture cannot be left solely to sociologists, anthropologists, and other experts on human cultures and societies. Humans are, among other things, animals, so even if culture were a distinctively human phenomenon, it would be essential to understand it at the biological and psychological levels—to find out where it comes from in evolutionary terms, and to identify the proximate biological and psychological processes that make it possible. Comparing human and nonhuman cultures (or, if you prefer, human cultures with animal traditions) helps us to understand what Thomas Huxley, "Darwin's bulldog," called "Man's place in nature" (1863). Each of us is part of at least one human culture, and usually we belong to many. For example, I am soaked in English culture, but I'm also influenced by Western culture, the culture of science, and, as a result of my upbringing, by Roman Catholic culture. Because each of us is embedded in the matrix of one or more human cultures, it can be difficult for us to get an aerial view of what culture really is and how it works. Comparing ourselves with other animals can give us this aerial view. It can reveal the fundamental processes that make culture possible, the ingredients that are and are not needed to make cultural transmission "take off" to become a system of cultural inheritance, analogous to that of genetic inheritance. It might turn

out that the full set of ingredients is present only in humans, but on the way to that conclusion we would have learned a great deal, not only about culture, but about a type of learning —social learning—that can have a profound influence on behavioral adaptation.

There is a good deal of contention about how to define culture in animals. What is your take on this issue?

I think it may be too soon to be using the term "culture" to describe examples of social transmission or traditional behavior in nonhuman animals. The risk is that, if we categorize them as examples of culture too soon, we'll forget that the critical ingredients of culture have not yet been identified, and then we won't prioritize the research that would enable us to answer this important question. This kind of maladaptive shortcut is made surprisingly often in the study of animal behavior. For example, field primatologists in the

1980s were so confident that they had seen examples of intentional deception that they claimed quite emphatically that nonhuman apes have "theory of mind"—the capacity to think about the thoughts and feelings of others. As a result, it has been hard in the last 20 years for researchers such as Daniel Povinelli and Michael Tomasello to get the animal behavior community to recognize that more careful research was needed to find out whether animals can really attribute mental states to themselves and others.

So, I'm uneasy about calling socially transmitted behavior "culture." Having said that, I should also point out that I don't think the exact content of a definition is terribly important. What's essential is that a definition should be explicit and reasoned. If it isn't clearly stated, then there will be cross-talk and confusion. I might say "I believe that fruit bats have culture," and, if I haven't said what I mean by culture, you might think I'm claiming that fruit bats go to the opera. When definitions aren't reasoned—for example, if I describe the behavior of my favorite species as "cultural" without thinking, or just because it sounds more exciting that way—then it's hard to make real scientific progress. Much of pre-Darwinian biology was about giving arbitrary names to things; it involved the kind of cataloging that goes on in a library. But contemporary biology is about understanding structures and processes. A definition without a reason is a throwback to cataloging science, but a reasoned definition usually represents or leads to a testable hypothesis. For example, if a researcher chooses to call all social transmission in animals "culture" because he believes that the nongenetic transmission process is the most important ingredient of culture, then his definition represents a testable hypothesis, and therefore contributes to progress in the field.

If you had to make an educated guess, how common would you say that cultural transmission is in nonprimates?

There are many kinds of social learning and, although most of them do not require the learner to be especially "clever," they all have the potential to yield very substantial adaptive advantages. Therefore, if "culture" is understood liberally to mean behavior affected by social learning, then I think it's very common in nonprimate as well as primate taxa. The phenotype of any animal that lives in a social group, and in an environment that is sufficiently variable to warrant adaptation through learning, is likely to be influenced by social learning.

When I was a graduate student, I had the bright idea that adult Syrian hamsters may have poor social learning ability because they are "solitary"; except when mating, they are highly intolerant of even the presence of mature conspecifics. However, my attempts to show this experimentally, by comparing the social learning ability of adult and pre-dispersal juvenile hamsters, were a rank failure. In each experimental task, the adult hamsters cheerfully learned from their "demonstrators," and thereby heartlessly proved me wrong.

If culture is defined more strictly—for example, as a system of inheritance that allows cumulative,

selection-based evolution—then I'm not yet convinced that it is present in any nonhuman species. To answer this intriguing question we would need much more information about the dynamics of social transmission in animals, and particularly about the fidelity with which behaviorial variants are copied across successive links in a transmission chain. If adaptive innovations are not transmitted faithfully, then an inheritance system based on social learning cannot have effects comparable to those of gene-based selection.

How do you see advances in neurobiology impacting the study of animal culture over the next five years?

The discovery of "mirror neurons" in the premotor cortex of macaque monkeys has caused a huge stir among those who study imitation and related processes in humans. These cells fire when the animal executes an action—for example, grasping an object—but also when the animal passively observes a human performing the same action. Curiously, the discovery of mirror neurons does not seem to have had such a dramatic impact on those studying social learning in animals. Part of the reason for this may be that there are still many gaps between research on the functions and mechanisms of animal behavior. The work of neurobiologists, psychologists, and ethologists is becoming ever more integrated, but these are still, to some extent, three separate scientific cultures.

However, there may be another, more specific reason why those studying social learning and culture in animals have not run with the lead provided by mirror neurons.

At first glance, it looks like mirror neurons could mediate imitation or copying of very specific features of behavior—the shape or topography of body movements. But, due to doubts that monkeys are able to copy at this level of specificity, many people have rejected this idea, and instead focused on the possibility that mirror neurons are involved in action understanding, theory of mind, or empathy, processes that are not so closely related to culture. I think that was a mistake. Looking into the crystal ball, I predict that the connection between imitation and mirror neurons—in the premotor cortex and elsewhere in the brain, in monkeys and in other taxa—will be "rediscovered," and that well-integrated behavioral and neurobiological studies will begin to answer important questions about mirror neurons. This will be greatly assisted by more widespread availability of scanners for functional magnetic resonance imaging (fMRI) of primates and rodents. The most important question, in my mind, is: Where do mirror neurons come from? Are some animals born with mirror neurons for a range of behaviors, or are mirror neurons made through associative learning? The answer to this question will tell us a great deal about the origins of the capacity to imitate and, insofar as imitation is involved in cultural transmission, about the origins of culture.

Dr. Cecilia Heyes is a professor at University College London in England. Her research focuses on the evolution of cognition. She is a co-editor of Social Learning in Animals: The Roots of Culture *(Academic Press, 1996), and* Evolution of Cognition *(MIT Press, 2000).*

SUMMARY

1. Cultural transmission involves the transfer and acquisition of information via social learning and teaching and may represent a powerful force for the acquisition and spread of behaviors both within and between generations of animals.

2. Cultural transmission differs from learning about other parts of the environment. Unlike other environmental influences, what is learned via cultural transmission is passed on from individual to individual. This can translate into the behavior of a single individual shifting the behavior patterns seen in an entire group. Furthermore, when cultural transmission is in play, what is learned by one individual may be passed down through many generations.

3. Cultural transmission involves a "model" individual and an "observer" who learns a specific behavior or response from the model. There are situations, however, that involve an interaction between observers and models, but that do *not* constitute cultural transmission because observers do not learn any particular behavior or response from models. Two examples of this are local enhancement and social facilitation.

4. Cultural transmission can occur through learning from other individuals via social learning (copying or imitation) and/or teaching.

5. To demonstrate imitation, there must be some new behavior learned from others, and that behavior must involve some sort of new spatial (topographic) manipulation as well as lead to the achievement of some goal. Copying differs from imitation in that what is copied need not be novel and need not involve learning some new topographical action.

6. Teaching, when rigorously defined, implies that one individual serves as an instructor and at least one other individual acts as a student who learns from the teacher. Teaching entails providing an immediate benefit to the student but not to the teacher, instructing naive "students," and imparting some new information to students faster than they would otherwise receive it.

7. Cultural transmission may occur via vertical, horizontal, or oblique transmission. Vertical cultural transmission involves the transfer of information from parent to child, horizontal cultural transmission occurs when information comes from peers, and oblique cultural transmission is the transfer of information from older to younger individuals, excluding transfers from parents to offspring.

8. Genetic and cultural transmission can operate independently on animals, but often they interact in interesting ways, as exhibited in the cultural transmission of birdsong in finches and the evolution of mate choice in guppies.

9. Data on more than 100 species of nonhuman primates have shown that there is a significant positive correlation between brain size and both innovation and tool-use frequency. It appears that it is the absolute size of the primate brain, not brain size in relation to body size, that correlates best with social learning, tool use, and innovation. A similar trend between large brain size and an increased propensity toward innovation was found for birds in North America, Britain, and Australia.

DISCUSSION QUESTIONS

1. Why do you suppose it took so long for ethologists to focus on the possibility that cultural transmission was an important force in animals? Can you imagine any biases—scientific, ideological, and so on—that might be responsible for this?

2. Suppose I run an experiment in which I take a bird (the observer) and let him view another bird (the demonstrator) opening a sealed cup by pecking at a circle on the cover of the cup. I then test the observer and see that he now opens the cup by pecking at the circle. What can I infer about social learning here? What other critical treatment is missing from this experiment?

3. Imagine that adults in some population of monkeys appeared to pick up new innovations (for example, potato washing, stone play) from observing others. How might you disentangle vertical, horizontal, and oblique cultural transmission as possible explanatory forces?

4. List the pros and cons of Hauser and Caro's definition of teaching. How might you modify this definition to address what you listed on the "con" side of your ledger?

5. Suppose that after extensive observations, you determine that certain animals in a population appear to rely on social learning much more often than other individuals, and that such differences are due to genetic variation. How might you use the truncation selection technique described in Chapter 2 to examine the heritability of the tendency to employ social learning?

SUGGESTED READING

Bonner, J. T. (1980). *The evolution of culture in animals.* Princeton: Princeton University Press. One of the earliest books looking at culture from an evolutionary perspective. This is a fun read and informative as well.

Boyd, R., & Richerson P. J. (1985). *Culture and the evolutionary process.* Chicago: University of Chicago Press. Probably the best book on the evolution of culture. This book can get very technical, but it is worth the effort to work through it.

Brass, M., & Heyes, C. (2005). Imitation: Is cognitive neuroscience solving the correspondence problem? *Trends in Cognitive Sciences, 9,* 489–495. An interesting paper on the role of neuroscience in explaining a long-standing "perspective-taking" problem in the study of imitation.

Heyes, C. M. (1994). Social learning in animals: Categories and mechanisms. *Biological Reviews of the Cambridge Philosophical Society, 69,* 207–231. Also Heyes C. M., & Ray E. D. (2000). What is the significance of imitation in animals? *Advances in the Study of Behavior, 29,* 215–245. Two overviews on social learning and cultural transmission.

Lefebvre, L., Reader, S. M., & Sol, D. (2004). Brains, innovations and evolution in birds and primates. *Brain Behavior and Evolution, 63,* 233–246. A nice review paper that compares published data on brain size, innovation, and cultural transmission in both primates and birds.

6

Sexual Selection

In each of the first five primer chapters, we have focused on a fundamental issue in animal behavior (natural selection, learning, and so on), identified basic theory, and then examined the issue across a whole suite of behaviors. In the remaining twelve chapters, we will once again return to theoretical, empirical, and conceptual questions, but each chapter will focus on a specific behavior, or more generally a specific set of related behavioral issues (sexual selection, mating systems, foraging, predation, cooperation, and so forth). We begin with the topic of **sexual selection**.

In his book, *The Descent of Man and Selection in Relation to Sex*, Charles Darwin provided the first detailed evolutionary theory of sexual selection, defining this process as one that "depends on the advantage which certain individuals have over other individuals of the same sex and species in exclusive relation to reproduction" (Darwin, 1871). Darwin's work on sexual selection encompasses a theory of: (1) **intrasexual selection**, whereby members of one sex compete with each other for access to the other sex, as well as (2) **intersexual selection**, whereby individuals of one sex choose which individuals of the other sex to take as mates. As we saw in our Chapter 1 discussion of cricket songs and parasites, this process of intersexual selection can get complicated, because traits that make an individual attractive to the opposite sex can also make it obvious to predators and parasites.

Recall that from the perspective of genetics, the number of copies of a gene passed down to the next generation is the currency of importance. Aspects of sexual selection are clearly important in measuring that currency, and by beginning here we have an excellent portal through which we can examine the processes that lead to the differential success of one gene over another.

In this chapter, we shall examine sexual selection from both proximate and ultimate perspectives, with particular emphasis on: (1) the evolution of mating preferences, (2) learning and sexual selection, (3) cultural transmission and female mate choice, and (4) male-male competition.

Intersexual and Intrasexual Selection

Darwin proposed that one factor that leads to differences in reproductive success is competition for mates—intrasexual selection. Competition for mates is ubiquitous in the animal kingdom, and in most species, it is males that compete for females as mates and not vice versa.

This fundamental difference between the sexes is due to a number of factors, but ethologists and evolutionary biologists believe that the primary one centers on the different type and number of gametes produced by males (sperm) and females (eggs). By definition, females produce fewer, but larger gametes (Figure 6.1). In a sense, then, each egg is extremely valuable, both because of its size and its relative rarity. Each sperm, on the other hand, requires much less energy to produce, and sperm are usually found in prolific quantities. Male reproductive success is limited by the much lower rate of gamete production of females compared with that of males. Thus, while males often produce millions of sperm, creating the possibility that some males will have extraordinary

FIGURE 6.1. Natural selection and gamete size. Natural selection has favored two types of gametes: small and quick (sperm) and large (egg). For gametes to be successful, they must be able to find another gamete and produce a healthy zygote. Small gametes (sperm) specialize in the former, while large gametes (eggs) specialize in the latter. Medium-sized gametes do neither and are selected against. *(From Low, 2000)*

reproductive success, females' eggs are often, but not always, few and far between, causing severe competition for this scarce resource (Trivers, 1985). The idea that (1) females should be the choosier sex because eggs are expensive and because a female's reproductive success is limited compared with that of a male, and (2) this should translate into greater variance in the reproductive success of males is known as **Bateman's principle**, after A. J. Bateman and his work on sexual selection among fruit flies (Bateman, 1948).

According to Darwin, all else being equal, any male trait that confers mating and fertilization advantages on its possessor, and is passed down across generations, will, over time, increase in frequency in a population, because males with such traits will simply produce more offspring than their competitors. Darwin's idea about the struggle among males for mating opportunities forms one basic foundation of our current understanding of sexual selection. Naturally, from a proximate perspective, the ways in which hormones, neurobiology, development, environment, and many other factors operate on any particular behavior play a very important role in the sexual selection process as well. We will return to some of these factors shortly, but it is worth noting that Darwin's theory of sexual selection predated much of what we know today about endocrinology, neurobiology, and so forth. This statement says much about the generality and power of the theory of sexual selection.

Competition for mates can take many forms, depending on such factors as ecology, demography, and cognitive ability. For example, males may fight among themselves, occasionally in dramatic "battles to the death," but often in less dangerous bouts, to gain mating privileges with females (Figure 6.2). This latter form of male-male sexual competition is illustrated by male stag beetles and red deer (*Cervus elaphus*), which use their "horns" (enlarged jaws) and antlers, respectively, in physical fights over females; the winners of such contests mate more often than the losers.

Until about thirty years ago, much of the work on mate selection focused almost exclusively on intrasexual competition, rather than mate choice, or intersexual selection (Andersson, 1994; Andersson and Simmons, 2006). Exactly why this was so is difficult to assess, but part of the explanation may be that male-male competition is very easy to observe in nature. In addition, some prominent evolutionary biologists of the 1930s dismissed mate choice as unimportant and directed research toward male-male competition (Huxley, 1938).

Mate choice is, in a sense, a much more subtle form of sexual selection than is competition between males because intersexual selection directly involves both males and females in the decision-making process. Just as intrasexual selection, in principle, could involve either males fighting for females or females fighting for males, so too does intersexual selection encompass female choice of a male and male choice of a female. Both clearly occur in nature, but female mate choice is much more prevalent. This is likely due to the fact that females stand to lose much more than males by making a bad choice of mates. In the first place, as mentioned above, females invest much more energy in each gamete they produce, and hence they should be choosier than males in terms of who has access to their gametes. In addition, in species with internal gestation, females typically devote much more energy to offspring before they are born, and hence they should be under strong selection pressure to choose good mates who will produce healthy offspring.

Above and beyond the physical genitalia that are necessary for the act of mating, males often possess other traits that play an important role in attracting mates. These traits are referred to as secondary, or epigametic, sexual characteristics. As we shall see, many conspicuous secondary sexual traits in males, such as ornamental plumage, bright colors, and courtship displays, have been favored by natural selection because of their effect on female mate choice. What's more, the underlying genetics of such secondary sexual characteristics

A   B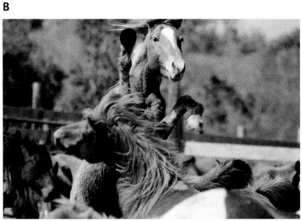

FIGURE 6.2. Competition for mates. (A) Male deer battle with their antlers. **(B)** Male horses compete for females. *(Photo credits: Manfred Danegger/Photo Researchers, Inc.; Rich Pomerantz)*

are the subject of much experimental work. For example, male fruit flies "sing" to females during courtship by vibrating their wings. This courtship song influences not only female mate choice, but may also be important in the process whereby new species are formed (speciation) in fruit flies (Spieth and Ringo, 1983; Tomaru and Oguma, 1994).

One particular form of song in fruit flies, called "pulse song," is quite conspicuous during courtship, and the interval between pulses (the interpulse interval, or IPI) appears to be critical in terms of the mate choice of female fruit flies (Ewing and Bennet-Clark, 1968; Ritchie et al., 1999; Schilcher, 1976a, 1976b). Early work on the genetics of courtship song in *Drosophila* suggested pulse song might be controlled by a large number of different genes, each of which would contribute a small amount to the expression of the song. More recent work, however, suggests that the genetics of song appear to involve three loci that account for a good deal of variance in courtship song (Gleason et al., 2002).

Both intersexual and intrasexual selection play a role in virtually all mating systems (see Chapter 7). Whether the system is *monogamous* (where a single male pairs up with a single female), *polygamous* (where some subset of males mates with many females), or *polyandrous* (where some subset of females mates with numerous males), sexual selection plays a role. Generally speaking, sexual selection will be stronger in polygamous and polyandrous systems than in monogamous systems. In polygamous and polyandrous systems, some individuals obtain many mating opportunities and some obtain no mating opportunities, while there is generally less variation in reproductive success in monogamous systems (see Chapter 7). That being said, sexual selection acts in monogamous systems as well, just not as strongly.

Evolutionary Models of Mate Choice

Studying how females choose their mates has become one of the most active areas in the field of ethology. As mentioned earlier, male-male competition took center stage in the sexual selection theater until approximately thirty years ago. The tables have clearly turned of late, and female mate choice is now the most studied of the processes leading to sexual selection (Andersson, 1994; Ord et al., 2005). Until recently, one unifying theme running through virtually all such studies was that they assumed that a female's choice of mates is under some sort of genetic control (Fisher, 1958). That is, genetic variation in mate-choice behavior in females was assumed to be responsible for variation in mate choice seen in nature. Of course, the environment played a huge role in determining *which* genes were chosen, and proximate factors played a role in determining *how* genes affected mate choice, but at the bottom of it all there was assumed to be a set of genes that controlled the process of mate choice. We will begin by working within this framework and in so doing discuss four evolutionary models of sexual selection that examine female preferences, as well as the traits that females prefer in their mates. Subsequent to this, we will spend time discussing the idea that learning and cultural transmission also play an important role in sexual selection.

FIGURE 6.3. Evolutionary models of mate choice. Evolutionary models of mate choice can be broken down into (1) "good genes" models, (2) "direct benefits" models, (3) "runaway selection" models, and (4) sensory exploitation models.

Evolutionary models of female mate choice can be broken down into four classes: "direct benefits," "good genes," "runaway selection," and "sensory exploitation" models (Figure 6.3). We will examine the logic of these models, and then look at case studies for each. It is important to note that we will focus on case studies in which the evolution of a sexually selected trait is best as explained by one of our four models. In many species, of course, the evolution of sexually selected traits might best be explained by a combination of two or more models. The logic of focusing on the more clear-cut cases, where a single model best explains the evolution of a sexually selected trait, is to provide a basic understanding of the dynamics of female mate choice, so that we do not put the cart before the horse. Once each model is understood on its own, students of animal behavior are better prepared to understand the more complex ways that sexual selection operates in nature.

DIRECT BENEFITS AND MATE CHOICE

The direct benefits model of female mate choice is the most basic of the evolutionary models we will examine (Kirkpatrick and Ryan, 1991; Møller and Jennions, 2001; Price et al., 1993). In this model, natural selection favors females who have a genetic predisposition to choose mates that provide them with tangible resources—above and beyond sperm—that increase their fecundity (Andersson, 1994; Figure 6.4). That is, any female who has the tendency to choose males that provide her with some important resource—food, safe shelter, assistance with parental care, and so on—will do better than her counterparts that are less choosy, and through time we should see more acutely picky females. One fascinating case of direct benefits centers on nuptial gifts in scorpionflies.

DIRECT BENEFITS AND NUPTIAL GIFTS. Randy Thornhill and his colleagues have examined female direct benefits and mate choice in the scorpionfly (*Hylobittacus apicalis*) in both the laboratory and the field (Thornhill, 1976, 1980a). They found that female scorpionflies choose their mates using a very basic rule: choose males that bring relatively large prey items—primarily aphids,

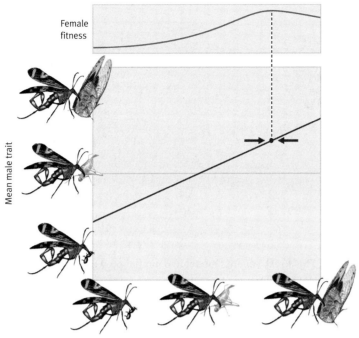

FIGURE 6.4. A graphical representation of the direct benefits model of female mate choice. Here males provide a direct benefit (in this case, food), and females choose males based on how the resource affects their fitness. (Based on Kirkpatrick and Ryan, 1991)

flies, beetles, and so on—during the courtship process (Figure 6.5). These **nuptial gifts**, which are consumed during courtship, provide females with a direct tangible benefit—food.

Males that bring no prey are immediately rejected by females (Cordero, 1996). But females do more than simply choose a mate based on nuptial gifts, they also determine how long they will mate with a given male based on the size of his gift—that is, based on the direct benefit they receive. When the nuptial gift is small (between 3 to 19 mm^2), there is a positive relationship between prey size and copulation time. When nuptial gifts are in this size range, it is the female that always terminates copulation, by pulling her abdominal tip away from the male. When the nuptial gift size is larger (greater than 19 mm^2), copulations last much longer (Figure 6.6A). Copulation time is important, because there is a strong positive relationship between it and the number of sperm transferred during such matings—indeed, copulation times of less than approximately seven minutes often involve no sperm transfer (Figure 6.6B).

Given that females can clearly distinguish males with large gifts from other males, what benefits do they receive by doing so? A female who actively chooses males that bring large nuptial gifts produces *more* eggs and, in all likelihood, has a longer life span, both because of the nutrition she receives directly and the decreased amount of time she must allocate to hunting (Thornhill, 1976, 1979b, 1980a, 1980b; Thornhill and Alcock, 1983).

The fact that nuptial prey size has such a strong effect on mating opportunities (and ultimately sperm transfer) creates strong selection pressure on males to bring large nuptial gifts to females. Finding prey that are large enough (greater than 19 mm^2) to result in long copulations with a female is both time consuming (many prey are much smaller) and quite dangerous (increased foraging time exposes males to greater risks of predation). Indeed, at any given time, only about 10 percent of the males in a population are in possession of such prey. This has led to some rather remarkable adaptations in male foraging behavior. Males will often sample, but then discard, prey that are too small to result in

FIGURE 6.5. Scorpionflies and nuptial gifts. To obtain mates, male scorpionflies present females with nuptial gifts, which are prey items that the females consume during courtship or mating. The male (top) provided the female (bottom) with a blowfly (at arrow), which she eats as they copulate. This system of nuptial gifts illustrates the direct benefits model of sexual selection, as the nuptial gifts provide the females with the direct benefit of nourishment. (Photo credit: Randy Thornhill)

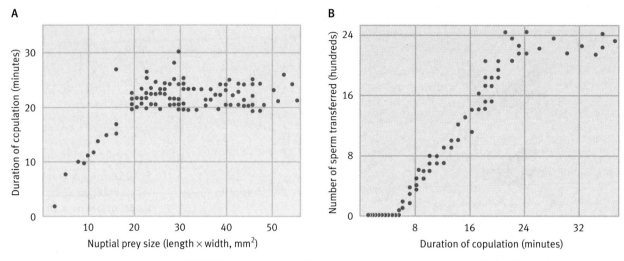

FIGURE 6.6. The direct benefits model and nuptial prey gifts. (A) Copulation time as a function of direct benefits. Male scorpionflies provide females with a nuptial prey gift. The greater the value of the gift, the longer a male is allowed to copulate with the recipient. **(B)** Longer copulation time leads to greater sperm transfer in scorpionflies. When males provide large nuptial gifts to females, the added copulation time translates into more sperm transferred to the female. *(From Thornhill, 1976, 1980b)*

long copulation opportunities with females. On the other hand, when females are hunting on their own, they almost never discard small prey.

Selection pressure on males to bring large nuptial gifts has also resulted in males stealing large prey from one another. In one study, Thornhill recorded such prey theft on 345 occasions; a follow-up study discovered that one way that males manage such thefts is to mimic the behavior of a female and then subsequently steal prey brought to them by other males (Thornhill, 1976, 1979a).

Thornhill's work not only provides evidence that females select among males based on resources that provide direct benefits, but it also illustrates the way that such choice shapes male behavior (both foraging and mating).

GOOD GENES AND MATE CHOICE

Females get more than direct resources such as food and shelter from their mates; they also get sperm, and with it genes that are passed on to offspring. Much theory, and some empirical work, now suggests that females are favored to choose mates that possess "good genes" (Andersson, 1994; Fisher, 1915; Kodric-Brown and Brown, 1984; Kokko et al., 2003; Mays and Hill, 2004). Good genes are those that code for some suite of favorable traits—traits that can be inherited by offspring of the appropriately choosy female. In **good genes models**, females who choose the males with genes best suited to their particular environment receive "indirect" benefits (Cameron et al., 2003), in the sense that their offspring receive some of the good genes—for example, genes associated with superior foraging skills or the ability to fend off predators—that led their mother to choose a male as a mate in the first place. As such, good genes models are sometimes called "indirect benefit models" of sexual selection.

Good genes models of sexual selection apply to mating systems in which the benefit(s) received by females lies in the genes residing on male sperm.

For example, in pronghorn antelopes (*Antilocapra americana*), males provide females with no direct benefits, and they do not appear to coerce females in any measurable way. Instead, female pronghorns undertake a long and energetic search to find mates with good genes by visiting different males that have harems of females. Early work had shown that females select males as mates based on a male's ability to defend his harem (Byers et al., 1994). Eventually, most females end up mating with a small subset of males in their population. This leads to high variance in harem size among males, and to males with large harems in prior years siring a disproportionate number of offspring. John Byers and Lissete Waits hypothesized that such males possessed good genes (and so they labeled them as "attractive" males). But how could a female know about a male's prior reproductive success? Here, the researchers assumed that females were using current harem defense as an indicator of good genes in males. If this is the case, then males with large harems (attractive males) should have offspring that are more likely to survive than offspring from other (nonattractive) males (Byers and Waits, 2006).

To test their hypothesis, Byers and Waits worked with a population of individually marked pronghorns that live in the National Bison Range in northwestern Montana. They followed females during the mating season and noted which males were selected as mates. When offspring were born, they too were marked (usually the first day they were born) and their survival was measured as a surrogate for fitness. Byers and Waits found that, in accordance with predictions from most good genes models, offspring from attractive males—males that most likely possessed superior genes leading to faster growth rates—had higher survival rates than offspring from other males. These findings suggested that females were selecting males based on some measure of a male's genetic quality (Figure 6.7).

Good genes models are somewhat controversial, for all such models must overcome two potentially difficult hurdles. First, how can females determine which males possess "good" genes? This is clearly a more daunting task than distinguishing among males in some more direct fashion (for example, by seeing how much potential for providing food males display during courtship). In pronghorns, females use harem defense as an indicator of good genes in males, but this is one of the few instances where ethologists and evolutionary biologists have good evidence of what male traits females use to infer good genes in

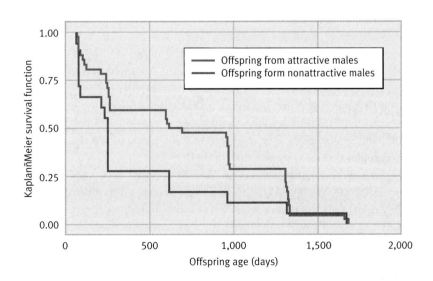

FIGURE 6.7. Indirect benefits in pronghorns. Offspring from attractive males—males that had large harems, high prior reproductive success, and that most likely possessed superior genes (green line)—had higher survival rates than offspring from other (nonattractive) males (orange line), suggesting that females were selecting males based on some measure of a male's genetic quality. *(From Byers and Waits, 2006, p. 16344)*

FIGURE 6.8. Peacock's tail. An example of an elaborate, costly trait that evolved in males as a result of sexual selection. *(Photo credit: Royalty-Free/ Corbis)*

potential mates. Second, how can females determine whether males have cheated in indicating that they possess good genes, given that natural selection would be likely to favor males that cheat in such a manner? That is, wouldn't males attempt to give the impression that they possess appropriately good genes, even if they don't? The answer is yes—natural selection should favor males who do just this. This, in turn, creates new natural selection pressures on females. Now only traits that are true and **honest indicators** of male genetic quality should be used by females when choosing mates. If females focus on such honest indicators, they can overcome the male cheater problem—at least temporarily.

PARASITE RESISTANCE AND GOOD GENES. Even if choosing honest indicators of male genetic quality is beneficial to females, they still face a difficult task. Which male traits should females accept as honest indicators of a male's genetic quality? One theory is that honest indicator traits should be generally "costly" to produce—the costlier the trait, the more difficult it is to fake, and hence the more likely it is that this trait is a true indicator of good genes (Zahavi, 1975; Zahavi and Zahavi, 1997; Figure 6.8). A costly trait that has been studied in the context of honest advertising is parasite resistance.

Females who choose males with strong resistance to parasites—a trait that would be difficult to fake—may receive indirect benefits in that they may be mating with individuals with "good genes." In this case, good genes refer to the genes conferring parasite resistance. The predictions of honest advertising models, when applied to parasites, go under the name of the "Hamilton-Zuk" hypothesis, after Bill Hamilton and Marlene Zuk, who first applied the idea of good genes to parasite resistance (Hamilton and Zuk, 1982).

Given that parasites that reside within their hosts (so-called endoparasites) can't be seen, how do females know which males have good genes with respect to endoparasite resistance? The answer to this dilemma must in some way lie in the female's ability to use some other male trait that correlates with the ability of a male to avoid being parasitized. If possessing trait X also means that males are good at fighting endoparasites, females can use trait X as a proxy for judging what they really need to know. That is, if information on internal parasitization is unavailable, using some other trait (X) that correlates well with the one of interest should be favored by natural selection. One such proxy cue appears to be body coloration (Figure 6.9). This has been studied extensively in many

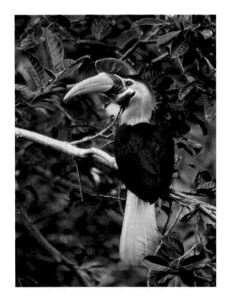

FIGURE 6.9. Elaborate coloration in males. In many birds, such as the red-knobbed hornbill (*Rhyticeros cassidix*), males are much more colorful than females as a result of different sexual selection pressures. *(Photo credit: Mark Jones/Minden Pictures)*

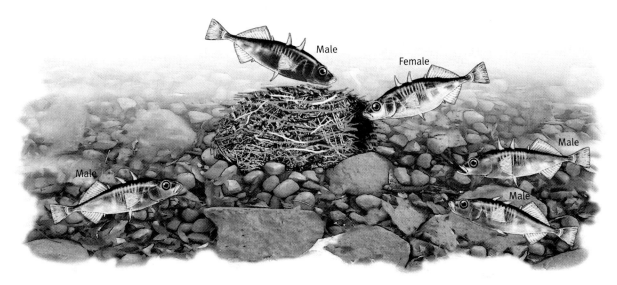

FIGURE 6.10. Color, parasites, and good genes. One reason stickleback females may prefer the most colorful (red) males is that color indicates resistance to parasites.

animal species, most prominently in birds and fish. Healthy males tend to be very colorful, while infected males have much duller colors (Milinski and Bakker, 1990; Figure 6.10). Although still the subject of some heated debate, numerous studies undertaken in birds and fish produce results that are consistent with the predictions of the Hamilton-Zuk hypothesis, in that females often choose the most colorful (and least parasitized) males (Figure 6.11).

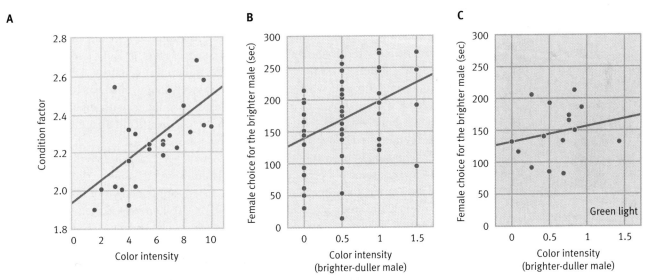

FIGURE 6.11. Female sticklebacks prefer brighter males. More colorful (redder) male sticklebacks were in better health **(A)** and were preferred by females **(B)**. Milinski and Bakker were able to show that it was color that females preferred, not other traits that bright-colored males might possess. **(C)** When females were given a choice between colorful and duller males, but red color was filtered out (using a green filter sheet), females did not prefer the brighter of the two males. *(From Milinski and Bakker, 1990, p. 331)*

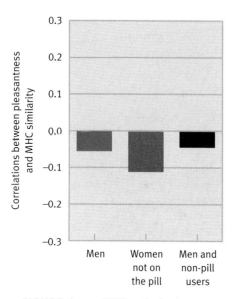

FIGURE 6.12. MHC and odor in humans. Subjects were asked about the "pleasantness" of the odor associated with a T-shirt worn by someone of the opposite sex. With the exception of women on oral contraceptives, men and women found the odor associated with MHC that was dissimilar from their own to be the most pleasant, and so there was a negative correlation between pleasantness and MHC similarity. *(From Wedekind and Furi, 1997)*

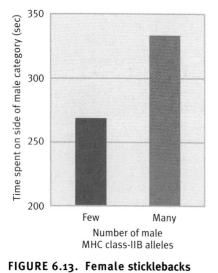

FIGURE 6.13. Female sticklebacks prefer males with more MHC alleles. Female sticklebacks spent more time on the side of the tank with males that had many different MHC alleles than with males that had few MHC alleles. *(From Reusch et al., 2001)*

MHC AND GOOD GENES. As we have seen above, if females are searching for honest indicators of good genes in males, honing in on traits associated with disease resistance should be favored by natural selection. One set of genes that is involved in disease resistance in many animals is known as the Major Histocompatibility Complex (MHC) (Milinski, 2006; Penn and Potts, 1998, 1999). Proteins produced by MHC genes guide the body in identifying "self" versus "foreign" cells (Wills, 1991).

A unique aspect of the MHC is that it is the most variable set of genes ever uncovered. Very few (if any) individuals have exactly the same MHC. Given this incredible genetic variability, biologists have predicted that animals may prefer mating with others who have a dissimilar MHC (Edwards and Hedrick, 1998; Ziegler et al., 2005). Such a preference could arise because offspring resulting from a mating between individuals with very different MHCs will have a new combination of MHC genes. Such new MHC combinations may be particularly good at providing immune system protection, since diseases evolve so rapidly that it is as if animals are trying to hit a moving target in trying to combat them. In this case, their weapon against such a moving target is a set of MHC genes that is constantly changing across generations.

Once again, females are faced with a problem—identifying which males have MHCs that differ from their own. Work using mice and rats suggests that females use odors to determine if another individual is a good MHC match— that is, whether he or she has sufficiently different MHC genes (Penn and Potts, 1998). This work in rodents has spurred experiments on odor, MHC, and mate choice in humans. To test the hypothesis that humans use MHC when choosing mates, and that odor plays a role in the process, male and female undergraduate students in Switzerland were tested by Claus Wedekind (Wedekind and Furi, 1997; Wedekind et al., 1995). In Wedekind and Furi's (1997) study, men were instructed to wear a cotton T-shirt for two nights. Blood samples from each of these males were then analyzed to determine MHC. Females also had blood samples taken for MHC analysis. These women were then given T-shirts from males with MHCs similar or dissimilar to their own. Women not on oral contraceptives consistently found the odors of the T-shirts from males with dissimilar MHCs sexier, suggesting that odor and MHC have a significant effect on female mate choice in humans (Figure 6.12). Wedekind found similar results when the men were subjects and women wore the T-shirts. Indeed, it seems that not only do females choose males with dissimilar MHC alleles, but they themselves use perfumes that specifically magnify their own MHC-mediated odors (Milinski and Wedekind, 2001).

Thorston Reusch and his colleagues have suggested that, in order to produce disease-resistant offspring, individuals should prefer mates with many MHC alleles, rather than choosing a mate that is dissimilar in MHC-related genes (Edwards and Hedrick, 1998; Reusch et al., 2001). They tested their "MHC allele counting" hypothesis using wild-caught stickleback fish from three populations of fish that reside in interconnected lakes. Reusch and his team used molecular genetic tools to sequence genes at a number of MHC loci in their sticklebacks. Sticklebacks from these three lakes varied in the number of MHC (class IIB) alleles they possessed, ranging from two to eight such alleles. When females were given a choice between males—some of whom had few MHC alleles and some of whom had many such alleles—they consistently preferred males with a greater number of MHC alleles (Figure 6.13).

In a fascinating series of experiments, Manfred Milinski and his colleagues (including Reusch) examined the proximate cues that female sticklebacks may be using to assess the MHC qualities of potential mates (Milinski et al., 2005). These researchers knew from prior work that females can assess the number of MHC alleles a male has using chemical cues alone. The question, then, was how do female sticklebacks do this? The answer may be related to the fact that the greater the number of MHC alleles found in an individual, the greater the number of MHC peptides, which are short strings of amino acids displayed at the cell surface (Rammensee et al., 1997). Milinski and his collaborators hypothesized that female sticklebacks were able to use odor to assess the diversity of MHC peptides for a particular male. More specifically, they proposed that MHC peptide ligands—that is, molecules that bind to proteins—were the key underlying proximate mechanism that females were assessing during mate choice.

Milinski and his team tested their ideas by simultaneously exposing a female to two different water columns. One column had water drawn from a tank that had male X swimming in it, and the other column also had water from male X's tank, but the water in this column was supplemented with MHC peptide ligands. The MHC peptide ligand diversity of both the male and the female were known, and a given pair together had either the optimal number of peptide ligands (producing offspring with intermediate MHC diversity and better disease resistance) or a suboptimal number of MHC peptides (Kurtz et al., 2004; Wegner et al., 2003a, 2003b).

What Milinski and his colleagues found was that when a pair had a less than optimal number of MHC peptide ligands, the addition of synthetic ligands to one side of the water column made the odor on that side more attractive, suggesting that the number of peptide ligands was the proximate cue being used by females to select males with good genes. Conversely, when a male and a female had the optimal number of MHC peptide ligands, the addition of ligands to one of the water columns made the odor associated with that column less attractive (Figure 6.14).

In a powerful follow-up experiment, Milinski's group tested a correlated prediction regarding odor and MHC peptide ligands and good genes. Soon after

FIGURE 6.14. Female sticklebacks use peptides to assess MHC. Female sticklebacks were given a choice between water from a tank containing a lone male, or water from a tank with that same male plus a certain number of added MHC peptides (x-axis). When the male and female had a combined number of MHC alleles that was below the optimum (left side of graph), the female preferred the water from the tank with the male and the added peptides. As the number of combined MHC alleles in the male and female increased to some level above the optimum (middle), female preference shifted to the water that contained only the male and no additional MHC peptides (right side). *(From Milinski et al., 2005)*

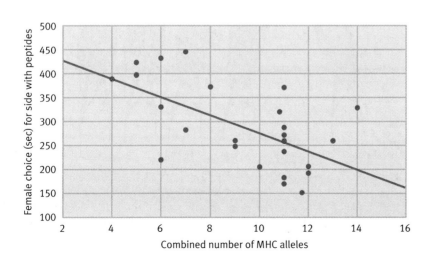

females give birth, they avidly forage, often raiding nests of other sticklebacks and eating their eggs. Males guard nests from such female attacks. What this means is that a female should be repelled by the very male MHC peptide ligand odor she was attracted to prior to mating, because such a repulsion would reduce the chance that she accidentally raids the nest of her mate and cannibalizes her own eggs. When Milinski and his team tested whether foraging females were repelled by the MHC peptide ligand odor of their former mates, they found strong evidence that this was indeed the case.

SYMMETRY AND GOOD GENES. Over the last decade, a considerable literature has developed on "symmetry" in the way traits are expressed, and what role this symmetry may play in sexual selection. The work on symmetry is the result of a long search for generalizable traits that can be used as indicators of the overall health and vigor of an individual. Wouldn't it be wonderful, the argument goes, if there were a simple cue, or set of cues, that individuals could hone in on and use to determine the underlying genetic quality (with respect to health, resistance to disease, and so on) of potential mates? Symmetry may be such a cue (Figure 6.15).

Evolutionary biologists have focused their search for some measure of health and vigor by examining what is called **developmental stability** (Møller and Swaddle, 1998; Swaddle, 2003). Developmental stability is a measure of how well an organism handles changing environments as it matures. The underlying premise here is that organisms that can handle changing environments may well be those favored by the process of natural selection. Suppose that individuals do in fact differ in their ability to respond to the changing (and often adverse) conditions they face throughout their development. How would an individual be able to assess which potential mates handle changing environmental conditions during development well and which potential mates don't handle such changing conditions during development well? Symmetry may be one way.

In most animals, **symmetry** is a measure of the similarity of the left and right sides of an organism. For example, consider the human face. One way to measure facial symmetry would be to calculate the distance from the middle

FIGURE 6.15. Symmetry and good genes. If males differ in the symmetry of their tail feathers, and this is a reflection of underlying genetic quality, females may select more symmetric males.

Symmetrical facial features

Less symmetrical facial features

FIGURE 6.16. Symmetry in the human face. The face on the left is more symmetrical than that on the right. Symmetry may be a cue of developmental homeostasis and is used as one cue in human mate choice.

of the nose to the corner of each of the eyes (Figure 6.16). If the distance to the corner of the right eye and the distance to the corner of the left eye were the same, this one component of the human face would be perfectly symmetrical.

When the symmetry of a trait can be assessed by others, then symmetry might be used in mating decisions. Why? Because if symmetry indicates that a potential mate has the genetic constitution to weather developmental perturbations (for example, disease, mutation, injury), then choosing such a mate increases the probability that your offspring will also be able to handle developmental perturbations (Møller and Thornhill, 1998). Such choices will be favored by natural selection.

While the work on good genes, symmetry, and mate choice is fairly controversial (Gangestad and Simpson, 2000; Rowe et al., 1997; Simmons et al., 1999; Swaddle and Cuthill, 1995), it is thought-provoking, and so we will examine one case study here. In a 1998 paper, Steve Gangestad and Randy Thornhill posed the following question: Do human females change their reliance on symmetry as a function of menstrual cycle? Their hypothesis was straightforward: If symmetry is important to females as a way of assessing male genetic quality, then they should be much more attuned to this when ovulating than at other times during the month (Gangestad and Thornhill, 1998). To test this, Gangestad and Thornhill began by giving women T-shirts worn by different males.

Using forty-one college women as subjects, Gangestad and Thornhill distributed "smelly" T-shirts that had been worn by males for two days (using a protocol similar to the one described earlier for MHC and human mate choice). Females were asked to rank the scent of a given T-shirt in terms of the attractiveness of the donor. The researchers also measured the symmetry of the male T-shirt donors and the reaction of females to the males' T-shirts at different periods during a normal ovulation cycle. Women did indeed show a stronger preference for the T-shirts of symmetric males—males that they never saw—just at the time when they were most fertile (Figure 6.17). In a follow-up study, Gangestad and his colleagues found that during their fertile periods, women with spouses showing a high degree of asymmetry were more attracted to other men than were women whose husbands were more symmetric (Gangestad et al., 2005).

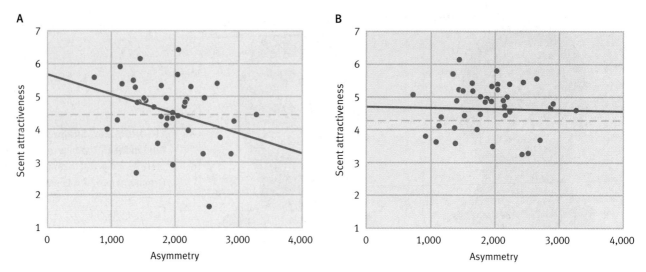

FIGURE 6.17. Smell, attraction, and fertility in women. College females smelled T-shirts worn by males for two days, and then the women rated the attractiveness of the scent of forty-one T-shirts worn by the men. **(A)** Women who were close to ovulation in their menstrual cycle preferred the scent of more symmetric males, while **(B)** women at a low fertility point in their cycle showed no such preference. The dashed line in the two graphs depicts the mean attractiveness rating, given a clean, unworn T-shirt. *(From Gangestad and Thornhill, 1998, p. 930)*

RUNAWAY SEXUAL SELECTION

Of all the evolutionary models we have explored, models of **runaway sexual selection** are probably the most difficult to understand. These models, first proposed by Sir Ronald Fisher, assume that two genes exist: a gene that codes for a particular trait in males, and a gene that codes for mating preference in females. Such models can be expanded to consider the case of numerous genes controlling for male and female traits, but it will be easiest to follow the case of two genes. In runaway selection models, specific alleles from our two genes become *associated with each other through time*—when one allele is present in male offspring in a clutch, the other allele is likely to be present in female offspring from that clutch (Andersson, 1994; Fisher, 1958; Kirkpatrick, 1982; Mead and Arnold, 2004).

To see how this runaway selection process works, imagine a population in which some fraction of the females have a heritable preference for brightly colored males, and the remainder of the females choose males randomly with respect to color. In this population, the degree of male coloration is also a heritable trait—some males are more colorful than others. So, we have a group of females, some of whom prefer brightly colored males and some of whom don't, and a group of males, some of whom are more colorful than others. Now, we will make an important assumption that is critical to many good genes models—the genes coding for both male color and female preference are present in both males and females, but they are only expressed, that is, "switched on," in the appropriate sex (preference genes in females, color genes in males).

Females that mate with colorful males should not only produce colorful sons but also daughters that possess their mother's genetically coded *preference* for colorful males. Over time, the alleles in females that code for the preference for colorful males and the alleles in males that code for color in males become linked in the sense that, as the frequency of one changes, the frequency of the other changes as well. Once this positive feedback loop is set in motion, it can, under certain conditions, "run away," like a snowball rolling down a snowy mountain. Across generations, selection may produce increasingly exaggerated male traits (for example, male color pattern) and stronger and stronger female preferences for such exaggerated traits.

STALK-EYED FLIES AND RUNAWAY SELECTION. Empirical evidence of runaway sexual selection comes from Jerry Wilkinson and his colleagues' work on the stalk-eyed fly (Wilkinson, 1993; Wilkinson and Reillo, 1994; Wilkinson et al., 1998a). In stalk-eyed flies, females prefer to mate with males possessing eyes that are at the end of long eye "stalks" (Figure 6.18). In one treatment of an experiment that spanned over thirteen generations of flies, males with the largest eye stalks were selected and allowed to breed with females. In a second treatment, males with the shortest eye stalks were allowed to breed. In neither case were females chosen for any particular trait; that is, females were selected randomly in these two treatments. Not surprisingly, in the treatment where long eye-stalk length was selected for thirteen generations, the average male eye stalk increased in length, producing a more exaggerated version of this trait. Conversely, in the case where individuals with short eye stalks were selected, the size of the average male eye stalk decreased in length.

The critical finding in this study, however, did not center on the length of male eye stalk per se. At the heart of the runaway sexual selection model was the discovery of a positive link between the length of the male eye stalk and the *female preference for this trait*. Recall that in both treatments—the long eye stalk and the short eye stalk male treatments—the females who mated with males were selected at random. All of the selection pressures were with respect to male eye-stalk length. Yet, after just a few generations, when females were given the choice between mating with males with short and long eye stalks, females from the short eye-stalk line preferred males with short eye stalks (Figure 6.19). This preference for short male eye-stalk length by females in the short eye-stalk line changed directly in response to selection pressure on *males*, in accordance with the prediction of the runaway selection model. In the long eye-stalk line, females preferred males with long eye stalks, but then so did females who had not been subject to any selection treatment (that is, females in a control line of flies). In other words, contrary to predictions of the runaway selection model, Wilkinson and his colleagues did not find evidence that selection on males in the long eye-stalk treatment produced significant changes in female preference for eye-stalk length. While there were a number of possible reasons why results were similar in the long eye-stalk length treatment and the control, Wilkinson and Reillo believe that female preference might very well have been detected had the experiment gone on for a longer period of time. Whether or not that is the case can only be ascertained by further experimentation.

SENSORY BIAS AND THE EMERGENCE OF MATE CHOICE

Before we complete our discussion of evolutionary models of mate choice, we need to consider one last model known as the **sensory exploitation, sensory bias**, or **preexisting bias** model of mate choice (Endler and McLellan, 1988;

FIGURE 6.18. Stalk-eyed flies and runaway selection. Male stalk-eyed flies show marked variation in the length of their eye stalks. Wilkinson bred lines of flies with long and short eye stalks to test the runaway model of sexual selection. *(Photo credit: Mark Moffett)*

FIGURE 6.19. Genetic correlation of male trait and female preference in stalk-eyed flies. Wilkinson and Reillo selected for males with long (L males) and short (S males) eye stalks. In both selection lines, females that mated were selected at random. When females in the long and short eye treatments, however, were given a choice between males, they preferred males from their own selection treatment group (females from the long line chose males with long eye stalks, as did unselected [control] females, but females from the short line did not choose males with long eye stalks but instead chose males with short eye stalks), suggesting that female preference was genetically linked to the male trait being selected (stalk length). *(From Wilkinson and Reillo, 1994)*

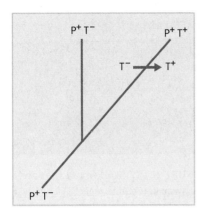

FIGURE 6.20. Sensory exploitation model. In the sensory exploitation model, female preference (P+) is assumed to predate the male trait (T) that is preferred. In one lineage here (shown in orange), the male trait is immediately preferred once it appears (T+). *(From Ryan and Rand, 1993, p. 189).*

FIGURE 6.21. Primate preference for red. There is growing evidence from work on sexual selection in primates that females prefer males with red fur coloration and/or red facial skin, as seen in this red uakari. *(Photo credit: Claus Meyer/Minden Pictures)*

Ryan, 1990; West-Eberhard, 1979, 1981). The idea here is that females initially prefer male traits that elicit the greatest amount of stimulation from their sensory systems (Ryan and Keddy-Hector, 1992). This often means that neurobiological systems that are already in place in the female are "tapped into" and used by males in the context of sexual selection.

To better understand sensory biases, consider the following example. Suppose that, for whatever reason, red berries are the most nutritious food source available to a fruit-eating, blue-feathered songbird species. Females who are best able to search out and subsequently eat red berries survive and reproduce better (Rodd et al., 2002; Smith et al., 2004). Thus, natural selection will operate on the neurobiology of females so that they will be acutely aware of the color red, and hone in on red things in their environment (Kirkpatrick and Ryan, 1991).

Once a preference for all things red is in place, if red feathers should suddenly arise in males of this normally blue-feathered species, birds with these red feathers may be chosen as mates because the female's nervous system is already designed to preferentially respond to red objects. Males with red feathers, then, are exploiting the preexisting neurobiologically based preferences of females—preferences that evolved as a result of other selection pressures.

The sensory bias model leads to a clear prediction regarding phylogenetic history. When we look at a phylogeny that includes information on both female preference and the male trait preferred by females, the female preference trait should predate the appearance of the male trait (Figure 6.20). In our case of red berries, the preference for red should be in place before red feathers are present. In a moment, we shall examine two case studies that test this sort of prediction.

One thing to keep in mind as we discuss the sensory bias hypothesis is that it was designed to elucidate the *origin*, not the long-term maintenance, of female preference. That is to say, the sensory bias hypothesis postulates how a female preference initially arose in a population, not how it was maintained in a population by natural selection over evolutionary time. So, as we walk through the sensory bias model, remember that the three other models we have discussed (direct benefits, good genes, and runaway selection) focus on how natural selection acts on mate choice, but the sensory bias model focuses on the emergence of mate choice.

TRICOLOR VISION, FRUITS, AND SENSORY BIASES IN PRIMATES. Let's continue with our discussion of red food and a possible sensory bias for red coloration, but now move from a hypothetical bird example to a real study involving primates. There is growing evidence from work on sexual selection in primates that females prefer males with red fur coloration and/or red facial skin (Sumner and Mollon, 2003; Figure 6.21). The question with respect to sensory bias is whether female preference for red coloration in males arose because of a sensory system that favored such coloration (Fernandez and Morris, 2007). To answer that question, we begin with a discussion of the primate visual system, particularly with regard to foraging.

Whereas other mammals have two types of photoreceptor cones in the eye (dichromatic vision), many, but not all, primate species have three types of cones—that is, they possess trichromatic vision. Possessing a third type of cone allows some primates to detect red-orange colors, whereas many other mammals are colorblind in this spectrum. Ethologists and others have suggested that trichromatic vision allows primates to more easily pick out red-orange fruits and edible ripe red leaves in a complex natural environment (Allen, 1879; Lucas et al., 1998; Mollon, 1989).

Peter Sumner and J. D. Mollon examined this possibility by measuring the visual (spectral) properties of the fruit and leaves eaten by six primate species (including chimps and two species of baboons) (Sumner and Mollon, 2000). When they compared the visual systems of these primates with the spectral properties of both the fruit and leaves these animals ate, they concluded that trichromatic vision provided primates with an enhanced ability to detect red foods (fruits and leaves) in a visually complex environment. Indeed, individuals in many (but not all) primate species with trichromatic color vision prefer red fruits and leaves as food (Lucas et al., 2003).

Returning to the sensory bias hypothesis, we can now ask whether the female mating preference for red coloration in males might have originated as a sensory bias associated with trichromatic vision and its effect on foraging for red food items (Allen, 1879). To address this question, Andre Fernandez and Molly Morris used already published data on both color vision and red fur/face color in primates and superimposed this data on a phylogenetic tree of more than 200 primate taxa (Fernandez and Morris, 2007). This phylogenetic data allowed them to test the sensory bias hypothesis by examining whether trichromatic vision that allows for the detection of red-orange colors predated a preference for red fur/face coloration. If trichromatic vision appeared after red fur/face coloration, the sensory bias hypothesis must be rejected. If trichromatic vision appeared before red fur/face coloration, however, then this is consistent with the sensory bias hypothesis.

Fernandez and Morris's phylogenetic analysis is consistent with the sensory bias hypothesis for the origination of female mate preference. They found that trichromatic vision evolved earlier than red coloration in males (Figure 6.22). This suggests that the *origin* of the female preference for red-colored males was linked to a sensory bias in females for foraging on red food items in their environment.

A Color Vision

B Skin Color

FIGURE 6.22. Color vision and red skin in primates. (A) A phylogenetic tree in which the presence of trichromatic color vision is shown to be ancestral for most modern lineages. The degree to which a pie graph is filled with black indicates the presence of color vision; white indicates dichromatic/monochromatic vision. **(B)** A phylogenetic tree for red skin color. The degree to which a pie graph is filled with black indicates the presence of red skin in males; white indicates the absence of red skin. In both phylogenetic trees, asterisks indicate that there is statistical confidence for reconstruction of the trait in that branch of the phylogeny. A comparison of these two phylogenies shows that trichromatic vision evolved earlier than red coloration in males. *(From Fernandez and Morris, 2007, p. 14)*

FIGURE 6.23. Frog calls and sensory bias. *Physalaemus pustulosus* males (one of whom is pictured here) add a unique "chuck" sound to the end of their advertisement calls. The calls of *Physalaemus coloradorum* males lack a whine. The calls of these two species have been used to test models of the sensory bias hypothesis. *(Photo credit: Michael Ryan)*

FROGS AND SENSORY BIASES.   One of the first studies of sensory exploitation involved two species of frogs—*Physalaemus pustulosus* and *Physalaemus coloradorum* (Ryan et al., 1990; Figure 6.23). Males in these two species use advertisement calls to attract females. As is the case for most species in the genus *Physalaemus*, males of both the *pustulosus* and *coloradorum* species begin such an advertisement with what is referred to as a high-frequency "whine." Females pick up the whine part of a male's call through the basilar papilla in the inner ear.

Pustulosus males are unique in that most add a low-frequency "chuck" sound to the end of their call. When *pustulosus* females choose between *pustulosus* males that chuck and those that don't, they prefer to mate with the former. Females detect the chuck through the amphibian papilla section of the inner ear, which is more sensitive to low-frequency sounds. Michael Ryan and his colleagues hypothesized that the preference for chucks in female *pustulosus* was the result of a sensory bias in favor of such low-frequency sounds.

Phylogenetic and behavioral evidence support the contention that the preference for chucks is due to sensory bias. To see this, we need to return to the *coloradorum* species. The chuck part of the call is absent in the call of *coloradorum* males. Indeed, when Ryan and his colleagues used molecular and morphological data to reconstruct the evolutionary history of the genus *Physalaemus*, they found that the common ancestor of *coloradorum* and *pustulosus* did not use a chuck call—that is, not only do male *coloradorum* not use the chuck call, but the chuck call was never used in any of the species that make up the evolutionary lineage leading to *coloradorum*. Yet, when modern computer technology is used to add a chuck call to the end of pre-recorded *coloradorum* male calls, *coloradorum* females show a preference for calls that include a chuck. In other words, Ryan's experimental manipulation of calls suggests that as soon as chucks appear in a *coloradorum* population, females prefer males that produce such calls. These studies suggest the auditory circuitry in *Physalaemus* frogs was designed in such a way as to prefer a certain class of sounds—low-frequency calls like chucks. The *coloradorum* studies provide evidence that the preference for chucks predated the actual appearance of chucks in the *Physalaemus* species, in accordance with the sensory bias hypothesis.

With an understanding of some of the basic evolutionary models of sexual selection that ethologists employ, we can now move on to a discussion of learning and mate choice.

Learning and Mate Choice

While evolutionary models of female mate choice have greatly expanded our understanding of sexual selection, these models do not usually incorporate the idea that individuals may *learn* various aspects of mate selection. To get a more complete understanding of mate choice, psychologists and ethologists have conducted many experiments examining the role of learning in selecting mates (Domjan, 2006). Some of the experimental work on learning and mate choice has been done in the field. But many experiments on mate choice have been undertaken in the laboratory under controlled conditions. Although they appear removed from the normal environment of the animal, the controlled stimulus-response experiments done in the lab can be quite instructive with respect to what they tell us about general aspects of animal mate choice. For example, controlled laboratory work on conditioned stimuli (see Chapter 4) and mating behavior across a number of species has found that, after exposure to a conditioned sexual stimulus, males are quicker to copulate, become better competitors with other males, display higher levels of courtship, and produce more sperm and progeny (Domjan, 2006; Figure 6.24).

SEXUAL IMPRINTING

One classic form of learning studied in the context of mate choice is **sexual imprinting** (Bateson, 1978; Lorenz, 1935; ten Cate and Vos, 1999). In sexual imprinting, young individuals quickly learn mating preferences from their interactions with adults (most often their parents). Normally, imprinting is restricted to some small time window during normal development, but the length of this window varies dramatically across species (including humans) and behavioral contexts (Bereczkei et al., 2004).

Ethologists have developed numerous ways to experimentally examine sexual imprinting, including:

1. Using the cross-fostering approach we discussed in Chapter 2. In the case of imprinting, the question of interest would be whether offspring raised by adoptive parents show different mating preferences than those raised by biological parents, and whether such preferences can be linked to something about the behavior or morphology of adopted parents (Cooke et al., 1972, 1976; Cooke and McNally, 1975).
2. Employing the "novel trait" approach, in which offspring are raised by parents that have some novel trait that an experimenter has introduced.

Let's examine the novel trait approach to studying sexual imprinting by focusing on Klaudia Witte and her colleagues' work on the mannikin bird, *Lonchura leucogastroides* (Witte et al., 2000). To study the role of sexual imprinting in this species, Witte added a novel trait to some adults in her population. The novel trait was a red feather that the researchers taped to the forehead of adult mannikins, so that the feather stood up like a crest. The key imprinting question for Witte and her colleagues was whether offspring that were raised in the presence of such adults adorned with a red head feather showed a sexual preference for individuals with red feathers when they matured. To examine this, Witte raised juvenile mannikins in one of four groups. Group 1 served as a control in which offspring were raised with their mother and father, both of whom lacked the red feather. In Group 2, offspring were raised with their mother and father, each of whom had a red head feather experimentally attached to their forehead by Witte and her colleagues. In Group 3, offspring were raised with an unadorned mother, but a father with a red feather; in Group 4, offspring were raised with an unadorned father, but a mother with a red feather.

When offspring reached sixty days of age, they were separated from their parents and their mate preferences were examined. These birds were given the choice between two members of the opposite sex—one of whom had a red head feather added, and one of whom did not. Witte and her team found results suggesting that young mannikins imprinted on the red head feather of

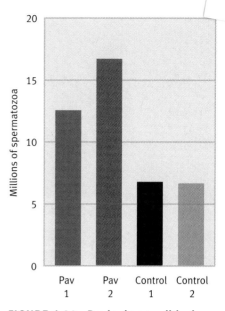

FIGURE 6.24. Pavlovian conditioning and number of sperm. Two different genetic lines of male quail (Pav 1 and Pav 2) learned to pair a distinctive experimental chamber with a chance to mate with a female. Males were then placed in the chamber with an artificial female. Subsequent to that, spermatozoa samples were taken. Males from both lines who had learned to pair the chamber with the chance to mate produced significantly more spermatozoa than control males (Control 1 and Control 2, which consisted of males from the two genetic lines who had not been given the chance to associate these two cues). (*From Domjan et al., 1998*)

their parents, and expressed a preference for such adorned birds when they themselves matured. Compared to the control groups (in which individuals often preferred unadorned mates), males raised with a mother with a red feather preferred females with red head feathers as mates, and females raised with a father with a red feather preferred males with red head feathers as mates.

Ethologists also examine the proximate underpinnings of imprinting. To see this, let's return to the dendritic spines that we first discussed in Chapter 3. Recall that neuroethologists have argued that an increase in dendritic spines is often associated with learning. If this is correct, it might also be true that when animals rely *less* on learning—including learning about potential mates—we might see a decrease in dendritic spine density. In the context of sexual imprinting, this might manifest itself as a decrease in dendritic spine density soon after an individual has imprinted on the phenotype of those of the opposite sex, since it has now completed learning about what traits to search for in a mate, and rarely changes such learned preferences after imprinting. Evidence has been found for such a decrease in spine density in the zebra finch.

Following up on early work by Klause Immelmann, behavioral studies have shown that when a male zebra finch is raised by its parents for the first month of life, but then kept in isolation for two months, he often imprints on the phenotype of the first female he encounters after isolation (Bischof and Clayton, 1991; Immelmann, 1972; Immelmann et al., 1991). When Hans Bischof and his colleagues measured dendritic spine density in one area of the zebra finch brain (the media neo/hypostriatum or MNH area), they found a decrease in the spine density after exposure to a female (Bischof and Rollenhagen, 1999; Rollenhagen and Bischof, 1991, 1994). That is, compared to spine density when males were in isolation, Bischof found fewer dendritic spines in males that had completed the process of sexual imprinting and hence were less reliant on learning about who to choose as a mate.

To further investigate what animals can learn about mate choice, we turn now to a discussion of mate choice in Japanese quail.

LEARNING AND MATE CHOICE IN JAPANESE QUAIL

Michael Domjan and his colleagues have been studying learning and mate choice in the Japanese quail for the better part of the last twenty years. With respect to mate choice, Domjan and his colleagues have found evidence that classical conditioning (see Chapter 4) in adults affects mate choice and that adult male Japanese quail will quickly learn to stay in areas in which they have the opportunity to mate with a female (Domjan et al., 1986; Mahometa and Domjan, 2005; Mills et al., 1997). While earlier work had demonstrated that sexual imprinting affects Japanese quail mate choice (Gallagher, 1976), Nash and Domjan found that learning can also play another role in mate choice. They examined whether adult classical conditioning might override the effects of sexual imprinting as a juvenile (Nash and Domjan, 1991).

Nash and Domjan began by using different strains, or varieties, of Japanese quail. Each trial in their experiment had three subjects—an adult male quail from the standard "brown" colored strain, an adult female quail from the brown strain, and an adult female quail from a lighter-colored "blond" strain of quail. The brown males used in this study were raised with other brown quail, and

FIGURE 6.25. **Overriding an imprinted sexual preference.** Male Japanese quail were raised in an environment with normal brown-colored quail and should have imprinted on brown females as future mates. These males were then put through a battery of tests in which experimenters measured the percentage of time they spent near a window. First they saw a blond female on the other side of the window followed by numerous chances to mate with her (Phase 1). Then they saw a brown female through the window, but they were not allowed to mate with her (Phase 2). Lastly, they were tested to see how much time they spent near blond and brown females (Phase 3). In Phase 3, B = exposure to a blond female, N = exposure to a normal (brown) female. A significant preference for blond females was uncovered. *(Based on Domjan, 1992, p. 53)*

these males had already sexually imprinted on the phenotype of brown females. All else being equal, when such males matured, they typically showed a strong preference for brown females as mates. But all else was not equal in Nash and Domjan's experiment.

In phase 1 of a trial, a brown male was allowed to see a blond female and was then given the opportunity to copulate with her. In phase 2 of a trial, the same male could see a brown female quail, but was never in physical contact with her. In other words, a given male learned that, in the laboratory, the presence of a blond female meant a mating opportunity, but the presence of a brown female did not. In the last phase of the experiment, males were tested to see how much time they spent near brown and blond females. The researchers found that blonds elicited a much stronger response (Figure 6.25). That is, adult-stage learning about who was likely to be a receptive mate overrode the effects of early sexual imprinting.

Cultural Transmission and Mate Choice

In addition to individual learning, the role of cultural transmission has also been examined with respect to mate choice and sexual selection. One area of sexual selection that has been explored is the extent to which **mate-choice copying** occurs—that is, when a female's mate-choice preference is affected by the preference of other females in her population (Dugatkin, 2000; Pruett-Jones, 1992; Westneat et al., 2000; see Chapter 5). Another area that involves cultural transmission and sexual selection is how song learning can affect mate choice in birds (Freeberg, 1998, 2004).

We will begin our discussion of cultural transmission and mate choice by providing an operational definition of mate-choice copying. We will then ask whether females copy the mate choice of others, and if so, under what conditions. Subsequently, we will examine some empirical aspects of mate-choice copying (see Chapter 5).

Following Stephen Pruett-Jones's definition, we will say that mate-choice copying has occurred when a male's probability of being preferred as a mate increases (or decreases) as the result of having been preferred (or not preferred) by a female in the past (Pruett-Jones, 1992). In other words, if a male has an X percent chance of mating if he has not recently mated, and a Y percent chance if he has recently mated, the effect of mate-choice copying is defined as the difference between Y and X. Mate-choice copying occurs if $Y - X > 0$; the greater $Y - X$, the stronger the effect of mate-choice copying. One nice feature of this operational definition is that these probabilities can be measured, and hence a mate-choice copying hypothesis can be supported or refuted by available data (Dugatkin, 1996a).

MATE-CHOICE COPYING IN GROUSE. Surrounded by Scotch pine, Norway spruce, and birch trees, black grouse mating arenas—technically referred to as **leks**—are interspersed throughout the bogs of central Finland, Wales, and Scotland (Figure 6.26). Many male black grouse (*Tetrao tetrix*) gather together at leks and occupy small territories, which they defend. Males then display—strutting about with their tail spread out, flapping their wings, jumping in the air, and hissing—to attract females to mate with them. As with many lek-breeding species, a single "top male" grouse obtains about 80 percent of all the matings at an arena. Before mating, females visit leks many times, often in groups that stay together and synchronize their trips to various male territories within an arena (Höglund and Alatalo, 1995). Jacob Höglund and his colleagues observed that males that had mated were likely to mate again fairly quickly, suggesting a possible role for mate-choice copying among females (Höglund et al., 1990). In addition, older females mated, on average, three days earlier than younger females, suggesting that mate-choice copying, if it occurred, was most common among younger females. This is what one would expect, as young and

FIGURE 6.26. Black grouse and mate-choice copying. Males try to attract females with whom to mate by displaying on leks. This involves strutting about, flapping their wings, jumping in the air, and hissing while females observe. Once some females have chosen mates, mate-choice copying will play a role in the mating decisions of other female black grouse, as they choose to mate with the males chosen by other females. *(Photo credit: Jan Smit/Foto Natura/Minden Pictures)*

inexperienced females stand to gain much more from watching older females than vice versa.

Höglund and his colleagues subsequently undertook a fascinating experiment using stuffed "dummy" females placed on male territories within a lek (Höglund et al., 1995). In this experiment, each of seven randomly chosen males on a particular lek had stuffed black grouse females (dummy females) placed on their respective territories early in the morning before real females arrived. Males courted these dummy females and even mounted them and attempted numerous copulations. After observing the males on the lek, females were more interested in mating with a male who had copulated with other females on his territory, even if they were dummy females. Because dummies were placed on the territories of randomly chosen males, this finding suggests that mate-choice copying, rather than some set of physical traits possessed by males, explains the skew in male reproductive success among black grouse.

Mate-choice copying likely plays a role in another species of grouse as well. In the early 1990s, Robert Gibson and his colleagues addressed the question of female mate-choice copying in sage grouse (Gibson et al., 1991). They examined the mating behavior of sage grouse females (*Centrocercus urophasianus*) in two different leks over a four-year period. One of their hypotheses regarding mate-choice copying behavior was that the unanimity of female mate choice would increase as more females mated on a given day, because more opportunities to observe and imitate would exist on such days.

To test this hypothesis, each day Gibson and his team arrived early in the morning before a lek formed and then observed all interactions on that lek—when females arrived, which males mated, which males courted, and so on—using telescopes. Gibson and his colleagues tested their mate-choice copying hypothesis using data from fifty-six days of observation. They began by using a computer simulation to estimate how often females would have chosen the same male on a lek if they had *not* been copying each other. Then they compared the results of their computer simulation with the data they had gathered on the relationship between the number of females visiting the lek and the unanimity of female mate choice. This comparison uncovered support for the mate-copying hypothesis, as the unanimity of female mate choice increased as more females appeared, and this increase occurred more quickly than expected by chance (Figure 6.27).

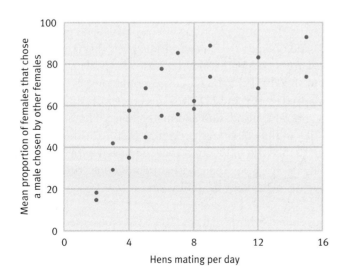

FIGURE 6.27. Female mate-choice copying in sage grouse. As predicted by models of mate-choice copying, when the number of hens mating per day increased, so too did the proportion of females choosing to mate with a male chosen by other females. The green points are the observed matings, and the orange points are the expected matings if the females had not been copying the mate choices of other females. *(From Gibson et al., 1991)*

MATE-CHOICE COPYING IN MICE. Recent work has examined the underlying endocrinological and genetic basis of mate-choice copying. Elena Choleris, Martin Kavaliers, and their colleagues studied mate-choice copying in mice, with a particular emphasis on the role of oxytocin in facilitating such copying. Oxytocin (OT) is a hormone secreted by the pituitary gland, and it appears to play an important role in social behaviors, including mate choice, maternal bonds, and individual recognition (Choleris et al., 2004; Ferguson et al., 2001; Pedersen and Boccia, 2002). Mice with deletions of the OT gene—so-called OT "knockout" mice—appear to learn normally, except in the context of *social learning* and mate choice (Choleris et al., 2003; Ferguson et al., 2000).

Choleris, Kavaliers, and their team studied mate-choice copying in three lines of mice, two of which were normal—that is, these mice had the OT gene—and one of which was an OT knockout line of mice. They allowed a female to choose between two healthy males, one of which had recently associated with an estrous female (and hence had traces of the odor of that estrous female in his area) and one of which had not. Females from the two normal lines of mice copied the mate choice of other females—they were attracted to males that had recently associated with estrous females. Females from the OT knockout line, however, did not copy the other females' mate choice. In conjunction with a number of control experiments run by Choleris and her team, these results: (1) suggest that knocking out the gene for oxytocin has the specific effect of inhibiting mate-choice copying behavior in mice, and (2) help us better understand the proximate underpinnings of copying.

SONG LEARNING AND MATE CHOICE IN COWBIRDS

Mate-choice copying is not the only means by which cultural transmission can affect mate choice in animals. Song learning in birds provides another good example of cultural transmission and sexual selection (see Chapter 5). One thing that is common to almost all songbirds is that they *learn* the songs they sing. In particular, much of the song-learning process involves learning songs from others, who are often referred to as tutors. Songs, in other words, are largely culturally transmitted.

Todd Freeberg undertook a series of experiments with cowbirds to learn more about the cultural transmission of birdsong and its long-term consequences for mate choice in this species (Freeberg, 2004). He collected juvenile and adult birds from two different populations of cowbirds—one population from South Dakota (SD) and one population from Indiana (IN) (Freeberg, 1998). Freeberg chose these particular populations because cowbirds display different social behaviors and sing different songs across populations.

Freeberg used the IN and SD birds in a cross-fostering experiment designed to examine cultural transmission and mate choice. He raised juvenile SD birds with either SD adults or IN adults (Figure 6.28). In Freeberg's experiment, if cowbirds behave like the individuals they are raised with, regardless of whether these individuals are from their native populations, then this would suggest a certain level of behavioral flexibility, and a role for cultural transmission of birdsong.

When juvenile cowbirds matured, they were observed in a large aviary that contained *unfamiliar* birds from both the SD and IN populations. Freeberg found that when placed into such groups, birds paired up and mated with others

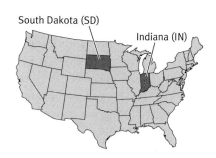
South Dakota (SD)
Indiana (IN)

Regime 1
Adults from SD
Juveniles from SD

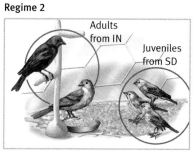
Regime 2
Adults from IN
Juveniles from SD

FIGURE 6.28. Cross-fostering. In Freeberg's cross-fostering experiments, juvenile cowbirds from South Dakota were raised with adults from South Dakota (regime 1) or adults from Indiana (regime 2).

who came from the same rearing regime (IN or SD) in which they were raised. That is, SD birds raised with SD adults preferred SD birds as mates, and SD birds raised with IN birds preferred IN birds as mates—the mating preferences of the SD birds were strongly dependent on the social environment in which the birds were raised.

Freeberg and his colleagues explored what it was about the social environment during development that might be responsible for SD birds preferring mates that were like the birds with which they were raised. The answer appears to involve copying and perhaps sexual imprinting. Males copied the songs of the adults with which they were raised, regardless of whether those adults were from South Dakota or Indiana (Freeberg et al., 2001). Furthermore, female SD birds prefer songs that are like those of the males with which they are raised (West et al., 1998). This preference might either be an example of females copying the song preferences of adult females in their population, or it might be a consequence of females imprinting on the songs of the males they were exposed to during development. Further work is needed to distinguish between these possibilities.

Male-Male Competition and Sexual Selection

As mentioned at the start of the chapter, once Darwin introduced the notion of sexual selection, much of the work in this area focused on *intrasexual selection*, which typically manifests itself in male-male competition for females (although female-female competition for males does occur in "sex-reversed" species such as the American jacana, *Jacana spinosa*, and the pipefish, *Syngnathus typhle*); (Berglund and Rosenqvist, 2003; Jenni and Collier, 1972). This form of sexual selection is often more dramatic than female mate choice, as it typically involves some sort of direct competition between males, as in the classic case of various males bashing horns to determine access to a female. But intrasexual selection need not be as dramatic as fierce fights between males. Competition may be less direct, as in the case of male cuckoldry or sperm competition (see Chapter 7).

RED DEER ROARS AND MALE-MALE COMPETITION

Some of the best-known studies of male-male competition are those of Tim Clutton-Brock and his colleagues on roaring in red deer (*Cervus elaphus*) (Clutton-Brock and Albon, 1979; Clutton-Brock et al., 1979). Clutton-Brock and Stuart Albon hypothesized that male red deer should use an honest indicator of each other's fighting ability to determine whether to compete for access to a female (Clutton-Brock and Albon, 1979). Male red deer stags on Rum Island, Scotland, form harems during the mating season (the rut) and fight off other males to defend their harems. While serious fighting is not common, 23 percent of harem holders show some sign of a fighting injury and 6 percent are permanently injured, suggesting strong selection pressure for accurately assessing an opponent's strength to avoid injury and possible death at the hands of a much stronger rival.

Clutton-Brock and Albon proposed that the main indicator of strength and fighting ability was roaring. Evidence suggesting that roaring was being used to assess an opponent's fighting ability in the context of harem holding included:

▸ Roaring and associated activities such as "parallel walks," in which males walk alongside one another to assess their size and fighting ability relative to others, were almost exclusively seen during the mating season (Figure 6.29).

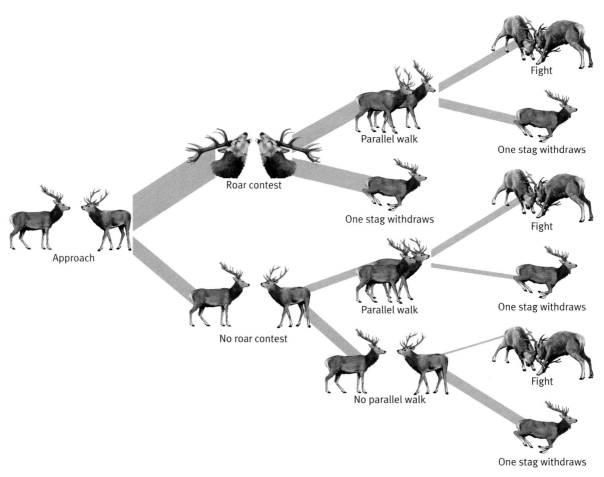

FIGURE 6.29. Approach and assessment in male red deer. When two male red deer approach within 100 m of each other during the mating season, any number of outcomes are possible. Thicker lines represent more likely outcomes. *(From Clutton-Brock et al., 1979)*

- During the rut, harem holders roared more than those without a harem (Figure 6.30).
- Roaring rates increased when a harem holder was approached by another male.
- By measuring the mean and the maximum roaring rates, as well as the outcome of fights, evidence was uncovered for a positive relationship between these variables. The more often a male roared, the more likely he was to win a subsequent fight.
- Roaring contests were much more common between mature stags of approximately equal fighting ability than between stags of unequal fighting ability, and roaring rarely escalated (via the "parallel walk" stage) to fighting except among the most closely matched stags, which suggested that roaring was a good indicator of fighting ability and one upon which stags often relied.

Clutton-Brock and his team experimentally manipulated red deer roars to examine the hypothesis that males use roar rate to assess opponents. Using stags of different sizes and abilities, the researchers played tapes for them of other males roaring at different rates. They then measured the responses of the stags to the different roars on the tapes. When playback tapes included sounds indicating a longer vocal tract, and hence presumably a larger opponent, male red deer responded by being more attentive to such calls and increasing their own rate of roaring (Reby et al., 2005).

Together, all of the data above suggest that male-male competition for females has led to an extraordinary social system involving fine-tuned communication designed to maximize access to females while minimizing injuries that result from serious fights.

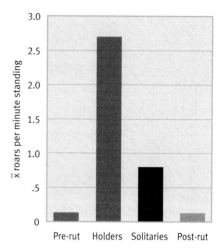

FIGURE 6.30. Roaring rates in red deer. Clutton-Brock and Albon found that males in possession of a harem (holders) roared much more than males not holding a harem (solitaries), as well as more often than males in the pre-rut or post-rut periods. *(Based on Clutton-Brock and Albon, 1979)*

MALE-MALE COMPETITION BY INTERFERENCE

Although many examples of male-male competition involve males fighting *before* a female is present, this need not be the case. An interesting subset of male-male interactions consists of males interfering with another male *while that male attempts to mate with a female*. This sort of behavior is common in amphibians and insects (Duellman and Trueb, 1994). For example, in the European earwig (*Forficula auricularia*), heavier males often succeed in interrupting copulation between lighter males and females by displacing lighter males to gain access to females (Forslund, 2000).

In at least some cases of male-male interference, females appear to solicit males to try to remove a rival during the actual mating event. Cox and Le Bouef hypothesized that females incite male-male competition because it increases the probability of mating with the highest-ranking male in a group (Cox and Le Boeuf, 1977). They tested their hypothesis on the elephant seal (*Mirounga angustirostris*), a species in which males form large harems of females and in which the males are much larger than the females (Figure 6.31). Harems of up to forty females are exclusively defended by a single dominant (large) bull seal, and there is consequently huge variation in reproductive success among males. In one long-term study, only 8.3 percent of males mated, but some individual males inseminated 121 different females (Le Boeuf and Reiter, 1988).

FIGURE 6.31. Elephant seal fights. Male elephant seals are much larger than females and fight for access to females during the breeding season. *(Photo credit: François Gohier)*

TABLE 6.1. Female seal elephants protest when mounted by nondominant males. Cox and Le Boeuf found that not only did alpha (dominant) males mount females more often, but that the females protested their mounts less often than mounts by nondominant adults or subadults (SA3, SA4). *(From Cox and Le Boeuf, 1977, p. 324)*

AGE OR SOCIAL RANK OF MOUNTING MALE	MOUNTS OBSERVED* (N)	TOTALLY PROTESTED (%)	PARTIALLY PROTESTED (%)	NOT PROTESTED (%)
Alpha	74	37	43	20
Adult	70	49	34	17
SA4	9	78	22	0
SA3	4	100	0	0

*Interrupted mounts are excluded.

Cox and Le Bouef marked 271 estrous female elephant seals and tracked attempted matings (mounts) with these females. Approximately 87 percent of the attempted mounts were "protested" to some degree or another by the females. Protesting included a large suite of behaviors, most prominently loud calls and constant back-and-forth movement to prevent the male from copulating. These protests seem quite effective, as 61.4 percent of protested mounts were interrupted, as opposed to 25 percent of mounts that went unprotested. Female protests appeared to be designed to solicit more dominant males to interrupt mounts, as the probability that a female would protest a male's attempt to mount her was a function of that male's rank. Females rarely protested dominant male mounts, but they often protested mounts attempted by subordinates (Table 6.1). This led to an increased probability of copulation between the highest-ranking males in the vicinity and the females who had protested mounts with subordinate males.

The elephant seal example shows how difficult it can be to completely disentangle female mate choice from male-male competition. Clearly, interruption of the copulation attempts of males by other males qualifies as male-male competition, but in the elephant seal example, this competition is initiated by a female to increase her probability of mating with the highest-ranking male in the area.

SEXUAL SIZE DIMORPHISM AND MALE-MALE COMPETITION FROM A PHYLOGENETIC PERSPECTIVE. Sexual selection via intense male-male competition has also been examined from a phylogenetic perspective. For example, Patrik Lindenfors and his colleagues have studied the relationship between sexual size dimorphism and male-male competition in the pinnipeds (seals, walruses, and sea lions), including the elephant seals described above (Lindenfors et al., 2002). They hypothesized that in species in which harem size is large, and hence where male-male competition is most intense, sexual size dimorphism (males larger than females) should be greatest. In addition, since sexual selection for large body size in pinnipeds should act strongly on males but not females, Lindenfors and his team predicted that, as harem size increased,

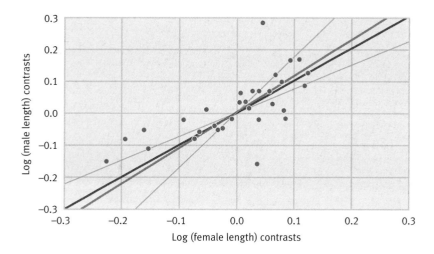

FIGURE 6.32. Harem size and sexual selection. In pinnipeds, there is a positive relationship between harem size and the relative difference in size between males and females. Each point represents a comparison between two species of pinnipeds. *(From Lindenfors et al., 2002, p. 189)*

female body size would remain fairly constant. The researchers wanted to make certain, however, that if this relationship was uncovered, it was a result of sexual selection pressures, rather than the fact that pinnipeds share a phylogenetic history, and hence share behavioral and morphological attributes because of evolutionary history. To distinguish between these possibilities, they used a phylogenetic technique called independent contrasts, which removes the effects of phylogeny from patterns found among related species. To test their hypotheses, the researchers first gathered together published data on harem size, male size, and female size for thirty-eight species of pinnipeds. They incorporated this data into a phylogenetic analysis, using a well-established phylogeny of pinnipeds as their base. Their analysis uncovered a significant positive correlation between harem size and sexual size dimorphism—the larger the average harem size in a species, the larger the relative size of males compared to females. This analysis also found that the relative size of males increased as harem size increased, but the relative size of females stayed fairly constant (Figure 6.32). The independent contrast analysis allowed the researchers to ascertain if it was selection pressure, rather than similar phylogenetic histories in pinnipeds, that explained their results.

MALE-MALE COMPETITION BY CUCKOLDRY

In many species of fish, ethologists have uncovered different male reproductive types, or morphs, that are distinct in structural, physiological, endocrinological, and behavioral traits (Gross, 1985; Gross and Charnov, 1980). In bluegill sunfish (*Lepomis macrochirus*), three male morphs—parental, sneaker, and satellite—co-exist within populations (Gross, 1982; Neff et al., 2003). Parental males are light-bodied in color (with dark yellow-orange breasts), build nests, and are highly territorial, chasing off any other males that come near their territory. It takes between six to thirteen days for their eggs to hatch, and males exert significant amounts of energy fanning the eggs (which oxygenates them) and defending the nest against predators during this time (Coleman et al., 1985; Figure 6.33).

Sneaker males look and act very different from parental males. These males are smaller, less aggressive, and do not hold territories. Instead, they lurk in hiding

FIGURE 6.33. Parental male bluegill sunfish tending his eggs. Parental male sunfish build nests and care for their eggs by fanning them and defending them against predators. *(Photo credit: Byron Neff)*

places near a parental male and zip into a territory while the parental male and female are spawning. Sneakers then shed their sperm and swim away, with the whole process taking less than ten seconds (Gross, 1982). Male-male competition here then involves sneakers trying to outcompete others by a "hit-and-run" type strategy in which they sneak into the parental male's territory and cuckold the parental male (Figure 6.34). Without the parental male present, sneakers would have no chance to cuckold anyone, for without the parental male, females would not be drawn to the area where sneakers are lurking. Using molecular genetic analysis, researchers have found that, depending on their relative numbers in a population, sneaker males fertilize between 0 to 58.7 percent of all bluegill eggs laid in Lake Opinicon, Canada (Philipp and Gross, 1994).

A third male morph, labeled satellite males, also exists in some bluegill populations. Satellite males tend to look like females. Disguised as such, they position themselves between a spawning pair. If the parental male is duped into believing that the satellite male is another female, he will attempt to spawn with both the female and the impostor satellite male, at which point the satellite male will release his own sperm.

Because of the very different reproductive behaviors seen among these three bluegill morphs, Byron Neff and his colleagues examined whether there are also differences in sperm production and sperm quality across morphs (Neff et al., 2003). In particular, they predicted that because of their hit-and-run mating strategy, sneaker males might invest most heavily in sperm production. Results are consistent with this prediction. Although parental males are larger than sneakers, and have testes that are larger, when Neff and his colleagues examined the ratio of testes size to body size—that is, the relative investment in testes—sneaker males had the highest ratio, followed by satellites and then parentals.

The relative investment in testes size is an indirect measure of sperm production. A more direct measure would be the number of sperm produced per ejaculate. Given that the sperm produced by sneakers are always competing with

FIGURE 6.34. Bluegill morphs. (A) Bluegill parental male preparing a nest. **(B)** Sneaker males hiding behind plants awaiting a chance to quickly sweep into a parental nest. **(C)** A satellite male swimming over a nest containing a male and female. **(D)** A satellite male swimming between a parental male and a female. **(E)** A composite of A–D. *(Based on Gross, 1982)*

parental sperm (sneakers are always in competition with the parental male they are attempting to cuckold), but parental sperm are not always competing directly with sneaker sperm (not all parentals are cuckolded), a high density of sperm per ejaculate should be more strongly favored in sneaker males. When Neff and his team looked directly at the density of sperm per ejaculate, they found that sneakers produced more sperm per ejaculate. Sneakers do, however, pay costs for investing so heavily in sperm production. First, their sperm are shorter lived than parental sperm. Second, when Neff and his colleagues stripped sperm from both sneakers and parentals, and then released the same number of parental and sneaker sperm over eggs, parental sperm were more likely to fertilize eggs than were sneaker sperm. If we focus on the sneaker and parental morphs, the work on testes and sperm production show two very different reproductive strategies—sneakers invest in producing many short-lived, lower-quality sperm, while parentals invest in producing fewer, but higher-quality sperm.

Few topics in animal behavior have fascinated ethologists to the extent that sexual selection has. In this chapter, we have examined many of the proximate and ultimate underpinnings of sexual selection. We are now ready to examine a related question: How can animal behaviorists understand the wide variety of mating systems seen in nature?

INTERVIEW WITH

Dr. Anne Houde

You've done extensive research on sexual selection in guppies. Why have you studied that species? How did you first get interested in working with these small fish?

An aspiring scientist can choose a study system in two different ways. First is to sit at your desk and read the literature for a while, find a research question, and then find a study system to help answer it. Second is to start by getting involved with organisms that interest you, either in the field or in the lab. Once you know your system, you can start asking questions. This is what I did: started with the system and then thought of the questions. Of course, to think of good research questions, I needed to have a good grounding in my field, animal behavior, and its literature.

I started out working on birds— terns—but found them to be so long-lived that it was hard to answer questions that interested me in a reasonable amount of time. Then I went in the opposite direction and started looking at the sexual behavior of *Drosophila*, but I did not find flies very exciting (I did not know about their songs and pheromones). When David Reznick came to study life history evolution in my department and gave me some guppies, I started looking at their sexual behavior. I soon realized that I could address some important questions about sexual selection simply by recording male color patterns and observing behavior. I turned out to be correct about this, and have been working on guppies for the last twenty-five years!

Back in 1871 Darwin proposed that females might exert some choice in choosing their mates. Why do you think it took so much longer to study this form of sexual selection compared to studying male-male combat?

The study of mate choice by females did not really get going until

the late 1970s, more than 100 years after Darwin's book about sexual selection. I think there are a few reasons for this. People did not take the idea of natural selection seriously until decades later; people had difficulty imagining that nonhuman animals could do things like choose their mates; and science itself has had a long history of being biased toward a male perspective.

When most people think of male-male competition they envision two rams butting heads. Is it possible for male-male competition to be more subtle?

Just as "survival of the fittest" does not only mean that the strong

survive by beating up the weak, male-male competition can take many forms. Darwin's classic distinction says that sexual selection (differences in mating success) can occur if female behavior results in greater mating success of some males than others (female choice), or if interactions between males lead to differences in mating success (male-male competition). So yes, two rams might butt heads until one emerges the victor and the other leaves the area. Presumably the winner then has greater access to reproductive females while the loser risks being beaten up if he comes near the females again. But the combat does not need to be overtly physical.

What else can males do to increase their own success at the expense of others? In many species, male-male interactions are mediated by signals such as coloration, visual displays, or songs and calls rather than fighting, which can be very costly. Males are able to communicate their prowess and likelihood of winning in physical combat through signals like these. Amazingly, these signaling systems seem to work in lieu of combat, perhaps because the signals evolve to be "honest." Animal behaviorists have been fascinated by the seeming paradox of how signals can be "honest"—evidently, males who "bluff" still face the risk of getting beaten up.

The effect of symmetry on mate choice has proven to be quite a contentious issue. Where do you come

down on the importance of symmetry when it comes to choosing mates?

There certainly seems to be something to the idea that mate choice can be based on symmetry—the question is why? There are plenty of empirical studies in which the researchers have related mate choice to some measure of symmetry, including studies of humans. The implication is that there must be some benefit to choosing a symmetrical mate if this preference has evolved. The argument goes that an individual with "good genes" will be developmentally stable and be more symmetrical than an individual with lower genetic quality. Thus, an animal choosing a mate should be able to use symmetry as a signal of good genes, and a preference for symmetry should be favored. Perhaps certain sexual ornaments like tail plumes or bright color patterns have evolved because they show off symmetry particularly well.

The problem I see is that there can be circularity in this reasoning. Let's suppose that "good genes" do result in greater symmetry (a point that needs more study). But individuals with good genes might show other signs of this too. Perhaps they are especially vigorous and athletic and potential mates can detect this. So, in studies that find a correlation between symmetry and attractiveness, choice might just be based on a different, unrelated correlate of good genes so that the correlation with symmetry is spurious. A case in point is a study of scorpionflies by Randy Thornhill showing that females prefer the odor of more symmetrical males, even with no chance to assess male symmetry. There is a way out of this problem, and there are studies that convince me that there are preferences for symmetry per se. What kind of study would convince you?

How far can we extrapolate from animal studies of mate choice to human mate choice? Are there warning signs one can look for that tell us we have crossed some line we shouldn't cross?

We can learn a great deal from animal studies to understand mate choice in humans. The now-famous "sweaty T-shirt" studies, in which mate choice based on odors has been detected in humans, are a good example. These are adaptations of studies done on rodents, and they reach similar conclusions about, for example, the role of relatedness or MHC genotype in mate choice, despite humans' notoriously poor sense of smell. So mate choice, narrowly defined, has some clear similarities between humans and other species. What are the pitfalls?

First of all, it is too easy to forget that the role of culture in human behavior is vastly more complex and important than in any other species. Studies of classified ads reveal that men prefer youth and beauty in women, while women prefer wealth in men. Do these preferences maximize reproductive success by identifying women with high reproductive value and men who are good resource providers, similar to many animal species? Maybe, but we need to think harder about the interplay of biological and cultural evolution in how men and women construct classified ads.

Second, there is a danger of falling into the "naturalistic fallacy," especially when thinking more generally about patterns of sexual behavior in humans. Yes, most animal species show the stereotype of macho males and choosy females. The same stereotype in humans probably has an evolutionary origin. Does this mean oppression of women by men is morally justified and inescapable? No, of course not. The answer to this paradox is to think more deeply about human moral systems (themselves the product of natural selection) and also the interplay of natural selection and cultural evolution in shaping the roles of men and women in human society.

How do you think the current focus on brain function will affect our understanding of the evolution of mate choice over the next five years?

It is always hard to see into the future, so let me start with two areas I think are especially promising right now. For several years, we have been seeing studies using various kinds of brain scans (e.g., PET scans), in which "active" parts of the brain are visualized. Mostly these are studies of humans, comparing brain activity in different contexts or between different people. I think this approach could be potentially useful in studies of sexual behavior and mate choice. For example, we might be able to look at the interplay between attraction, fear, and aggression when an individual responds to different potential mates.

An even more powerful genomic approach to understanding brain function during mate choice involves directly assessing gene expression in the brain. Scientists are beginning to use this method to understand which genes are involved in a variety of behavioral activities and contexts, including mate choice. Ultimately, perhaps, we will be able to combine both of these techniques to look at how in situ gene expression patterns in different parts of the brain depend on behavioral context.

Dr. Anne Houde is a professor at Lake Forest College. Her work on sexual selection in guppies has had a profound impact on the way ethologists think about the process of natural selection, and is summarized in her book, Sex, Color and Mate Choice in Guppies *(Princeton University Press, 1997).*

SUMMARY

1. When developing his theory of sexual selection, Darwin outlined two important processes—intersexual selection and intrasexual selection.
2. Intrasexual selection involves competition among one sex, usually males, for access to the other sex.
3. Intersexual selection involves mate choice, wherein individuals from one sex, usually the female sex, choose their mates from among members of the opposite sex.
4. Evolutionary models of female mate choice can be broken down into four classes: "direct benefits," "good genes," "runaway sexual selection," and sensory exploitation models.
5. Females learn how to select mates through sexual imprinting and classical conditioning in which they are rewarded with the opportunity to mate.
6. Mate choice is one of the more active areas of ethology in terms of studying the cultural transmission models of behavior. Work in this area includes studies of mate-choice copying as well as song learning and mate choice in birds.
7. Male-male competition for access to females with whom to mate can be exhibited through fighting, roaring, interfering with another male as he attempts to mate a female, and cuckolding another male by fertilizing his mate's eggs.

DISCUSSION QUESTIONS

1. Suppose that a group of males was engaged in a series of fights, and male A emerged as the dominant individual. Now suppose that a female assessed all the males involved in fights and chose male A. Why might this example blur the distinction between intersexual selection and intrasexual selection?
2. Secure a copy of Kirkpatrick and Ryan's 1991 paper "The evolution of mating preferences and the paradox of the lek," in *Nature* (vol. 350, pp. 33–38). Drawing from this paper, list the similarities and differences between sexual selection models in terms of both assumptions and predictions.
3. Why do you suppose it is so difficult to demonstrate mate-choice copying? Choose a species and design an experiment that would examine whether mate-choice copying is present in that species. How many controls did you need to construct to rule out alternative hypotheses to mate-choice copying?
4. Pick any of the numerous "reality" shows on television that focus on dating, and watch a series of episodes. As you watch, imagine yourself as an ethologist studying mate choice. What traits do males prefer in females? What traits do females prefer in males? Can you say anything about how your observations match up against current models of sexual selection?
5. Explain how the sensory bias hypothesis and the good genes model might both be important in explaining mating preferences among females in some species of birds. Distinguish between the origins of a female mating preference and its subsequent evolution.
6. Read over Lindenfors, Tullberg, and Biuw's 2002 paper entitled "Phylo-genetic analyses of sexual selection and sexual size dimorphism in

pinnipeds" in *Behavioral Ecology and Sociobiology* (vol. 52, pp. 188–193). Explain why pinnipeds are such an excellent group for a phylogenetic analysis that examines the relationship between sexual dimorphism and sexual selection.

SUGGESTED READING

Andersson, M. (1994). *Sexual selection*. Princeton: Princeton University Press. This book is considered the modern reference guide for work on sexual selection.

Darwin, C. (1871). *The descent of man and selection in relation to sex*. London: J. Murray. This is the book that started it all. It was in this book that Darwin outlined his theory of sexual selection.

Fisher, R. A. (1915). The evolution of sexual preference. *Eugenics Review, 7,* 184–192. One of the earliest models of the process of sexual selection.

Houde, A. E. (1997). *Sex, color and mate choice in guppies*. Princeton: Princeton University Press. A book-length case study of sexual selection in a model system: the guppy (*Poecilia reticulata*).

Kirkpatrick, M., & Ryan, M. (1991). The evolution of mating preferences and the paradox of the lek. *Nature, 350,* 33–38. This *Nature* article provides a nice view of the contrasting models in the sexual selection literature.

7

Mating Systems

A Monogamy

B Polygyny

C Polyandry

D Polygynandry

FIGURE 7.1. Four basic mating systems. These are: **(A)** monogamy (1 male, 1 female), **(B)** polygyny (1 male, more than 1 female), **(C)** polyandry (1 female, more than 1 male), and **(D)** polygynandry (more than 1 male, more than 1 female). Each mating system can be further subdivided in a number of ways.

In Chapter 6, we examined intersexual and intrasexual selection, and spent a significant amount of time on how and why individuals end up with particular types of mate(s). In this chapter, we will look at a related question: How can we understand the *mating systems* that we observe in nature? Why, for example, do some animals choose a single mate for life, while others mate with a single partner each breeding season, but switch partners across breeding seasons? And, why, for that matter, do some mating systems involve a male (or female) having two (or more) opposite-sex partners during a single breeding season?

Mating systems can occur in many forms and gradations. For example, we tend to think of our own species as being fairly monogamous. In general, monogamy means "having one mate," but this definition sometimes fails to capture important aspects of mating systems. For example, people in most modern industrial societies are better characterized as serially monogamous, since, with the high divorce rate, many individuals will in fact be married to more than one person during their lifetime (serial monogamy), just not at the same time.

Different Mating Systems

Before examining a series of questions regarding the evolution of mating systems, let us do a quick survey of different forms of mating systems. In order to do so, we begin by tackling a definitional question. There has been some debate in the mating systems literature as to whether "pair bonds" between males and females—that is, long-term relationships that often involve rearing offspring—are important in defining a classification of mating systems (Davies, 1991; Emlen and Oring, 1977; Thornhill and Alcock, 1983). Here we will avoid having our broad-scale classification of mating systems depend on identifying pair bonds, and instead simply use the number of copulatory partners as the critical variable in defining our mating systems (Figure 7.1). Occasionally, when subdividing mating systems, however, it will be helpful to examine the role of pair bonding, and we will do so when needed.

With some definitional issues behind us, we can now return to a general classification of mating systems (Table 7.1).

TABLE 7.1. Mating combinations. Various mating combinations and how they map onto potential mating success for males and females. *(From Davies, 1992, p. 29)*

	MATING SUCCESS	
MATING COMBINATION	**FOR A MALE**	**FOR A FEMALE**
Polyandry (e.g., 2 ♂ 1 ♀)	Share one female	Sole access to several males
Monogamy (1 ♂ 1 ♀)	Sole access to one female	Sole access to one male
Polygynandry (e.g., 2 ♂ 2 ♀)	Share several females	Share several males
Polygyny (e.g., 1 ♂ 2 ♀)	Sole access to several females	Share one male

MONOGAMOUS MATING SYSTEMS

As we touched on above, **a monogamous mating system** is normally defined as a mating system in which a male and female mate with each other, and only each other, *during a given breeding season.* As such, we can have animal societies in which pairs mate only with one another during season 1, but in subsequent years find new mates (serial monogamy)—indeed, this sort of mating system is very common in territorial animals.

In some animal populations, a given male and female will mate only with one another during their entire life span (or more precisely, the life span of the individual that dies earliest), although this form of monogamy is relatively rare compared to serial monogamy. As an example of this type of lifetime monogamy, let us look at the oldfield mouse, *Peromyscus polionotus* (Dewey and Dawson, 2001; Foltz, 1981; Figure 7.2).

Early work suggested that monogamy was rare in mammals (Eisenberg, 1966; Kleiman, 1977). In the early 1980s, however, David Foltz hypothesized that while monogamy was uncommon in large, conspicuous, diurnal species (those active in the daytime), it was much more common in smaller diurnal groups, particularly rodents (Foltz, 1981). Behavioral work suggested that Foltz might be correct, even though the genetic evidence for monogamy in rodents at the time was much weaker (Kleiman, 1977). To remedy this dearth of genetic support for monogamy in rodents, Foltz studied the breeding system of the oldfield mouse, in part because these rodents were relatively easy to study in both the laboratory and the field, and in part because other work suggested that a great deal of genetic variation existed in this species (Selander et al., 1971).

Foltz excavated more than 500 oldfield mouse burrows, captured the individuals in each burrow, and then brought them into the laboratory. One hundred and seventy-eight families were collected from these burrows, and a genetic analysis was conducted. From a subset of these families, Foltz calculated that 90 percent of the offspring found in a family group were fathered by the male in their burrow (Figure 7.3). Furthermore, behavioral observations of both males and females found that most females remained with the same mates across litters, suggesting long-term, perhaps lifetime, monogamy to be the rule, rather than the exception, in this species.

Despite the fact that long-term monogamy appears to be the most common mating behavior seen in oldfield mice, Foltz found that approximately 13 percent

FIGURE 7.2. Long-term monogamy in the oldfield mouse. From data on 500 oldfield mouse burrows, Foltz found that 90 percent of the offspring in a family group were fathered by the male in their burrow. Behavioral observations also suggest that many females remained with the same mates across litters, suggesting long-term monogamy. *(Photo credit: © James F. Parnell)*

FIGURE 7.3. Who fathers whom? In the oldfield mouse (*Peromyscus polionotus*), the male found in the burrow, on average, fathers 90 percent of the pups in that burrow.

of the burrows excavated contained only an adult female, rather than the typical male and female. When this small subset of females without live-in mates was analyzed, they were found to be more likely to switch mates across litters, compared to females that were already paired with a mate in the field. Whether these females were choosing a more polygamous mating strategy, or whether their mates had simply died, and hence made them polygamous by necessity, remains to be tested.

MONOGAMY AND FITNESS CONSEQUENCES. From an adaptationist perspective, one would expect that in mating systems like that of the oldfield mouse, where most individuals pair with a mate for life, there would be strong fitness consequences associated with choosing a high-quality mate—that is, a mate that would give their partners high relative reproductive success by siring attractive offspring, offspring with strong immune systems, and so on. Karen Ryan and Jeanne Altmann tested this idea in a series of fitness-related mate-choice trials involving oldfield mice (Ryan and Altmann, 2001). A male was given the choice between two virgin, but sexually mature, females, and the male's preference was recorded. Then, in one treatment, males were paired with the female for which they had expressed a preference, and in a second treatment, males were paired with the female that they had not preferred.

When Ryan and Altmann examined the number of pups that survived in each treatment, they found significantly more pups were born to pairs made up of a male and his preferred mate (Figure 7.4A), documenting the strong fitness consequence of mate choice in a species in which lifelong monogamy was the norm. The researchers then ran a fascinating set of follow-up experiments. They again let a male choose between two females, and they recorded which female the male preferred—let's call this part I of the experiment. Then, in part II, a naive male—a male who had no experience with either of the females—was paired with either the female that had been preferred (in one treatment) or the female that had been rejected (in a second treatment). The researchers found that the number of offspring raised in these two treatments was approximately equal, suggesting that what constituted a good mate was different for each individual oldfield mouse—otherwise we would have expected to see more offspring from matings involving females that been preferred in part I of the Ryan and Altmann experiment (Figure 7.4B).

FIGURE 7.4. Fitness consequences of choice in monogamous systems.
(A) Males sired more pups with females they preferred as compared to the case when the males were mated to females that they did not prefer. **(B)** No differences were found in the number of pups sired when a male was paired with a female that was preferred by *another* male compared to the case when a male was mated with a female rejected by *another* male. *(Based on Ryan and Altmann, 2001, pp. 438, 439)*

A

B

Animal behaviorists continue to examine the costs and benefits associated with monogamy. It is difficult to understand why males would ever choose to engage in monogamous pairings when they could potentially inseminate many different females over a short period of time. From an adaptationist perspective, ethologists predict that monogamy should occur in ecological situations that create significant fitness advantages to a male who opts to remain with a single female. Later in the chapter, we will see some research that suggests what those circumstances may be. In general, when resources are relatively scarce, a male's fitness may be highest when he is part of a monogamous pair and provides some sort of care for the offspring. In such situations, males may help raise offspring by bringing food to the nest and defending the offspring from potential predators. This is often referred to as the mate-assistance hypothesis of monogamy (Emlen and Oring, 1977).

PROXIMATE UNDERPINNINGS OF MONOGAMY. Animal behaviorists have made much progress in understanding the proximate underpinnings of monogamous mating systems (Young et al., 2005). One species that has proven quite useful for understanding the neurobiology of monogamy and pair bonding is the prairie vole (*Microtus ochrogaster*). In this species, males and females who are courting approach one another, and this affiliative ("friendly") behavior is a prerequisite to partner choice. Once individuals mate and form a strong pair bond, they are actively aggressive to other members of the opposite sex (Carter et al., 1995). Brandon Aragona and his colleagues studied how this transformation from affiliative to aggressive behavior in a monogamous species takes place (Aragona et al., 2006).

Aragona and his team focused on male prairie voles and the transmission of the neurochemical dopamine in a section of the brain called the nucleus accumbens (n.a.), because earlier work had found dopamine transmission in the n.a. was linked to both affiliative (friendly) and aggressive behavior in the prairie vole (Aragona et al., 2003; Liu and Wang, 2003). These researchers began by examining which area of the nucleus accumbens was associated with pair-bond formation. By injecting a chemical that is known to stimulate pair bonding, they established that a specific area of the n.a. called the rostral shell was associated with affiliative, mating-related behavior. Within the rostral shell, activation of two dopamine-related receptors—labeled D1 and D2—was critical to the formation of long-term monogamous relationships. When D2 receptors were activated by dopamine, pair bonding was facilitated, whereas when D1 receptors were activated, pair bonding was inhibited. This suggested to Aragona and his colleagues that D2 receptors mediated pair-bond formation, while D1 receptors were critical to the aggression seen toward unfamiliar, opposite-sex individuals once two individuals had formed a pair bond.

To test their theory, Aragona and his team looked at D1 receptors in males that had recently formed pair bonds with females. These males showed a surge in D1 receptor activation, as well as aggression toward any female that was not their mate. Moreover, when Aragona and his team experimentally blocked D1 receptor activation in the male prairie voles, aggression toward unfamiliar females disappeared.

Aragona and his team's work demonstrates how D1 and D2 dopamine receptors are critical for both the affiliative and aggressive behaviors exhibited by male prairie voles in long-term monogamous relationships. Their studies are also a good example of how the proximate underpinnings of monogamy can be

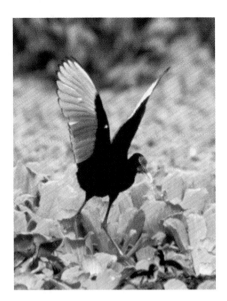

FIGURE 7.5. Polyandrous birds. In the wattled jacana (*Jacana jacana*), polyandry is the typical mating system. The male bird incubates the eggs and cares for the young after they hatch. Here we see a male bird defending his two young chicks. *(Photo credit: © Natalie Demong)*

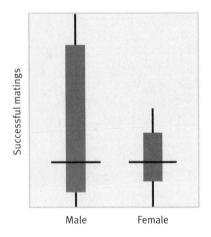

FIGURE 7.6. Variance and polygyny. Since each and every successful mating involves a male and a female, the average reproductive success must be equal in both sexes. In polygynous mating systems, however, the variance in reproductive success is often much higher in males than in females, with some males having very high reproductive success and others faring much more poorly (horizontal lines represent average reproductive success). *(Based on Low, 2000, p. 55)*

experimentally examined, even down to the level of brain receptors and their role in mating behaviors.

POLYGAMOUS MATING SYSTEMS

A **polygamous mating system** is defined as one in which either males or females have more than one mate during a given breeding season/cycle. Polygamy includes **polygyny**, wherein males mate with more than one female per breeding season, and **polyandry**, in which females mate with more than one male per breeding season. Polygamy can be also be subdivided temporally, in that polygamy can be simultaneous or sequential. Simultaneous polygamy refers to the case in which an individual maintains numerous mating partners in the same general time frame, whereas sequential polygamy involves individuals forming many short-term pair bonds in sequence during a given breeding season.

Polyandry has been particularly well studied in jacanas—a group of sex-role-reversed shorebirds in which the males incubate the eggs and care for the young, and the females compete aggressively for multiple mates. Stephen Emlen and his colleagues studied one of these species, the wattled jacana (*Jacana jacana*) in Panama (Emlen et al., 1998; Figure 7.5). While polyandry in some species of jacanas is simultaneous, and females nest with numerous males at one time, wattled jacana females are usually sequentially polyandrous. In this species, males have small territories (40 meters in diameter) that abut one another. Female territories are considerably larger and contain anywhere from one to four male territories.

In the wattled jacana, a female lays clutches of eggs sequentially, after mating with males on her territory, with intervals of less than two weeks often separating the production of sequential clutches. Given that a female's territory encompasses a number of male territories, it was rather surprising that the probability was very high that a chick in a nest on a particular male's territory was his genetic offspring. That is, given the possibility that a female was also engaging in copulations with other males in her territory, the fact that there was a 92.5 percent probability that a given chick in a nest was the offspring of the male guarding that nest was rather remarkable. Not surprisingly, this figure went down dramatically when males in surrounding nests were not incubating eggs or tending young chicks and had more time available for mating attempts.

One important thing to keep in mind with respect to polygamy is that this type of breeding system increases the variance in reproductive success in the sex that has more than one mate per season (see Chapter 6). For example, in polygynous systems, there is often intense competition among males to mate with as many females as possible, and this typically produces a distribution of mating success in which a few individuals do extraordinarily well, but many males obtain no mates whatsoever (Figure 7.6). The converse holds true for the case of polyandry, although variance in reproductive success is usually less dramatic in this situation.

FEMALE DEFENSE POLYGYNY. We shall return to the evolution of polygamy later, but for the time being, let's examine one species characterized by a polygynous mating system—a very small Australian wasp in genus *Epsilon* (Smith and Alcock, 1980). In this species of wasps, males mature earlier than females. When they mature, males search for unopened brood cells from which females will emerge. Such cells are often clustered together, and males are very territorial once they uncover such a potential gold mine of reproductive opportunities that they can easily defend as a unit. Once a virgin female wasp emerges from her cell, the closest male present climbs on her back and mates with her. The rewards to males who guard against intruders may be mating opportunities with as many as two dozen virgin females (Figure 7.7). Because males mate with many females (that is, they are polygynous) and they defend females from mating attempts by other males, the mating system of these wasps is referred to as **female defense polygyny**.

Randy Thornhill and John Alcock have argued that three characteristics are often present in insects displaying female defense polygyny: (1) females are short-lived and have low fecundity, receiving all the sperm they will ever use from a single male, (2) females mate shortly after becoming adults, and (3) females are grouped close together in space (Thornhill and Alcock, 1983). These three characteristics apparently make female defense polygyny adaptive for males. Its relative effect on female fitness remains less well understood.

LEKS. One well-studied form of polygyny is called **lekking**, or **arena mating** (see Chapter 6). Lekking, which has been studied in birds, mammals, amphibians, fish, and insects, occurs when males set up and defend small arenas called leks—temporary territories specifically for mating—that typically contain no apparent resources (no food or shelter, for example). Females then come to these leks and select mates from among the males present. Often a single male will obtain a very large proportion (sometimes more than 80 percent) of all the matings at that lek, making this sort of system a classic case of polygyny (Hoglund and Alatalo, 1995; Mackenzie et al., 1995). If, for example, a single male did receive 80 percent of the matings at a lek, only 20 percent of the matings would be with other males, and some males might not succeed in mating at all.

Leks have long fascinated ethologists, and they have been studied from many different perspectives. Here we shall focus on two questions: (1) What benefit(s) do females obtain from this form of polygyny, and (2) what benefit(s) do males obtain?

The benefit(s) that females may receive from choosing among males on a lek has been a contentious issue in ethology, in part because females appear to receive sperm, and only sperm, from males—that is, females appear to receive few direct, material benefits (see Chapter 6). One possibility is that females select among males using indicators of male condition—for example, size, number of parasites, and other indicators of health and vigor—and that such choice will lead to offspring with higher survival probabilities because they possess "good genes" with respect to health. An alternative explanation is that females may use these same indicators to select among mates because such choice will lead to the production of male offspring that are attractive to the next generation of females—an idea sometimes referred to as the **sexy-son hypothesis**. Through a series of experiments using the sandfly (*Lutzomyia longipalpi*), Theresa Jones and her colleagues attempted to distinguish between these two hypotheses regarding the benefits that females receive in polygynous lek mating systems (Jones et al., 1998).

Sandflies form leks in which males defend small arenas that measure about 4 cm in diameter. Females can choose freely among courting males, who emit a chemical attractant called a pheromone. As in many lekking species, a single male on a lek will often obtain all matings with visiting females, and neither males nor females will provide parental care to the young.

FIGURE 7.7. Epsilon wasps and female defense polygyny. Male wasps in this species wait at the nest for females to emerge from their brood cells so that they can mate with them and defend them against mating attempts by other males. Pictured here is one male (left) on the nest and a female (at arrow) that is starting to emerge from a hole in the mud nest, and with whom he will mate. *(Photo credit: Bonnie Heim)*

Jones and her team set up experimental sandfly leks in the laboratory, and they undertook a two-part experiment. In the first part of the experiment, five randomly selected males were put together in an arena, and once a lek was established, a single, virgin female sandfly was allowed to choose among these males. Once that female mated with a male, she was removed from the lek, and a second female was allowed to select a mate. This process went on until ten females had selected mates and had been inseminated in a given lek. Then, for the second part of their experiment, Jones and her colleagues took the males that had rarely been selected by females in the first part of their experiment, and they put them in new leks. The researchers then allowed a sequence of ten females to select among males at these new leks. Thus, in the second part of the experiment, females were forced to select among males that were unattractive. By comparing the results obtained in the two halves of the experiment, the experimenters could begin to decipher what benefits females might receive when selecting males in a highly polygynous mating system.

To distinguish between the good genes and sexy-son hypotheses, the researchers first compared the survival of offspring that were the product of females choosing among a random sample of males (part 1) and the offspring of females that were forced to choose between less attractive males (part 2). No evidence for the good genes model was uncovered, as offspring from both part 1 and part 2 survived with approximately the same probabilities. Jones and her team, however, did find support for the sexy-son hypothesis. When male offspring from part 1 and part 2 were placed in a lek, females showed a strong mating preference for the former, suggesting that first-generation females were receiving sexy-son benefits as a result of their choice among lekking males.

To examine the benefits that males might obtain from a lek mating system, we will examine lekking in birds (also see Chapter 6, where we discuss lekking in grouse). From the perspective of a male on a lek, the fitness benefits are huge *if* you are the individual chosen as a mate by most females. Consider an extreme case of polygyny in which one male out of all the males on a lek obtains all the matings at that lek. The benefits of being that one male are clearly enormous, and they might make up for the fact that the odds that you are in fact the male that all females choose is very low. If you aren't the male chosen, your reproductive success for that round of lekking approaches zero. But we can also ask whether there are other potential benefits that males on a lek might receive—that is, we can examine whether males who receive few mating opportunities may still obtain some sort of benefits from being at a lek. For example, a male may receive benefits from helping his genetic relatives on a lek (Hoglund, 2003; Hoglund et al., 1999; Kokko and Lindstrom, 1996; Petrie et al., 1999).

One avian species that makes use of leks is the peacock (*Pavo cristatus*). Peacocks generally have many different leks that females can visit, and the females are often drawn to leks that contain the most males (Alatalo et al., 1992; Kokko et al., 1998; Figure 7.8). If only one or a few males at a given lek obtain matings, and the lek is composed of lots of males that are genetic relatives, these relatives may receive indirect benefits from the matings that their kin receive.

Marion Petrie, Andrew Krupa, and Terry Burke studied a group of 200 peacocks living in Whipsnade Park in England (Petrie et al. 1999). These peacocks divide up into many different leks, and males defend their arenas within the leks all day during the breeding season. Petrie and her team did a molecular genetic analysis to determine whether individuals in a lek were genetic kin, and

A B

FIGURE 7.8. Peacocks on leks. The benefits to mating on leks have been measured in the peacock. **(A)** Four males gather on a lek before any females arrive to observe them (one of the males is under the brush in the top left corner). **(B)** When a female appears on the lek, the male displays his tail in an attempt to get her to choose him as her mate. *(Photo credits: Marion Petrie; Frans Lanting/Minden Pictures)*

they found that indeed they were, with the average genetic relatedness within the groups being equivalent to that of half-siblings. Petrie and her colleagues then ran an experiment in which they released into Whipsnade Park a group of peacocks raised elsewhere. These males were raised in such a way that they did not interact with their genetic relatives any more than they interacted with strangers during their development. Petrie's group found that when the birds who had been raised without interactions with their genetic relatives formed their own leks, genetic relatives set up their arenas much closer to one another than one would expect by chance. That is, even without the opportunity to learn about who is kin and who isn't during their development, the peacocks were able to gauge genetic relatedness and clustered near genetic kin within their leks. And again, in such leks of genetic kin, even males who did not mate received direct benefits from their genetic relatives who did mate.

PHYLOGENETIC HISTORY OF POLYGYNY IN WARBLERS. Animal behaviorists who study polygyny have also undertaken phylogenetic studies on the origin of this type of mating system (Searcy et al., 1999). Consider, for example, the family of birds known as Acrocephaline warblers, a group that includes such species as the Seychelle warbler, the moustached warbler, and three species of reed warblers. To construct a phylogenetic history of mating systems in warblers, it's important to know the following about warblers and their territories: First, mating systems in these species vary from monogamous to polygynous. Second, warblers in monogamous systems show much higher levels of parental care than do warblers in polygynous systems, with monogamous males providing much more food to chicks than do polygynous males. And third, warbler species in this family of birds also differ in terms of the quality of the habitats they inhabit, ranging from poor habitats with little food, to much better habitats that contain significantly more and better food types for warblers.

To examine the evolution of mating systems in warblers, Bernd Leisler and his colleagues used molecular genetic data to build a phylogeny of seventeen

A

B

FIGURE 7.9. Warbler mating systems. The phylogeny of mating systems has been studied in warblers, including **(A)** the polygynous great reed warbler (*Acrocephalus arundinaceous*), and **(B)** the monogamous Seychelle warbler (*Acrocephalus sechellensis*). *(Photo credits: John Hawkins/FLPA; M. D. England/www.ardea.com)*

warbler species (Leisler et al., 2002). They also gathered published data on habitat quality, parental care, and mating system (monogamous versus polygynous) in warblers (Figure 7.9). Habitat quality was scored from poor (few, poor-quality food items) to medium (more, larger prey) to good (highly productive areas with quickly renewing food sources), and paternal care was scored as "full paternal care," "reduced paternal care," or "no paternal care." Finally, they took the data on habitat quality, male parental care, and mating system and superimposed them onto their phylogenetic tree.

From an ecological and behavioral perspective, Leisler's work found a strong correlation between mating system and habitat quality. Most monogamous systems were found in poor habitats, and most polygynous systems were found in better habitats. In addition, males were much more likely to provide significant parental care to developing chicks in poor habitats. These two findings together suggest that monogamy is associated with poor habitat quality because in such habitats food is scarce enough that it takes two parents to gather enough food to provision developing chicks.

Leisler and his team's phylogenetic analysis also examined which type of mating system—monogamy with male parental care or polygamy with reduced male parental care—was ancestral, and which was derived (see Chapter 2). To do this, they used a statistical technique called maximum likelihood analysis, which allowed them to take data from their phylogenetic tree and calculate probable ancestral states of various traits. Leisler and his colleagues found evidence that the ancestral state in warblers in this family was a monogamous system, in which males displayed parental care and the birds lived in poor habitats. Polygynous systems with reduced care evolved from this ancestral state. What this phylogenetic analysis allows us to do is reconstruct the evolution of polygyny. In warblers, it appears that, through evolutionary time, some species began inhabiting better-quality habitats. Once this occurred, and it was possible for chicks to receive enough food from a single parent, males were freed from parental care duties and the evolution of polygyny was facilitated (Figure 7.10).

A

B
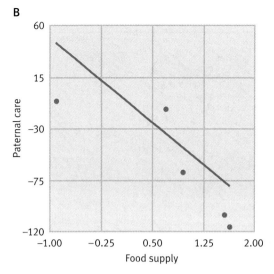

FIGURE 7.10. **Phylogeny of warbler mating systems. (A)** Paternal effort is represented as the proportion of a pie chart that is green. This paternal effort was mapped onto the warbler phylogeny. **(B)** The relationship between paternal care and food supply in several species of warblers is shown by the data points. Where there was less food, there was greater paternal care; where there was more food, there was less paternal care. Values on the x-axis and the y-axis can be negative because of statistical transformations associated with this phylogenetic analysis. *(From Leisler et al., 2002, p. 384)*

POLYANDRY IN SOCIAL INSECTS. Recall that polyandry refers to a mating system in which females mate with more than one male per breeding season. Polyandry has been well-studied in social insects, where a single queen will often mate with many worker males. Compared to cases of nests where a single male mates with a queen, polyandrous nests often have greater levels of within-group conflict.

The reason that there is less within-colony harmony in the nest of polyandrous queens is the presence of numerous "patrilines"—that is, offspring descended from different fathers. When polyandry is absent, all workers have the same mother and father, and hence the same genetic interest. With the creation of patrilines, genetic interests are more divergent, with each patriline competing with the others for greater representation in the next generation (Seeley, 1995, 1997; Figure 7.11). While it increases within-group conflict, the decreased genetic relatedness among offspring that comes from polyandry does provide queens with at least one benefit—her offspring, as a group, are likely to survive when the hive is infected with disease. This is because high genetic diversity among a queen's offspring increases the odds that some of those offspring will have a genotype that allows them to survive attack by some disease-causing agent (Seeley and Tarpy, 2007).

Thornhill and Alcock have listed a number of other possible benefits that female insects accrue by adopting a polyandrous mating strategy (Thornhill and Alcock, 1983). These benefits include:

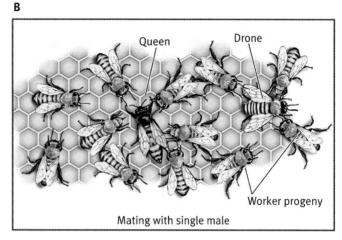

FIGURE 7.11. Polyandry and within-hive harmony. (A) When a queen mates with two different drones (denoted by red and blue), two patrilines (red and blue) exist in a single hive. Such hives have greater within-hive conflict than those in which **(B)** a queen mates with a single male (red).

1. Sperm replenishment
   - Female adds to depleted or low sperm supply.
   - Female avoids the cost of storing sperm.
2. Material benefits
   - Nutrients
   - Reduced predation
   - Protection from other males
3. "Genetic benefits"
   - Replacement of "inferior" sperm
   - Increased genetic variance in offspring
4. Convenience
   - Female avoids the costs of fending off copulation attempts by male.

Of these, Thornhill and Alcock hypothesize that "material benefits" account for most of the polyandry seen in insects. These material benefits include: (1) seminal fluid that sometimes contains chemicals that a female can sequester and use in various contexts, (2) nutritious spermatophores— sperm-encompassing packets filled with nutrients and produced by male insects such as moths and butterflies, (3) "nuptial gifts" such as prey items presented by courting males, (4) access to superior feeding sites and oviposition (egg-depositing) sites, and (5) male parental care (as in some waterbugs).

PROMISCUOUS MATING SYSTEMS

When polyandry and polygyny are occurring in the same population of animals, the breeding system is said to be **promiscuous**. Yet, there are two very different kinds of promiscuity, which vary dramatically as a function of the presence or absence of pair bonds between mating individuals. In one form of promiscuity, both males and females mate with many partners and no pair bonds are formed.

FIGURE 7.12. Versatile dunnocks. The dunnock mating system is extremely versatile and includes monogamy, polyandry, polygyny, and polygynandry. Here we see **(A)** a female with a newly hatched offspring (just visible in egg), and **(B)** a female feeding her brood. *(Photo credits: Nick Davies; W. B. Carr)*

For example, a male may defend a territory that contains food, and females may visit such territories, obtain food, mate with a male, and then repeat this sequence many times (Davies, 1991).

The type of promiscuity outlined above need not be tied to male territoriality. In many primate species, when females are in estrous, both males and females mate repeatedly, often in rapid succession, with many opposite-sex partners. Take the case of the Barbary macaque (*Macaca sylvanus*) (Taub, 1980, 1984). During their estrous period, female Barbary macaques search for new male mating partners after each copulation, which has the effect of minimizing the chances that a female will mate with just one male (Whitten, 1987). At the same time, this pattern of female behavior results in males having numerous female sexual partners, producing a promiscuous breeding system.

In the second type of promiscuous breeding system, **polygynandry**, several males form pair bonds with several females simultaneously. For example, in the dunnock (*Prunella modularis*), pairs of males will often jointly defend the territory(ies) of a pair of females (Figure 7.12). Nick Davies has studied the dunnock mating system and the help provided by males to females (Davies, 1986). He observed cases in which one or two males were resident on a female's territory, and he found that females either received help from one of the males, both, or neither of them, but that, on average, polygynandrous females received the equivalent help that a female with only a single mate would receive (Davies, 1992; Figure 7.13). The more help a polygynandrous female received, the higher the mean nestling weight of the chicks in the brood and the lower the chick mortality rate due to starvation. We will examine Davies's work on polygynandry in the dunnock in more detail later in the chapter.

DISEASE AND PROMISCUITY. Margie Profet has added an interesting dimension to the study of promiscuous breeding by examining this type of breeding system in relation to female reproductive health (Profet, 1993). Her basic argument goes as follows: Sperm are known to be vectors—that is, carriers—of sexually transmitted diseases, some of which are quite dangerous to females (Ewald, 1994). During insemination, bacteria and other disease-causing agents

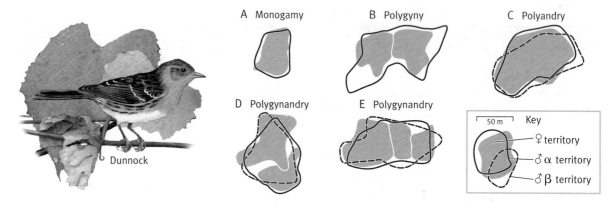

FIGURE 7.13. Incredible variation in dunnock breeding systems. Female territories are shown in green, while alpha male territories are depicted by solid red lines and beta male territories are shown by dashed red lines. In a single dunnock population, we can find mating systems ranging from monogamy to polygamy, polyandry, and polygynandry. *(From Davies, 1992, p. 27)*

from both male and female genitalia hitch a ride on sperm tails and work their way to the uterus (Profet, 1993).

Menstruation, Profet argues, is a defense that has evolved in females to rid the female reproductive tract of pathogens carried in by sperm. As such, menstruation should be most common in promiscuous breeding systems, as the probability of disease transfer via sperm should be highest in systems where both males and females engage in sexual activity with numerous partners. Promiscuous breeding systems not only expose females to greater quantities of sperm, but to a greater diversity of sperm, and hence to a greater diversity of diseases that use sperm as vectors. And both of these factors increase a female's risk of infection (Figure 7.14). While Profet suggests that a qualitative test of the data on breeding systems and menstruation supports her hypothesis (Profet, 1993), a more quantitative analysis by Beverley Strassmann did not find any link between promiscuity and copiousness of menstruation in primates (Strassmann, 1996). Clearly, further work needs to be undertaken to better elucidate the evolutionary relationship between promiscuity and menstrual bleeding.

FIGURE 7.14. Sperm, breeding systems, and menstruation. Margie Profet has argued that promiscuous breeding systems deliver not only more sperm to females, but a greater diversity of sperm (denoted by different colors). As the probability of sperm-transported disease increases, Profet predicts that menstruation should become more common.

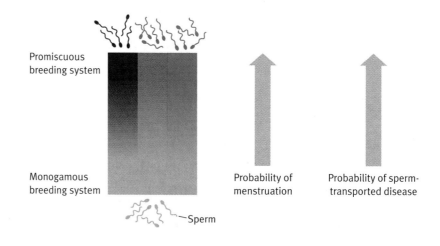

The Ecology and Evolution of Polygynous Mating Systems

With a survey of different mating systems in hand, we can now address questions about the ecology and evolution of these different mating systems. We will first look at the role of resource dispersion on female mating decisions and then at a model to predict when polygyny is favored by natural selection.

POLYGYNY AND RESOURCES

The study of animal mating systems has long been tied to female dispersion patterns—that is, how females move about in relation to one another and their environment (Bradbury and Vehrencamp, 1977; Emlen and Oring, 1977). The basic argument goes as follows: A female can often fertilize all her available eggs by mating with one or a very few males. That being the case, female fecundity is not so much tied to the availability of mates as it is to the availability of resources—for example, food, defense, and so forth (Krebs and Davies, 1993). The more resources that are available, the more offspring females can produce. Males, on the other hand, can potentially fertilize large numbers of females, and so male reproductive success is more tightly associated with access to females than with access to resources. As such, female dispersion patterns should track the distribution of resources, whereas male dispersion patterns should track the dispersion of females.

If females track resources and males track females, then the mating system in a population is intimately tied to the distribution of resources because resource distribution will affect whether males can defend more than one female at a time. If resources are dispersed fairly homogeneously and/or if females must cover large areas to obtain enough resources to survive, it may not be economically feasible, in terms of costs and benefits, for males to mate with and potentially defend more than one female.

When resources are clumped—for example, when food is located in discrete groupings—the economics of mating systems may shift, and males may be able to mate with and defend several females at once. Moreover, when females live together for easier access to resources and for protection from predators, it may be easier for a male to mate with multiple partners. For example, seal populations can be found aggregating on both ice packs and beaches. On ice packs, females are widely dispersed, and males typically guard and mate with anywhere from one to a few females. In contrast, when the seals are on land, females cluster tightly in particularly safe areas on the beach, and males are able to defend herds of females against the approach of other males, leading to a more polygynous mating system (Le Boeuf, 1978).

The effect of female dispersion on male mating patterns can be examined experimentally. To see this, let us examine the mating system of the grey-sided vole (*Clethrionomys rufocanus*). Rolf Ims found that when he experimentally manipulated food distribution, female dispersion patterns changed in the predicted manner—when resources became more clumped, females clustered themselves together in the area of their resources (Ims, 1987). Ims then undertook an ambitious experiment in which he introduced the grey-sided vole to a small island in Norway. In one treatment, he used caged female voles to simulate an environment in which females moved about a home range and were fairly spaced out. In a second treatment, caged females were clustered together. As a control, Ims ran a reverse experiment in which males were in cages and their distribution was manipulated. As predicted, Ims found that males tracked the distribution of caged females across treatments, but female dispersion was unaffected by the distribution of caged males.

THE POLYGYNY THRESHOLD MODEL

The idea that females often track resources and males track females does not mean that decisions regarding polygyny are made strictly by males. For example, in systems where males have territories that can sustain numerous mates simultaneously, females will often have to decide which territory they settle on by choosing between alternative male territories. In 1969, Gordon Orians created the **polygyny threshold model (PTM)** to predict the behavior of females in just such a scenario (Orians, 1969).

HOW THE PTM WORKS. To see how the PTM works, imagine that ten males each have their own territory, and that these territories vary with respect to some resource that is valuable to females. Let's say the resource in question is food, with male 1's territory representing the area with the most food, and male 10's territory that with the least food. The first female arriving to choose a male territory on which to settle can base her choice simply on what territory is optimal with respect to food intake, and so she should choose male 1's territory. A second female choosing between male territories now faces the same landscape as the first, except that male 1's territory is occupied by a male and another female. If this female chooses male 1's territory, she will only get some fraction of the food available there. If the food still available on male 1's territory, even though it is already occupied by another female, is greater than the food available on any of the other nine male territories, our second female should choose to settle there (on male 1's territory) anyway. In so doing, she has passed the "polygyny threshold"—that is, she opts to stay on a territory with another female and thus to be part of a male's polygynous relationships (Figure 7.15).

Now let's say that the second female does not pass the polygyny threshold for staying on territory 1, and she settles on male 2's territory. Our third female now comes in and chooses between male 1's territory (another female present), male 2's territory (another female present), and the territories of males 3–10 (no other females present). Her situation is slightly different from that of female 2 when she arrived, however, because the best open territory is now male 3's territory, and that isn't as profitable (in terms of fitness effects) as male 2's territory. If female 3 chooses to settle on territory 1 or 2, then the polygyny threshold has been crossed for whichever of these she settles on. This sort of logic can be applied to all subsequent females, and it allows us to make a few clear-cut predictions with respect to territory settlement (J. Brown, 1982).

One prediction is that polygyny should often occur in "patchy" environments, where resources such as food are clumped in discrete patches that are spread out over the landscape. In such patchy environments, males can defend territories that have these valuable resources and the quality of a male's territory will affect his mating success—males with better territories (more food, better safety,

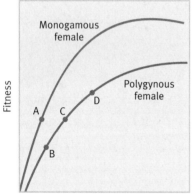

FIGURE 7.15. Female choice of territories. Imagine a female deciding among territories. She should choose the territory with the highest quality, that is, with the most food available or the most shade and so on, regardless of whether she would be the lone female (monogamous territory) or one of several females (polygynous territory), because such a choice would provide her with the greatest fitness. If she had to choose between monogamous territory A and polygynous territory B, our female should choose to settle on territory A because she would have a higher fitness there. If polygynous territory D was available, however, she should opt for territory D over territory A, for now the polygynous territory (D) would provide her with greater fitness. If she had to choose between polygynous territory C and monogamous territory A, she should be equally likely to choose territory A or territory C, for each would provide her with approximately the same fitness.

and so on) should have higher reproductive success than males with poorer territories. A second prediction the PTM makes relates to female fitness. When two females settle at about the same time, and hence face the same sort of economic decisions regarding the availability of resources and where to settle, a female that opts to settle on a territory on which she is the lone mate of the male (a territory with a monogamous mating pair) and a female that decides to settle on a territory that already contains a male and one or more females (a territory in which we see polygamy) *should have about equal fitness* (Krebs and Davies, 1987). It is this equivalency of fitness among monogamous and polygamous females that makes the PTM stable. Because monogamous females and females in polygamous relationships settle in such a way as to produce approximately equal fitness, there is no temptation for females to move from territory to territory once this state has been reached, as any such move would in fact lower an individual's reproductive success (see Borgerhoff-Mulder, 1990, for some limitations of the PTM).

THE PTM AND MATE CHOICE IN FEMALE BIRDS. Wanda Pleszczynska used lark buntings (*Calamospiza melanocorys*) in one of the first experimental tests of the PTM. In lark buntings, the resource that primarily determines female settlement onto male territories is shade cover, as the main cause of nestling mortality in lark buntings is overheating—the more shade on a territory, the better the territory. This shade effect can be shown experimentally by artificially increasing the shade in a given territory and demonstrating that such a manipulation increases nestling survival (Pleszczynska and Hansell, 1980).

Because shade protection is such a critical resource, it will often be the case that the male territories that are best suited to provide shade have already been settled by other females (Figure 7.16). Settling on such a territory anyway

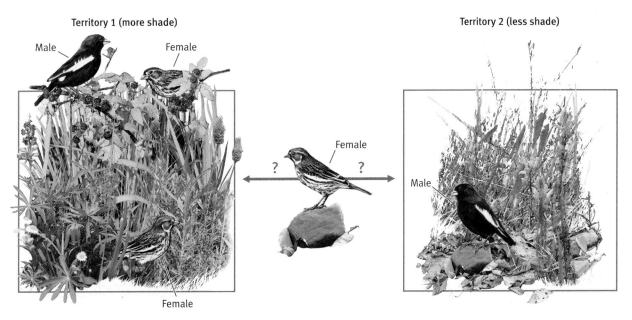

FIGURE 7.16. The polygyny threshold model. In the lark bunting, shade is a limiting resource, as it affects nestling survival. Females may choose the territory of a male with good shade cover (Territory 1) over a territory with less shade cover (Territory 2), even if this means entering a polygynous relationship rather than a monogamous one.

and becoming a "secondary" female—that is, settling on a territory that already contains a male and a female—allows access to shade. The cost of becoming such a secondary female is that a male only provides paternal care to the nestlings of his "primary" female (the mate that arrived first) (Krebs and Davies, 1987). Pleszczynska and Hansell found that increasing shade availability on a territory not only made it much more popular, but that as the PTM predicts, secondary females who bred in areas with shade cover (but who did not receive male aid) had about the same reproductive success as did monogamous females who bred on territories with less shade cover (but who did receive male aid).

THE PTM AND HUMAN FEMALE MATE CHOICE. While much of the experimental work on the polygyny threshold model has been undertaken in birds, Monique Borgerhoff-Mulder, an evolutionary anthropologist, has applied this model to mate choice in tribal human societies (Borgerhoff-Mulder, 1990). Borgerhoff-Mulder looked at polygamy among the Kipsigi tribe of Kenya, and she tested the basic prediction that when females are choosing between males with territories that differ in resource value, there should be a positive correlation between territory quality and female preference for males on superior territories.

One consequence of the European colonization of parts of southwestern Kenya was the emigration of a pioneer group of Kipsigis who moved to areas traditionally associated with the Masai tribe (Figure 7.17). Borgerhoff-Mulder obtained the settlement records of this migration, and she was able to determine when Kipsigi males settled on specific territories, how large each territory was, how many wives a male had at settlement time, and how many wives he obtained after settlement (Table 7.2). She found that the number of wives a male had *prior* to settlement did not affect the size of his territory at the time of settlement in the Masai area, suggesting that a male's prior success did not determine his territory size. The number of wives, however, that a male obtained *subsequent* to territory settlement was strongly affected by the size of his territory—with larger, and presumably more resource-rich, territories came an increase in the number of wives (Borgerhoff-Mulder, 1988, 1990), as predicted by the PTM.

A   **B**   **C**

FIGURE 7.17. Polygynous Kipsigis. In the Kipsigi population, polygyny is the norm. Kipsigi "co-wives" both relax **(A)** and work **(B)** together. **(C)** A man with many wives will have numerous huts, grain stores, strips for maize, and so on. Here we see the plot of a man with three wives. *(Photo credits: Monique Borgerhoff-Mulder)*

TABLE 7.2. Polygyny in Kipsigi tribes. Kipsigi males are often polygynous. The number of wives a male obtains *after* settling in a new territory is a function of territory size. The husband's "total wives" consists of the sum of his "previous wives" (wives taken before settling the new territory), "pioneer wives" (wives taken during the initial period of settling the new territory—1930–1949), and "subsequent wives" (wives taken after the initial settlement period—that is, after 1949). *(From Borgerhoff-Mulder, 1990, p. 258)*

YEAR OF ARRIVAL	HUSBAND	SIZE OF PLOT SETTLED	PREVIOUS WIVES	PIONEER WIVES	HUSBAND'S TOTAL WIVES
1930	O	150	3	1	4
1932	D	100	2	2	4
	A	160	3	1	4
1933	C	100	0	2	4
	B	300	0	6	8
1935	F	50	2	1	3
1936	E	30	0	2	3
1937	I	70	2	1	4
1938	S	100	4	0	4
1939	H	60	1	1	2
	G	120	0	3	3
1940	P	60	1	1	3
1942	L	40	1	1	4
1943	J	180	0	2	4
	K	32	2	1	3
1944	M	40	1	1	3
	T	20	2	0	3
1945	U	20	2	0	3
1946	V	8	1	0	2
	N	36	1	1	2
1947	W	20	4	0	4
	X	20	2	0	3
1949	Q	29	0	1	2
	R	20	1	1	3
	Y	10	1	0	1

Female Kipsigis did pay a cost of polygyny, however, in that there was a negative relationship between the number of wives a male had and female reproductive success, even when controlling for territory size. This cost to polygyny may help explain why, as predicted by the PTM, in addition to preferring males with large territories, women also preferred bachelors (monogamous) to married men (polygynous), all else being constant.

EXTRAPAIR COPULATIONS

Most species of birds nest during their breeding season, and some sort of pair bond is formed between a male and female at the nest. It was often thought that such pairings were truly monogamous, in the sense that members of a given pair only mated with their nesting partner during a breeding season. Starting in the

FIGURE 7.18. Indigo buntings. (A) A female indigo bunting. Although socially monogamous, female indigo buntings are often involved in extrapair copulations. **(B)** A male indigo bunting. Males defend their territories against intruders. Even so, an average of 13 percent of all matings in indigo buntings involve extrapair copulations. *(Photo credits: David Westneat)*

early 1980s, however, ornithologists interested in bird mating patterns began to uncover more and more instances of what are now referred to as **extrapair copulations**, or **EPCs** (Ford and McLauglin, 1983; McKinney et al., 1984). Ethologists were finding that males and females were leaving their territories during the mating season and mating with other individuals, usually those in nearby territories. The occurrence of such EPCs prompted some animal behaviorists to make a distinction between social monogamy and genetic monogamy. Most bird species in which EPCs were recorded formed pair bonds with just a single partner during a mating season, and as such displayed what is referred to as social pair bonding, or social monogamy. Yet, genetically, these systems resembled promiscuity more than monogamy, as mating occurred both with the social partner and with other individuals during the mating season.

The increased reproductive success of males who leave territories and engage in EPCs is clear, as they can fertilize more females. But why would a female be involved in EPCs? The answer depends on the particular species and its ecology and demographics, but in general females engaging in EPCs may (1) increase the probability that all their eggs are fertilized (the fertility insurance hypothesis), (2) maximize genetic diversity in their offspring, thereby increasing the chances that some of the offspring will be well adapted to the environment in which they mature, (3) use EPCs to select males who have good genes (see Chapter 6) but who might not be willing to form a pair bond and provide direct benefits to their offspring (Griffith et al., 2002; Neudorf, 2004), and (4) increase the amount of direct benefits—food, protection, and so on—that they receive from males.

Among those studying mating dynamics in birds was David Westneat. His behavioral observations of indigo buntings suggested that about 13 percent of all matings were EPCs (Westneat, 1987b; Figure 7.18). Westneat was worried, however, that such observations might underestimate the actual percent of all offspring that were sired via extrapair copulations. This worry stemmed from the fact that the buntings were hard to observe, and hence a significant number of EPCs may have been overlooked. Furthermore, it was not clear how many extrapair *matings* translated into extrapair *fertilizations*. For example, indigo bunting females generally resisted EPCs to a greater extent than mating with their nesting partner, with the females resisting EPCs in 34 out of 43 attempts, while only resisting mating with their pairmates in 72 out of 320 attempts (Westneat et al., 1987). And so not all EPCs would result in offspring.

To examine what impact EPCs had on mating dynamics in buntings, Westneat ran one of the first genetic analyses of parentage done in conjunction with a detailed behavioral study (Westneat, 1987a; Figure 7.19). This study was conducted before DNA fingerprinting techniques were widely available, and instead relied on a technique called electrophoresis, which, although less powerful than DNA fingerprinting, does allow one to rule out a particular adult individual as the parent of a particular offspring.

Over the course of two years, Westneat biopsied (took genetic samples from) hundreds of individually recognizable buntings. Using electrophoretic comparisons, and plugging that data into existing mathematical models, he found that, of the 257 young that were biopsied, 37 had genotypes that were *not* consistent with the genotype of one of their presumed parents (Westneat, 1987a), and so at least 14 percent (37 out of 257) of all young were sired via an extrapair copulation—right in line with the 13 percent Westneat had predicted based on his behavioral observations. Subsequent to that analysis, however, updated mathematical models showed that electrophoretic estimates of the percent of young fathered by extrapair fertilizations in buntings were an underestimate. Plugging Westneat's numbers into these newer models uncovered extrapair fertilization rates from 27.2 to 42.1 percent (depending on the year) in buntings (Westneat et al., 1987).

Since Westneat's pioneering work, many studies have documented EPC frequency in birds, with EPCs accounting for 76 percent of all young in one population of the superb fairy wren (*Malurus cyaneus*; Mulder et al., 1994; Webster and Westneat, 1998; Westneat et al., 1990). Given that monogamy was long considered to be the norm in birds, these are staggering numbers—numbers that are only available because of the revolution in molecular genetics that is still underway today.

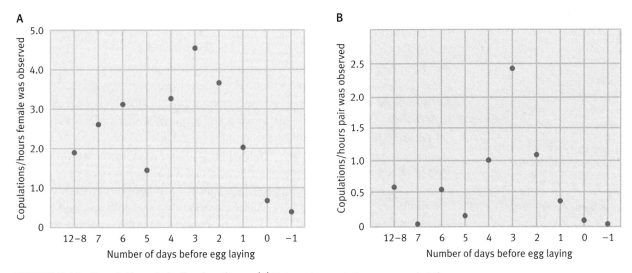

FIGURE 7.19. Copulations in indigo buntings. (A) Extrapair copulations occurred at the highest rate three days before egg laying (the day the egg was laid is zero on the x-axis), as was the case for within-pair copulations **(B)**. *(Based on Westneat, 1987b)*

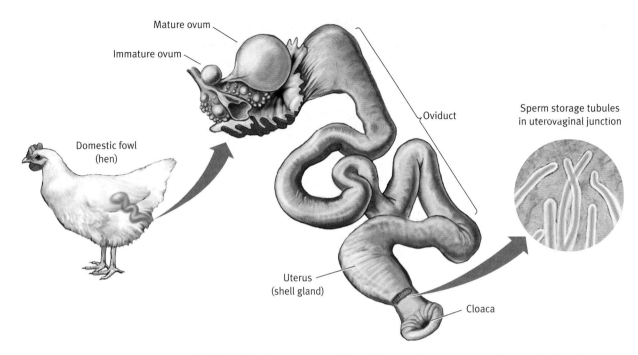

Mature ovum

Immature ovum

Domestic fowl
(hen)

Oviduct

Sperm storage tubules
in uterovaginal junction

Uterus
(shell gland)

Cloaca

FIGURE 7.20. Sperm competition. The reproductive system of domestic fowl. Sperm storage occurs in sperm storage tubules (SST) at the uterovaginal junction. Females in many species can store sperm from multiple males, setting the stage for sperm competition. Only a small proportion of sperm makes it into the SST. *(Based on Birkhead and Møller, 1992)*

SPERM COMPETITION

In many promiscuous breeding systems, there are big winners and big losers in terms of reproductive success. With respect to males, a few individuals will obtain the vast majority of matings in a population, and many males will fail to obtain even a single mating opportunity. In Chapter 6, we saw how both male-male competition and female mate choice can affect which males are on the upper and lower ends of this mating curve distribution. Here, we will look at the effect of **sperm competition**—that is, the direct competition between the sperm of different males to fertilize a female's eggs—on mating success and the evolution of mating systems.

In some promiscuous (as well as some polyandrous) mating systems, males compete not only for access to mating opportunities with females, but directly for access to eggs. In these systems, competition occurs *after* a female has mated with numerous males. If females store sperm from numerous matings, sperm from different males may compete with one another over access to fertilizable eggs (Figure 7.20). When sperm competition exists, selection can operate directly on various attributes of sperm, such as sperm size and shape. In many ways, an adaptationist approach to sperm competition predicts that such competition should be under the strongest selection pressure imaginable. After all, if a male wins a physical fight with an opponent, this *may* provide him with access to an estrous female, which *may* lead to a mating opportunity, which *may* lead to fertilization. In sperm competition, if sperm fertilizes an ova—then in terms of fitness, that's all that matters.

SPERM COMPETITION IN DUNGFLIES. Sperm competition has been extensively documented in many groups of animals, and an analogous sort of competition, known as "pollen competition" is known to occur in plants as well (Delph and Havens, 1998). In fact, numerous books and edited volumes are now dedicated to sperm competition and its implications for both sexual selection and mating systems (Birkhead and Møller, 1992, 1998; Smith, 1984). One of the leaders in this field, in terms of both empirical and theoretical aspects of sperm competition, is Geoff Parker, whose initial work on sperm competition in dungflies is regarded as the origins of modern research in this area (Parker, 1970b, 2001).

Dungflies use the droppings of large, often domestic, animals as their choice site for breeding. While in most insects, copulations often last a matter of seconds, in dungflies they can last on the order of thirty minutes or more. After a detailed analysis of the natural history of mating in dungflies in British pastures, Parker was faced with a number of unresolved issues regarding dungfly mating (Simmons, 2001). Here we shall focus on one of these, namely, why did dungflies copulate for so very long? Sperm competition theory, first developed by Parker himself, provided the answer to this and many other questions surrounding the mating system of dungflies (Parker, 1970b).

When a new dung pat is created and females begin to arrive, there ensues intense male competition for mating opportunities. A thousand or so males can descend on a single dung pat, all in search of females. Males that are lucky enough to find a female and begin copulating are under constant physical attack from other males trying to break up their pairing and start their own round of copulating (Figure 7.21).

To test for the role of sperm competition in this mating system, Parker relied on a technique that entomologists of the day had been using in various biocontrol programs (Parker, 1970a). He irradiated the sperm of certain males, creating males whose sperm would then fail to produce eggs that hatched. As such, Parker could take pairs of males, irradiate one of them, and then examine

A

B

C

D

FIGURE 7.21. Dungfly mating. In dungflies, sperm competition can be intense, with the last male copulating with a female fathering up to 80 percent of her offspring. The images show: **(A)** dungflies copulating, **(B)** a male passively guarding a female against other males, **(C)** a male actively guarding a female from another male, and **(D)** a male struggling with an intruder attempting to displace him. *(Photo credits: Geoff Parker)*

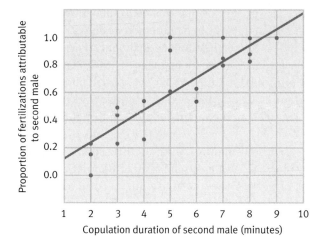

FIGURE 7.22. Sperm competition in dungflies.
The longer a male dungfly mates with a female dungfly, the greater his fertilization success. *(From Simmons, 2001)*

the relative success of each male by simply determining the proportion of eggs that failed to hatch—that is, the proportion of fertilizations attributable to the irradiated male.

Parker found that the number of eggs that were fertilized by the last male to mate with a female was proportional to how long such a mating lasted. The longer the last mating, the greater the reproductive success of the male. More specifically, the longer such a copulation, the greater the extent to which the last male's sperm displaced the sperm of males who had copulated with the female earlier (Figure 7.22). Such "last male precedence" is common when sperm competition is in play, but it is not ubiquitous (in some mating systems, sperm competition appears to favor the first, rather than the last, male to mate with a female).

In the dungfly system, the last male to mate with a female copulated on average for thirty-six minutes, and this resulted in his fathering approximately 80 percent of the young in the clutch of eggs deposited by a female (Parker, 1970a). If copulation time correlates with greater displacement of a competitor's sperm, why don't males copulate for even longer periods and thereby attempt to displace 100 percent of a competitor's sperm? The answer appears to be that males must weigh such an option against what else could be done with the time in question. While increasing the time spent with female A will increase the displacement effect, it is also time that the male could have used to find another female with whom to mate. Given that the rate of sperm precedence slows down with time, it will often benefit a male to use such additional time to find other potential mates (Parker, 1974b; Parker and Stuart, 1976).

SPERM COMPETITION IN SEA URCHINS. While sperm competition is often thought of in terms of its effect in utero, it can also play an important role in species that do not have internal fertilization. To get a better sense of the importance of sperm competition in such systems, let's consider Don Levitan's work on sperm velocity and fertilization rates in the sea urchin (Levitan, 2000).

Levitan began his work by asking whether variation in the speed at which sperm traveled correlated with fertilization rate. Using sea urchin sperm makes this task a bit easier than using sperm from birds or mammals, because sea urchins secrete their sperm and eggs into seawater. With a video camera that can tape sperm swimming along and a microscope to see which eggs are fertilized, Levitan was able measure the sperm's swimming speed and fertilization success.

Levitan found that to fertilize the same number of eggs, males who produced slow-moving sperm needed to release up to 100 times more sperm than males who produced fast-moving sperm (Figure 7.23). Levitan then examined what happens to sperm as they age. In so doing, he was examining a predicted trade-off between the speed at which a sperm moves and how long that sperm survives. Basic natural selection thinking suggests that since swimming fast and swimming for a long time both require energy, and since individuals only have so much energy, fast-moving sperm shouldn't live as long as slow-moving sperm.

When examining the expected trade-off between speed and longevity, Levitan first found that *all* sperm slow down as they get older (Figure 7.24). Not only did sperm decrease their swimming speed with age, but as they aged, they were much less likely to fertilize an egg, even when they encountered one. For example, sperm that were only an hour old could be as much as 100 times less likely to fertilize an egg as were newly released sperm. After two hours, sperm fertilized no eggs at all. Clearly, then, time is of the essence when trying to fertilize sea urchin eggs.

With data on longevity and speed in hand, Levitan could return to the question raised earlier: Is there a trade-off between sperm speed and sperm life span for individual sea urchins? The answer is a definitive yes, as Levitan found a negative correlation between velocity and endurance. Individuals who produced fast-moving sperm had their sperm become ineffective at much quicker rates than other individuals. The energy used up in swimming fast resulted in less energy for swimming for a long time, as well as a shorter life span for sperm.

OTHER EFFECTS OF SPERM COMPETITION. Sperm competition not only affects the speed at which sperm swim, but it also affects the various shapes and functions that sperm can take (Bellis et al., 1990; Gomendio et al., 1998; Holman and Snook, 2006; Moore et al., 1999). For example, Roger Baker and Mike Bellis's **kamikaze sperm hypothesis** suggests that natural selection

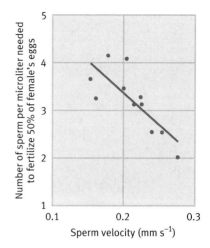

FIGURE 7.23. Sperm velocity and fertilization. In sea urchins, slower sperm fare poorly. The slower the sperm, the more sperm needed to fertilize a female's eggs. *(Based on Levitan, 2000)*

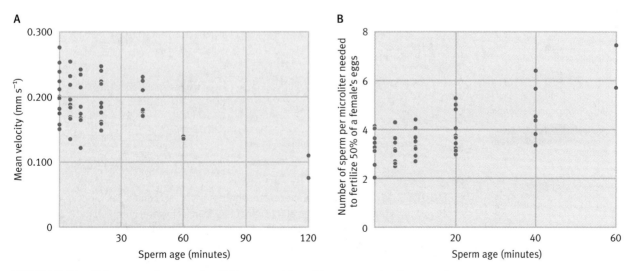

FIGURE 7.24. Older sperm fare poorly. (A) In sea urchins, older sperm swim slower, and **(B)** a greater quantity of such sperm is needed to achieve high fertilization rates. *(Based on Levitan, 2000)*

might favor the production of some sperm types that are designed to kill other males' sperm rather than fertilize eggs (Baker and Bellis, 1988).

While the evidence is equivocal in humans, sperm competition has had clear effects on sperm morphology in insects, frogs, mammals, birds, fish, and worms (Birkhead and Møller, 1992, 1998; Eberhard, 1996; Stockley et al., 1997; Figure 7.25). For example, in a phylogenetic analysis of 100 species of Australian (myobatrachid) frogs, Philip Byrne and his colleagues found that species under intense sperm competition had males that produced sperm with relatively long tails (Byrne et al., 2003). While the exact advantage of longer-tailed sperm in these frogs is not yet known, other studies have found that sperm with longer tails swim faster than their shorter-tailed competitors, and hence have an increased probability of fertilizing an ova (Oppliger et al., 2003).

Sperm competition also has effects on the number of sperm produced per ejaculate. One prediction from sperm competition theory is that the number of sperm per ejaculate should be a function of the probability that a female has recently mated with other males (Baker and Bellis, 1993). To see this, consider two males that we will call M1 and M2. Suppose that M1 is about to copulate with a female. The greater the chance that such a female has mated with M2 in the recent past and that his sperm are still present, the greater the chance that M1's and M2's sperm will be in direct competition to fertilize the eggs of the female. To counter the continuing presence of M2's sperm, sperm competition theory predicts that M1 will ejaculate more sperm in an attempt to increase the chances that he will fertilize the female's eggs.

Baker and Bellis tested this hypothesis in humans. They obtained data on the interval between copulations in a given pair of individuals, and assumed that the longer this interval, the greater the chances that a partner would have been unfaithful. Then, they obtained sperm samples from individuals the next time they copulated with their partner. Baker and Bellis found that not only did sperm number increase as a function of time since last copulation, but that even when absolute time was statistically removed from the equation, the relative

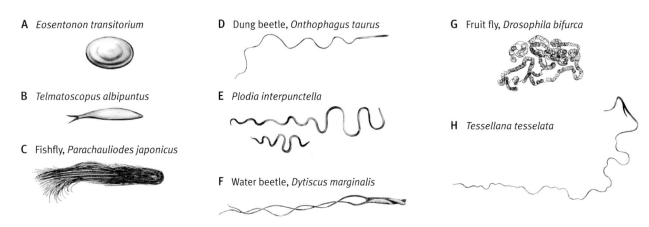

FIGURE 7.25. Variability in sperm morphology. Sperm competition is one of the many forces that have led to incredible variability in insect sperm morphology. Pictured here are: **(A)** sperm from *Eosentonon transitorium*, **(B)** fishlike sperm from *Telmatoscopus albipuntus*, **(C)** sperm bundle from the fishfly *Parachauliodes japonicus*, **(D)** 1 mm sperm from the dung beetle *Onthophagus taurus*, **(E)** short and long sperm from *Plodia interpunctella*, **(F)** paired sperm from the water beetle *Dytiscus marginalis*, **(G)** giant 58 mm sperm from *Drosophila bifurca*, and **(H)** hook-headed sperm from *Tessellana tesselata*. *(Based on Simmons, 2001)*

FIGURE 7.26. Sperm number in humans. In human males, the number of sperm ejaculated during a copulation is a function of the time since a pair last copulated. Note that the y-axis is a measure of "residuals"; hence negative values are possible. *(Based on Baker and Bellis, 1993)*

amount of time couples spent together predicted sperm volume as well (Figure 7.26). When couples spent more time together, and hence the risk of extrapair copulations was low, sperm count was significantly lower than when couples spent less time together.

With respect to sperm competition, it is important to keep in mind that females are not simply "inert environments" that serve as receptacles of male sperm (Parker, 1970b). Rather, females themselves may play an active role in sperm competition via **cryptic choice**—that is, female mate-choice behavior that is not obvious to males. William Eberhard, for example, suggests that, among other things, cryptic choice may affect how much sperm a female allows a copulating male to inseminate her with, how she goes about transferring such sperm to the organs where sperm are stored, and which sperm she may select for actual fertilization (Eberhard, 1996). Precisely how females select among sperm remains unknown in most cases, but this is an active area of study within animal behavior research (Birkhead and Pizzari, 2002; Holman and Snook, 2006).

Multiple Mating Systems in a Single Population?

There is some contention in the ethological literature as to whether mating systems should be defined in terms of the behavior of individuals or of the overall population. For example, if some individuals—let's say some males—in a population have more than one mate, while others have just a single mate, how do we define the mating system? One way would be to argue that there are monogamous individuals and polygynous individuals. Alternatively, mating could be defined at the population level. Here, if a significant proportion of males are polygynous, than the mating system is considered to be polygynous.

Ethologists often adopt the second definition, primarily because in polygynous populations most individuals attempt to obtain more than one mate, even though some end up with only a single mate and some with no mate at all. Nonetheless, sometimes we must move away from a population-level analysis. In the case of dunnocks, which we discussed earlier in the chapter, we see monogamous, polygynous, polyandrous, and polygynandrous mating groups all in the same population. Let's return to this mating system, and examine it in a bit more detail.

DUNNOCKS

For more than two decades, Nick Davies and his colleagues studied a population of about eighty dunnocks that reside in the Botanical Gardens of Cambridge University, and their work has provided a rare detailed portal into a very complex mating system (Davies, 1992). What makes the dunnock breeding biology so fascinating from a mating systems perspective is the long-term persistence of monogamy, polygyny, polyandry, and polygynandry *in the same population*. For Davies, unraveling the story behind the dunnock mating system is akin to detective work: "The puzzle is the dunnock's extraordinary breeding behavior and variable mating system. The job of the nature detective is to understand alternative options facing individuals, to assess their reproductive payoffs, and then to discover whether different mating strategies might emerge as a result of individuals competing to maximize their reproductive success" (Davies, 1992, p. 21).

Underlying much of the variance in mating systems, including that of the dunnock, is the fact that the fitness of males and females are affected in different ways by the mating system. For a male, reproductive success will often be lowest when he shares access with other males to a single female (polyandry), and then increase in the following order: sole access to a single female (monogamy), joint access to two females (polygynandry), and access to numerous females (polygyny). In other words, male reproductive success increases as a function of both the number of mates and the degree to which a male has sole reproductive access to such mates.

On the other hand, female reproductive success increases in precisely the opposite direction, with polyandrous and polygynandrous females having the highest reproductive success. As such, a conflict of interest between the sexes—sometimes referred as a "battle of the sexes"—exists with respect to what constitutes the optimal breeding system (Arnqvist and Rowe, 2005). In dunnocks, females appear to be winning this battle of the sexes (at least for now), as over the course of ten years, 75 percent of females and 68 percent of males observed by Davies and his team were involved in either polyandrous or polygynandrous mating groups (Davies, 1992).

The battle of the sexes, in conjunction with the dispersal patterns of dunnocks, helps us better understand the complex breeding system found in this bird. Early in the breeding season, females compete with each other to establish territories, and such female territories are chosen independently of the position of males. Males then attempt to delineate their own territories so that they overlay as many female territories as possible. Given this, Davies argues that the difference between monogamy and polygyny is a function of *male* territory size. Polygynous males had larger territories than monogamous males, but when comparing these two breeding systems, the territory size of females remained constant. On the other hand, the difference between polyandry and polygynandry was a function of female territory size. Male territory size remained constant across these systems, while female territory size was significantly larger in the former.

TABLE 7.3. Food and territory size. Supplementing the food on dunnock territories led to a decrease in female territory size but not male territory size. *(From Davies, 1992, p. 63)*

	TERRITORY SIZE (m²)						
	WITH FEEDER			CONTROL			
	MEAN	(SE)	*n*	MEAN	(SE)	*n*	SIGNIFICANCE OF DIFFERENCE
Females	2,776	(379)	28	4,572	(456)	39	$P < 0.01$
Males							
Territory defended by one male	2,864	(340)	11	2,642	(416)	13	NS
Territory defended by two males	5,276	(797)	14	6,614	(674)	17	NS

In Davies's population of dunnocks, because all individuals were marked (with color rings) and rarely strayed more than two miles from the Botanical Gardens, he was able to undertake experiments designed to more precisely gauge how resource defense and territoriality influenced the dunnock mating system. Davies and Arne Lundberg reasoned that since females were in strong competition with one another for territories with the best resources, if the resources available on a territory were experimentally supplemented, territory size should shrink, as females would then be able obtain the same amount of resources without having to defend as large an area (Davies and Lundberg, 1984).

To test their hypothesis, Davies and Lundberg placed artificial feeders on a randomly selected set of female territories, and they did indeed find that the female territories shrank as predicted. Moreover, they found that the male territories that overlay the manipulated female territories did not change in size (Table 7.3). What did occur, however, was a shift in the distribution of mating systems, in such a manner as to favor males. When female territory size shrank as a result of supplemental resources, males were better able to monopolize more than one female, and a shift away from polyandry and toward polygynandry occurred. This finding nicely supports Davies's argument that, in the dunnock, females track resources, males track females, and the resulting interaction helps us to better understand the incredible variation in mating systems in this small brown bird.

In both this chapter and in Chapter 6, we have examined how ethologists study ultimate and proximate questions associated with mate choice and mating systems. Within this chapter, for example, we asked what factors led an animal to remain with one mate or to have many mates and found that the availability of resources and the production and survival of healthy offspring were key factors. In Chapter 8, we will focus on another very actively researched area in ethology, namely, the role of genetic relatedness in shaping social behavior. Indeed, we have seen examples of how genetic relatedness plays an important role in behavioral decisions throughout the first seven chapters. We are now ready to examine this in much greater detail.

Dr. Nick Davies

The dunnocks you work with have proven to be a model system for so many questions in behavioral ecology and animal behavior. Why did you choose to work with this species?

In 1979, when I started as a young University lecturer at Cambridge, I was excited by the new theoretical ideas of Bill Hamilton, Robert Trivers, John Maynard Smith, and Geoff Parker. They were beginning to explore the evolutionary consequences of individual conflicts of interest, not only the long-recognized conflicts among rival males, but also those between the male and female of a breeding pair and between parents and their offspring. These ideas led to a profound change in how we interpret individual adaptations. For example, the classical work on clutch size (pioneered by David Lack) had considered what would be optimal from a pair's point of view. Once genetic conflicts within families were recognized, a whole new world of possibilities was opened up, involving deception, manipulation, cheating, and compromise. Likewise, previous studies of mating systems had emphasized ecological pressures (food, nest sites, predation) that might lead to one system rather than another. But now we began to consider social conflicts as important selection pressures too.

So I was on the lookout for a field study which would allow me to take a fresh look at bird mating systems. While wandering in the University Botanic Garden, I noticed the dunnocks chasing around the bushes in pairs, threes, and fours

and decided to color-band them for individual recognition to see what was going on. Once I had this initial excuse to begin the study, I then discovered more interesting new questions from the bird watching rather than from the theoretical literature.

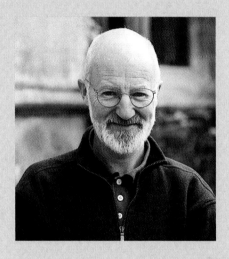

Your work on the dunnock suggests these birds have an incredibly plastic mating system. Why do you think that is?

It is clear from watching behavior that males and females have different mating preferences. These conflicts make good sense in relation to individual reproductive payoffs from the different mating combinations. For a female, polygyny (one male plus two females) was the least successful option, because she had to share the help of one male with another female, and her chicks often starved. In polygyny, females often chased and fought each other. If one of them could drive the other away,

then she could claim the male's full-time help and so enjoy the greater success of monogamy. A polyandrous female (one female with two males) was even more successful: if she shared copulations between both her males, then both helped to feed her brood. With this extra help, more chicks survived. This explained why a female encouraged both alpha and beta males to copulate with her. Our experiments showed that she maximized total male help by sharing copulations equally between the two males.

By contrast, a male fared least well in polyandry. Although more young were raised, there was the cost of shared paternity. Our DNA fingerprinting results showed that an alpha male did better with full paternity of a pair-fed brood. This explains why alpha males acted against the female's wishes, and tried to drive beta males away, or at least prevent them from copulating. A male did best of all in polygyny, the system in which a female did worst. Although each female was less productive, the combined output of two females in polygyny exceeded that of a monogamous female. So once again there was conflict—the male intervened in the squabbles between his two females in an attempt to retain them both.

The variable mating system thus reflects the different outcomes of sexual conflict. Where a male can prevent the conflicts between two females, we find polygyny. Where a female can escape the close guarding of her alpha male, and give a mating share to the beta male, we observe polyandry. Monogamy occurs when neither sex can gain a second mate. Polygynandry—for example, two males with two females can be viewed as a "stalemate": the alpha male is unable to drive the beta male off and so claim both females for himself, and neither female can evict the other and so claim both males for herself.

So the interesting question is: What determines whether particular individuals can get their best option despite the conflicting preferences of others? This is influenced by individual competitive ability and various practical considerations, such as vegetation density (which determines how easily an alpha male can follow a female). The main point is that the social conflicts are played on an ecological stage, which may affect the likely outcomes.

Sexual selection and mating systems are often presented as two distinct topics. Is it possible to understand one without the other?

Darwin's theory of sexual selection aims to explain the evolution of traits that increase an individual's mating success: size, weapons, ornaments, mate choice, and so on. Mating systems are the outcomes of this competition for mates. So you need to think about both process and outcome for a full understanding.

Why do you think polyandry is rare compared to polygyny?

When you look at social groups, it is certainly true that you more often see one male defending a group of females rather than the converse, namely one female defending a group of males. In theory, this is exactly what you would expect, because a male usually has a greater potential reproductive rate than a female. This means that an increase in the number of mates leads to a much greater increase in male reproductive success than it does in female reproductive success. Thus, males often go for quantity, while females seek quality, when they search for mates. Nevertheless, until recent years we underestimated the frequency with which females seek matings with multiple males. They often do this surreptitiously, sometimes outside their social groups, to increase their access to resources, to increase male care, to reduce male harassment, or to improve the genetic quality of their offspring.

> **Males often go for quantity, while females seek quality, when they search for mates. Nevertheless, until recent years, we underestimated the frequency with which females seek matings with multiple males. They often do this surreptitiously. . . .**

Recently there has been some debate as to who calls the shots when it comes to mating systems—males or females? Clearly any given mating requires both a male and female, but are there certain situations in which you expect males to be controlling the mating system, and others where mating systems are primarily under the control of females?

Darwin's theory of sexual selection aimed to explain how individuals competed for mates. He proposed two processes: people readily accepted the first, namely male-male competition (Darwin's "law of battle"), but were reluctant to believe the second, namely female choice. We now have good evidence for this, of course. It is interesting to see reactions to Parker's theory of sperm competition (sexual selection after the act of mating) follow the same history. At first, everyone focused on males—mate guarding, frequent copulation, mating plugs, sperm removal, testis size, and so on. Consideration of female roles ("cryptic female choice" of sperm) came later, and it is still controversial. My guess is that female roles will be crucial, simply because females should be better able to control events inside their own bodies.

In some cases, the act of mating seems to be under male control; for example, where female insects lay their eggs in localized patches (e.g., cow pats), powerful males can monopolize the laying sites, and a female is forced to mate in order to gain access. In other cases, females can more easily escape males; for example, insects that lay their eggs in more dispersed sites can often refuse matings, and in birds (where females can often easily escape males by flying off) mating rarely occurs without female consent. It will be interesting to see whether cryptic female choice of sperm is more likely in cases where females have less control over the act of mating.

Dr. Nick Davies is a professor at Cambridge University in England. His long-term work on dunnocks, summarized in Dunnock Behaviour and Social Evolution *(Oxford University Press, 1992), elegantly shows the complexity of animal mating systems and how one goes about testing fundamentally important hypotheses in such a system.*

SUMMARY

1. Animal mating systems are typically classified as monogamous, polygynous, polyandrous, polygynandrous, or promiscuous, depending on the number of mates that males and females take and the timing of such mating in relation to breeding season.

2. A female can often fertilize all her available eggs by mating with one or a very few males. That being the case, female fecundity is not so much tied to the availability of mates as it is to the availability of resources, such as food, defense, and so on. The more resources available, the more offspring females can produce.

3. Males can potentially fertilize many, many females, and so their reproductive success is tied more to access to females than to access to resources. As such, female dispersion patterns should track the distribution of resources, whereas male dispersion patterns should track the dispersion of females.

4. Recent work in neurobiology and endocrinology has provided animal behaviorists with a better understanding of the proximate underpinnings of both monogamy and polygamy.

5. Phylogenetic work has shed light on the relationship between mating systems and habitat quality. Monogamous systems are often found in poor habitats, and polygynous systems are found in better habitats.

6. The polygyny threshold model predicts under what conditions polygyny should occur in nature. In this model, females weigh the costs and benefits associated with being in a polygynous relationship on a good territory versus a monogamous (or more precisely, a less polygynous) relationship on a poorer territory.

7. While extrapair copulations and extrapair matings were once thought to be rare in birds, genetic evidence suggests that this is far from true in many species.

8. In some mating systems, males compete not only for access to mates, but directly for access to eggs. If females store sperm from numerous matings, sperm from different males compete with one another over access to fertilizable eggs in what is known as sperm competition.

DISCUSSION QUESTIONS

1. Define and distinguish among serial monogamy, serial polygyny, simultaneous polygyny, promiscuity with pair bonds, and promiscuity without pair bonds.

2. Read Jenni and Colliers's 1972 article "Polyandry in the American jacana (*Jacana spinosa*)" in *Auk* (vol. 89, pp. 743–765). What selective forces favored polyandry in jacanas, and how did ecological factors affect selection pressure?

3. Why do you think that polygamous mating systems more strongly favor the evolution of virulent diseases in animals and humans than do monogamous breeding systems? Think about this from the perspective of the disease-causing agent.

4. Define an EPC. How does this differ from an extrapair mating? Why did it take ethologists so long to recognize the extent of EPCs in nature? How has molecular genetics revolutionized the way we think of mating systems in birds?

5. How has natural selection via sperm competition shaped both sperm morphology and male behavior? Create a list of potential ways in which females may affect sperm competition and its outcome.

6. What is a lek, and why is that form of polygyny especially interesting to ethologists? How has knowledge of kinship bonds contributed to an understanding of why males form leks?

SUGGESTED READING

Arnqvist, G., & Rowe, L. (2005). *Sexual conflict*. Princeton: Princeton University Press. A book-length treatment of sexual conflict and the way that it shapes mating systems.

Birkhead, T., & Parker, G. (1997). Sperm competition and mating systems. In J. R. Krebs & N. B. Davies (Eds.), *Behavioural ecology: An evolutionary approach* (4th ed., pp. 121–145). Oxford: Blackwell. A nice overview of sperm competition and its effects on the evolution of mating systems.

Davies, N. B. (1992). *Dunnock behaviour and social evolution*. Oxford: Oxford University Press. This is a delightful book about Davies's long-term work on dunnock behavior, with an emphasis on dunnock mating behavior.

Orians, G. (1969). On the evolution of mating systems in birds and mammals. *American Naturalist, 103*, 589–603. This is the paper in which Orians lays out the idea for the polygyny threshold model.

Parker, G. (1970). Sperm competition and its evolutionary consequences in insects. *Biological Reviews of the Cambridge Philosophical Society, 45*, 525–567. The seminal paper (no pun intended) of sperm competition and animal behavior.

Searcy, W., Yasukawa, K., & Lanyon, S. (1999). Evolution of polygyny in the ancestors of red-winged blackbirds. *Auk, 116*, 5–19. A nice paper on the phylogenetic approach to mating systems.

8

Kinship

onsider the following scenario: In an open field somewhere, a group of ground squirrels feed and go about their normal daily activities. Seemingly out of nowhere, a long-tailed weasel (*Mustela frenata*) appears, targeting the squirrels in the field for its next meal. Suddenly a piercing alarm call given by one squirrel alerts others of the impending danger. The field comes to life with squirrels making mad dashes everywhere, doing whatever they can to reach their burrow, or at least some safe haven. Later, when the predator has clearly set its sights elsewhere, the squirrels reemerge.

If we think about this type of alarm calling in the light of natural selection, it seems counterintuitive. Why should an individual squirrel be the potential "sacrificial lamb" and give off an alarm cry? After all, screaming alarm calls as loud as possible, if nothing else, should make the alarm caller the single most obvious thing in the entire field. Why would the alarm caller do anything to attract a predator in its direction and make itself the predator's most likely next meal? Why not let another squirrel take the risks?

Paul Sherman has been addressing these sorts of questions in long-term studies of alarm calls in Belding's ground squirrels (*Spermophilus beldingi*; Sherman, 1977, 1980, 1981, 1985; Figure 8.1). Sherman has found that genetic relatedness affects animal behavior in important ways, playing a large role in whether or not a squirrel will emit an alarm call when a predator is detected.

In this chapter, after an introductory section demonstrating the power of kinship to affect animal behavior, we will examine:

▸ the theoretical foundation underlying "inclusive fitness," or kin selection models of social behavior,
▸ the evolution of the family unit,
▸ parent/offspring conflict and sibling rivalry,
▸ how animals recognize kin.

A   **B**

FIGURE 8.1. Alarm calling in squirrels. In Belding's ground squirrels, females **(A)** are much more likely than males to emit alarm calls when predators are sighted. Such alarm calls warn others, including female relatives and their pups **(B)**. *(Photo credits: George D. Lepp and Paul Sherman)*

Kinship and Animal Behavior

Belding's ground squirrels, like many other species—for example, prairie dogs—give alarm calls when a predator is spotted (Hoogland, 1983, 1995; Figure 8.2). These calls warn nearby individuals that a predator is in the vicinity, leading to a mass exodus toward places of safety. To begin to answer why Belding's ground squirrels give alarm calls at the risk of their own lives, we need to recognize that alarm calls in these squirrels are most often emitted by females. That is, female squirrels give alarm calls when a predator is in the vicinity more often than expected by chance, while males give fewer alarm calls than expected by chance (Figure 8.3). This is a critical piece of information, as it changes the question from "Why are alarm calls emitted?" to "Why do females give alarm calls so often?" The answer lies in gender differences in where the squirrels live and their proximity to their kin.

In Belding's ground squirrels, males leave home to find mates, but females mature in their natal area (that is, their place of birth). This male-biased dispersal creates an imbalance in the way males and females are related to the individuals who live around them—females find themselves surrounded by relatives, while adult males are generally in groups that do not contain their genetic relatives (Figure 8.4). What this means is that when females give alarm calls, they are warning close kin. Any alarm calls given by adult males, however, primarily warn unrelated individuals. Kinship, then, lies at the heart of female alarm calling. Further support for the kinship-based alarm-calling hypothesis includes Sherman's finding that, in the rare instances in which adult females do move away from their natal groups and into groups with far fewer relatives, they emit alarm calls less frequently than do native females.

Kinship not only promotes prosocial behavior—indeed, most of this chapter will focus on cooperation between genetic relatives—but it acts as a force in deterring antisocial behavior as well. As an extreme case, consider homicide in humans. Martin Daly and Margo Wilson examined 512 homicide cases occurring in 1972 in Detroit, Michigan (Daly and Wilson, 1988). In the police records, 127—a full 25 percent—of these murders were committed by what the

FIGURE 8.2. Calling out danger.
Black-tailed prairie dogs are also often on the lookout for predators. Alarm calls in this species help kin escape potential danger. *(Photo credit: John Hoogland and Wind Cave National Park)*

First squirrel giving an alarm call to a predatory mammal

FIGURE 8.3. Ground squirrel alarm calls.
When comparing the observed (orange bars) versus the expected (green bars) frequencies of alarm calls in Belding's ground squirrels, females clearly are responsible for emitting such calls at a rate greater than that expected by chance ($p < .001$). As a result of dispersal differences across sexes, females, but not males, are often in kin-based groups. *(From Sherman, 1977)*

FIGURE 8.4. Kin selection and ground squirrels. Belding's ground squirrel groups are typically made up of mothers, daughters, and sisters who cooperate with one another in a variety of contexts. Males that emigrate into such groups cooperate to a much smaller degree. *(Based on Pfennig and Sherman, 1995)*

police records denote as "relatives." The police, however, classify in-laws, and even boyfriend-girlfriend pairs, as relatives, rather than limiting this category to genetic kin. When Daly and Wilson considered only genetic kin, rather than these other categories, only 6 percent of the murders involved relatives. Genetic kin don't kill each other all that often because harming genetic relatives is selected against for the very same reason that dispensing altruism to relatives is favored—they both have indirect consequences on those who share the same genes.

With respect to Daly and Wilson's homicide data from Detroit, it might be argued that the reason that homicide rates among genetic kin are low is that, in modern society, people encounter unrelated individuals much more often than genetic kin. For example, if killers spent 94 percent of their time with unrelated individuals and 6 percent with genetic kin, then the 6 percent murder rate among genetic kin would be expected simply by chance, and this would not indicate that genetic relatedness reduces homicide. Yet, Daly and Wilson found that, even when the amount of time spent with genetic kin versus everyone else is taken into account, genetic relatives rarely kill each other (Table 8.1). Few forces have the power to shape animal behavior the way that genetic kinship can.

Kinship Theory

The modern study of animal behavior and evolution began in the early 1960s, when W. D. Hamilton, one of the leading evolutionary biologists of the twentieth

TABLE 8.1. Risk of homicide in cases where the victim and offender were cohabitants in Detroit in 1972. Observed values indicate the number of homicides that were actually committed. Expected values indicate the number of homicides in each category that we would expect if genetic kinship were not playing a role. Relative risk rates were much higher for individuals who were not genetic relatives. These numbers are underestimates since the "parent" and "offspring" categories include some stepfamily members and some in-laws. *(From Daly and Wilson, 1988)*

THE AVERAGE DETROITER ≥ 14 YEARS OLD IN 1972 LIVED WITH 3.0 PEOPLE	NUMBER OF VICTIMS		RELATIVE RISK (OBSERVED/EXPECTED)
	OBSERVED	EXPECTED	
0.6 Spouses	65	20	3.32
0.1 Nonrelatives	11	3	3.33
0.9 "Offspring"	8	29	0.27
0.4 "Parents"	9	13	0.69
1.0 Other "relatives"	5	33	0.15

century, published his now famous papers on genetic kinship and the evolution of social behavior (Hamilton, 1963, 1964). These papers formalized the theory of "inclusive fitness" or "kinship" theory and revolutionized the way scientists understood evolution and ethology (Kuhn, 1962). You will recall from Chapter 1 that inclusive fitness theory conceptualizes an individual's total fitness as based both on the number of its own offspring and the contribution it makes to the reproductive success of its genetic relatives.

Simply knowing which individuals in a population are genetic relatives provides ethologists and behavioral ecologists with enough information to make some basic, but important, predictions about social behavior. With this in mind, we can now address the question of *why* kinship is so powerful an evolutionary force in promoting social behaviors like cooperation and altruism (in Chapter 9 we will discuss other paths leading to such behaviors). Hamilton had this to say in his seminal mathematical model tying together genetic kinship and the evolution of altruism:

> In the hope that it may provide a useful summary we therefore hazard the following generalized unrigourous statement of the main principle that has emerged from the model. *The social behavior of a species evolves in such a way that in each distinct behavior-evoking situation the individual will seem to value his neighbors' fitness against his own according to the coefficients of relationship appropriate to that situation* [Hamilton's italics]. (Hamilton, 1964, p. 19)

Although rightly credited with being the father of modern kinship theory, Hamilton was not the first to recognize the power of kinship to shape behavior (Dugatkin, 2006). Before Hamilton, Charles Darwin suggested that the suicidally altruistic defense behavior that he observed in social insects like bees may have evolved as a result of bees' defending hives of their genetic kin—that is, under certain conditions, natural selection could favor such extreme altruism

FIGURE 8.5. Helping offspring. One classic case of helping genetic relatives is that of mothers feeding their young. In bank swallows, young chicks remain at the nest, and mothers remember the location of their nests so that they can return after foraging to feed youngsters there. When chicks learn to fly, mothers learn to recognize their offspring's voices. *(Based on Pfennig and Sherman, 1995)*

if the recipients of the altruistic act were genetic relatives (Figure 8.5). About seventy-five years later, a famous population geneticist, J. B. S. Haldane, also weighed in on the subject of altruism and genetic kinship. It has been rumored that Haldane once said that he would risk his life to save two of his brothers or eight of his cousins. Haldane, who was quite versed in mathematics, made this rather bold statement by counting copies of a gene that might code for cooperative behavior. Such a gene-counting approach to kinship and the evolution of cooperation has been extended by theoreticians, but in its most elementary form, it is the heart and soul of kinship theory. So, let's see how it works.

RELATEDNESS AND INCLUSIVE FITNESS

The *Random House Dictionary* defines kinship as "family relationship," but the evolutionary definition is much more restrictive. In evolutionary terms, relatedness centers on the probability that individuals share genes that they have inherited from common ancestors—parents, grandparents, and so on. Genes that are shared because of common ancestry are referred to as "identical by descent." For example, you and your brother are kin because you share some of the same genes, and you inherited them from common ancestors—in this case, your mother and father. In a similar vein, you and your cousins are kin because you share genes in common; only now your most recent common ancestors are your grandparents. In general, most recent common ancestors are those individuals through which two (or more) organisms can trace genes that they share by descent.

Once we know how to find the common ancestor of two or more individuals, we can calculate their relatedness, labeled *r*, which is equal to the probability that they share genes that are identical by descent. For example, two siblings are related to one another by an *r* value of 0.5. To see why, recall that all of the genes that siblings share come from one of two individuals—their mother or father. As such, there are two ways, *and only two ways*, that siblings can share a copy of gene X—via mother or father. If sibling 1 has gene X, then there is a 50 percent chance she received it from her mother; if sibling 2 has gene X, there is again a 50 percent chance that her mother passed this gene to sibling 2. What that means is that there is a 1 in 4 chance that the siblings share gene X through their mother. The same argument can be made to demonstrate that there is a 1 in 4 probability that the father is the reason that the siblings share gene X. To calculate the chances that the siblings share gene X through *either* their mother or their father, we add the probabilities for each and obtain 1/4 + 1/4 = 1/2, or 0.5. This value—labeled *r*—can be calculated for any set of genetic relatives, no matter how distant. For example, the genetic relatedness between cousins is 1/8 (that is, *r* = 0.125), between grandparent and grandchild is 1/4 (that is, *r* = 0.25), and between aunts/uncles and their genetic nieces and nephews is also 1/4 (that is, *r* = 0.25; Figure 8.6).

Calculating relatedness starts the process that allows us to see why kinship is such a powerful force in animal behavior. The next step in the process is to recall that natural selection favors those genes that get the most copies of themselves into the next generation. To this point, we have been thinking about a gene in terms of the effect it has on the *individual* in which it resides, but kinship calculations suggest that this is a somewhat restricted view. Given that relatives, by definition, have a higher probability of sharing gene X through common descent than do strangers, then gene X may increase its chances of getting copies of itself into the next generation by how it affects not just the individual in which it resides, but that individual's genetic relatives as well.

Think about it like this: Clearly, when an individual reproduces (and its offspring survive), copies of that individual's genes make it into the next generation. But that is not the *only* way that genes can increase their representation in future generations. If a gene—let's call it gene G—codes for preferentially aiding genetic kin, then that gene can increase its representation in the next generation because it is coding for aid to individuals that are likely to have G as well (Hamilton, 1963). How likely a recipient is to have a copy of G is equal to the genetic relatedness of the donor and recipient (50 percent probability for siblings, 25 percent probability for uncle and nephew, and so on). When we depict fitness in this manner, and consider both direct and indirect components to fitness, we are talking about **inclusive fitness**.

With an understanding of how *r* is calculated, we can now examine inclusive fitness theory in more detail. Hamilton tackled the question of kinship

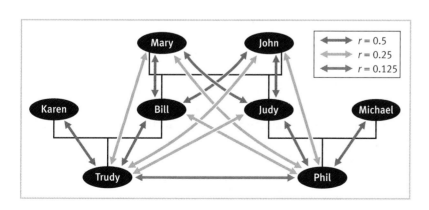

FIGURE 8.6. **Genetic relatedness.** Family trees can be used to calculate *r*, the genetic relatedness between individuals. Take this family tree of relatives. Mary and John are married and have two children: Bill and Judy. Bill marries Karen, and they have one child: Trudy. Judy marries Michael, and they have one child: Phil. Orange arrows represent an *r* of 0.5, yellow arrows an *r* of 0.25, and the green arrow an *r* of 0.125.

and animal behavior in a now famous pair of papers, "The Genetical Evolution of Social Behavior, I and II" (Hamilton, 1964). The essence of inclusive fitness models is that they add on to "classical" models of natural selection by considering the effect of a gene, not only on the individual in which it resides, but on individuals (genetic kin) carrying genes that are identical by descent. The equations in some of Hamilton's papers on kinship can be daunting, even to those with a mathematical background. Fortunately, these equations can be captured in what is now referred to as "Hamilton's Rule." This rule states that gene X increases in frequency whenever:

$$\left(\sum_{1}^{A} rb \right) - c > 0$$

where b = the benefit that others receive from traits associated with gene X (recall the benefit that squirrels received when they heard one of their group-mates give an alarm call), c = the cost accrued to the individual expressing the trait (think of the alarm caller and its risk of being taken by a predator), r is our measure of relatedness ($r = 0.5$ for siblings, $r = 0.125$ for cousins, and so on), and A is a count of the individuals affected by the trait of interest (those who hear the alarm call and head to safety; Grafen, 1984). In other words, the decision to aid family members is a function of how related individuals are, and how high or low the costs and benefits associated with the trait turn out to be. When genetic relatedness is high, then r times b is more likely to be greater than c than when genetic relatedness is low. What this means is that natural selection more strongly favors kin helping one another when r is high. In addition, as the benefit that recipients obtain (b) increases, and/or the cost (c) to the donor decreases, the probability that r times b is greater than c increases—in other words, natural selection should strongly favor kin helping one another when b is high and/or c is low. Finally, as A—the number of relatives helped by an act of altruism—increases, selection more strongly favors altruism.

Hamilton's theory has had a profound impact on the work of ethologists, behavioral ecologists, and comparative psychologists. Moreover, the impact of Hamilton's ideas has been even greater as a result of Jerram Brown's refor-mulation of Hamilton's equation. Fieldworkers in animal behavior had found the b and c terms of Hamilton's model difficult to measure in nature, but Brown solved the problem by coming up with the "offspring rule," which used the number of offspring that were born and survived as the currency of measure (Brown, 1975). This formulation set up the possibility of field manipulations in which Hamilton's and Brown's ideas could be tested by counting the number of offspring across different experimental treatments. For example, if an ethologist wanted to know the positive effects that young "helpers-at-the-nest" might have on raising their siblings, she could examine the difference in the average number of chicks that survive in the presence and absence of such helpers (Brown et al., 1982; Figure 8.7). In terms of measuring the costs to the helper of helping, ideally ethologists would measure the number of offspring produced by individuals who did not help versus those who did help. All else being equal, the difference between these values would allow for an estimation of the cost of helping. It is possible that the difference might be negative—helpers could have more offspring than those who did not help—in which case helping would entail no real fitness costs.

FIGURE 8.7. The effects of helping kin. Using groups of gray-crowned babblers that ranged from an initial size of six to eight individuals, Brown and his colleagues removed all but one of the nonreproductive helpers from the experimental groups, while leaving the number of nonreproductive helpers in the control groups unchanged. Reproductive success, as measured by the number of fledglings, was significantly lower in the experimental groups because they had fewer helpers. *(Based on Brown et al., 1982)*

FAMILY DYNAMICS

While Hamilton's Rule makes some very general predictions about animal social behavior, subsequent work by animal behaviorists and behavioral ecologists has generated more specific predictions about what can be called "family dynamics" (Emlen, 1995a). In particular, Stephen Emlen has developed an "evolutionary theory of family" that aims to test specific predictions regarding "the formation, the stability, and the social dynamics of biological families" (Emlen, 1995a, p. 8092).

The building blocks for Emlen's work on family dynamics are: (1) inclusive fitness, which is also known as kin selection theory; (2) ecological constraints theory, which examines dispersal options of mature offspring, and specifically the conditions that favor dispersal from home rather than remaining on a natal territory (Brown, 1987; Emlen, 1982a, 1982b; Koenig et al., 1992; Koenig and Pitelka, 1981); and (3) reproductive skew theory, which examines how reproductive opportunities are divided among potential breeders by predicting conditions that should favor conflict or cooperation over breeding decisions (Figure 8.8).

In an important paper in 1995, Emlen made fifteen specific predictions about animal family dynamics, and for each of these, he reviewed the evidence from the animal literature, both for and against his predictions (Table 8.2). Two years after publication of Emlen's paper, Jennifer Davis and Martin Daly tested Emlen's fifteen predictions as they relate to human families (Davis and Daly, 1997). While Emlen's data are from a wide variety of animals, Davis and Daly's analysis is necessarily restricted to one species—*Homo sapiens*. Most of their data came from the 1990 Canadian General Social Survey, a telephone survey that amassed information on family dynamics in 13,495 households. Such a survey is probably reflective of modern Western society, but it is important to recognize that it does not necessarily represent all societies that live in more ancestral human conditions, such as hunter-gatherer societies.

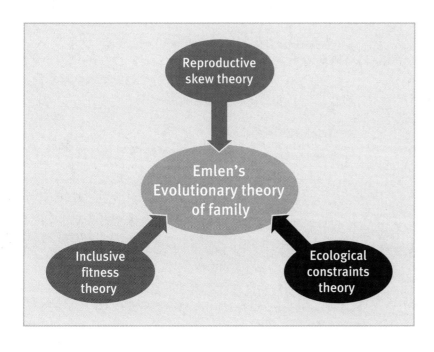

FIGURE 8.8. Evolutionary theory of family. Emlen's theory is generated by combining inclusive fitness, reproductive skew, and ecological constraints theory.

TABLE 8.2. Biological families. The table lists the fifteen hypotheses associated with Emlen's evolutionary theory of the family. *(From Emlen, 1995b, p. 8093)*

NO.	ABBREVIATED PREDICTION	EVIDENCE
1	Family groupings will be unstable, disintegrating when acceptable reproductive opportunities materialize elsewhere.	**Supportive:** 7 avian species; 2 mammalian species
2	Family stability will be greatest in those groups controlling high-quality resources. Dynasties may form.	**Supportive:** 5 avian species
3	Help with rearing offspring will be the norm.	**Supportive:** 107 avian species; 57 mammalian species **Counter:** 5 avian species; 6 mammalian species
4	Help will be expressed to the greatest extent between closest genetic relatives.	**Supportive:** 5 avian species; 3 mammalian species **Counter:** 1 avian species
5	Sexually related aggression will be reduced because incestuous matings will be avoided. Pairings will be exogamous.	**Supportive:** 18 avian species; 17 mammalian species **Counter:** 1 avian species; 3 mammalian species
6	Breeding males will invest less in offspring as their certainty of paternity decreases.	**Supportive:** 1 avian species (many additional studies, some supportive, others counter, have been conducted on nonfamilial species)
7	Family conflict will surface over filling the reproductive vacancy created by the loss of a breeder.	**Supportive:** 6 avian species
8	In stepfamilies, sexually related aggression will increase because incest restrictions do not apply to replacement mates. Offspring may mate with a stepparent.	**Supportive:** 4 avian species
9	Replacement mates (stepparents) will invest less in existing offspring than will biological parents. Infanticide may occur.	**Supportive:** 2 avian species; 2 studies summarizing mammalian data (Hausfater and Hrdy, 1984; Hrdy, 1999)
10	Family members will reduce their investment in future offspring after a parent finds a new mate.	**Supportive:** 2 avian species **Counter:** 2 avian species
11	Stepfamilies will be less stable than biologically intact families.	No data currently available
12	Decreasing ecological constraints will lead to increased sharing of reproduction.	**Supportive:** 2 avian species
13	Decreasing asymmetry in dominance will lead to increased sharing of reproduction.	**Supportive:** 2 avian species; 1 mammalian species
14	Increasing symmetry of kinship will lead to increasing sharing of reproduction.	**Supportive:** 4 avian species
15	Decreasing genetic relatedness will lead to increased sharing of reproduction. Reproductive suppression will be greatest among closest kin.	**Supportive:** 5 avian species; 2 mammalian species

A review of the papers by Emlen and by Davis and Daly provides us with a unique opportunity to examine and test evolutionary theories of family in both humans and nonhumans. To do this, we will examine a subset of four of Emlen's predictions (his predictions numbered 1, 2, 4, and 9) in more detail. These four predictions were chosen to show the diversity of issues that kinship touches upon within animal and human behavior.

PREDICTION 1. "Family dynamics will be unstable, disintegrating when acceptable reproductive opportunities materialize elsewhere."

This is the most basic prediction made by Emlen, as it focuses on fundamental costs and benefits associated with family life. Broadly speaking, individuals who have a higher inclusive fitness when remaining with their family should stay as part of the family unit, while those who have better opportunities for increasing their inclusive fitness elsewhere should depart and avail themselves of that opportunity. Evidence in support of this prediction in animals comes from many studies of birds and mammals.

One technique for experimentally examining prediction 1 is to create new, unoccupied territories and examine whether mature offspring leave their natal area to live in such newly created areas (Komdeur, 1992; Pruett-Jones and Lewis, 1990; Walters et al., 1992). To see how such an experiment is undertaken, consider Stephen Pruett-Jones's work with superb fairy wrens (*Malurus cyaneus*), an insectivorous (insect-eating) Australian bird species (Pruett-Jones and Lewis, 1990; Figure 8.9). In superb fairy wrens, a breeding pair is often helped by its nonbreeding young male offspring, who provide their siblings with such resources as additional food and protection. In contrast, female superb fairy wrens emigrate from their natal territory and hence do not help to raise siblings at their parents' nest. To test the prediction that families will break down when suitable territories emerge for young helper males, Pruett-Jones and Lewis removed the breeding males from twenty-nine superb fairy wren territories. All in all, they performed forty-six removals over time, as some territories had a resident removed more than once.

By removing breeding males from their natal territories, new breeding opportunities arose for male helpers in nests in new areas that were near the area of the removals. All but one of the thirty-two potential male helpers who could have dispersed to the newly opened territories did so, and, they did so quickly—new territories were usually occupied by former male helpers within six hours. But why? Why did males immediately leave home when reproductive opportunities emerged? Apparently, a shortage of females and breeding territories created a scenario in which reproductive opportunities were exceedingly rare, and so selection favored male helpers who instantly seized the opportunity for a breeding territory and thus disbanded family life when the chance arose (Figure 8.10). As such, Pruett-Jones and Lewis's work suggests that helping-at-the-nest may raise the inclusive fitness of young males when territories are limited, but not otherwise.

Not surprisingly, the picture is not as clear-cut when it comes to testing Prediction 1 in humans. In their analysis of the data from the Canadian General Social Survey, Davis and Daly found that married individuals were much more likely to live away from their parents than were single individuals in the same age/sex category. This suggests that new marriages—that is, new opportunities for reproductive success—cause existing family units to dissolve. It is important to understand that it need not have turned out that way, however. Davis and

FIGURE 8.9. Superb fairy wren. In superb fairy wrens, young males often act as helpers-at-the-nest. When Pruett-Jones removed breeding males from their territories, almost all potential male helpers who could have dispersed to newly opened territories did so. *(Photo credit: Graeme Chapman)*

FIGURE 8.10. Family breakup. In the superb fairy wren, male helpers often assist their parents. If a vacant territory opens up, however, male helpers are quick to leave the family unit and attempt to start their own family.

Daly *might* have discovered that married individuals were *more* likely than single individuals to live with one set of parents, but instead the data supported Emlen's first prediction.

While the above data on dispersal and residence patterns suggest that marriage causes the dissolution of existing family units (and, of course, creates new such units), Prediction 1 was not supported when Davis and Daly used another set of relevant data to test this prediction. When they asked whether married and single individuals living away from their parents differed in terms of contact with parents or grandparents, very few differences emerged—differences we might expect if marriage did break up already existing families. For most age/sex categories, married individuals living apart from either set of parents were just as likely to stay in contact (via phone, visits, letters) with parents and grandparents as were single individuals living away from home, in clear contrast to Prediction 1.

Davis and Daly tested Prediction 1 in other ways as well, and they argue, that as a whole, the data from the Canadian GSS do not support Emlen's first prediction. Davis and Daly note, "at best Emlen's first prediction holds only for some demographic groups with some types of relatives" (Davis and Daly, 1997, p. 415). Rather, Davis and Daly believe that, with some exceptions, it appears that human parents act as post-reproductive helpers to their own offspring, which may select for strong family bonds that do not easily dissolve when offspring get married.

PREDICTION 2. "Families that control high-quality resources will be more stable than those with lower-quality resources. Some resource-rich areas will support dynasties in which one genetic lineage continuously occupies the same area over many successive generations."

Inclusive fitness theory predicts that individuals may remain in their natal territory if there are enough resources for them to mate and provide for their own offspring. That is, if the benefits associated with remaining on a territory of birth are sufficiently great—lots of food and the space to attract a mate and breed, for example—then that, in conjunction with the indirect benefits of helping relatives, produces a strong force to keep families intact. On the other hand, individuals will tend to leave their family if there are not enough resources at their natal territories.

Emlen argues that offspring from families that control high-quality resources are likely to be much more reluctant to vacate the natal territory, as few alternative territories provide the resources that are available at home. Over the long run, this will create dynasties in families that occupy the very highest-quality territories (see Chapter 13). Not only are the offspring that remain on high-quality territories receiving a benefit, but their parents are as well, since they then pass down the best-quality territories to their genetic kin (Brown, 1974).

Data from six species of birds support the dynasty-building hypothesis in that birds from high-quality family territories are indeed less likely to disperse from the natal territory than their counterparts from families with inferior territories. For example, in cooperatively breeding acorn woodpeckers (*Melanerpes formicivorus*), the critical measure of territory quality is the number of storage holes (Figure 8.11). In a New Mexican population of acorn woodpeckers studied by Peter Stacey and David Ligon, territories varied from less than a 1,000 to greater than 3,000 storage holes for acorns.

Not surprisingly, individuals on territories with lots of storage holes produced a greater average number of offspring (Stacey and Ligon, 1987; Figure 8.12). More to the point, in areas with more than 3,000 storage holes, 27 percent of the young remained on their natal territories and helped their relatives, while only 2 percent of the young on territories with fewer than 1,000 holes stayed

FIGURE 8.11. Dynasty building in acorn woodpeckers. In cooperatively breeding acorn woodpeckers (*Melanerpes formicivorus*), the young not only survive better on territories with more storage holes, they are also more likely to remain on their natal territories throughout their life, creating a "family dynasty." Such dynasties enable kin groups to compete for superior territories. *(Photo credit: Steve & Dave Maslowski/Photo Researchers, Inc.)*

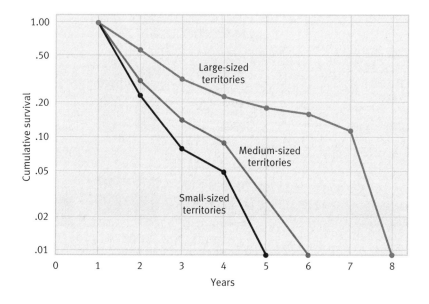

FIGURE 8.12. Territory quality and survival in acorn woodpeckers. Increasing territory size, and hence increasing number of storage holes, led to increased rates of survival. *(Based on Stacey and Ligon, 1987, p. 663)*

and helped, despite the fact that many open territories were available to all young individuals. The benefits of remaining on a high-quality territory appear to be real, as (male) birds who served as helpers had a relatively high probability of eventually entering the breeding population, often breeding in turn on their natal territory, either at the same time as their parents or after their parents had died (Stacey and Ligon, 1987).

In terms of human family dynamics, Prediction 2 translates into well-to-do families being more stable than poorer families. Davis and Daly found that if a stable family is defined in terms of co-residence (as in the nonhuman case), then this prediction is not supported. To cite just one of Davis and Daly's examples, young adults from rich (First World) families tend to be *less* likely to be living with their parents than are same-aged individuals from poorer families (White, 1994a). Nonetheless, since resources are much more mobile than ever in today's Western economies, it might be argued that familial co-residence is an inappropriate yardstick for measuring family stability. If the measure of stability is defined in terms of maintaining family contacts and providing social support during adulthood, the data are more supportive of Prediction 2.

At the most general level, data suggest that contact and support are indeed found more often in wealthy families (Eggebeen and Hogan, 1990; Taylor, 1986; White and Reidmann, 1992). Davis and Daly used GSS data to address the more detailed question of whether contact with kin is not only more likely, but more frequent, as a function of wealth. Using letter, phone, or face-to-face conversations as a measure of contact, they examined whether individuals in wealthier families kept in contact more often with parents, grandparents, and siblings than did individuals in poorer families. The GSS data suggest that for most age/sex cohorts, wealthier individuals did keep in touch with relatives more often than did lower-income individuals (Figure 8.13). But Daly and

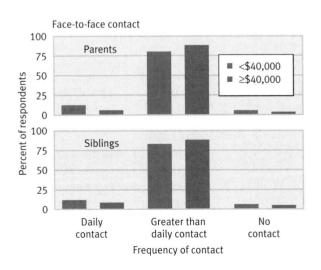

FIGURE 8.13. Wealth and familial contact. Based on Emlen's dynasty building hypothesis, Davis and Daly hypothesized that familial contact would be greater in wealthy human family units. The data from the 1991 Canadian General Social Survey support this general prediction. *(From Davis and Daly, 1997)*

FIGURE 8.14. White-fronted bee-eater kinship. Inclusive fitness models of behavior have been tested extensively in white-fronted bee-eaters. *(Photo credits: N. J. Demong)*

Wilson offer an important caveat that emerged from the massive data set they examined (only a small fraction of which we see in the figure). They note that while "the available evidence indicates that high-income families are more likely to maintain social ties at some level and to engage in exchange . . . the present analysis also suggests that the strength of these ties may be weaker" (Davis and Daly, 1997, p. 420).

PREDICTION 4. "Assistance in rearing offspring (cooperative breeding) will be expressed to the greatest extent between those family members that are the closest genetic relatives."

As mentioned earlier, under Hamilton's Rule, when genetic relatedness is high, we predict increasing levels of cooperative and altruistic interactions between related individuals. In addition, Hamilton's Rule suggests that, all else being equal, when given the choice between helping individuals who differ with respect to r (the coefficient of relatedness), more aid should be dispensed to the closest genetic kin than to more distantly related kin.

Emlen reports that of the nine studies published on cooperation in birds or mammals that live in extended families, eight of the studies revealed individuals who preferentially extended aid as a function of genetic relatedness. For example, in white-fronted bee-eaters (*Merops bullockoides;* Figure 8.14), helpers chose to aid individuals they themselves were most closely related to in 108 of 115 opportunities (Figure 8.15).

In addition to supporting a basic prediction of kinship theory, Emlen's results helped resolve a thorny issue surrounding Hamilton's Rule. Beginning in 1975, a number of researchers, including Mary Jane West-Eberhard and David Barash, had suggested that individuals should dispense altruistic aid to relatives in *direct proportion* to their genetic relatedness (Barash, 1975; West-Eberhard, 1975). Let's label this the "proportional altruism" model. For example, imagine that an individual has nine units worth of aid that it can dispense to relatives. Suppose then that this individual interacts with one sibling ($r = 0.5$) and one uncle ($r = 0.25$). Since siblings share an r value twice as great as that between uncle and nephew, the proportional altruism model predicts that six units of aid

FIGURE 8.15. Helping close relatives. In white-fronted bee-eaters, individuals are more likely to help those to whom they are more closely related (as indicated by r, the coefficient of relatedness). For example, when interacting with genetic kin with $r = 0.5$, birds dispensed aid 80 percent of the time, but that percentage drops to less than 20 percent when $r = 0.125$. *(Based on Emlen, 1995b)*

should be dispensed to the sibling and three units of aid should be dispensed to the uncle.

Stuart Altmann argued that the proportional model was based on faulty logic, because an individual always increases its inclusive fitness most when it is altruistic toward its closest genetic relative (Altmann, 1979). Instead, Altmann predicted that an individual should dispense *all* of its aid to the recipient that is its closest genetic relative (let's call this the "all-or-nothing" model). In our hypothetical case, Altmann's model predicts that all nine units should be dispensed toward the donor's sibling. In principle, Altmann is right, but the question really is whether animals actually do behave in accordance with Altmann's predictions. Emlen's work on white-fronted bee-eaters enables us to answer this question, for it allows behavioral and evolutionary biologists to determine which of these two models better fits data gathered in the wild. In support of Altmann's model, Emlen found that helpers not only overwhelmingly chose to help their closest genetic relative, but that once a helper made a choice, it dispensed all of its aid toward the chosen individual.

In many ways, kinship and aiding relatives is best exemplified by social insects, who show extreme levels of cooperation in conjunction with an odd genetic architecture that creates sisters that are "super relatives." These super relatives come about because many social insects have a haplodiploid genetic system. Normally, we think of all individuals in a species as being either diploid (possessing two copies of each chromosome) or haploid (possessing only one copy of each chromosome). Haplodiploid species defy this convention in that males are haploid, while females are diploid.

As a result of the genetics underlying haplodiploidy, sisters are related to one another on average by a coefficient of relatedness of 0.75, which has the effect of making females more related to their sisters than to their own offspring. This value differs from the standard average relatedness of sisters in diploid species ($r = 0.5$), because in haplodiploids, full sisters inherit exactly the same genes from their father, while in diploid species, females have only a 50 percent chance that a gene that they inherited from their father is identical to a gene that their sister inherited from their father.

With an r of 0.75 between sisters, one would expect high levels of aid giving—just the sort of thing for which social insects are well known. It is, of course, the female workers in many species who go to suicidal lengths to defend a hive full of their sisters. A bee's stinger is designed for maximal efficiency, and this often entails having the stinger ripped from the body of the bee doing the stinging, in a way that causes the death of the stinging individual. Kinship need not, however, produce such ultra-altruism. If individuals are able to gauge their relatedness to others, then social insects may be influenced by kinship in any number of ways. Consider the fascinating case of **worker policing** in honeybees (*Apis mellifera*), in which sterile worker bees use information associated with genetic relatedness to "police" their hive, and destroy eggs that are less related to them so that their inclusive fitness is increased (Ratnieks and Visscher, 1989).

In honeybee hives, queens produce most of the offspring, but workers can also produce unfertilized eggs that always develop into males. Using the mathematics of inclusive fitness theory, Francis Ratnieks and P. Kirk Visscher found that in honeybee colonies with a single queen who mates one time, female workers are more related to their nephews (their sisters' sons, $r = 0.375$) than to their brothers (the queen's sons, $r = 0.25$) (Ratnieks and Visscher, 1989). But this

A

B

FIGURE 8.16. Honeybee policing. (A) While the queen (designated by the red dot on her back) typically lays the eggs in a honeybee colony, workers also attempt to lay unfertilized eggs. **(B)** When an egg laid by a worker is detected by worker police, it is eaten or destroyed. Workers are much more likely to destroy eggs produced by other workers than eggs produced by the queen. Such "policing" has inclusive fitness benefits associated with it. *(Photo credits: Francis Ratnieks)*

inequality switches when the queen mates multiple times. And indeed, honeybee queens typically mate with ten to twenty different males. When multiple mating takes place, workers may be more closely related to brothers (males produced by the queen) than to nephews (males produced by their sister workers), with the exact values of relatedness depending on the number of different males with whom a queen mates. Under such conditions—when female workers are more related to brothers than to nephews—Ratnieks has hypothesized that worker policing of honeybee reproduction may evolve (Ratnieks and Visscher, 1988, 1989). Such policing, for example, may take the form of workers favoring those eggs to which they are most highly related (Figure 8.16).

Ratnieks and Visscher examined the possibility that honeybee workers may favor brothers over nephews. They found that honeybee workers showed remarkable abilities to discriminate between worker-laid eggs, which produce nephews, and haploid queen-laid eggs, which produce brothers. After twenty-four hours, only 2 percent of the worker-laid eggs remained alive, while 61 percent of the haploid queen-laid eggs remained alive (Figure 8.17). Workers

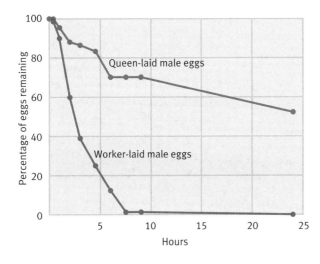

FIGURE 8.17. Worker policing in honeybees. In honeybees, where queens often mate with ten to twenty males, workers are more related to the male offspring of the queen (their brothers) than to offspring of other workers (their nephews). Workers police the hive and search out and eat the eggs of other workers. *(From Ratnieks and Visscher, 1989)*

A

B

FIGURE 8.18. Wasp policing. Policing occurs in wasps, as well as in honeybees. In the wasp *Dolichovespula saxonica*, workers often lay (haploid) eggs, both in nests with single-mated and multiply mated queens. Such eggs are often eaten when detected by other workers. **(A)** The wasp in the middle of the photo is a worker who has just laid an egg. **(B)** Here a worker is eating another worker's egg. Policing is much more common in wasp colonies where the queen has mated with many males. *(Photo credits: Kevin Foster)*

appear to use a specific egg-marking pheromone produced only by queens to distinguish which eggs to destroy and which eggs to leave unharmed, and in so doing, they police the hive in a manner that increases their inclusive fitness (Ratnieks, 1995; Ratnieks and Visscher, 1989).

Tom Wenseleers and Ratnieks extended the logic of policing behavior to further explore the relationship between kinship and reproduction in insects (Wenseleers and Ratnieks, 2006; Figure 8.18). If policing was effective at removing the eggs laid by workers, they reasoned, then this should create strong selection pressures against worker reproduction in the first place. They tested this idea by examining policing behavior in ten species—nine species of wasps and the honeybee. They predicted, and subsequently found, that the more effective policing was at removing worker eggs, the less often workers attempted to reproduce (Figure 8.19).

FIGURE 8.19. Effective policing. The more effective that policing was at removing worker eggs, the fewer the workers that attempted to produce eggs. *(From Wenseleers and Ratnieks, 2006)*

Unfortunately, in Davis and Daly's examination of Prediction 4 in humans, the GSS data were not collected in a way to address this question. For the most part, individuals in the GSS study were either related by an *r* value of 0.5 or 0.0, and thus the distinction between how different relatives, that is, individuals with different positive values of *r*, are treated could not be addressed.

PREDICTION 9. "Replacement mates (stepparents) will invest less in existing offspring than will biological parents. . . ."

This prediction stems from an extension of kinship theory to the case of stepfamilies. Inclusive fitness theory predicts that when stepparents decide how to distribute benefits to offspring, they should favor their biological offspring ($r = 0.5$) over their stepchildren ($r = 0$). The extreme version of this hypothesis predicts that, under certain conditions, a stepparent may opt to harm, potentially in a fatal manner, their mate's offspring by previous mates, as such offspring are unrelated to the stepparent (in genetic kinship terms), and as such are a drain on resources that return no kin-based benefits (Blaffer-Hrdy, 1979; Hausfater and Blaffer-Hrdy, 1984; Hrdy, 1999; Parmigian and Vom Saal, 1995; Figure 8.20). Further, as a result of the fact that in most species males are physically dominant to females, Emlen and Sarah Blaffer-Hrdy argue that such violence to stepchildren—even in humans—will be more common when the stepparent is a male (Blaffer-Hrdy, 1977; Emlen, 1995a).

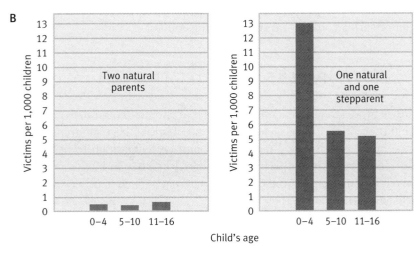

FIGURE 8.20. **Child abuse and genetic relatedness. (A)** The per capita rates of child abuse reported in 1980 by the American Humane Association in the United States. Rates of child abuse were significantly greater in households where one parent was not genetic kin. **(B)** The same relationship between child abuse and family type was also uncovered in Canada, as reported in 1983 by a provincial registry in Hamilton, Ontario. *(From Daly and Wilson, 1988)*

With respect to human behavior and Prediction 9, cross-cultural data demonstrate that stepparents invest less in their stepchildren than in their biological children, and children from stepfamilies leave home significantly earlier and have more behavioral problems than children from biologically intact families (Bray, 1988; Daly and Wilson, 1996; Emlen, 1995b; Hofferth, 2006; Hofferth and Anderson, 2003; White, 1994b). Some of the strongest data on human behavior comes from comparisons of biological families versus stepfamilies. Stepchildren suffer up to 100 times more child abuse than do biological children (Daly and Wilson, 1988, 1999). The extreme version of such abuse translates into stepchildren being murdered at a much higher rate than biological offspring in most, but not all, large-scale studies (Daly and Wilson, 1988, 1994, 1999; Kaplun and Reich, 1976; Temrin et al., 2000). Such abuse and murder are predominately at the hands of the stepparent, and because custom and law around the world favor a mother's rights—when a couple separates, mothers generally have custody of the children—the abusing parent is typically a stepfather.

The case for the lack of genetic relatedness driving stepfamily violence in humans is not constrained to interactions between stepparents and stepchildren. In addition to stepparents having no genetic connection to their stepchildren, stepsiblings and half-siblings also have a lower r (respectively 0 or .25) than full biological siblings ($r = 0.5$), and indeed some data suggest that conflicts are more common among half-sibs (Aquilino, 1991; Zill, 1988).

Data from rodents, carnivores, and primates also support the hypothesis that stepparents invest less in stepchildren. Moreover, infanticide on the part of male, as well as female, stepparents has been uncovered in numerous species in these groups (Hausfater and Blaffer-Hrdy, 1984).

Conflict within Families

As is obvious from the above, genetic relatedness plays a pivotal role in understanding how animal social behaviors evolve. Most often, inclusive fitness theory is used to better understand why relatives are more cooperative as a function of genetic relatedness. But, as we have seen in the case of child abuse, inclusive fitness theory can also be used to understand conflicts within families. To examine this phenomenon more closely, we will now turn to the subjects of parent-offspring conflict and sibling-sibling conflict.

PARENT-OFFSPRING CONFLICT

Inclusive fitness theory generally predicts that parents should go to great lengths to help their offspring because parents and offspring have an average r of 0.5. Furthermore, parents are almost always in a better position to help offspring than vice versa. As such, parental aid should be seen in many contexts. And indeed it is. Hundreds of studies have shown that parents, mothers in particular, provide all sorts of aid to their offspring.

A relatedness value of $r = 0.5$ creates strong selection pressure for parents (especially mothers; see Chapter 7) to provide aid to their offspring. Yet, there are limits to this aid, as first conceptualized by Robert Trivers in his parent-offspring conflict theory (Trivers, 1974). This theory recognizes that **parent-offspring conflict** arises with respect to a parent's decisions about how much aid to give to any particular offspring. From the perspective of the parent, these decisions are affected by how much energy is available for helping current offspring, and by how many offspring it is likely to have in the future.

In principle, a parent could dispense every ounce of energy it has to provide offspring X with all the benefits at its disposal. But if such an effort kills the parent or severely hampers the parent from producing other offspring in the future, then natural selection may not favor such behavior, as it might not maximize the *total number of offspring* that the parent is able to produce over the course of his or her lifetime. To see why, remember that every offspring has an r of 0.5 to its parent, and natural selection should favor parents who raise as many healthy offspring as possible over the course of their lives. So, there are limits on parental investment with respect to any given offspring X.

Now, let us look at **parental investment** from offspring X's perspective. Offspring X will receive some inclusive fitness benefits when its parent provides aid to both current and future siblings, each of whom has an average r of 0.5 to offspring X. Yet, offspring X is more related to itself ($r = 1$) than to any of its siblings. As such, in terms of inclusive fitness, offspring X values the resources it receives from its parent more than the resources that its parent provides to its siblings (current or future). The conflict between parent and offspring arises because, although each offspring will value the resources it receives more than those dispensed to its siblings, all offspring are equally valuable to a parent, in terms of its own inclusive fitness. This then sets up a zone of conflict between how much offspring X wants a parent to give to him, and how much a parent is willing to give (the former always being greater than the latter). This zone is where parent-offspring conflict takes place.

PARENT-OFFSPRING CONFLICT AND MATING SYSTEMS IN PRIMATES. The degree of parent-offspring conflict predicted in any population is in part a function of the mating system (see Chapter 7) that exists in that population (Hain and Neff, 2006; Long, 2005). To see why, recall that in any parent-offspring conflict situation, natural selection favors offspring that weigh (1) the inclusive fitness benefits associated with receiving continued parental assistance versus (2) the inclusive fitness benefits of curtailing the degree of parental assistance received, and leaving a parent with more resources to produce future offspring.

The degree of relatedness between current offspring and future offspring is not fixed, but rather is a function of the mating system. In long-term monogamous species, current offspring and future offspring will have an average genetic relatedness of $r = 0.5$, because they are likely to have the same mother and the same father. But suppose the mating system is polyandrous (see Chapter 7), with a female mating with many males. Then the genetic relatedness between current and future offspring will be somewhere between 0.5 (for full siblings) and 0.25 (for half-brothers or half-sisters). Compared to the case of monogamous mating systems, in polyandrous mating systems, natural selection will favor offspring who attempt to extract more in the way of parental assistance. Parent-offspring conflict should then be more intense in polyandrous versus monogamous mating systems (Macnair and Parker, 1978; Mock and Parker, 1997; Parker and Macnair, 1979; Trivers, 1974).

Tristan Long tested the hypothesis that offspring will attempt to extract more resources from parents in polyandrous systems than in monogamous systems. He did this by asking whether there was evidence that fetuses grew faster in utero—taking more maternal resources—in polyandrous primate species. In-utero parent-offspring conflict is particularly fascinating, as it shifts the balance of power between parent and offspring. In most cases of parent-offspring conflict, a mother has the upper hand, as she is almost always behaviorally dominant to her offspring. When the offspring is still in utero, however, it is more difficult (but not impossible) for mothers to deprive offspring of resources without depriving themselves too, thus shifting the balance of power away from the mother and toward the developing fetus.

To examine this possible in-utero parent-offspring conflict, Long used the independent contrast phylogenetic method we discussed in Chapter 6 (Felsenstein, 1985, 2004). Long asked whether, if he controlled for phylogenetic effects, strong parent-offspring conflict would be more likely to occur in polyandrous or in monogamous primate species.

Long began by using a well-established phylogenetic tree for primates. From this tree, he was able to find sixteen pairs of primates to use in his independent contrast analysis. Each pair was made up of species that had diverged from a recent common ancestor—one of these species was monogamous, and the other was polyandrous. Long then compared already published data on fetal growth rates for each of the species in his pairwise comparison (Long, 2005). He predicted that in polyandrous mating systems, a fetus would attempt to sequester more resources during development, and hence would show faster rates of growth than fetuses in species that were monogamous. Long's independent contrast analysis found just such a relationship.

Long also examined how mating systems were connected to parent-offspring conflict in a slightly different way. Because sperm competition (see Chapter 7) is more intense in polyandrous species, males in such species tend to have larger testes. Testes size, then, can often be used as a proxy for the degree of polyandry. When Long examined the relationship between testes size and parent-offspring conflict (measured by fetal growth rate), his phylogenetic analysis again found a positive relationship, showing nicely how the extent of parent-offspring conflict can be mediated by the type of mating system in place (Figure 8.21).

FIGURE 8.21. Parental investment and testes size. Testes size tends to be larger in males from polyandrous vs. monogamous species. The relationship between testes size (a proxy measure of polyandry) and parent-offspring conflict (measured by fetal growth rate) was positive in Long's analysis of primates. The x and y axes measure residual log values of testes size and fetal growth rate, respectively. *(Based on Long, 2005)*

A

B

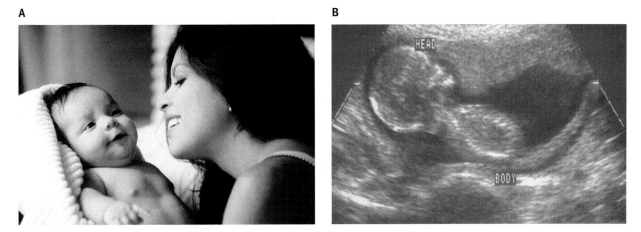

FIGURE 8.22. Mothers and babies. While the parent-offspring relationship is usually cooperative **(A)**, parent-offspring conflict can occur, even in utero as shown by an ultrasound **(B)**. *(Photo credits: Ariel Skelley/Corbis; Visuals Unlimited)*

IN-UTERO CONFLICTS IN HUMANS. David Haig has hypothesized that parent-offspring conflict may also occur in humans (Haig, 1993; Figure 8.22). Parent-offspring conflict in pregnant women occurs because, as mentioned earlier, mother and fetus do not have identical interests in terms of how to maximize inclusive fitness. Using published medical literature, Haig argues that, in humans, fetal cells have "invaded" the maternal endometrium—the membrane lining the mother's uterus—during implantation, and that such cells are designed by natural selection to manipulate maternal spiral arteries in such a way as to make constriction of the arteries (which would make fewer resources available to the fetus) much more difficult. Such an invasion benefits the fetus in two ways: (1) by providing the fetus with direct access to maternal arterial blood and allowing the fetus to release hormones and other substances directly into the maternal bloodstream, and (2) by putting the volume of blood—and hence the nutrients it contains—under fetal, rather than maternal, control.

Haig suggests that placentally produced hormones, such as human placental lactogen and human chorionic gonadotropin, change the in-utero environment in a manner that benefits the fetus at the cost of the mother. For example, a fetus may use human placental lactogen to manipulate insulin (a hormone produced in the pancreas, which helps the body use glucose) in such a manner that sugar would remain in the blood a longer time than normal. This manipulation would provide the fetus with more time to access such sugar for itself. The maternal counterresponse is to increase the production of insulin. If this countermeasure is unsuccessful, the fetus obtains extra sugar, but the mother suffers from gestational diabetes (Wells, 2007).

Gestational diabetes may thus be a possible outcome of parent-offspring conflict, and how it is viewed may have serious implications for the treatment of pregnancy-related medical conditions. If, for example, medical doctors viewed gestational diabetes as a "disease" that needed to be cured, they might act differently than if they viewed gestational diabetes as an evolutionary measure selected by fetal genes to increase sugar flow to the fetus. These sorts of issues are being studied by researchers in the field of evolutionary medicine (Ewald, 2000; Nesse and Williams, 1995; Stearns and Ebert, 2001).

SIBLING RIVALRY

Most readers are probably familiar with **sibling rivalry** from basic psychology classes, but animal behaviorists have been fascinated with such rivalries as well, and they have developed a substantial empirical and theoretical literature on this subject (Mock and Parker, 1997). The logic underlying the models of sibling rivalry is in many ways similar to that of parent-offspring conflict. Instead of imagining the world from the viewpoint of genes in parents versus genes in offspring, however, we now shift perspectives and focus on genes in siblings.

Mathematical models of sibling rivalry are constructed to consider sibling rivalry among many different siblings, but here we'll provide a simplified model by focusing on the evolution of this sort of behavior when only two siblings are involved. Consider two siblings that we will label sib 1 and sib 2. From the viewpoint of sib 1, sib 2 is a valuable addition to family life, as sibs 1 and 2 share an *r* of 0.5. Such genetic relatedness means that what is good for sib 1 is *usually* good for sib 2, but it also means that in a situation in which resources are limited and the siblings must compete for these resources, each individual will act as if it is more important to receive resources for itself than to have the same resources go to its sibling (Figure 8.23). We have adopted this sort of logic in our discussion of parent-offspring conflict, but here the competition is directly between siblings in a clutch of offspring, rather than between parent and offspring per se.

Imagine an extreme environment in which there is only enough food for one sibling to survive. Because of their genetic relatedness to one another, each

Abundant resources

Scarce resources

FIGURE 8.23. Sib-sib conflict. Kin selection theory predicts that individuals generally should not be very aggressive toward kin such as sibs. This is especially true when there are abundant resources. But if there are limited resources, conflict over the resources will increase as each individual is more related to itself ($r = 1$) than to its sib ($r = 0.5$).

sibling values the other at a level that is half of that at which it values itself. In such a resource-poor environment, we would expect intense, perhaps even lethal, competition to emerge among siblings. If we made the environment less harsh by adding more food, we would expect sib-sib interactions to be less competitive, but since each values itself more than the other, some level of competition should still be the norm, rather than the exception. We should simply expect the rivalry to emerge in less lethal ways when resources are not as limited.

Sibling rivalry is illustrated nicely in the ongoing study of egrets by Douglas Mock and his colleagues (Mock, 2004; Mock and Parker, 1997). As idyllic as the interactions of downy chicks in a bird nest may seem to the casual observer, the interactions among egret chicks actually resemble prizefights more closely than some picturesque scene of nature taken from a Disney film (Figure 8.24). Consider the following summary of work on sib-sib interactions:

FIGURE 8.24. Sib-sib competition in birds. In nests of egrets, sib-sib competition can be intense and result in the death of smaller, less dominant chicks. Sibling rivalry can be seen in the fights between siblings in the nest, as shown here, where one of the chicks is preparing to bite its sibling on the back of its head. *(Photo credit: Millard H. Sharp/Photo Researchers, Inc.)*

> Sibling fights take many forms, depending mainly on how the loser concedes and how quickly it does so. The simplest fights, which usually occur while the participating dyad has had a series of increasingly one-sided battles, are those in which the attack inspires no retaliation. At the next level, return fire is brief until the loser is tagged with several unanswered shots and crouches low. From there, the severity of the beating is left largely to the victor's discretion. Sometimes it continues to jab at its opponent, causing the latter to screech and hide its face. As an alternative to jabbing, a dominant chick may seize the cowering victim by its head or neck, lift that part a few centimeters and then slam it down forcefully against the nest cup. If the attack persists for more than a few extra blows, the loser is likely to flee, sometimes squawking loudly and racing about the nest dodging behind the other nest occupants while being hit. During such chases, the primary target is the back of the head. Frequently bullied chicks soon develop a characteristic baldness, dotted with fresh and crusted blood, where the nape feathers have been plucked forcibly during fights. (Mock and Parker, 1997, pp. 103–104)

When egret chicks first hatch, parents bring back enough food to fill all the chicks' guts, thus removing any impetus for sib-sib aggressive interactions. As the chicks grow, however, a point is quickly reached at which the food brought to the nest is not enough to feed everyone, and an intense battle scene emerges when a parent returns to the nest with a juicy bolus (a soft chewed mass) of partially digested fish. Parents regurgitate such boluses in the nest, and most are grabbed before they hit the ground. The key to obtaining access to a bolus is positioning within the nest, and specifically vertical positioning (the higher the better when mom returns). Even a chick tilting its head up above horizontal is a cue likely to spark aggression in egrets' nests.

Egrets, like most birds, hatch eggs asynchronously—that is, they lay their eggs in sequence, rather than all at one time. Thus, hatching order produces chicks that can differ in age by many days. Such age differences play a critical role in determining who emerges as the victor in sib-sib interactions, since chicks that hatch first start to feed sooner and hence receive more food, which leads to a weight advantage over chicks that hatch later. As a result, a very clear age-related dominance hierarchy exists among chicks. First-hatched chicks are often much larger than second-hatched chicks, who may themselves tower over those

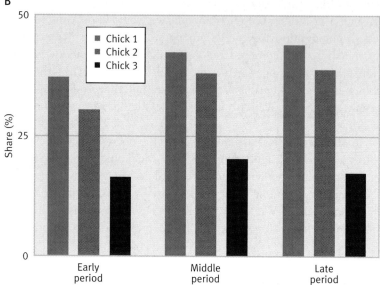

FIGURE 8.25. Birth order and food intake. (A) Normal broods of little blue herons include four to five chicks that are hatched asynchronously. The three eldest chicks (chicks 1, 2, and 3) are heavier than the youngest chicks (chicks 4 and 5). If a younger chick is part of a brood in which one of its older sibs has died (lost sib), its average weight is less than that of its older sibs but more than it would be if it were in a brood in which no sibs had died (no loss). **(B)** In egret broods, the oldest, dominant chick (1) receives more food than the middle chick (2), who in turn gets more than the youngest chick (3). This holds for the early period after hatching (1–13 days), the middle period (14–21 days), and the late period (21–30 days). *(Based on Mock and Parker, 1997)*

hatched later (Figure 8.25A). In sib-sib interactions, large size means better fighting ability, which translates into significantly more food (Figure 8.25B).

Kin Recognition

Given the power of kinship to affect social interactions, ethologists and behavioral ecologists have a long-standing interest in how kin recognize one another (Fletcher and Michener, 1987; Hepper, 1991; Hepper and Cleland, 1998; Holmes, 2004; Pfennig and Sherman, 1995). Early in this chapter, we went through a general procedure to show how to calculate relatedness (*r*). Of course, animal behaviorists don't assume that nonhumans are able to calculate genetic relatedness in the manner we described. We need only assume that natural selection favors individuals who act in a manner that makes it appear as though they are making such calculations.

Some examples of kin recognition in animals are nothing short of incredible. And, not surprisingly, these cases typically involve situations in which there are important fitness benefits for recognizing kin, but in which the task of kin recognition is difficult—for example, when individuals live in very large groups. Consider, for example, the remarkable kin recognition abilities seen in some species of penguins. Parents travel long distances to the sea to obtain food to

A

B

FIGURE 8.26. Kin recognition in penguins. Kin recognition via vocal signatures has been examined in **(A)** the emperor penguin (*Aptenodytes forsteri*) and **(B)** the king penguin (*Aptenodytes patagonicus*). Both species of penguins live in large colonies, and parents returning from foraging with food for their chicks use vocal cues to find their offspring in the midst of numerous other chicks. *(Photo credits: Hans Reinhard/Photo Researchers, Inc.)*

take back to the inland areas where their chicks have hatched. When parents return from their journey, they must find their young among scores—sometimes thousands—of screaming, hungry chicks in a colony (Aubin and Jouventin, 2002; Brumm and Slabbekoorn, 2005). How do parents returning from a foraging bout (that might last weeks) reunite with their own young? For species like the emperor penguin (*Aptenodytes forsteri*) and the king penguin (*Aptenodytes patagonicus*) (Figure 8.26), the answer appears to center on complex vocal cues that allow for kin recognition via "vocal signatures" emitted by the young (Aubin and Jouventin, 1998; Aubin et al., 2000; Jouventin et al., 1999; Lengagne et al., 2000).

Yet, not all penguin species are as proficient as the king and emperor penguins at recognizing the vocal signatures of their offspring. Studies indicate that penguins that build nests are not as adept at recognizing the vocal calls of their young as are individuals who live in dense colonies and do not nest (Jouventin and Aubin, 2002; Searby et al., 2004). Parents in nest-building species can find their offspring by remembering the location of their nests, presumably because any chick in their nest is their offspring (see below), and hence natural selection to recognize offspring by vocal cues in these species is weak. When the problem of kin recognition is more difficult—in dense colonies with no nests—natural selection favors the evolution of more complex vocal recognition systems.

MATCHING MODELS

Many models of kin recognition center on individuals having some "internal template" against which they match others and gauge relatedness (Reeve, 1989). These **kin recognition matching models** differ in their specifics, but the basic idea is that individual 1 determines if individual 2 is kin or nonkin, depending

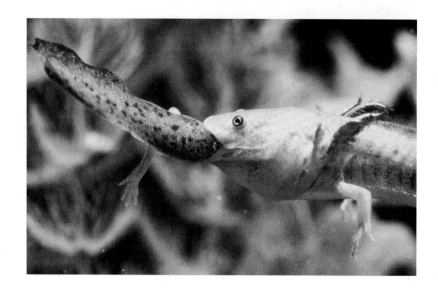

FIGURE 8.27. Tadpole cannibals. As in the spadefoot toad, two different tadpole morphs—a carnivorous cannibal and an herbivorous omnivore—exist in a number of amphibian species. Here a tiger salamander *(Ambystoma tigrinum)* cannibal morph (right) is eating an omnivore morph (left). *(Photo credit: David Pfennig)*

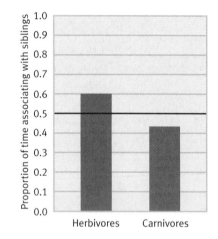

FIGURE 8.28. Kin recognition in spadefoot toads. Spadefoot toad tadpoles come in two morphs: carnivorous and herbivorous. Individuals from each tadpole morph were placed between two groups of tadpoles, one of which contained sixteen unfamiliar siblings, the other of which was composed of unfamiliar nonsiblings. Herbivorous morphs preferred unfamiliar sibs, while carnivorous morphs (who cannibalize other tadpoles) preferred nonkin. The solid horizontal line represents the value expected if tadpole behavior was random with respect to kinship. *(Based on Pfennig et al., 1993)*

on how closely individual 2 matches the internal template of individual 1. The internal template may be generated genetically, via learning, or via social learning, but in all cases, the animal infers the degree of kinship as some function of the extent to which others match its own template (Alexander, 1979, 1991; Boyse et al., 1991; Crozier, 1987; Robinson and Smotherman, 1991). Templates can range from dichotomous "kin/nonkin" classification systems to more graded systems of kinship, in which individuals can distinguish among kin at a finer level (sibling, cousin, and so on).

TEMPLATE MATCHING IN TADPOLES. David Pfennig and his colleagues have uncovered a fascinating case of template matching in the cannibalistic behavior of spadefoot toad tadpoles (*Scaphiopus bombifrons*) (Elgar and Crespi, 1992; Pfennig et al., 1993; Figure 8.27). In nature, two feeding morphs of spadefoot toads exist: juveniles that feed on detritus (small, often drifting vegetative clumps of food) typically develop into herbivorous omnivores, while those that feed on shrimp tend to mature into carnivorous cannibals.

Pfennig and his team examined kin recognition abilities in the herbivore and cannibal spadefoot morphs by testing both morphs in the presence of either *unfamiliar* siblings or *unfamiliar* nonrelatives. When visual cues (behavior and morphology, for example) and chemical cues (odors, for example) were both in play, herbivores preferred associating with their siblings over unrelated individuals, presumably because of the inclusive fitness benefits associated with interactions with genetic kin. Carnivorous individuals that cannibalize other tadpoles were taken from the same sibship as the omnivores that were being tested. When these cannibals were tested by Pfennig and his colleagues, they spent more time near unrelated individuals, presumably to avoid the costs of killing their genetic kin (Figure 8.28).

Pfennig and his colleagues also offered carnivores a choice between unfamiliar siblings and unfamiliar nonrelatives in a protocol that allowed carnivores to actually eat other tadpoles. Carnivores were not only more likely to eat unrelated individuals, but they were able to distinguish between relatives and nonrelatives by some sort of taste test. That is, carnivores were equally likely to suck relatives and nonrelatives into their mouths, but they released their relatives much more frequently than unrelated individuals. Being able to recognize kin has clear advantages, as ingesting kin would generally be selected against whenever alternative food sources were available. But as the costs and benefits of eating kin change, we expect the tadpoles' behavior to change. And indeed, the researchers found that cannibalistic toads were much less picky when they had been starved for twenty-four hours or more—that is, when they were very hungry, they would occasionally eat even genetic kin (Figure 8.29).

MHC, KINSHIP, AND TEMPLATES. In Chapter 6, we learned that animals sometimes use potential partners' Major Histocompatibility Complex (MHC) genes, which they identify by odor, to determine which mate to choose. MHC also plays a role in kin recognition (Frommen et al., 2007; Manning et al., 1992). Jo Manning and her colleagues examined this role in house mice (*Mus musculus domesticus*), a species in which females nest together and nurse all offspring at their nest (Manning et al., 1992). When the female mice nest together, they all receive a benefit, which is protection from infanticidal males that sometimes attack and kill offspring that are not their own (Manning et al., 1995). At the same time, communal nesting creates a situation in which females can be "cheated"— this occurs when other females at their nest are protected from danger, but do not nurse all pups present. One way to minimize the cheater problem, and to maximize inclusive fitness benefits, would be for females to form communal nests with their genetic relatives. And because MHC differences are correlated with differences in odor, one way that females may discriminate among kin and nonkin is through odors associated with the MHC (Packer et al., 1992).

Manning and her colleagues worked with six wild populations of house mice, individually marking each mouse and determining its MHC "haplotype" (similar to a genotype). They observed pregnant females and examined whether females who had just given birth opted to nest alone or in a communal nest. Ninety percent of the females chose to nest communally. With respect to kin recognition, when females selected which communal nests to join, they chose nests with individuals who had an MHC similar to their own. While this does not definitively show that females use MHC as a cue for kinship, it is consistent with such a hypothesis.

RULE-OF-THUMB MODELS OF KIN RECOGNITION

As we saw in the penguin studies discussed earlier, in species in which individuals do not raise their offspring in dense colonies, but instead live in discrete nests that are physically separated, a second, and in some sense simpler, form of kin recognition may evolve. In such scenarios, natural selection might favor a kin recognition rule of the form "if it lives in your nest/cave/territory, then treat it like kin" (Blaustein, 1983; Holmes and Sherman, 1983; Sherman and Holmes, 1985; Waldman, 1987).

To see how such a rule of thumb might work, imagine a population of animals in which family units live in a fixed area—let's call it a nest—that is set apart from other nests. In such a population, all of the machinery (cognitive, genetic, sensory) necessary to distinguish kin from nonkin may be superfluous. It may be that a rule that instructs individuals to treat all individuals in their nest as kin works just as well in terms of kin recognition as the more complicated rules associated with matching. After all, if everyone in a nest is almost always kin,

FIGURE 8.29. Hunger and carnivorous toads. The carnivorous morph of spadefoot toads prefers to eat nonkin over kin. When starved for 24 hours (A), only a little more than 10 percent of individuals eaten were kin. If starved for 48 hours, this figure rises. As a control, toads were again starved for 24 hours (C), and results were similar to the original 24-hour deprivation treatment (A). The solid horizontal line represents the value expected if cannibalism were random with respect to kinship. *(Based on Pfennig et al., 1993)*

Dr. Francis Ratnieks

Why has so much work on animal behavior and kinship been done in the social insects? How did you decide to work with this group?

Becoming a social insect biologist was literally plan B. On completing my BSc in Ecology at the University of Ulster in Northern Ireland, I decided to study pest management. I felt this would be useful and would combine my interests in insects and ecology. I applied to do a Ph.D. in the Department of Entomology at Cornell University as this seemed the best place for studying insects. The professor of apiculture, the late Roger Morse, offered me a studentship. Although studying honeybees was something I had never thought of, I accepted. I quickly became enthusiastic about honeybees and beekeeping. More gradually, I developed interests and ideas about social evolution and behavior, and taught myself how to model social evolution. I also expanded into wasps and ants.

Social insects have been the most important group of organisms for testing predictions arising from William Hamilton's inclusive fitness theory. It has been a two-way street. Social insects have played a key role in validating the theory, and the theory has revolutionized our understanding of social insects, especially how eusociality evolved and the reproductive behavior of insect societies.

Social insects can be used to study practically any question. They are literally a gateway to biology. An immense number of important discoveries have been made with the honeybee alone, which is only one of 20,000 social insect species. Social insects have been very useful for testing Hamilton's theory because relatedness, the theory's central parameter, varies both within and

between species because queens can be mated to one or more males, because there can be different numbers of queens per colony, and because haplodiploidy (in ants, bees, and wasps) causes relatedness to differ between the sexes. Insect colonies are also very practical to study. A colony of ants can be kept in a plastic box. A colony of honeybees can be kept in a hive. Honeybees are easy to study once you know how. Some honeybee studies are even based on decoding waggle dances by viewing the dancing bees through the glass walls of an observation hive. This is the only case in animal behavior where the animals "talk to" the researchers.

I often tell students that Hamilton's inclusive fitness theory is as important to the field of evolution and behavior as Einstein's e=mc² is to physicists. Is that an overstatement?

It is not an overstatement. Both are elegant and concise mathematical representations of a fundamental underlying relationship. Hamilton's Rule tells us the condition under which any behavior or trait that affects other individuals of the same species will be favored or disfavored by natural selection. Einstein's equation tells us the relationship between mass and energy. The relationship in Einstein's equation is inviolable. Technically speaking, Hamilton's Rule is not inviolable because gene frequencies, and therefore the traits they code for, can also be affected by genetic drift as well as by natural selection. Does that make Einstein's equation more important? I don't think so. It just reflects a difference between physics and biology.

How is it that a simple mathematical rule can be so important? The reason is simple. Many biological processes can be represented mathematically. For example, population growth can be represented by multiplication. The relatedness term in Hamilton's Rule comes from the simple fact that each gene in an organism has a precise probability of being passed on to an offspring. The probability is usually 0.5, but can be 1, for example, from a haploid male bee to his daughter.

Hamilton's Rule is also a good example of the importance of mathematics in biology. The mathematics is not hard. High school algebra is enough to understand it. The hard part for the student is combining the mathematics with the biology. The best way is to jump in and have a go!

Kinship isn't the only factor that promotes social behavior and altruism in animals—is it?

Kinship is very important. Consider the evolution of eusociality. The problem is to explain altruism—how can natural selection select for individuals to forego reproduction to help others? Eusociality evolved within families, with offspring helping their parents rear more brothers and sisters. Helpers are as closely related to the individuals reared (brothers and sisters) as to their own sons and daughters. (Although many queen bees, wasps, and ants mate to several males, which diminishes relatedness, this evolved after eusociality.)

But if all that is needed for eusociality to evolve is high relatedness, why is eusociality not more common? Two other things are needed. First, a nest or some way of keeping the family together, so that help is directed to kin. Second, some way of helping, such as by providing food or by defending. Eusociality arose many times in the *Hymenoptera* because many species have nests to which the mother brings food for her offspring. Helpers can help simply by bringing more food. In termites food was not needed as the family was living inside its food—a log. Here, defense was the key.

In many modern-day insect societies, worker altruism is also caused by social pressure. Workers in most bee, wasp, and ant species have ovaries and can lay eggs. But in many such species, worker reproduction is rare. In the honeybee, fewer than 0.1 percent of the workers lay eggs.

Egg laying by workers is deterred by an effective policing system that kills worker-laid eggs. This means that worker honeybees are better off working rather than laying eggs, given that almost all their eggs will be killed if they lay any.

Do the terms "kinship" and "family" differ in meaning when discussed in ethology as opposed to when they are used by nonscientists in the course of normal conversation? How so?

I don't think there is much difference. Sometimes people will refer to other individuals as a brother or sister when they are not true relatives. But the people using these words probably know the difference. By referring to someone unrelated to you as brother or sister is often a way of showing that you have a common interest because you belong to the same group within society. The fact that we humans have what seems like a keen natural understanding of kinship suggests that it is important to us and is a human universal. That is, it is something innate in being human, rather than something that is purely cultural. Given the importance of relatedness in social behavior, this is not surprising.

Can you envision a day when sociologists and animal behaviorists will be using a common framework for studying kinship and behavior? What might such a framework look like?

A common interdisciplinary framework is something that is possible. However, even if this is established, the subjects and goals of the different disciplines may be sufficiently different that they may be using very different parts of a large and unwieldy framework. This is especially true when studying humans, given the vast number of disciplines involved, including history,

economics, anthropology, sociology, political science, criminology, psychology, and biology. What insights would a historian studying the Tudors take from evolutionary biology, for example?

The value of a common framework can be seen when some important insight from one discipline is ignored in another discipline. For example, studies by evolutionary biologists Martin Daly and Margo Wilson have shown that kinship may influence abuse of children by parents and stepparents. This idea, which comes from Hamilton's theory (and is also part of common knowledge, given well-known stories like Cinderella), ran counter to the way that sociologists were trained. The question then is, why were sociologists not trained to consider this and are they now doing so?

The debate triggered by the publication of the book *Sociobiology* by E. O. Wilson in 1975 is a good example of the friction that can be caused when disciplines and ideologies collide. It is easy for more heat than light to be generated. The value of ideas or theories originating in one discipline and exported to another can be gauged by the new insights they give and the degree that they unify previously disparate fields when tested with real data. Interdisciplinary cross-pollination is not just one way, from biology to social science. The study of animal behavior has greatly benefited from insights from game theory, which was originally developed within the social sciences.

Dr. Francis Ratnieks is a professor at Sussex University, England. His seminal work on social behavior has focused on the role of genetic relatedness in shaping insect societies.

FIGURE 8.30. Kin recognition breakdown. While adopting an "if it's in your nest, it is your offspring" rule often works for mothers, the system can be sabotaged by "nest parasites." Here a mother dunnock is feeding a baby cuckoo that has been dumped into her nest. *(Photo credit: Eric and David Hosking/ Corbis)*

selection should favor the simplest possible kin recognition rule. Of course, such kin recognition rules are subject to cheating. Cowbirds and cuckoo birds, for example, lay their eggs in the nests of other species, who then raise those chicks as if they were their own (Ortega, 1998; Figure 8.30). Such "nest parasites" are in an evolutionary arms race with their hosts—hosts are selected to detect and reject foreign eggs, and nest parasites to circumvent any detection system that might evolve in their host (Dawkins and Krebs, 1979).

Spatial cues and kin recognition rules can often change through the lifetime of an individual. For example, in bank swallows (*Riparia riparia*), parents *initially* feed any chick in their nest, thus adopting the rule "if it is in my burrow, it is likely kin" (Hoogland and Sherman, 1976; see Figure 8.5). This makes good sense, because for the first three weeks of life chicks cannot fly, and it is therefore extremely likely that any chick in a burrow is kin. At three weeks, however, chicks learn to fly and there is consequently much more mixing among young. Michael Beecher has found that when their chicks are about twenty days old, bank swallow mothers switch from their rule of thumb (feed what is in your nest) to using distinctive vocal cues (that is, a template-based system) to recognize and feed their offspring (Beecher et al., 1981a, 1981b, 1986).

The study of animal behavior was revolutionized by the introduction of inclusive fitness models. Since W. D. Hamilton introduced these models in the early 1960s, almost every animal behaviorist who has studied social behavior has at one time or another thought about whether kinship plays a role in the system that he or she is studying. As we have seen, kinship theory not only allows researchers to make predictions about when animals should be cooperative and altruistic toward their kin, but it also makes predictions about when they should not be so (as in parent-offspring conflict, sibling rivalry). Inclusive fitness continues to be one of the most actively researched areas in ethology, with modern work employing molecular genetic and phylogenetic analyses to expand the frontiers of research in this area.

SUMMARY

1. W. D. Hamilton's "inclusive fitness" or "kinship" theory has revolutionized the way that scientists understand evolution and ethology.
2. In evolutionary terms, relatedness centers on the *probability* that individuals share genes that they have inherited from some *common ancestor*—parents, grandparents, and so on. The essence of inclusive fitness models is that they add on to "classical" models of natural selection by considering the effect of a gene not only on the individual that bears it, but also on those sharing genes that are identical by descent (that is, genetic kin).
3. The decision to aid family members is a function of how related individuals are, and how high or low the costs and benefits associated with the trait turn out to be. When individuals are highly related and a gene codes for an action that provides a huge benefit at a small cost, selection strongly favors this trait.
4. Parents should be particularly willing to go to great lengths to help their offspring. But a zone of parent-offspring conflict is also predicted under basic kinship theory.
5. While sibling rivalry is most often associated with the field of psychology, basic kinship theory also defines the conditions under which sibling rivalry should be favored, including competition for food.

6. Many models of kin recognition center on individuals having some "internal template" against which they match others and gauge relatedness.
7. In a species in which kin groups are spatially segregated from one another over relatively long periods of time, a second, and in some sense simpler, form of kin recognition may evolve. In such scenarios, natural selection might favor a kin recognition rule of the form "if it lives in your nest/cave/ territory, then treat it like kin."

DISCUSSION QUESTIONS

1. Why would it be an advantage for animals to gauge very small differences in genetic kinship relationships? Why, for example, would it be better able to distinguish relatives at the level of cousin ($r = 0.125$) than simply sibling ($r = 0.5$)? What sorts of benefits might be possible when small differences in relatedness could be gauged?
2. Read Emlen's 1995 "An evolutionary theory of family," in *Proceedings of the National Academy of Science* (vol. 92, pp. 8092–8099). List the evidence for and against three of the predictions that we did not examine in this chapter.
3. Try to find some statistics on the rate of child abuse in families where children are adopted. What might you expect based on the logic adopted by Daly and Wilson? What do your data show?
4. Based on the parent-offspring conflict model, what differences in weaning behavior would you expect to see between younger and older mammalian mothers?
5. How might both kin selection and kin recognition rules be useful in understanding cases of "adoption" in animals?
6. How does a phylogenetic comparison of mating systems in primates shed light on kinship and parent-offspring conflict?

SUGGESTED READING

Crozier, R. H., & Pamilo, P. (1996). *Evolution of social insect colonies: Sex allocation and kin selection*. Oxford: Oxford University Press. A book-length treatment of kin selection in social insects.

Emlen, S. T. (1995). An evolutionary theory of the family. *Proceedings of the National Academy of Sciences, U.S.A., 92*, 8092–8099. Here Emlen lays out all fifteen predictions derived from his "evolutionary theory of family."

Hamilton, W. D. (1963). The evolution of altruistic behavior. *American Naturalist, 97*, 354–356. Hamilton's ideas on kinship, boiled down to their main ingredients.

Reeve, H. K. (1998). Game theory, reproductive skew and nepotism. In L. A. Dugatkin & H. K. Reeve (Eds.), *Game theory and animal behavior* (pp. 118–145). New York: Oxford University Press. An overview of how kinship is incorporated into a family of models known as "reproductive skew" models.

Sherman, P. W. (1977). Nepotism and the evolution of alarm calls. *Science, 197*, 1246–1253. This paper on kin selection and alarm calls in Belding's squirrels is perhaps the most well-cited empirical study in all the inclusive fitness literature.

9

Cooperation

In the last chapter, we focused our attention on the strong role that genetic relatedness plays in promoting prosocial behavior. Animals that are not genetic relatives, however, cooperate with each other in many contexts. Here we shall examine such cooperation among unrelated individuals. As a case in point, consider the following scenario: In many streams of the Northern Mountains of Trinidad, the water is clear, and during the dry season, the behavior of guppies (*Poecilia reticulata*) can be seen from the riverbank. If you sit beside such streams, you will eventually see some guppies—perhaps a pair of them—break away from their group and approach a potentially dangerous predator, such as a pike cichlid, *Crenicichla alta*. This behavior is called predator inspection (see Chapter 2). These guppies are not necessarily genetic relatives, and they could just as easily have headed for cover (and many others probably did just that). Instead, they approached the predator and did so in what looks like a coordinated fashion (Pitcher et al., 1986; Figure 9.1).

How can such cooperative behavior emerge among animals? The risk-taking guppies described above are in what appears to be a no-win situation. Think about it like this: The best thing that could happen for guppy 1 is that guppy 2 takes all the risks and passes the information it receives onto guppy 1, cost-free. But, of course, the same holds true for guppy 2, as its highest payoff comes when guppy 1 approaches the predator alone, and then passes the information it receives to guppy 2. Yet, if both fish opt to wait for the other to inspect the predator, each may be worse off than if they had inspected the predator as a pair.

Is there a solution to this dilemma? Is any sort of cooperation possible in such a scenario? The answer is yes, and we will examine exactly how later in this chapter. But before we do, we need two things under our belt—a definition and a broader overview of cooperation.

The word **cooperation** typically refers to an *outcome* from which two or more interacting individuals each receives a net benefit from their joint actions, despite the potential costs they may have to pay for undertaking such actions. For example, jointly hunting prey may provide each of two hunters with a food bonanza, even though there are costs (possible injury, energy expended) associated with hunting. In addition to looking at outcomes (that is, successfully capturing prey), it is also important to examine cooperation in terms of individual action. Suppose, for example, that to successfully hunt prey, a pair of hunters

FIGURE 9.1. Risk taking and cooperation in guppies. Two male guppies (lower left and lower center of photo) inspect a pike cichlid predator. Guppies cooperate during such risky endeavors. *(Photo credit: Michael Alfieri)*

needs to both (1) flush the prey into an open area, and (2) pounce on the prey when it is flushed into the open. A successful hunting strategy might be for hunter 1 to flush out the prey, and for hunter 2 to follow up by pouncing on the prey. If hunter 1 flushes the prey into the open, then we can say it acted cooperatively, in that hunter 1's behavior made a successful capture possible.

An individual could cooperate by acting in a way that would benefit itself and its partner, even if its partner didn't—that is, even if its partner cheated (deriving a benefit from the actions of its partner without taking any action itself). In our case, hunter 1 could flush out the prey, but hunter 2 might not pounce. What this means is that, in addition to defining cooperation as an outcome, it is necessary to define what it means "to cooperate." Here "to cooperate" means to behave in such a way as to make the benefits that could be obtained from joint action possible, even though they may not necessarily be achieved (Dugatkin et al., 1992; Mesterton-Gibbons and Dugatkin, 1992).

Cooperation occurs in many species and is manifested over a wide variety of behaviors. To better understand the origins and the benefits of cooperation among unrelated individuals, we will examine the following questions in this chapter:

- What paths leading to cooperation have been identified by ethologists? What theory lies behind each? What empirical evidence supports each of these paths?
- What do we know about both the ultimate and proximate underpinnings of cooperation?
- What role does phylogeny play in explaining the distribution of animal cooperation?
- What role does cooperation play in coalition formation?
- How can we explain *interspecific* cooperation (that is, cooperation among animals from different species)?

The Range of Cooperative Behaviors

Although cooperation is far from ubiquitous in the animal kingdom, it does occur in many contexts: foraging, predation, antipredator behaviors, mating, play, aggressive interaction, and so forth. To give you a sense of the sorts of cooperation seen in animals, we will discuss: (1) helping in the birthing process, and (2) social grooming in primates.

HELPING IN THE BIRTHING PROCESS

Thomas Kunz and his colleagues describe an interesting case of cooperation in the Rodriques fruit bat (*Pteropus rodricensis*). In this bat, unrelated female "helpers" assist pregnant individuals in the birthing process (Kunz et al., 1994). To study this form of cooperation, Kunz and his team observed females for three hours before the start of the birthing process to its completion, and found that

FIGURE 9.2. Bat midwives. (A) A nonpregnant female helper bat assumes the "feet down" birthing position as it "tutors" the pregnant female. **(B)** A pregnant female in a cradle position during birth is being groomed by a helper. **(C)** As the wing and foot of the pup emerge, the helper continues to groom the female that is giving birth. *(Based on Kunz et al., 1994)*

helpers were integrally involved at almost every stage (Figure 9.2). To begin with, pregnant Rodriques fruit bats must assume a "feet down" position in order to give birth. Yet, expectant mothers do not take the feet down position until they observe the helper female assume this position. This sort of tutoring on the part of helpers is remarkable—helpers themselves are not pregnant, and hence would normally not assume such a position.

During the birthing process, the helper continues providing assistance by grasping the wings of the pregnant females, thereby providing both protection and warmth, and subsequently cleaning (licking) newborn pups upon their emergence. Once pups are born, helpers guide the newborns into a suckling position, where they can obtain milk from their mother. These bat "midwives" cooperate with pregnant mothers during virtually every stage of the birthing process. Although not nearly as well documented, other anecdotal evidence for assistance during birth has been recorded in marmosets (*Callithrix jacchus*), Indian elephants (*Elephas maximus*), African hunting dogs (*Lycaon pictus*), raccoon dogs (*Nyctereutes procyonoides*), and bottle-nosed dolphins (*Tursiops truncatus*) (Essapian, 1963; Gaffrey, 1957; Lucas et al., 1937; Poppleton, 1957; Yamamoto, 1987).

SOCIAL GROOMING

Many animals groom, or clean, themselves in an attempt to remove external parasites. This sort of grooming might involve scratching an area of skin or licking it. **Social grooming**, or **allogrooming**, wherein one individual grooms another, is one of the most obvious and frequently observed cooperative behaviors recorded by primatologists. From the time of the earliest experimental work on primates, primatologists have recognized that, while social grooming often serves the function of removing parasites from the body of a partner, it may also have many other functions as well—indeed, social grooming has been considered a large part of the glue that holds primate troops together (Carpenter, 1942; Zuckerman, 1932; Figure 9.3).

One benefit linked to social grooming is "tension reduction" within primate groups (Schino et al., 1988; Sparks, 1967; Terry, 1970). Aggression, especially aggression by top-ranking individuals as they seek to achieve or maintain their dominance in a troop of primates, can be very dangerous. In addition to the serious costs associated with fighting-related injuries, aggression among top-ranking members can often cause disruption of normal everyday group living, with all group members suffering. One manner in which primates reduce the chances of escalating violence in a group is through social grooming, which has the effect of lowering the level of tension between putative combatants. From a proximate perspective, one means by which social grooming lowers tension levels is through increasing the circulating levels of affiliative hormones such as endorphins and opioids (Keverne et al., 1989; Martel et al., 1993). This sort of tension reduction through social grooming may play a role in nonprimate species as well, as recent work has found that social grooming on the part of subordinate meerkat females placates dominant meerkats (Kutsukake and Clutton-Brock, 2006).

Many studies have suggested that primates are capable of exchanging one sort of resource—for example, social grooming—for another resource in what amounts to a "biological marketplace" (de Waal, 1997; Noe and Hammerstein, 1995; Noe et al., 2002). For example, consider the ability to groom another individual as one resource, and providing aid to an individual that is involved in some sort of aggressive interaction as another resource. In terms of biological markets, social grooming can be exchanged for aid during aggressive interactions. If individual 1 groomed individual 2, individual 2 might "pay back" the act of grooming by aiding individual 1 when it is involved in an aggressive interaction with individual 3 (we shall explore these sorts of coalitions in more depth later in this chapter).

Numerous experiments in primates have examined whether individuals cooperate with one another by exchanging social grooming for aid during aggressive interactions. To test for such an exchange system, Gabriele Schino ran a statistical analysis of thirty-six published studies that examined both aid

FIGURE 9.3. Primate grooming.
Primates of many different species engage in various forms of grooming behavior. Such behavior may serve numerous functions simultaneously. *(Photo credit: Chris Crowley/Visuals Unlimited)*

giving and social grooming (Schino, 2007). When Schino summarized the data from these thirty-six studies—studies that involved both wild and captive primate populations—she found a positive correlation between aid dispensed during combat and social grooming, suggesting an exchange-based system of cooperation.

Other work suggests that grooming can be "exchanged" for currencies besides aid during combat. Primates also appear to exchange social grooming for access to scarce resources such as water or food, entrance into new groups, aid in chasing potential predators away, and future association with individuals with "special skills" that others do not possess (de Waal, 1989; Stammbach, 1988). Grooming others, however, can also have associated costs, as evident in both captive and wild populations. In both rhesus macaques (*Macaca mulatta*) and blue monkeys (*Cercopithecus mitis*), individuals involved in social grooming were less vigilant, thereby subjecting themselves or their offspring to increased rates of aggression from other troop members and possibly increased predation rates (Cords, 1995; Maestripieri, 1993).

Paths to Cooperation

Within animal behavior and evolutionary biology, work on the evolution of cooperation can be traced at least as far back as Darwin's interest in cooperation and altruism in insects and other groups (Darwin, 1859, 1871). Darwin was well aware that social insects were often hypercooperative. Although he was unable to completely explain why, Darwin did come close to explaining the "riddle" of such behavior via kinship. After Darwin, the study of cooperation was primarily (but not exclusively) kept alive first by Petr Kropotkin, a Russian prince and naturalist, and later by such researchers as W. C. Allee, A. E. Emerson, and others that were part of what was called "the Chicago School of Animal Behavior" (Dugatkin, 2006; Mitman, 1992). Although these natural historians, ethologists, and population biologists amassed a good deal of data that documented cooperation among animals, they did little in the way of advancing any theory on how cooperation evolved (Allee, 1951).

A theoretical foundation for studying the evolution of cooperation has emerged over the last forty years (Dugatkin, 1997a; Lehmann and Keller, 2006; Nowak, 2006b; Sachs et al., 2004). From Hamilton's innovative work in 1963 (see Chapter 8) to the present, four paths to the evolution and maintenance of cooperation in animals have been developed—kin-selected cooperation, reciprocity, byproduct mutualism, and group selection (Axelrod, 1984; Brown, 1983; Hamilton, 1964; Wilson, 1980a; Figure 9.4). There is now ample empirical evidence available to put some of the models underlying these paths to the test. Since we focused on kin selection in Chapter 8, we will only consider the remaining three paths to cooperation here.

PATH 1: RECIPROCITY

Robert Trivers tackled the problems associated with the evolution of cooperation between unrelated individuals in an important paper entitled "The Evolution of

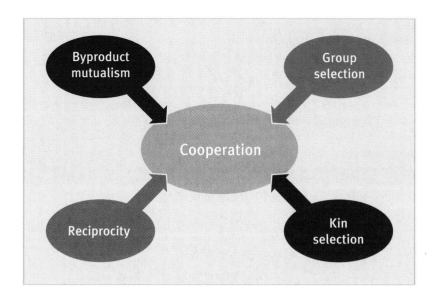

FIGURE 9.4. **Four paths to cooperation.** Reciprocity, byproduct mutualism, kin selection, and group selection can all lead to cooperative behavior.

Reciprocal Altruism" (Trivers, 1971). Trivers argued that if individuals benefited from exchanging acts of cooperative and altruistic behavior—what Trivers referred to as **reciprocal altruism**—then this sort of reciprocal exchange system might be favored by natural selection. That is, if individual A pays some cost to help individual B, but this cost is made up for at some point in the future, when B helps A, then natural selection might favor behaviors that lead to this type of reciprocity. Reciprocal altruism will be more likely to occur among individuals that live in groups and therefore expect to have continuing interactions with the same partners, as well as among individuals with the ability to recognize in the future those who had helped them in the past.

Trivers addressed the question of the evolution of reciprocity in a theoretical framework called "game theory." Game theory is a mathematical tool that is used when the "payoff"—some resource such as food, mating opportunities, and so on—that an individual receives for undertaking an action is dependent on what behavior others adopt. In particular, Trivers, with some help from W. D. Hamilton (see Chapter 8), suggested that the evolution of cooperation could best be understood by employing a mathematical game called the **prisoner's dilemma**.

To understand how the prisoner's dilemma game works, we will begin with a human example, and then examine this game in terms of animal behavior. Imagine the following scenario: While in separate rooms, two criminal suspects are interrogated by the police in the hope of getting a confession from one or both of them. Cooperation and defection (that is, not cooperating, which is also called cheating) are now defined from the perspective of the suspects. To defect means to "squeal" and tell the authorities that the other suspect is guilty, and to cooperate is to stay quiet (and not betray the other suspect). Imagine that the police have enough circumstantial evidence to put both suspects in jail for one year, even without a confession from either. But if each suspect informs on the other, both go to jail for three years. Finally, if only one suspect (the defector) informs on the other suspect (the cooperator, who does not inform on the other suspect), such behavior allows the defector to walk away a free man, but causes the cooperator to go to jail for five years.

Table 9.1 depicts the payoffs to each suspect as a function of how he behaves, and how the other suspect behaves. If both suspects cooperate, they both receive

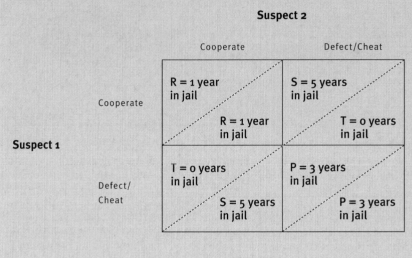

TABLE 9.1. The prisoner's dilemma game. In this game, each player can either cooperate or defect. For the matrix to qualify as a prisoner's dilemma game, it must be true that T > R > P > S. T = "Temptation to cheat" payoff, R = "Reward for mutual cooperation" payoff, P = "Punishment for mutual defection" payoff, and S = "Suckers" payoff. Each cell shows the payoff to suspect 1 (above the dashed diagonal line) and the payoff to suspect 2 (below the dashed diagonal line). For example, in the lower left cell, when suspect 1 defects and suspect 2 cooperates, the former gets 0 years in jail, while the latter gets 5 years in jail. There are other technical requirements for a matrix to be a prisoner's dilemma, but we will ignore them here.

a payoff of R (the Reward for mutual cooperation; 1 year in jail), and if they both defect, each one receives P (the Punishment for mutual defection; 3 years in jail). If suspect 1 defects, but suspect 2 cooperates, the former receives a payoff of T (the Temptation to cheat payoff; 0 years in jail), and the latter receives S (the Sucker's payoff; 5 years in jail). If we order the payoffs in this matrix from high to low, we see that T > R > P > S. It is this series of inequalities that defines our game as a prisoner's dilemma. That is, for a game to be a prisoner's dilemma, the payoff structure of the matrix must be T > R > P > S.

Suspect 1 will receive a higher payoff individually (serving fewer years in prison) if he defects regardless of what suspect 2 does. As such, suspect 1 should always defect. The same holds true individually for suspect 2, and he should also always defect. So, both suspects should defect. The *dilemma* in the prisoner's dilemma is that while each suspect receives P (3 years in prison) when they mutually defect, both suspects would receive a higher payoff (R, which is only 1 year in prison) if they had both cooperated (Poundstone, 1992).

As we shall see in a moment, the prisoner's dilemma game can be used to model certain types of animal, as well as human, cooperation. As long as each animal does better individually to defect regardless of the action of the other player, but both do better when there is mutual cooperation rather than mutual defection, the prisoner's dilemma game can be used to model animal cooperation. Before we look at animal examples, let us explore the prisoner's dilemma in more depth, and examine what sort of predictions about behavior emerge from this model.

Robert Axelrod and W. D. Hamilton used both analytical techniques and computer simulations to examine what sorts of behavioral strategies fared well—obtained high payoffs—when individuals were trapped in a prisoner's dilemma game. They examined the success of an array of behavioral strategies in an *iterated*, or repeated, prisoner's dilemma game (Axelrod and Hamilton, 1981). In the iterated version of the prisoner's dilemma game, two individuals (let's call them partners) play the prisoner's dilemma game with one another many times, and the exact end point is unknown. Thus, this type of game tends to mimic certain natural situations, since social, group-living animals generally encounter each other more than once. In addition, the iterated version of the game allows for the possible emergence of fairly complex strategies. If a pair of individuals plays the prisoner's dilemma game just once, then on that one play of the game, the only strategies possible are "cooperate" or "defect." In the iterated prisoner's dilemma game, however, when players encounter each other many times, more complex rules, including "if-then" rules of the form "if the other individual does X, then I will do Y," can be employed—for example, "if she cooperates, I will cooperate; otherwise I will defect."

Axelrod and Hamilton searched for the **evolutionarily stable strategy** (**ESS**) to the iterated prisoner's dilemma game (Maynard Smith, 1982; see Math Box 9.1 for explanation of an ESS). They demonstrated that if the probability of

---

MATH BOX 9.1

Evolutionarily Stable Strategies (ESS)

An evolutionarily stable strategy is defined as "a strategy such that, if all the members of a population adopt it, no mutant strategy can invade" (Maynard Smith, 1982). Here "mutant" refers to a new strategy introduced into a population, and successful invasions center around the relative fitness of established and mutant strategies. If the established strategy is evolutionarily stable, the payoff from the established strategy is greater than the payoff from the mutant (new) strategy. To see this more formally, let's consider two strategies, I and J. We will denote the expected payoff of strategy I against strategy J as $E(I, J)$, the payoff of J against I as $E(J, I)$, the payoff of I against I as $E(I, I)$, and the payoff of J against J as $E(J, J)$. Strategy I is an ESS if the following two conditions are met:

Either

$$E(I, I) > E(J, I) \tag{1}$$

or

$$E(I, I) = E(J, I), \text{ but } E(I, J) > E(J, J) \tag{2}$$

If condition (1) holds true, then I does better against other I's than J does. Since we start with a population full of I's (except for one J mutant), this condition assures that I is an ESS.

Condition (2) addresses what happens when I and J have the same fitness when interacting with I. If this is true, then J may now reach higher frequencies by chance, since when J occurs as a mutant it does just as well as I. I is then an ESS if it does better than J when paired up against J, that is, when $E(I, J) > E(J, J)$.

meeting a given partner in the future was sufficiently high, then in addition to the success of a simple strategy of "always be noncooperative" (labeled "always defect" or ALLD), a *reciprocity-based* strategy called **tit for tat (TFT)** was one solution to the iterated prisoner's dilemma (see Math Box 9.2).

TFT is a strategy in which an individual cooperates on the initial encounter with a partner and subsequently copies its partner's previous move. Thus, after

---

MATH BOX 9.2

An ESS Analysis of TFT and the Prisoner's Dilemma Game

Axelrod and Hamilton (1981) examined whether tit for tat (TFT) and the "always defect" (ALLD) strategy were evolutionarily stable—that is, whether they could resist invasion from mutants if they themselves were at a frequency close to 1. They began this task by proving that if the strategy ALLD or a strategy that alternates D and C (ALTDC) could not invade TFT, then no single pure strategy could invade. They then considered whether ALLD or ALTDC could in fact invade TFT.

Recall the payoffs of the prisoner's dilemma (T, R, P, and S). If we let w equal the probability of interacting with the same player on the next move of a game, then the moves of the game can be represented as a geometric series, and the expected number of interactions with a given opponent is equal to $1/(1 - w)$. So, for example, if $w = 0.9$, the expected number of interactions with a given partner is 10 $[1/(1 - 0.9)]$. This being the case, when TFT is close to being at a frequency of 1, virtually all TFT players meet other TFT players, and their payoff is:

$$R + wR + w^2R + w^3R + \ldots, \text{ which sums to } R/(1 - w) \tag{1}$$

An ALLD mutant would have all its interactions with TFT, and its payoff would be:

$$T + wP + w^2P + w^3P + \ldots, \text{ which sums to } T + wP/(1 - w) \tag{2}$$

and so TFT can resist invasion from ALLD when:

$$R/(1 - w) > T + wP/(1 - w) \tag{3}$$

Solving the inequality for w, ALLD fails to invade TFT when:

$$w > (T - R)/(T - P) \tag{4}$$

Now, when playing TFT, ALTDC gets a payoff when:

$$T + wS + w^2T + w^3T \ldots, \text{ which sums to } (T + wS)/(1 - w^2) \tag{5}$$

TFT is thus resistant to invasion when:

$$R/(1 - w) > (T + wS)/(1 - w^2) \tag{6}$$

Solving the inequality for w, ALTDC fails to invade TFT when:

$$w > (T - R)/(R - S) \tag{7}$$

Hence, Axelrod and Hamilton (1981) concluded that TFT is resistant to any invasion when:

$$w > \text{maximum of these two values: } (T - R)/(T - P) \text{ and } (T - R)/(R - S). \tag{8}$$

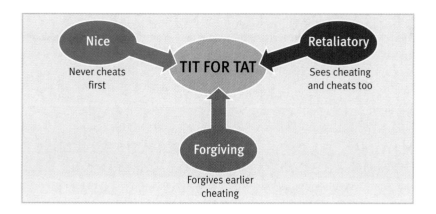

FIGURE 9.5. Tit for tat. The tit-for-tat strategy has three fundamental characteristics. The individual using TFT is (1) nice—it never cheats first, (2) retaliatory—it always responds to a partner that is cheating by cheating itself, and (3) forgiving—it only remembers one move back in time, and hence is capable of "forgiving" cheating that is done early in a sequence.

the first move, it operates under an if-then rule: if the partner cooperates, then cooperate; if the partner defects, then defect. It thus should reciprocate acts of cooperation, as well as acts of defection. This behavioral rule incorporates social learning into our cooperation paradigm, as individuals copy what their partners do, and such behavior can potentially ripple through an entire population.

Axelrod hypothesized that the TFT strategy's success is attributable to its three defining characteristics: (1) "niceness"—a player using TFT is never the first to defect, as it initially cooperates with a new partner, and then cooperates as long as its partner cooperates, (2) swift "retaliation"—an individual playing TFT immediately defects on a defecting partner since it copies its partner's previous move and so, if its partner defects, it defects, and (3) "forgiving"—because TFT instructs players to do what their partner did on the last move, those using a TFT strategy have a memory window that is *only one move back in time* (Axelrod, 1984). As such, the player using TFT forgives prior defection if a partner is currently cooperating—that is, those using a TFT strategy do not hold grudges (Figure 9.5). Since the original models of TFT have appeared, dozens of variants of this strategy have been examined, but most share the essential characteristics we have just discussed (Dugatkin, 1997a).

Numerous studies have examined reciprocity in animals: here we will focus on three of these studies. The first examines the prisoner's dilemma and the use of TFT during antipredator behavior in guppies, the second addresses reciprocity (but not necessarily TFT) in the context of vampire bat food sharing, and the third looks at the proximate underpinnings of human reciprocity.

PREDATOR INSPECTION AND TFT IN GUPPIES. Let's return to the scenario outlined at the start of the chapter—that of guppies inspecting a potentially dangerous predator. Here, inspecting a predator would be acting cooperatively, while failing to inspect, or just lagging behind during inspection, would be a form of cheating. Before addressing whether guppies use TFT while inspecting a predator, we first need to examine whether a pair of fish inspecting a predator are indeed trapped in a prisoner's dilemma game (Dugatkin, 1997a). As mentioned earlier, for a payoff matrix to be a prisoner's dilemma, it must be true that $T > R > P > S$. What evidence is there that these inequalities hold true for inspecting guppies?

IS T > R? Manfred Milinski has argued that a fish that trailed behind its partner while inspecting a possible predator would do better than its co-inspector, as it could assess how dangerous the predator was by observing whether the lead

TABLE 9.2. The payoffs for predator inspection. When T > R > P > S, predator inspection is a prisoner's dilemma.

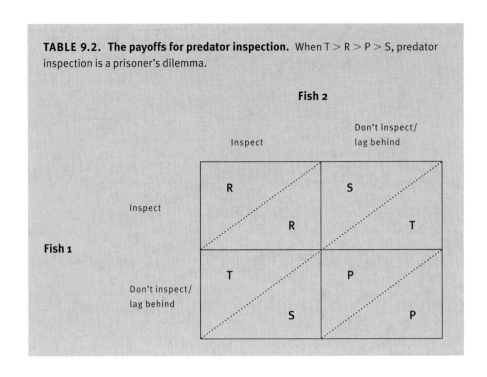

fish was attacked (Milinski, 1987). The trailing fish would receive a payoff of T if it stayed behind, but a payoff of R if it swam beside its partner (Table 9.2). Two pieces of evidence suggest that the payoff of T—that is, the payoff to lagging behind, while another fish inspected—is in fact greater than the R payoff associated with mutual inspection. First, inspectors are more likely to get eaten the closer they approach a predator (Figure 9.6), so it is more dangerous to be leading an inspection than lagging behind. Second, inspectors transfer the information that they receive during an inspection, so that any fish lagging behind would still receive the benefits associated with inspection (Dugatkin, 1992b; Magurran and Higham, 1988; Milinski et al., 1997; Figure 9.7).

IS R > P? Here we will rely on an argument that adaptationists make in regard to predator inspection. If P is greater than R—if the payoff for inspecting in a group is less than the payoff when no one inspects—it would not pay for any individual to inspect, and the phenomenon of inspection would be rare and maladaptive when it occurred. Given that inspection is a well-known phenomenon, however, that is documented in many species, this is unlikely to be the case, and so R, the payoff for mutual cooperation, is probably greater than P, the payoff for mutual defection (Dugatkin and Godin, 1992; Pitcher, 1992; Figure 9.8).

IS P > S? If predator inspection is to qualify as a prisoner's dilemma, it must also be true that the payoff to mutual cheating (P) is greater than the payoff associated with inspecting alone (S). While it appears to be the case that having no inspectors in a shoal is dangerous for all group members (no one obtains information on danger levels), the most perilous situation for a single fish is to be the lone inspector in a group. Evidence from a number of experiments indicates that single fish (stragglers) suffer very high rates of predation, suggesting that P > S (Milinski, 1977).

FIGURE 9.6. The risk of inspecting predators. Ten groups of six guppies each—two low inspectors, two medium inspectors, and two high inspectors—were placed with a predator in a pool that was one meter in diameter. The probability of surviving thirty-six hours was a function of inspection tendencies, with those inspecting most often suffering the highest mortality. *(From Dugatkin, 1992b)*

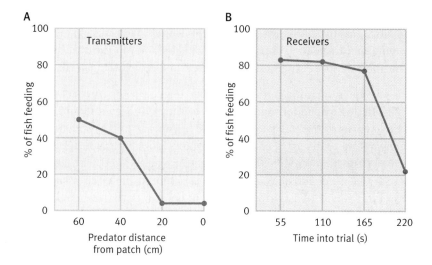

FIGURE 9.7. Information transfer in minnows. Magurran and Higham designed an experimental protocol in which some fish (transmitters) were allowed to inspect, while others (receivers) could see the transmitters, but not the predators. As the predator approached the transmitters, the latter fed less often **(A)**, as did the receivers **(B)**, suggesting that receivers were getting information about danger from the transmitters. *(Based on Magurran and Higham, 1988, p. 157)*

Precisely measuring T, R, P, and S in controlled experiments is difficult, and there is contention in the published literature over whether the payoff matrix associated with inspection meets the prisoner's dilemma requirement that T > R > P > S (see Dugatkin, 1997a, for a summary of these sometimes heated debates). We can't settle this debate here, but what we can say is that it is at least possible, and perhaps probable, that the payoff matrix is such that inspectors are trapped in a prisoner's dilemma. Working under the assumption that this is the case, theory suggests that we should examine inspection behavior to see whether individuals use a strategy akin to TFT (Croft et al., 2006).

The dynamic nature of inspection behavior in guppies and sticklebacks (but not mosquitofish) supports the idea that inspectors do, in fact, use the TFT strategy when inspecting potential predators (Dugatkin, 1997a; Stephens et al., 1997). As predicted by TFT, fish that inspect predators appear to be:

FIGURE 9.8. Inspection behavior in the wild. Researchers placed a model predator into a tributary of a river in Trinidad, and they recorded inspection behavior. Inspectors clearly recognize the head region of a predator as most dangerous. **(A)** There were fewer inspections of the predator's head than of its trunk and tail. **(B)** Inspector group was smallest when inspecting the head region of a predator. **(C)** Approach distance was a function of the part of the predator's body that was being inspected, with inspectors staying the farthest away when they were inspecting the predator's head. *(Based on Dugatkin and Godin, 1992b)*

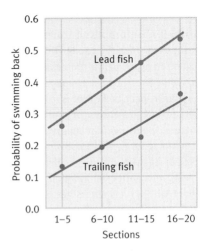

FIGURE 9.9. "Retaliation" in guppies? When pairs of guppies inspect a predator, lead fish in a given section of a tank are more likely to turn back to safety than are trailing fish (at about the same distance). This might be interpreted as lead fish "retaliating" against trailing fish, who fail to stay by their side. *(Based on Dugatkin, 1991, p. 130)*

FIGURE 9.10. Blood-sucking reciprocators. To survive, female vampire bats require frequent blood meals. Individuals often regurgitate part of their blood meals to others, but they are much more likely to do so for those who have shared a meal with them in the past. *(Photo credit: Jerry Wilkinson)*

FIGURE 9.11. Vampire bat cooperation. Vampire bats need frequent blood meals. If a hungry bat approaches a satiated bat, she is much more likely to get a regurgitated blood meal if she has fed the satiated bat in the past.

- "nice," as each starts off inspecting at about the same point in time,
- "retaliatory," as inspectors cease inspection if their partner stops (Figure 9.9),
- "forgiving"—if inspector A's partner has cheated on it in the past, but resumes inspection, A then resumes inspection as well (Dugatkin, 1991).

The prisoner's dilemma game can be used to make some further predictions. If the payoffs for inspection match those of the prisoner's dilemma, then the payoffs shown in Table 9.2 suggest that everyone should prefer to associate with cooperators. This is because cooperators do better when paired with other cooperators, and defectors also do better when paired with cooperators, and hence, whenever possible, all individuals should prefer to associate with cooperators. Evidence exists that inspectors do in fact remember the identity and behavior of their co-inspectors. When an individual fish is given the choice between associating with a fish that has been cooperative during prior encounters versus a fish that has not been cooperative, it prefers to associate with cooperators over defectors, at least when it is in a small group (Dugatkin and Alfieri, 1991a, 1992; Dugatkin and Wilson, 2000; Milinski et al., 1990).

Overall, game theory has proven to be a powerful tool for animal behaviorists (Dugatkin and Reeve, 1998; Nowak, 2006a; Sigmund, 1993). The prisoner's dilemma game, in particular, sheds light on the evolution of cooperation in numerous behavioral contexts. For example, other work has shown that the prisoner's dilemma game can help explain the (reciprocal) exchange of grooming bouts in impala, wherein individuals use their rough tongues to lick parasites off the body of another impala (Hart and Hart, 1992; Mooring and Hart, 1992). When the payoffs in nature match those of the prisoner's dilemma, as is likely the case for predator inspection in fish and grooming in impala, researchers can generate and test specific predictions regarding cooperative behavior.

RECIPROCITY AND FOOD SHARING IN VAMPIRE BATS. One of the first well-documented cases of reciprocity was uncovered in the food-sharing behavior found in vampire bats (*Desmodus rotundus*). A typical group of vampire bats is composed largely of females, with a low average coefficient of relatedness (between 0.02 and 0.11) (Wilkinson, 1984, 1990; Figures 9.10 and 9.11).

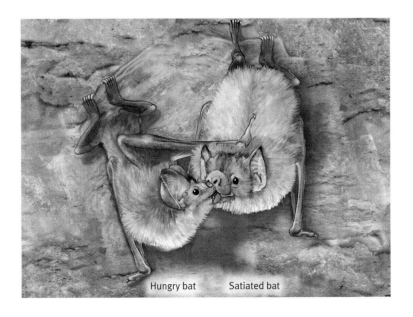

Hungry bat   Satiated bat

Females in a nest of vampire bats regurgitate blood meals to other bats that have failed to obtain food in the recent past (Wilkinson, 1984, 1985). This sort of food sharing can literally be a matter of life or death, as individuals may succumb to starvation if they don't receive a blood meal every sixty hours (McNab, 1973). Jerry Wilkinson examined whether relatedness, reciprocity, or some combination of the two best explained the evolution and maintenance of blood sharing in this species.

When Wilkinson examined which individuals were involved in food sharing, it was indeed the case that, despite the fact that the average relatedness in groups was low, genetic relatives were still more likely to swap blood meals than were other individuals (Figure 9.12). To examine whether reciprocity per se

FIGURE 9.12. Vampire bat blood meals. Wilkinson used twenty-one regurgitation events not involving mothers and their offspring to examine the role of relatedness and reciprocity in blood sharing. The graphs show: **(A)** all possible association patterns (a measure of when the recipient bat and some other bat are together) that could be found between the recipient bat and others in the nest, **(B)** the actual association patterns found between donors and recipients, **(C)** the genetic relatedness between recipients and all other roost members, and **(D)** the actual relatedness between a recipient and a donor. Bats were much more likely to regurgitate a meal to close kin and to those with whom they associated more often. Follow-up laboratory work found that bats were capable of keeping track of who fed them in the past and who didn't. *(From Wilkinson, 1984)*

was also important, Wilkinson created what he called an "index of opportunity for reciprocity." When analyzing the data with this sort of index, Wilkinson suggested three lines of evidence that reciprocity per se is important in blood sharing in vampire bats: (1) the probability of future interaction between group members in a nest of vampire bats is high as predicted by TFT models, (2) blood meals provide a huge, potentially life-saving benefit for recipients, while the cost of giving up some blood may not be as great to the donor, and (3) vampire bats are able to recognize one another and are more likely to give blood to those that have donated blood to them in the past—that is, they reciprocate acts of food sharing. So, while the vampire bats don't necessarily play a strict version of TFT, they are clearly employing some sort of reciprocal altruistic strategy.

NEUROBIOLOGICAL AND ENDOCRINOLOGICAL UNDERPINNINGS OF HUMAN RECIPROCITY. In addition to work on the evolution of cooperation, recent studies have shed light on the proximate underpinnings of cooperation, including reciprocity. As a case in point, we will examine the neurobiological and endocrinological underpinnings of reciprocity and trust in humans.

Much of this proximate work on the neurobiology of human cooperation has been undertaken by researchers in the new field of **neuroeconomics**—a collaborative research effort between economists and neurobiologists who specialize in brain science (Glimcher, 2004; Glimcher and Rustichini, 2004; Montague, 2006; Sanfey et al., 2006; Zak, 2004).

Experiments in neuroeconomics typically involve subjects who are making some economic decision—in our case, the focus will be on the economics of reciprocal altruism—while they are hooked up to a magnetic resonance imaging machine (fMRI) or a positron emission tomography (PET) device. In other words, subjects have their brain activity monitored as they make some sort of decision associated with reciprocal altruism.

To see how neuroeconomics can shed light on one proximate component of human cooperation, let us examine a study done by James Rilling and his colleagues (Rilling et al., 2002). Rilling and his team had women subjects play the prisoner's dilemma depicted in Table 9.3. Subjects were hooked up to an fMRI

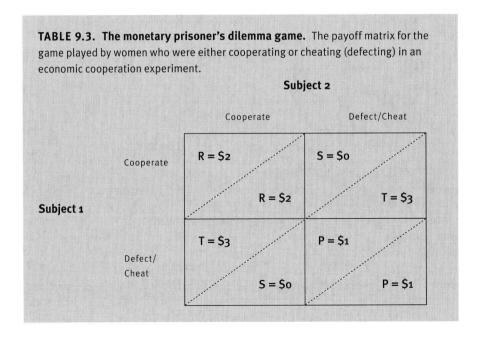

TABLE 9.3. The monetary prisoner's dilemma game. The payoff matrix for the game played by women who were either cooperating or cheating (defecting) in an economic cooperation experiment.

	Subject 2	
	Cooperate	Defect/Cheat
Subject 1 Cooperate	R = $2 / R = $2	S = $0 / T = $3
Defect/Cheat	T = $3 / S = $0	P = $1 / P = $1

A

B

FIGURE 9.13. The prisoner's dilemma game and social cooperation. To study whether there was a neurobiological basis of reciprocal altruism and cooperation, researchers had subjects play an iterated prisoner's dilemma game. **(A)** One of the subjects played from inside an fMRI machine that monitored her brain activity as she played, while the other subject played the game on a computer in another room. Each subject saw the payoff matrix that represented her own payoffs. Depicted above is a situation in which both subjects cooperated, as indicated by the red highlighting seen in the upper left square of each game matrix. **(B)** The fMRI scans showed that, when both subjects cooperated, brain areas associated with reward processing—the ventromedial/orbitofrontal cortex (OFC), the rostral anterior cingulate cortex (rACC), the anteroventral striatum (including the caudate nucleus and the nucleus accumbens), and the subgenual anterior cingulate cortex (ACC)—were activated. *(Based on Rilling et al., 2002; photo credit: James Rilling; reprinted by permission of Cell Press)*

machine and played the iterated prisoner's dilemma game over a networked computer with another subject who was in another room (Figure 9.13).

What Rilling and his team found was that even though the highest monetary reward in this game ($3) was obtained when an individual cheated and her partner cooperated, the fMRI scan of players' brains as they made their economic decisions indicated that the most emotionally rewarding payoff was that associated with mutual cooperation (which yielded $2 to each individual). That is, not only did subjects say that they found mutual cooperation to be the most rewarding outcome, but it was the mutual cooperation payoff that caused the greatest activation of brain sections associated with reward processing in humans, namely the ventromedial/orbitofrontal cortex (OFC), the anterior cingulate cortex (ACC), and the nucleus accumbens.

Work in neuroeconomics has not only examined emotions and rational behavior with respect to reciprocity per se, but it has also examined what sections of the brain are active when we punish those who fail to act cooperatively during economic interactions. Punishing those who violate social norms is of particular interest to those behaviorists, including animal behaviorists, who wish to understand how social norms evolved before modern legal codes came into place. In particular, such behaviors often entail a *cost* to those who dole out the punishment, and a *benefit* to others not even involved in the interaction. Dominique de Quervain and his colleagues at the University of Zurich hypothesized that one proximate mechanism involved in maintaining this sort of punishment lies in the pleasure that we derive from enforcing social norms (de Quervain et al., 2004), and that this can indirectly be measured through neurobiological scans of the brain.

To test this hypothesis, de Quervain and his colleagues had pairs of subjects play what is sometimes called the trust game. In the trust game, two players—who are not allowed to communicate with each other—begin with 10 units of money (called monetary units, or MUs, in this experiment). Player A—who was hooked up to a PET scanner—starts the game by deciding whether to give his 10 MUs to player B or to keep them for himself. A is told that, if he gives his money to B, the investigator will quadruple the gift to 40 MUs, so that B now has 50 MUs, and A is broke. Then player B is given a choice. He can send half his MUs back to player A, or he can keep everything for himself. So if A "trusts" B to send the money back, and B does send back the money, A and B each end up with 25 MUs; while if A opts to give nothing, they both end up with 10 MUs.

De Quervain hypothesized that if A does trust B to play fairly, and gives him the money, but B then turns around and keeps all the MUs, A should view this as a violation of trust and social norms. He hypothesized that, in such a case, A should then wish to punish B. To allow for this possibility, one minute after B makes his decision, A can opt to "punish" B by revoking some of the MUs that he initially gave B. In one treatment of the experiment, A paid a cost in MUs for doing so, and in other treatments punishing player B did not have any cost associated with it.

If A trusts B, but B violates that trust, A will indeed punish B, even if it costs monetary units to do so. More to the point, not only did subjects say that they enjoyed punishing those who violated their trust, PET scans of their brains demonstrated that one section of the brain associated with *reward* (the dorsal striatum, which includes the caudate nucleus) is most active when A undertakes its act of retribution. That is, individuals derived *pleasure* from punishing cheaters. Indeed, results suggest that the more intense the punishment doled out to cheaters was, the more active was the dorsal striatum of the individual exacting retribution (Figure 9.14). In an interesting twist to the original experiment, A was sometimes told that B's decision was determined by the equivalent of an electronic coin toss, and so it was out of B's hands. In that condition, when B did not send money back to A, A did not view this as a violation of trust and did not respond by punishing B, nor did the researchers see the increased activity in the dorsal striatum that was observed when A was punishing B.

Research has also examined the endocrinological underpinnings of reciprocity and trust in humans. As we learned in Chapter 6, oxytocin (OT) is a hormone that has been associated with numerous affiliative behaviors like pair bonding and parental care in nonhumans. Because there are dense accumulations of OT receptors in the amygdala of the human brain, a region associated with social behavior (Loup et al., 1991), Paul Zak and his colleagues hypothesized that OT would also play a role in affiliative interactions in humans (Kosfeld et al., 2005; Zak et al., 2005). In particular, they ran a series of experiments that examined the role of OT in the trust game we described in the de Quervain neuroeconomics experiment.

Zak's version of the trust game was slightly different from the one described earlier. In the Zak version, player A was given $10. He was then asked how much of that $10 he was willing to give to player B, with the understanding that whatever he gave to player B would be *tripled* by the experimenter. Then player B was given a choice to send back as much money as he desired (including $0) to player A.

FIGURE 9.14. The trust game and punishment. Two subjects played the trust game while one of them (player A) was hooked up to a PET scanner that monitored his brain activity. The caudate nucleus, which is part of the dorsal striatum of the brain—depicted in yellow—was very active when player A punished player B for failing to return some of the money that A had provided to B. *(From de Quervain et al., 2004; reprinted by permission of the AAAS)*

Rather than attaching their subjects to a brain-scanning device, Zak and his team drew blood from the subjects immediately after they had played the trust game, and they analyzed the blood sample to estimate OT levels. Subjects were tested in one of two treatments. In Treatment 1, player B was told that player A had made his choice voluntarily, and in Treatment 2, B was told that A was forced to send a randomly selected amount of money to him. The researchers hypothesized that B would feel more trust toward A when he received money that A had voluntarily sent, and that B would then send back more money and would show an increased level of OT (compared to Treatment 2). Results were consistent with these hypotheses.

Zak and his colleagues found that OT levels were significantly higher in Treatment 1, where player B believed that the money he/she had received from player A was sent voluntarily (Figure 9.15). Further evidence for the role of OT in human decisions about trust was also uncovered. Zak and his team found that the more money A sent B, the more money B sent back, and the higher B's OT levels—but this was only true when B believed A had sent the money voluntarily.

Together, the neuroeconomics work and the studies on hormones and trust are providing researchers with a much better understanding of the proximate basis for cooperation in humans.

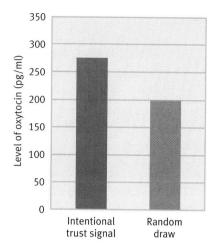

FIGURE 9.15. Oxytocin and trust. The level of oxytocin was higher when subjects believed money was sent to them voluntarily (versus sent as a function of a random draw). *(From Zak et al., 2005)*

PATH 2: BYPRODUCT MUTUALISM

A second path to the evolution of cooperation is **byproduct mutualism** (Brown, 1983; Connor, 1995; Rothstein and Pirotti, 1987; West-Eberhard, 1975). Cooperation here is a "byproduct" of the fact that an individual would incur an immediate cost or penalty if it did not act cooperatively, such that the immediate net benefit of cooperating would outweigh that of cheating. In other words, there would be no temptation to cheat, and so individuals would cooperate. So, for example, if you and a friend are trapped in a cave and the only way out is for you both to push the large boulder blocking the entrance, there is no temptation for you not to do so, as you will both pay a large cost if either of you fails to cooperate (Figure 9.16).

FIGURE 9.16. Byproduct mutualism. In the case of byproduct mutualism, there is an immediate cost paid for not cooperating. Here, neither person gains by failing to move a stone that neither can budge alone.

Byproduct mutualism differs from reciprocity in two fundamental ways. First, as alluded to in the cave example, there is no temptation to cheat under byproduct mutualism, while such a temptation always exists in systems involving reciprocity. In addition, while most (but not all) forms of reciprocity require some form of scorekeeping, with byproduct mutualism individuals need not keep track of the past behavior of partners because in such situations it is always in the best interest of all parties to cooperate, and hence past behavior is not relevant in this decision-making process.

SKINNERIAN BLUE JAYS AND BYPRODUCT MUTUALISM. One critique of the work on cooperation and the prisoner's dilemma is that it is very difficult for investigators to measure the precise payoffs (Clements and Stephens, 1995). A potential way around this problem is to use what are called Skinner boxes (as in operant psychology experiments), which allow precise control over the payoffs that animals encounter in the lab. Kevin Clements and David Stephens adopted this technique in their study of blue jay (*Cyanocitta cristata*) cooperation (Clements and Stephens, 1995; Figure 9.17).

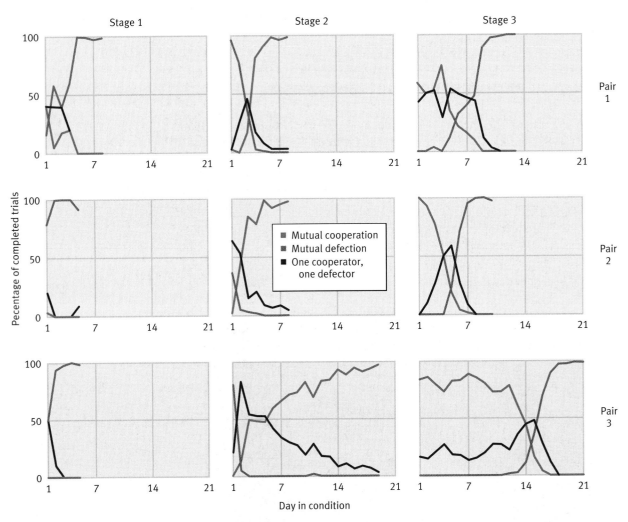

FIGURE 9.17. Byproduct mutualism and blue jays. Three pairs of blue jays were tested in a three-stage experiment: Stage 1 = prisoner's dilemma, Stage 2 = byproduct mutualism, and Stage 3 = prisoner's dilemma. Jays cooperated when the payoff matrix matched byproduct mutualism, but not when it matched the prisoner's dilemma. *(Based on Clements and Stephens, 1995)*

Clements and Stephens tested pairs of blue jays, each of whom could peck one of two keys—a cooperate key or a defect key. After the birds made their decisions, they were given a certain amount of food. The amount of food they obtained depended on what action they took (cooperate or defect), what action the other bird took, and which of two different payoff matrices the researchers had set up. The first matrix had payoffs that matched a prisoner's dilemma matrix (P matrix), while the second had payoffs that mimicked a byproduct mutualism matrix (M matrix), in which there was no temptation to cheat, since the birds always received more food for cooperating (Table 9.4). In each case, bird 1 would begin a trial by pecking one of the keys and bird 2 would end the trial (again by pecking either the cooperate or defect key). For example, if a

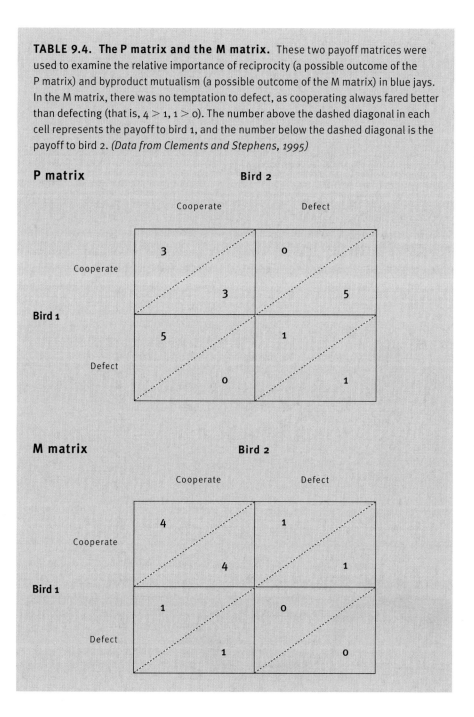

TABLE 9.4. The P matrix and the M matrix. These two payoff matrices were used to examine the relative importance of reciprocity (a possible outcome of the P matrix) and byproduct mutualism (a possible outcome of the M matrix) in blue jays. In the M matrix, there was no temptation to defect, as cooperating always fared better than defecting (that is, $4 > 1$, $1 > 0$). The number above the dashed diagonal in each cell represents the payoff to bird 1, and the number below the dashed diagonal is the payoff to bird 2. *(Data from Clements and Stephens, 1995)*

pair was in the P matrix part of the game and bird 1 cooperated when bird 2 defected, bird 2 obtained five food items, while bird 1 received no food items.

Birds were exposed to the P matrix, then to the M matrix, and finally to the P matrix once again, and on any given day a pair of birds would play these games with each other more than 200 times. Clements and Stephens found that, regardless of whether or not the jays could see each other, birds defected in the original prisoner's dilemma matrix, cooperated in the M matrix, and reverted to defection the second time they encountered the P matrix (see Figure 9.17 again). As such, blue jays appeared to cooperate via byproduct mutualism and not reciprocity, even when a payoff matrix (the prisoner's dilemma) that should promote reciprocity was presented. Why this is so remains unknown. What we do know is that reciprocity then failed to emerge as a stable solution, even when pairs of birds had more than a sufficient number of plays of the game to establish long-term mutual cooperation.

BYPRODUCT MUTUALISM AND HOUSE SPARROW FOOD CALLS. House sparrows (*Passer domesticus*) produce a unique "chirrup" call when they come upon a food resource (Summers-Smith, 1963). These calls appear to attract other birds to a newly discovered bounty, and as such, chirrup calls may be regarded as some type of cooperation. To examine just what type of cooperation, Marc Elgar tested whether the chirrup vocalization did in fact bring conspecifics to a newly discovered food source, and if so, under what conditions (Elgar, 1986). To do so, he recorded chirrup calls at artificial feeders containing either bread that was divisible among sparrows, or that was just enough food for a single bird.

To begin with, Elgar did find some evidence that those sparrows arriving at a patch of food first (labeled as "pioneers") were the most likely to produce chirrup calls. Furthermore, chirrup call rates were higher when the food resource was divisible (Figure 9.18). Elgar hypothesized that if the food items

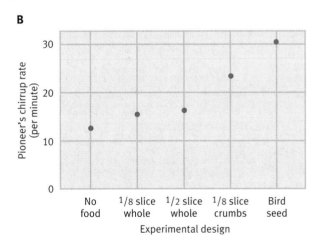

FIGURE 9.18. Food size and food calls in sparrows. (A) The first bird to arrive at a food patch (labeled the pioneer) was more likely to produce a "chirrup call" that attracted other birds when resources were more divisible. **(B)** Pioneers also called more often when food was easily divisible. *(Based on Elgar, 1986, p. 171).*

were small enough that sparrows could pick them up and fly away, which is what the sparrows did in one of his treatments, they would do so without producing chirrup calls. Chirrup calls were, however, associated with larger food items—that is, those that were too big to remove from the experimental area. It may be that given that sparrows needed to remain at a feeder with large food items, and that it is safer to do so in the company of other sparrows, the benefits associated with predator detection outweighed the costs of inviting other foragers to share food at the site. In that case, chirrup calls would be most easily understood in the context of byproduct mutualism. The calls are emitted when the immediate net benefit for calling (predator detection and some food) is greater than the net benefit for not calling (more to eat).

PATH 3: GROUP SELECTION

A third path to cooperation is via **group selection**. Ideas about group selection have a long history, but we can only touch on the most salient aspects of this theory here (Sober and Wilson, 1998; Wilson, 1980a; Wilson and Wilson, 2007). Although still controversial, modern group selection models of cooperation are quite straightforward. These models are often called trait-group selection models, where a trait group is defined as a group in which all individuals affect one another's fitness.

The kernel of trait-group selection models is that natural selection operates at two levels: within-group selection and between-group selection. In the context of cooperation and altruism, within-group selection acts *against* cooperators and altruists, since such individuals, by definition, take on some cost that others do not. Selfish types—those who do not cooperate—are always favored by within-group selection, since they receive any benefits that accrue because of the actions of cooperators and altruists, but they pay none of the costs.

As opposed to within-group selection, between-group selection favors cooperation if groups with more cooperators outproduce other groups—for example, by producing more total offspring or being able to colonize new areas faster. Consider the case of alarm calls. Alarm callers pay a cost within groups, as they may be the most obvious target of a predator honing in on such a call. But their sacrifice may benefit the group overall, as other individuals—including other alarm callers, as well as those that don't call—are able to evade predators because of the alarm call. Thus, groups with many alarm callers may outproduce groups with fewer cooperators. For such group-level benefits to be manifest, groups must differ in the frequency of cooperators within them, and groups must be able to "export" the productivity associated with cooperation (for example, more total offspring, faster colonization of newer areas, and so on).

Group selection models remain controversial. Many animal behaviorists argue that all group selection models (including trait-group selection models) can be mathematically translated into selfish gene models. That is, they posit that group selection models simply partition the effect of a trait into within- and between-group components, but that if you sum up the effects over all groups you get the same solution as a selfish gene model would produce (Dawkins, 1979; Queller, 1992). This is absolutely correct. One can always take a group selection model and translate the mathematics into a model in which natural selection favors one allele over another. Such mathematical equivalence, however, does not mean that group selection models do not shed new light on animal behavior, as trait-group selection models do instantly focus attention on what is happening within and between groups, and this is not necessarily the case for selfish gene models (Dugatkin and Reeve, 1994). Thus, under certain conditions, group selection models may spur investigators to construct experiments that would not be obvious if they were using selfish gene models.

To get a more comprehensive view of group selection, let's focus on the evolution of specialized foraging behavior in an environment containing many social insect colonies (Wilson, 1990).

WITHIN- AND BETWEEN-GROUP SELECTION IN ANTS. Cooperative colony foundation occurs in a number of species of ants where cooperating co-foundresses are *not* closely related (Bernasconi and Strassmann, 1999; Holldobler and Wilson, 1990). Cooperative colony foundation has been especially well studied in the desert seed harvester ant *Messor pergandei*. In terms of between-group selection, in many populations of *M. pergandei*, adult ants are very territorial, and "brood raiding"—wherein brood captured by ants from nearby colonies are raised within the victorious nests, and colonies that lose their brood in such inter-actions die—is seen among young starting colonies in the laboratory (Ryti and Case, 1984; Wheeler and Rissing, 1975). Within groups, all co-founding queens in a nest assist in excavating their living quarters, and each produces approx-imately the same number of offspring. As such, there exists a positive correlation between the number of cooperating foundresses in a nest and the number of initial workers (brood raiders) produced by that colony (Rissing and Pollock, 1986, 1991; Table 9.5). Nests with more workers—that is, those with more cooperating foundresses—are more likely to win brood raids (Rissing and Pollock, 1987).

TABLE 9.5. Cooperating co-foundresses. In the ant *Messor pergandei*, unrelated queens (here W, Y, B, and O) co-found nests. The reproductive output of queens within a nest tends to be approximately equal. Differences in all three measures across the four queens were not statistically significant. *(From Rissing and Pollack, 1986)*

NEST NO.	NO. OF EGGS	% LAID BY			
		W	Y	B	O
1	22	—	32	41	27
2	24	38	25	38	—
4	32	41	28	25	6
5	11	45	—	55	—
8	29	28	34	38	—
9	44	34	16	27	23
10	36	31	19	50	—
11	21	43	—	24	33
15	29	38	—	21	41

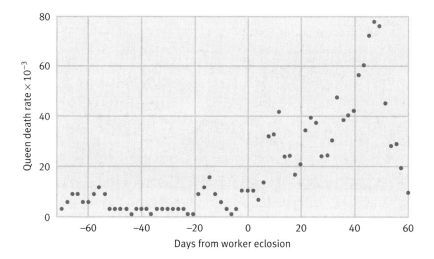

FIGURE 9.19. From cooperation to aggression. Co-founding *Messor pergandei* queens are cooperative during worker production, with very little queen-queen aggression during this phase of colony development. Once workers are produced—known as "worker eclosion," which is when they emerge from eggs— (starting at day 0), however, queen-queen aggression in nests escalates, as does the queen death rate. *(From Rissing and Pollock, 1987)*

Until workers emerge, queens within a nest do not fight, and no dominance hierarchy exists (Figure 9.19). After workers emerge and the between-group benefits of having multiple foundresses are already set in place with the presence of brood raiders, all that remains is within-group selection, which favors being noncooperative. It is at this juncture that queens within a nest often fight to the death.

The scenario depicted above is precisely what is necessary for group selection to operate, as group selection requires the differential productivity of groups based on some trait. In the case of *M. pergandei*, the trait is queen-queen cooperation. Such cooperation is selected against *within* groups because cooperators pay a cost not borne by noncooperators. At the same time, cooperation may be selected for between groups, since groups with many cooperators differentially survive brood raiding, which is the between-group component of group selection.

Yet, the results of these studies with respect to between-group selection have been challenged. David Pfennig constructed a field experiment contrasting single and double foundress associations in *M. pergandei*. Not only did double foundress nests not outlive single foundress nests in Pfennig's experiment, but no brood raiding at all was observed, calling into question all of the elements necessary for group selection to operate in the wild (Pfennig, 1995).

One of the strongest cases to date of group selection comes from Steve Rissing's work on another ant, *Acromyrmex versicolor* (Rissing et al., 1989). In this species, many nests are founded by multiple queens, no dominance hierarchy exists among queens, all queens produce workers, and brood raiding among starting nests appears to be common. Furthermore, the probability of the nest surviving the brood raiding period is a function of the numbers of workers produced.

A. versicolor differs from *M. pergandei*, however, in that queens in the former species forage after colony foundation (Figure 9.20). As a result of increased predation and parasitization, foraging is a dangerous activity for a queen. Foraging involves bringing back materials that increase the productivity of the nest's fungus garden, which is the food source for the colony. Once a queen takes on the role of forager, she remains in that role. After a queen becomes the sole forager for her nest, all queens share equally in the food produced

FIGURE 9.20. Extreme cooperation by foraging queen. In the ant *Acromyrmex versicolor*, a single queen (shown in the blowup circle) is the forager for a nest. Such foraging is very dangerous, but all food collected is shared equally among (unrelated) queens.

by the fungus garden. In other words, the forager assumes both the risks and the benefits of foraging, while the other queens in her nest simply assume the benefits but not the costs (Table 9.6). Once again, however, cooperation—in this case, extreme cooperation on the part of the forager—within nests appears to lead to more workers. This in turn affects the probability that a given nest will be the one to survive the period of brood raiding, thus providing the between-group component necessary for cooperation to evolve (Cahan and Julian, 1999; Rissing et al., 1989; Seger, 1989). Indeed, when Rissing and his team experimentally blocked the foraging queen's opportunity to leave the nest and gather food, the remaining queens often failed to choose a new forager, causing failure of the fungus garden and a decrease in the number of workers produced by the remaining queens (Pollock et al., 2004; Rissing et al., 1996).

TABLE 9.6. Harmony among *Acromyrmex versicolor* queens. In *A. versicolor*, unrelated queens co-found nests, with a single queen taking on the dangerous role of forager for everyone in the nest. All indications are that reproduction within nests is equal between foragers and nonforagers. *(Based on Rissing et al., 1989)*

	FORAGER	NONFORAGER
Mean number of primary eggs	8.6	8.5
Mean primary egg length	0.52	0.54
Mean number of total eggs	20.37	18.94

As always, we could analyze the cooperation described in both examples above in terms of selfish genes, and we would come to the same conclusions we arrived at from the trait-group perspective. That said, in both *M. pergandei* and *A. versicolor,* we see systems in which population biology and demographics may match those that are postulated in trait-group models. The multiple nests, intense competition between nests, and multiple foundresses in these species make them ideal for an analysis at both the within-group and between-group levels.

Coalitions

Much, but not all, of the cooperation we have addressed so far involves pairwise, or dyadic, interactions. In these **dyadic interactions**, two individuals interact in such a way that the fitness of each is affected by both its own action and the action of its partner. Cooperation can also occur in **polyadic interactions**—that is, interactions that involve more than two individuals. One example of polyadic interactions involving cooperation is **coalition** behavior, which is typically defined as a cooperative action taken by at least two other individuals or groups against another individual or group. When coalitions exist for long periods of time, they are often referred to as **alliances** (Harcourt and de Waal, 1992).

Coalitions have been documented in numerous primate species, hyenas (*Crocuta crocuta*), wolves (*Canis lupus*), lions (*Panthera leo*), cheetahs (*Acinonyx jubatus*), coatis (*Nasua narica*), and dolphins (*Tursiops truncatus*) (Harcourt and de Waal, 1992; Figure 9.21). In most instances, coalitions involve an animal intervening in a dyadic, usually aggressive, interaction between other group

A

B

FIGURE 9.21. Coalitions. (A) Three male dolphins swim together, forming a long-term coalition (or alliance). Such male coalitions "herd" females. A female is seen to the left of the three males. Occasionally different alliances join together to form superalliances that compete against other such superalliances. **(B)** Pairs of male chimps often form coalitions to act against larger, more dominant, individuals. *(Photo credits: Richard Connor; Frans de Waal)*

members (Harcourt and de Waal, 1992). Often, the intervening individual is dominant to others involved in the interaction. In primates, interventions often take the form of the intervener coming to the aid of one of the two other individuals involved in an interaction (Harcourt and de Waal, 1992). This need not be the case, however, as intervening animals may break up an interaction between two others, without favoring either combatant (Dugatkin, 1998a, 1998b; Johnstone and Dugatkin, 2000). This type of intervention has been found in various primate species (Harcourt and de Waal, 1992), as well as in the cichlid fish, *Melanochromis auratus* (Nelissen, 1985).

We will examine two examples of coalitions, one in primates and one in dolphins. In each of these cases, coalitions form among males to gain access to reproductively active females.

COALITIONS IN BABOONS

One of the most well-cited examples of coalition formation is Craig Packer's work on male reproductive coalitions in baboons (*Papio anubis*). In *P. anubis*, a male solicits coalition partners by rapidly turning his head between the solicited animal (that is, the individual from which he is requesting aid) and his opponent, while at the same time threatening his opponent (Packer, 1977; Figure 9.22). In his observation of coalition formation, Packer documented ninety-seven solicitations that resulted in coalitions being formed. On twenty of these occasions, the opponent was consorting with an estrous female, and this increased the probability of a coalition being formed between the other two individuals (the enlisting male and the solicited male). On six of these twenty occasions, the estrous female deserted the opponent and went to the enlisting male, suggesting a benefit to coalition formation, at least for the enlisting individual.

FIGURE 9.22. Baboon coalitions. A male baboon (middle) involved in an aggressive interaction (with male on left) will often solicit others to aid him by turning his head in the direction of a potential coalition partner (male on right).

What about the costs and benefits to the animal that is solicited into a coalition? Joining a coalition may be fairly costly to solicited individuals, who rarely ever obtain access to the estrous female but who risk being attacked by the opponent. Packer's study suggests that solicited males may overcome such costs by having the individual who enlisted them respond when they themselves need help (reciprocal coalitions). In fact, Packer discovered that baboons had "favorite partners," and that favorite partners solicited each other more often than they solicited other group members, suggesting that "alliance" rather than "coalition" may be the correct label for this sort of baboon interaction.

Other studies of coalitions and their effect on access to reproductive females in baboons have generally supported Packer's findings (Noe, 1986; Smuts, 1985). But Bercovitch found that in olive baboons (*Papio anubis*), males who enlisted others in coalitions were no more likely than males they had solicited to obtain mating opportunities with females, and baboons who declined to join a coalition were again solicited in the future (Bercovitch, 1988). The reason for the discrepancy between Packer's and Bercovitch's studies are as yet not clear, but Charlotte Hemelrijk suggests that it may be tied to the presence of a clear alpha male in the Bercovitch study, but not in the Packer study (Hemelrijk and Ek, 1991).

ALLIANCES AND "HERDING" BEHAVIOR IN CETACEANS

Richard Connor and his colleagues have uncovered an interesting case of alliance formation in bottlenose dolphins (*Tursiops truncatus*) (Connor, 1992; Connor et al., 1992, 2001; Krutzen et al., 2003). What makes this case particularly intriguing is that dolphins are notoriously difficult to track for long periods of time, and thus while ethologists have generally thought dolphins capable of sophisticated behavior in the wild, this has been very difficult to document in any scientific manner. Connor and his colleagues examined pairs and trios of males forming close associations in the bottlenose dolphin population of Shark Bay, in Western Australia. He and his colleagues found not one, but two different types of alliances between male dolphins, with both forms of alliances focusing among males who were "herding" reproductive females to keep them close.

"First-order" alliances in dolphins are composed of pairs or trios of males acting in a coordinated fashion to keep females by their side, presumably for the purpose of mating. Males in first-order alliances stay very close to one another, and alliances remain stable for many years. When females herded by an alliance of male dolphins try to swim away (which they often do), the males act in a very coordinated, aggressive manner to prevent the females from leaving (Connor et al., 1992).

What makes alliance formation in dolphins unique is that different first-order alliances also join together in "second-order" superalliances and aggressively attack and steal females from other alliances. Connor showed that on two occasions, a defending alliance was assisted by another alliance in its attempts to maintain the female it was herding, creating a battle of second-order alliances. Second-order alliances have been documented in only one other species—humans—and Connor argues that the complex social interactions inherent in dolphin superalliances, as well as in other aspects of dolphin society, may explain the evolution of large brain size in dolphins (Connor, 1992).

Phylogeny and Cooperation

In conjunction with inclusive fitness theory (see Chapter 8), the work we have examined so far provides the conceptual foundations for predicting when natural selection favors cooperation. We can now examine other aspects of cooperative behavior, including a phylogenetic component, which provides a window through which to examine how evolutionary history may affect cooperative behavior.

Recall that phylogenetic analysis allows us to test whether a trait may be common in a group of animal species as a result of common descent rather than independent selection regimes. In other words, phylogenetic analysis lets us ask whether one reason that a trait is common within a taxa is that all members of that taxa share a common ancestor that possessed this trait. For example, if we find cooperation in species 1, 2, 3, and 4, and all of these species evolved from species 5, which also displayed cooperation, then species 1–4 may not represent independent data points with respect to the origin of cooperation. Natural selection may very well be maintaining a trait in many related species, even when such a trait originated in a common ancestor, but phylogenetic logic suggests that to count all such cases as originating independently in all these species is questionable.

PHYLOGENY AND COOPERATIVE BREEDING IN BIRDS

Cooperative breeding in birds is common enough that numerous adaptationist hypotheses have been put forth to explain its selective value and distribution (Brown, 1987; Stacey and Koenig, 1990; see Chapter 8). Early studies of cooperative breeding in birds, however, were quite different from the adaptationist approach discussed in Chapter 8, and gave much more weight to phylogeny's role in cooperative breeding (Brown, 1974; Davis, 1942; Fry, 1977; Hardy, 1961).

Employing newly developed phylogenetic analyses made possible by more powerful computers, Scott Edwards and Shahid Naeem examined cooperative breeding from a phylogenetic perspective (Edwards and Naeem, 1993). Using 166 species of cooperatively breeding passerine birds in ninety-seven genera, they began their work by testing whether the distribution of cooperatively breeding species was random within the genera of passerine birds on which they focused. Edwards and Naeem created a computer simulation to predict what the distribution of cooperative breeding species would be if they distributed into genera simply based on the number of species in that genera. They found that the distribution of cooperative breeding species in nature differed significantly from the random distributions generated by computer simulations, with some genera having more than the expected number of cooperatively breeding species, and others less than the expected number (Figure 9.23).

Edwards and Naeem followed this analysis by using already published phylogenetic trees to examine the distribution of cooperative breeding. For example, their phylogenetic analysis of jays, Australian songbirds, Australian treecreepers, and New World wrens suggests that cooperative breeding may have arisen a limited number of times in some common ancestor(s) of modern-day species. Phylogenetic analysis suggests that modern species displaying cooperative breeding had a common ancestor that had this type of mating

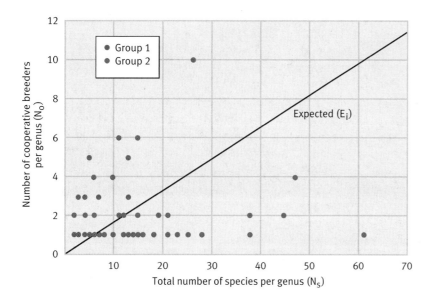

FIGURE 9.23. Phylogeny and cooperative breeding. The solid line represents the slope expected if the number of cooperators per passerine genus (seventy-one) were proportional to genus size. In group 1, cooperative breeding was overrepresented; in group 2, cooperative breeding was underrepresented. (Based on Edwards and Naeem, 1993, p. 761)

system, and modern species that do not display cooperative breeding had a common ancestor in which cooperative breeding was absent. In other words, common ancestry, rather than natural selection alone, may explain the origin and the distribution of cooperative breeding in some modern groups of birds.

The phylogenetic approach does not necessarily conflict with an adaptationist view of cooperative breeding, although it does emphasize the importance of history (phylogeny) in our understanding of the distribution of cooperative breeding. For example, it may be that a set of species derived from a single ancestor initially "inherited" the tendency toward cooperative breeding (a phylogenetic component), but that subsequent to this, natural selection favored continued cooperation in some species, but not others (a selective component).

PHYLOGENY AND COOPERATION IN SOCIAL SPIDERS

Most spiders are asocial, building individual webs and hunting alone. There are, however, a handful of social spider species—23 out of about 39,000 species—in which individuals display extreme levels of cooperation (Agnarsson et al., 2006). In these species, individuals build very large communal webs, jointly maintain these webs, cooperatively hunt for prey, and cooperate in raising brood born in their colonies (Figure 9.24). With respect to foraging, this sort of cooperation allows spiders to obtain more and larger prey (Uetz, 1992).

Ingi Agnarsson and his colleagues examined the phylogenetic history of social spiders to estimate the number of times sociality had independently evolved in this group (Agnarsson et al., 2006). That is, of the twenty-three species in which sociality has been recorded, how many of these represented independent evolutionary events? Their phylogenetic analysis found that sociality had evolved either eighteen or nineteen different times in spiders—this was evident because, except for one instance, sociality was scattered across the phylogenetic tree, and not clustered in species with a common ancestor that displayed sociality. This (eighteen or nineteen) is a remarkably high number of evolutionary origins for cooperation. And, indeed, the twenty-three social species that have been documented today appear to represent only a small fraction of the number of

FIGURE 9.24. Communal webs. A giant web built by a communal spider group. *(Photo credit: Piotr Naskrecki/ Minden Pictures/FLPA)*

social spider species that have existed through evolutionary time, as Agnarrson and her colleagues estimate that most of the spider species that evolved sociality have gone extinct.

This phylogenetic analysis of spider sociality has implications for other evolutionary/behavioral questions. For example, it seems that cooperative nest maintenance, cooperative foraging, and other components of social spider life may be "evolutionary dead ends" in the sense that they are associated with high rates of extinction. Why might this be so? Agnarrson and her colleagues argue that although the short-term benefits of sociality in spiders—increased foraging success and so on—may allow for social spider species to initially prosper, sociality has a long-term cost. It turns out that social spiders are very inbred, and display very skewed sex ratios, with females dramatically outnumbering males, sometimes in a 10:1 ratio (Aviles and Maddison, 1991; Aviles et al., 1999, 2000; Johannesen et al., 2002; Lubin and Crozier, 1985; Roeloffs and Riechert, 1988; Smith and Hagen, 1996). In the long run, as inbreeding and skewed sex ratios become more and more pronounced, the probability of extinction may increase, leading to the evolutionary dead-end scenario we see in social spiders.

Interspecific Mutualisms

We have been focusing on intraspecific cooperation (that is, cooperation among individuals within a particular species). There is, however, much evidence that *interspecific* cooperation (cooperation between individuals from different species) is important in shaping animal social behavior as well (Boucher, 1985; Bronstein, 1994; B'shary and Bronstein, 2004; Connor, 1995; Foster and Wenseleers, 2006; Kawanabe et al., 1993; Law and Koptur, 1986; McGill, 2005; Thompson, 1982; Vandermeer, 1984). Such cooperation *between species* is usually referred to as **mutualism** (instead of byproduct mutualism), and so I will use that label here. A classic case of mutualism is that between ants and butterflies. Below we will consider one aspect of this mutualism.

FIGURE 9.25. Butterflies and ants in a mutualistic relationship. In the mutualism between the butterfly *Jalmenus evagoras* and the ant *Iridomyrmex anceps*, butterfly larvae cannot survive in the absence of ants, and ants receive some of their food from the nectar produced by the butterfly larvae. *(Photo credit: Naomi Pierce)*

ANTS AND BUTTERFLIES—MUTUALISM WITH COMMUNICATION?

In numerous species of butterflies and ants, a mutualistic relationship has developed in which butterfly pupae and larvae produce a sugary secretion that ants readily consume, and ants protect the larvae from predators such as certain species of wasps and flies (Pierce et al., 2002). Such a mutualistic relationship constitutes a win-win scenario, with individuals in both species better off than they would be otherwise.

Naomi Pierce has been studying one such mutualistic relationship between the imperial blue butterfly (*Jalmenus evagoras*) and a species of ants (*Iridomyrmex anceps*) (Figure 9.25). The benefits to both parties in this mutualism are enormous. Pierce and her colleagues have found that when faced by predation in nature, butterfly larvae are much less likely to survive when ants are experimentally removed from their environment (Figure 9.26). While ants

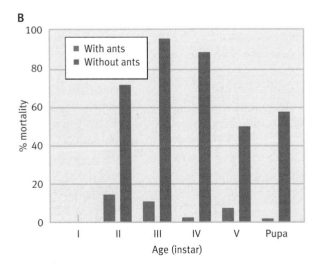

FIGURE 9.26. Butterflies need their ant partners. The probability of survival of *Jalmenus evagoras* larvae and pupae when faced by predation was much higher when ants were present than when they were experimentally excluded at two Australian field sites: **(A)** Mt. Nebo and **(B)** Canberra. *(From Pierce et al., 1987, p. 242)*

Dr. Hudson Kern Reeve

You've worked on cooperation in both wasps and naked mole rats. Isn't that a strange combination? How did you settle on these species?

Superficially, it is indeed a very strange combination—social paper wasps are aerial insects and naked mole rats are subterranean mammals! But there is a deep evolutionary connection between them that has stimulated my interest in both: I think that both manifest common principles of social evolution. The ways that the societies are organized are actually quite similar, with high reproductive skews (near reproductive monopoly by one or a few individuals) occurring among cooperating relatives. In both, the highest-ranking reproductive female behaviorally enforces her reproductive dominance.

I know you spend a good chunk of time engaged in fieldwork each year. Do you find that long hours of behavioral observation and tracking lead you toward new work on cooperation? Could you provide an example?

Yes, I think ultimately that all of the best evolutionary theories are rooted in field observation. (For example, Bill Hamilton, the architect of kin selection theory, was a superb naturalist.) My own view that social organisms, including social insects, engage in reproductive transactions (as embodied in "transactional skew theory") grew out of repeated observations of resource exchanges and *restraint* of aggression in social wasp colonies. Social wasps are constantly exchanging food and water

and are curiously nonaggressive when each is laying an egg, as if they had the equivalent of a "social contract" over the division of resources, and, ultimately, reproduction. I don't think that I ever would have seriously considered the idea that social wasps are reproductively paying each other to cooperate, had I not watched nearly

a thousand hours of videotapes of field colonies.

Perhaps more theory is devoted to the evolution of cooperation than to any other issue in ethology. Why do you think that is?

I think that it has attracted a great deal of theoretical interest because it represents an evolutionary puzzle that even had Darwin fretting: How could an organism ever achieve a reproductive advantage by enhancing the reproductive output of another organism at the expense of its own? Hamilton provided one important answer to this puzzle through his kin

selection theory. But this solution left unanswered the question of how cooperation could evolve between unrelated organisms—the latter, of course, has been the focus of intense theoretical activity. No doubt, we humans are especially interested in cooperation among nonrelatives, because each of us observes and experiences it regularly (to varying degree!) every day.

Do you ever encounter the sense that some in the scientific community simply believe animals are not cognitively sophisticated enough to undertake acts of cooperation and altruism?

Yes, unfortunately, this is still a pervasive view. I think that this view is highly questionable. An organism needn't have a huge brain in order to engage in high-order social interactions (I refer back to the notion that social wasps can have "social contracts" over reproduction!). I think that many behavioral biologists currently underestimate the cognitive complexity of their organisms, and the situation isn't helped by the fact that most theorists find it easiest to model simply behaving organisms!

In fact, there is now a major push to think of social organisms (especially social insects) as self-organizing robots whose rules of social interaction are very simple. I think that the latter view is headed in the wrong direction, because it ignores the evidence that organisms are highly conditional (context-specific) in their social behavior. I think that the evidence will eventually reveal that most social organisms are best viewed as proactive inclusive fitness maximizers, i.e., behave according to their cognitive *projections* of the inclusive fitness consequences of alternative social actions—and are not anything like toasters with a few settings determining simple input-output (stimulus-response) relationships. An inclusive fitness projector will always win evolutionarily over a self-organizing robot, provided that the neural machinery costs are not too great, and it is precisely the latter that I think has been systematically overestimated. Another way to put this is that the difference between a large brain and a small brain is not that the latter results in less sophisticated behavior; rather, the smaller brain still enables very sophisticated behavior, but over a somewhat narrower range of conditions (the ones regularly encountered by its bearers).

How have the fields of mathematical economics and political science contributed to our understanding of the evolution of cooperation?

The influence of economics and political science on evolutionary biology is immense, in large part because the theoretical apparatus of game theory was developed and refined in these two disciplines by people such as von Neumann and Nash and many others. Now, game theory is *the* central theoretical tool in understanding the evolution of social behavior.

Ironically, I think that evolutionary biology, now enriched by game theory, eventually will absorb human economics and political science as

part of itself, because the latter two disciplines are just two subfields of the study of human social behavior, and we evolutionary biologists believe that the only satisfying theory of any organism's social behavior ultimately must be evolutionary! I am sometimes criticized for thinking that social wasps have reproductive transactions on a human economic analogy—surely that is too anthropomorphic! But this criticism gets things backwards: If human economic behavior and wasp social behavior are evolved responses to similar selection pressures, then the connection between them is much

> Game theory is *the* central theoretical tool in understanding the evolution of social behavior.

deeper than a simple analogy, i.e., if they really are manifestations of the same evolutionary principles, then anthropomorphism is the correct stance!

Do you think that the rules governing cooperative behavior are sometimes transmitted culturally in nonhuman primates?

There is growing evidence that this is so, and the important consequence is that, for such primates (and certainly for humans), we need to understand how cultural and biological evolution will interact. Do they proceed independently of each

other, as some believe, or does one somehow entrain the other? This will be a hugely important focus for theoretical and empirical research in the years ahead.

How close are we to having a comprehensive understanding of animal cooperation? What, if anything, remains to be done?

My view is that we are still very far away. There is no shortage of theories, but I suspect the best ones have yet to be developed. What is most limiting are the data that cleanly discriminate among alternative theories. The latter is true in part because theorists have not always been clear about which predictions separate alternative theories and in part because empiricists have not always been good at deriving the right theoretical predictions for their study organisms (or for the contexts in which the latter are studied). This is not to sound pessimistic. On the contrary, it is an extremely exciting time to be a sociobiologist, as we are on the brink of beginning to solve many, many puzzles! In my view, what we cannot afford to lose is the conviction that these puzzles have general, elegant solutions.

Dr. Hudson Kern Reeve is an associate professor at Cornell University. His work integrates theoretical, empirical, and conceptual approaches to ethology to understand cooperation, kinship, aggression, and the distribution of reproductive opportunities within nonhuman and human groups.

can survive in the absence of the nectar they consume from larvae and pupae, they obtain a significant portion of their nutrients from their butterfly larvae partners (Fiedler and Maschwitz, 1988; Pierce et al., 1987, 2002).

This ant-butterfly mutualism involves costly investment in the other by both parties. Larvae raised in a predator-free laboratory environment pupate later at a much larger size (Pierce et al., 1987), as they are able to modify the amount they secrete and use the nutrients normally distributed to ants for their own development. Size in both male and female *J. evagoras* is correlated with reproductive success and, as such, pupating early represents a significant cost— smaller body size as a result of earlier pupating and hence less reproductive success—to the butterflies (Elgar and Pierce, 1988; Hill and Pierce, 1989; Hughes et al., 2000). Although the cost to ants for protecting butterfly larvae has not been quantified, it is likely associated with an increased risk of detection by their own predators and parasitoids, as well the metabolic costs associated with defense (Pierce et al., 1987).

Travasso and Pierce extended the study of the *J. evagoras/ I. anceps* mutualism one step further by examining whether there was interspecific communication in this system. It turns out that ants are almost deaf when it comes to airborne sounds, but they are quite sensitive to vibrational cues (Travasso and Pierce, 2000). Given this, Travasso and Pierce began by examining the role of vibrational cues in communication between ants and butterflies. They found that larval sound production (stridulation) was higher when ants were in the vicinity, suggesting that vibrational cues were designed to be used as a way to communicate with ant guards.

In a follow-up experiment, pairs of butterfly pupae were tested together, with one of the pair having been "muted" when the experimenters applied nail polish to its stridulatory organs. Then, using an elaborate "preference" testing device that included two bridges on which the ants could march, Travasso and Pierce examined whether ants were more attracted to the muted individual in a pair, or the individual who was free to produce vibrational communication. What they uncovered was that ants demonstrated a clear preference for associating with the pupae that could (and did) produce vibrations, providing further evidence that vibrational communication plays a real role in this ant-butterfly mutualistic relationship (Figure 9.27).

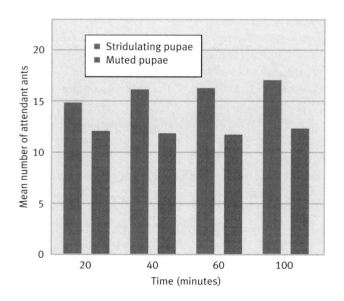

FIGURE 9.27. Stridulating attracts ants. Stridulating *J. evagoras* pupae attracted more ants than *J. evagoras* pupae that had been experimentally muted. *(Based on Travasso and Pierce, 2000)*

Few issues have engaged the attention of animal behaviorists more than understanding cooperative and altruistic behaviors, as these behaviors appear to be such a fundamental part of group living in social species. In Chapters 8 and 9, we have seen how both ultimate and proximate perspectives can shed much light on these topics. We are now ready to move on to another topic—foraging—that has also spurred much interest among both behavioral biologists and behavioral psychologists.

SUMMARY

1. Cooperation typically refers to an *outcome* in which two or more interacting individuals each receives a net benefit from their joint actions, despite the potential costs they may have to pay for undertaking such actions.

2. Cooperation has been studied in taxa ranging from insects and fish to birds and mammals. This work includes studies of cooperation in the context of foraging, predation, antipredator activities, and aggression.

3. In addition to kin-selected cooperation, which we discussed in Chapter 8, three paths to the evolution and maintenance of cooperation in animals have been developed—reciprocity, byproduct mutualism, and group selection. Many mathematical tools have been employed to model these paths, and, of these, game theory is the most often used tool.

4. Work on cooperation via reciprocity has centered on what is known as the prisoner's dilemma game and a strategy called tit for tat. Recent work in neuroeconomics has shed light on some proximate aspects of human reciprocity by examining which areas of the brain are associated with trust and how individuals respond to cheating by their partners in some economic games.

5. Cooperation via byproduct mutualism occurs when an individual would incur an immediate cost or penalty if it did not act cooperatively, such that the immediate net benefit of cooperating outweighs that of cheating.

6. Group selection models of cooperation have both a within- and between-group component. Within-group selection favors cheating, while between-group selection favors cooperation.

7. Cooperation can also occur in interactions that involve more than two individuals. One example of this type of cooperation is coalition behavior, which is typically defined as a cooperative action taken by at least two other individuals or groups against another individual or group.

8. Phylogeny can be used to help better understand the distribution of cooperation among related species. The phylogenetic approach does not necessarily conflict with an adaptationist view of cooperative breeding, although it does emphasize the importance of history (phylogeny) in our understanding of the distribution of cooperative breeding.

9. In addition to cooperation between members of the same species (that is, *intraspecific* cooperation), there is a great deal of evidence that *interspecific* cooperation (that is, cooperation between members of different species) is also important in shaping animal social behavior.

DISCUSSION QUESTIONS

1. Read G. Wilkinson's (1984) article "Reciprocal food sharing in vampire bats," in *Nature* (vol. 308, pp. 181–184). Then outline how Wilkinson was able to separate out the effects of kinship and reciprocity in his study of vampire bats.

2. Run a small prisoner's dilemma experiment with a few other students. In one group, using coins as payoffs, test pairs of subjects (who cannot communicate with each other in any manner) and tell them beforehand that they will only play this game once. In a second treatment, use pairs of subjects (who cannot communicate with each other), but inform them that they will play this game many, many times together, but do not tell them exactly how many times. In a third and fourth treatment, repeat treatments 1 and 2, but allow the subjects to communicate with each other before the game starts. What sort of differences and similarities do you predict across treatments? What do the data say?

3. Respond to the following statement: Animals aren't capable of human-like thought processes and therefore they cannot be cooperating.

4. Why do you suppose that work on animal behavior and cooperation draws more attention from other disciplines, such as mathematics, political science, and psychology, than any other area in ethology? What might we learn about human cooperation from studies of animal cooperation? What sorts of things would be difficult to glean about human cooperation by studying animal cooperation?

5. Work from neuroeconomics has shed light on the neurobiology of cooperation in humans. What sorts of evolutionary questions come to mind when you read about these proximate studies in neuroeconomics?

SUGGESTED READING

Axelrod, R., & Hamilton, W. D. (1981). The evolution of cooperation. *Science, 211,* 1390–1396. A classic paper that essentially introduced most ethologists to using game theory to address cooperative behavior.

Connor, R. C. (1995). The benefits of mutualism: A conceptual framework. *Biological Reviews of the Cambridge Philosophical Society, 70,* 427–457. A conceptual overview of work on mutualism and byproduct mutualism.

Dugatkin, L. A. (1997). *Cooperation among animals: An evolutionary perspective.* New York: Oxford University Press. A review of theoretical and empirical work on cooperation.

Kropotkin, P. (1902). *Mutual aid* (3rd ed.). London: William Heinemann. One of the first important books on cooperative behavior in animals.

Packer, C. (1977). Reciprocal altruism in *Papio anubis. Nature, 265,* 441–443. A highly cited study that was one of the first to experimentally tackle alliances and cooperation.

Wilson, D. S., & Sober, E. (1994). Re-introducing group selection to the human behavioral sciences. *Behavioral and Brain Sciences, 17*, 585–654. An overview applying group selection thinking to human communities.

Zak, P. J. (2004). Neuroeconomics. *Philosophical Transactions of the Royal Society of London Series B—Biological Sciences, 359*, 1737–1748. A concise introduction to this fascinating new subdiscipline at the cutting edge of biology, psychology, and economics.

10

Foraging

If the number of copies of genes making it into the next generation is the currency of natural selection, then it is an inescapable fact that searching for and consuming food—what behavioral biologists call **foraging**—is a critical part of every animal's existence. Depending on the circumstances, individuals can survive to reproductive age without being aggressive, they can survive to reproductive age without play, they can survive to reproductive age if they don't cooperate or find a territory; however, they can't survive to reproduce if they don't eat. As such, we expect that animals should spend a fair share of their available time foraging, whether their food is seeds, nuts, and berries (as in granivores), plants (as in herbivores), living animals (as in carnivores), or dead animals (as in scavengers). We further expect that natural selection should favor efficient foraging strategies; and all evidence indicates that this is in fact the case (Figure 10.1).

Consider the following incredible story of ant foraging. About fifty million years ago, ants began cultivating their own food by entering into a mutually beneficial relationship with certain species of fungi. The ants promote the growth of the fungi (good for the fungi), while also feasting on the vegetative shoots produced by their fungal partners (good for the ants). Aside from humans, ants are one of the few groups on the planet that grow their own food, and they do so in this rather spectacular way.

Cameron Currie and his colleagues have found that the ant-fungus relationship is even more complicated than scientists first believed (Cafaro and Currie, 2005; Currie et al., 1999a, 1999b). Researchers who study fungus-growing ants have long known of a whitish-gray crust found on and around many ants with fungus food gardens. It turns out that the substance is actually a mass of *Streptomyces* bacteria. This type of bacteria produces many antibiotics. Currie and his colleagues hypothesized that ants actually use the bacteria to produce antibiotics that kill parasites that grow in their fungal gardens (Figure 10.2). That is, they postulated that not only have ants evolved a complex relationship with their food source (fungi), they have even evolved a means to protect this food source from destruction.

Four lines of evidence support the researchers' claim. First, all twenty species of the fungus-growing ants they examined had *Streptomyces* bacteria

A   **B**

FIGURE 10.1. Foraging. Many animals spend a good deal of their waking hours foraging. Here **(A)** a black bear and **(B)** a Richardson's ground squirrel are foraging. *(Photo credits: Ron Erwin)*

associated with them. Second, ants actually transmit the bacteria across generations, with parents passing the bacteria on to offspring. Third, when male and female reproductive ants are examined (before their mating flights), only females possess the bacteria. This is critical, as only females start new nests that will rely on the bacteria to produce antibiotics, and only females are involved in "cultivating" fungus gardens. Fourth, and most important, the bacteria found on fungus-growing ants produce antibiotics that wipe out only *certain* parasitic diseases. When Currie and his colleagues tested the antibiotics produced by the bacteria, they found that they were potent only against *Escovopsis*, a serious parasitic threat to the ants' fungus garden. Other parasitic species (those not a danger to fungus-growing ants) were unaffected by *Streptomyces* antibiotics.

Recent work by Currie and his team continues to find remarkable new dimensions to the relationship between ants, their fungus food source, and the parasites that infect their fungal gardens. In addition to directly using the antibiotics produced by *Streptomyces* to clean their fungus gardens, the ants meticulously groom these gardens and physically remove fungus infected with *Escovopsis*. Ants actually pick up parasitic *Escovopsis* spores and hyphae and place them in areas of their body called infrabuccal pockets. Inside these pockets, the spores and hyphae are killed by the antibiotics that are also present in the infrabuccal pockets. The ants then take the dead spores and hyphae and deposit them in a separate pile away from the fungus garden (Little et al., 2003, 2006).

What makes the work on animal behavior and foraging so fascinating is that the examples can be as incredible as the ant story above. Of course, not all the examples of foraging we will touch on in this chapter are as dramatic as the ant and fungus garden case, but each example is interesting in its own way. In this chapter, we will touch on the following foraging-related questions:

- How do animals know what food items look like?
- How does foraging theory predict where animals will forage and what they will eat?
- How does group social dynamics affect foraging?
- How can we incorporate neurobiology, molecular biology, and endocrinology into our study of animal foraging behavior?
- What role does learning play in foraging decisions?

FIGURE 10.2. Tending the garden. A worker of the leaf-cutter ant *(Acromyrmex octospinosus)* tending a fungus garden. The thick whitish-gray coating on the worker is the mutualistic bacterium *(Actinomycetous)* that produces the antibiotics that suppress the growth of parasites in the fungus garden. *(Photo credit: Christian Ziegler)*

Finding Food and the Search Image

In a moment we will review some empirical and theoretical studies that examine whether animals forage in highly efficient, perhaps even optimal, ways. Before we do that, let us begin by addressing a very basic question about animal foraging behavior—namely, how do animals determine what specific food types look (smell, feel) like? While there are many ways one could begin to answer that question, we will focus on what is called **search image** theory. First proposed by Luke Tinbergen in 1960, the idea behind a search image is that when animals encounter a prey type more and more, they form some sort of representation of that target—the prey—and that this representation or image becomes more and more detailed with experience, which in turn translates into the forager becoming more successful at finding that type of prey (Tinbergen, 1960).

There is some debate as to the exact nature of the search image that animals form, with some researchers arguing that foragers are keying on one or two salient attributes of the prey (color, movement, pattern), while others argue that the search image formed is closer to some sort of representation of the entire prey item (Langley, 1996; Pietrewicz and Kamil, 1979; Reid and Shettleworth, 1992). In either case, the animals are learning something relevant about their prey, and most animal behaviorists argue that the search image—a learning-based, proximate mechanism for becoming more efficient at finding prey—likely evolved as a response to the difficulty of finding prey that blend into their background—that is, cryptic prey (Balda et al., 1998; Kamil and Balda, 1990; Zentall, 2005).

Optimal Foraging Theory

In this section, we will examine a class of *mathematical models* that are collectively known as **optimal foraging theory (OFT)** (Kamil et al., 1987; Sih and Christensen, 2001; Stephens and Krebs, 1986). These models use a form of mathematical analysis known as optimization theory to predict various aspects of animal foraging behavior within a given set of constraints. Optimal foraging theory began in earnest in 1966 with back-to-back papers in the *American Naturalist*, one of which was written by Robert MacArthur and the other by John Emlen (Emlen, 1966; MacArthur and Pianka, 1966). These papers set the stage for ethological and behavioral ecological models that followed in abundance, especially during the 1970s (for a nice review of these models, see Stephens and Krebs, 1986).

When animal behaviorists and behavioral ecologists build optimal foraging models, they begin by making a set of assumptions—for example, foragers can't search for more than one item at a time, they only have so many hours in a day to search for food—and then proceed to see which types of food a forager should take, given the constraints. While there are many optimal foraging models in the animal behavior literature, we will examine four such models, which address the following questions:

- What food items should a forager eat?
- How long should a forager stay in a certain food patch?
- How is foraging affected when certain nutrient requirements are in place?
- How does variance in food supply affect a forager's decision about what food types to eat?

WHAT TO EAT

One of the most basic foraging problems faced by an animal is deciding which type of food items should be in its diet, and which should be excluded (Stephens and Krebs, 1986). For example, imagine that a forager could search for, and potentially consume, food types 1, 2, and 3. Should the forager eat all three? Only one? Two of the three? If so, which ones? To tackle this question, animal behaviorists have developed optimality models specifically designed to handle prey choice. We will now examine the underpinnings of this first optimal foraging model and then review a classic test of it.

Let's first consider the simplest possible case—choosing between two different types of food (Caro, 1994a; Figure 10.3). For carnivores, this might be a choice between two prey species; for granivores, the choice would likely be between two different types of seeds. Indeed, the choice a forager might have could even be between two different size classes (small or large) of the same food. In our model, each prey item will have an energy value, encounter rate, and handling time associated with it. For example, let's say that during foraging bouts one prey type is encountered every three minutes (encounter rate), and once it is encountered, such a prey item takes two minutes to kill and ingest (handling time) and provides the forager with 300 calories (energy value). Next, we define the profitability of a prey item as its energy/handling time. The greater the energy/handling ratio, the greater the profitability of a prey type.

We will assume that the prey type with the highest profitability—let's call it prey type 1—is always taken by a forager. This means that the optimal diet problem boils down to two simple questions—should prey type 2 also be taken, and if it should, under what conditions? We begin by examining the assumptions that are made in the basic optimal prey choice model and then proceed to its main conclusion (Krebs and McCleery, 1984). The model assumes:

FIGURE 10.3. Foraging decision. Here a female cheetah (the forager) has killed a hare (the prey). In making the decision whether to take hares rather than some other prey into the diet, the animal will compare the energy value (the amount of calories provided to the forager by eating this prey), encounter rate (how often the prey is encountered by the forager), and handling time (time for the forager to kill and ingest the prey) for each putative prey. *(Based on Caro, 1994a)*

The Optimal Diet Model

Imagine a forager has only two prey types that it consumes (for example, two types of seeds, two types of herbivores, and so on). Within our model, a forager must eat one of these prey items (or it will starve) and so our question becomes: Which item does a forager always take, and under what conditions does a forager take both types of prey? To begin, let us define the following terms:

e_i = energy provided by prey type i
h_i = handling associated with prey type i (how long does it take to eat prey i , once it is caught)
λ_i = encounter rate with prey type i
T_s = amount of time devoted to searching for prey
T = total time

We will assume that an animal always takes the prey type that has a higher e_i/h_i value (called the profitability of a prey type), and we will label this prey type as prey 1. The question then becomes whether a forager should take prey 1 alone, or whether a forager should take both prey 1 and prey 2 upon encountering them.

We begin by calculating the total energy (E) associated with prey 1 divided by the total time associated w ith this prey (T).

For prey type 1:

$$\frac{E}{T} = \frac{T_s \lambda_1 e_1}{T_s + T_s \lambda_1 h_1} \tag{1}$$

The numerator here takes the total number of prey type 1 captured ($T_s \lambda_1$) and multiplies it by the energy value (e_1) of each prey, producing the total energy produced by prey type 1. The denominator adds together the total search time (T_s) and the total handling time ($T_s \lambda_1 h_1$), given such a search. This can be simplified to:

▸ Energy intake from prey can be measured in some standard currency (for example, calories).
▸ Foragers can't simultaneously handle one prey item and search for another.
▸ Prey are recognized instantly and accurately.
▸ Prey are encountered sequentially.
▸ Natural selection favors foragers that maximize their rate of energy intake.

With these assumptions in place, a bit of mathematical analysis (Math Box 10.1) produces a fascinating, and somewhat surprising prediction. Recall that we are asking whether a forager should add prey type 2 to its diet. Yet, what the model predicts is that the encounter rate with prey type 2—that is, how often a predator encounters this less profitable item—does *not* affect whether or not it should be added to the diet. Rather, the model predicts that there is a critical encounter rate with the most profitable item (prey type 1)—if the encounter rate the predator experiences for prey 1 is above this critical value, only prey type 1 is taken and, if it isn't, then both prey type 1 and prey type 2 are taken. That is, the decision of whether to add prey type 2 to the diet is not dependent on our forager's encounter rate with prey type 2; rather, it is related to its encounter rate with prey type 1. This basic prediction of optimal diet choice has been tested many times.

$$\frac{E}{T} = \frac{\lambda_1 e_1}{1 + \lambda_1 h_1} \tag{2}$$

Now, we can ask whether this value is greater than the E/T associated with taking both prey types. To find the E/T of taking both prey type 1 and prey type 2, we calculate the following:

$$\frac{E}{T} = \frac{T_s(\lambda_1 e_1 + \lambda_2 e_2)}{T_s + T_s \lambda_1 h_1 + T_s \lambda_2 h_2} \tag{3}$$

The numerator represents the total energy obtained from prey types 1 and 2, while the denominator adds together the total search time (T_s) and the total handling time for prey types 1 and 2. This can be simplified to:

$$\frac{E}{T} = \frac{\lambda_1 e_1 + \lambda_2 e_2}{1 + \lambda_1 h_1 + \lambda_2 h_2} \tag{4}$$

Our question then boils down to when the following inequality is true:

$$\frac{\lambda_1 e_1}{1 + \lambda_1 h_1} > \frac{\lambda_1 e_1 + \lambda_2 e_2}{1 + \lambda_1 h_1 + \lambda_2 h_2} \tag{5}$$

When this inequality holds true, our predator should take only prey type 1. When it does not hold true, our predator should take prey type 1 and prey type 2. Equation (5) can be shown to hold true when:

$$\lambda_1 > \frac{e_2}{e_1 h_2 - e_2 h_1} \tag{6}$$

From (6) we can derive two important predictions:

1. Once a critical encounter rate with prey type 1 is reached, it alone should be taken.
2. The decision about whether to take prey type 2 does *not* depend on how common prey type 2 is (that is, on prey type 2's encounter rate). This can be seen in (6) by the absence of λ_2 from our inequality.

John Krebs and his colleagues experimentally tested the predictions of this optimal prey choice model in great tit birds (*Parus major*) (Krebs, 1978; Krebs et al., 1978). In an ingenious laboratory experiment, great tits were placed in front of a moving conveyor belt (Figure 10.4). Krebs and his team used two different-

Great Tit

Conveyor belt

Mealworm pieces

FIGURE 10.4. Great tit foraging. One classic early experiment using optimal foraging theory had mealworms of different sizes presented on a conveyor belt to great tits.

sized pieces of mealworm as the two different prey item types, and they had precise control of the rate at which these two prey types were encountered by the tits, the exact energy provided by both types of prey, and the precise handling time associated with each size of mealworm. With these parameters measured, it was possible to use the model to predict when the birds should take only the most profitable prey types, and when they should take both types of prey.

Krebs and his fellow researchers found that the optimal prey choice model did a very good job of predicting how the tits would forage, in that it was the encounter rate of the most profitable prey, not the least profitable prey, that determined whether tits took the least profitable items (Figure 10.5A). Similar results have been found when testing the optimal prey choice model in foraging experiments with bluegill sunfish (Werner and Hall, 1974; Figure 10.5B). And

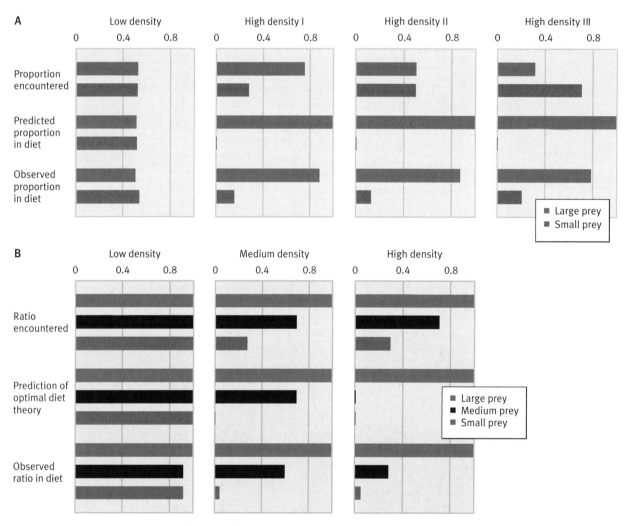

FIGURE 10.5. Optimal choice of diet. (A) Optimal foraging in great tits was examined by Krebs and his colleagues (1978) in four density conditions. With a knowledge of exact encounter rates, handling times, and energy values, they were able to predict the birds' optimal diet of large and small prey. **(B)** Optimal foraging in bluegill sunfish was studied by Werner and Hall (1974). They were able to predict the optimal foraging of the fish on three different size classes of *Daphnia*. The fit between expected and observed foraging is quite good, although the fish tended to oversample medium and small *Daphnia* in the high-density treatment. *(Based on Krebs, 1978, p. 31)*

this same mathematical model could be used for any type of forager deciding between two prey types—for example, the case of a carnivore predator choosing between two herbivore prey species.

WHERE TO EAT

Another critical decision a forager must make is how long to stay in a patch of food. For example, how long should a hummingbird spend sucking nectar from one flower, given that there are other flowers available, or how long should a bee spend extracting pollen from one flower before moving on to the next one? To address such questions, Eric Charnov developed an optimality model that generated a result known as the **marginal value theorem** (Charnov, 1976; Parker and Stuart, 1976).

To see how Charnov's model works, imagine a forager feeding in an area that contains different patches of a single type of food. A patch of food for a chimp could be a tree full of fruit, but for a bee it might be a flower (Figure 10.6). More generally, a patch is defined as a clump of food that can be depleted by a forager. Once a forager begins feeding in a patch, the *rate* at which it takes in food slows down, as the more the forager eats, the less food remains in the patch. Other less depleted patches will then be attractive, but in order to get to these patches, the forager must pay some cost—energy, lost time foraging while traveling, increased rate of predation during travel, and so forth—associated with traveling between patches. The question then becomes how long a forager should stay in a patch that it is depleting before moving on to another patch.

Charnov's model makes a few clear, testable predictions regarding patch residence time, assuming that we know the rate of food intake:

▶ A forager should stay in a patch until the marginal rate of food intake—that is, the rate of food intake associated with the next prey item in its patch—is equal to that of the average rate of food intake across all patches available.

FIGURE 10.6. Patch choice. For a bee, different flowers in a field of flowering plants might represent different patches.

In other words, a forager should stay in a patch x time units, where x is that point in time when its marginal rate of food intake in that patch is equal to the average amount of food it could get in other patches, given that it has to pay a cost to get to such other patches.

▶ The greater the time between patches, the longer a forager should stay in a patch. This makes sense, since increased travel time leads to an increase in the costs associated with such travel, and such costs need to be compensated—remaining in a patch longer is one means by which such compensation can be achieved.

▶ For patches that are already of generally poor quality when the forager enters the patch, individuals should stay longer in such patches than if they were foraging in an environment full of more profitable patches. Think of it this way: In order to make up for the travel costs associated with a move from a patch, a forager has to stay longer in a poor patch than in a good patch to obtain a fixed amount of energy (Figure 10.7).

Richard Cowie tested one of the predictions of the marginal value theorem using great tits as subjects. Inside a large aviary, Cowie built a series of artificial trees, each of which contained numerous branches (Cowie, 1977). Attached to some of the branches were sawdust-filled potting baskets. Under the sawdust were the mealworms for which the birds were searching (Figure 10.8A). Cowie was able to calculate the rate of gain in different types of sawdust-filled patches. In addition, he could manipulate the travel time between patches, because each

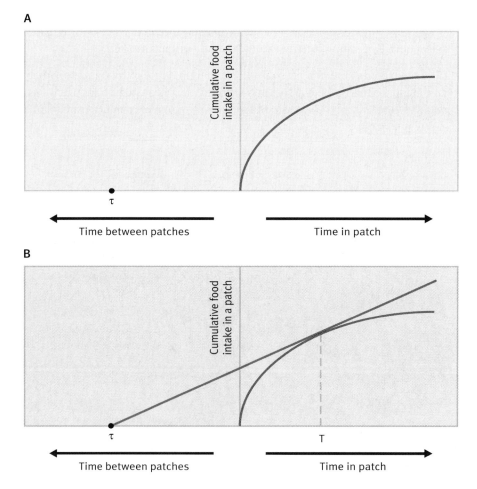

FIGURE 10.7. Graphical solution to marginal value problem. (A) To calculate the optimal time for a forager to remain in a patch, we begin by drawing a curve that represents the cumulative food gain in an average patch in the environment. Then, going west on the x-axis we find the average travel time between patches (τ). **(B)** We then draw a straight line from τ that is tangent to the food gain curve. From the point of tangency, we drop a perpendicular dashed line to the x-axis, which gives us an optimal time (T) for the forager to stay in the patch.

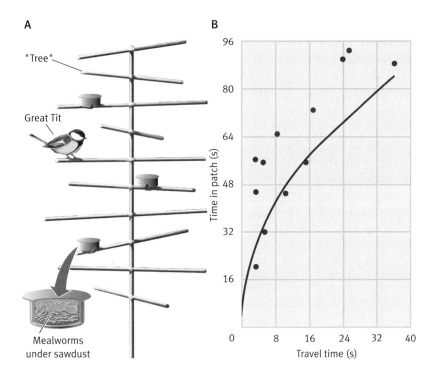

A

"Tree"

Great Tit

Mealworms
under sawdust

B

(y-axis: Time in patch (s), values: 16, 32, 48, 64, 80, 96)
(x-axis: Travel time (s), values: 0, 8, 16, 24, 32, 40)

FIGURE 10.8. Optimal time in patch and travel time. In a test of the marginal value theorem, Cowie (1977) constructed **(A)** an artificial tree that allowed him to control both patch quality and travel time. **(B)** The solid line is the predicted optimal time in a patch plotted against the travel time, which was calculated based on the marginal value theorem, while the data points are the observed times the birds stayed in the patch plotted as a function of travel time between patches. (*Based on Krebs, 1978, p. 44*)

pot had a lid, and the lids could be made to be easily dislodged—creating a short travel time between leaving one patch and starting to forage at another—or the lids could be constructed so as to be very difficult to open, simulating a long travel time. Based on all this, Cowie calculated the optimal time to stay in a patch as a function of travel time between patches. The results clearly demonstrate that the amount of time birds spent in a patch matched the optimal time predicted by the marginal value theorem (Figure 10.8B).

Any time a resource depletes as a function of use, and costs associated with traveling between patches of that resource are present, one can use the marginal value theorem to solve for optimal patch time. This approach has, for example, been used to calculate how long a male should search for and mate with a female (where the female is now the "patch") (Parker and Stuart, 1976).

SPECIFIC NUTRIENT CONSTRAINTS

In addition to maximizing their rate of energy intake, animals are constrained by a need to spend time foraging for specific nutrients that are essential for survival. For example, many animals need to take in very small quantities of trace elements like zinc in order to remain healthy, and this requirement may compromise their general foraging rules—rules designed to maximize energy intake per unit time. If looking for a trace element takes time away from other activities—searching for other foods, antipredator behavior, mating, and so forth—fulfilling minimum requirements can be very costly. These constraints appear to be particularly severe in herbivores, who often must take in large amounts of low-energy food to survive (Crawley, 1983; Roguet et al., 1998).

Let's examine this in more detail by focusing on Gary Belovsky's study of nutrient constraints in the moose (*Alces alces*)—a species in which the nutrient constraint is sodium intake (Belovsky, 1978; Figure 10.9). Sodium is a particularly good candidate for a nutrient constraint study because vertebrates

FIGURE 10.9. Moose foraging on a salt budget. Linear programming models of foraging have been used to predict the diet of salt-limited moose. (*Photo credit: Joe McDonald/Visuals Unlimited*)

require large amounts of sodium (this chemical is lost in urine), sodium is scarce, and besides water, sodium is the only nutrient for which a "specific hunger" has been documented in animals (Stephens and Krebs, 1986).

Moose have a particular problem in habitats where sodium is restricted to aquatic plants, because such plants are usually inaccessible in the winter when lakes are frozen. This, coupled with the fact that terrestrial plants provide much more energy per unit time than aquatic plants, presents a difficult problem for a foraging moose; namely, how much time to spend eating aquatic plants when the lakes are not frozen. Foraging for such aquatic plants during nonwinter months provides much needed sodium (which can be stored by the moose), but it takes time away from foraging for energy-rich terrestrial plants (Figure 10.10).

To predict foraging behavior in the above situation, animal behaviorists use a mathematical technique called linear programming. Linear programming models are designed to handle optimality problems, in which some optimum must be achieved in the face of a particular constraint. In our case, natural selection should favor any behavioral strategy that provides moose with the most energy per unit time, subject to the constraint that a certain amount of sodium must be ingested. In practice, we need to predict how much time during nonwinter periods a moose should devote to foraging for energy-poor, but relatively sodium-rich, aquatic plants.

Belovsky constructed a linear programming model to predict moose foraging behavior (Belovsky, 1978). The model included the minimum amount of food a day that a moose needs to survive, how quickly a moose digests its food, the energy value of aquatic and terrestrial plants, and the sodium constraint. It

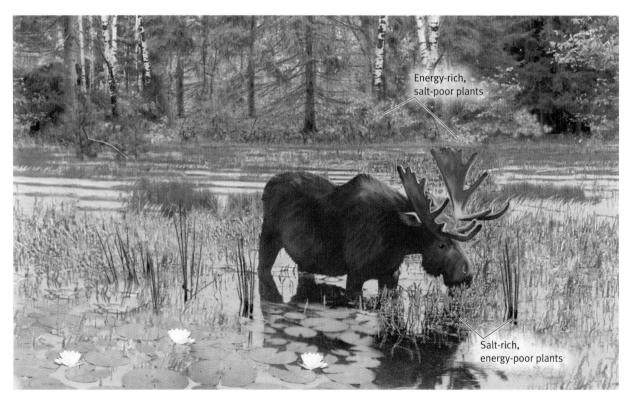

Energy-rich, salt-poor plants

Salt-rich, energy-poor plants

FIGURE 10.10. Specific foraging constraints. Moose need salt, and they acquire it from energy-poor plants. This takes time away from foraging on energy-rich terrestrial plants. Linear programming models can help predict the moose's foraging behavior.

turns out that a moose needs to take in about 2.57 grams of sodium a day in the summer to get enough sodium to make it through the winter. Based on all this, the linear programming model that Belovsky built predicted that moose should spend about 18 percent of their summer foraging time on aquatic plants. The actual percent of time spent foraging on aquatic plants, when such plants are accessible, closely matches the model's prediction. Because of the success of the sodium constraint model, Belovsky has extended his use of linear programming techniques to other herbivore foraging problems.

RISK-SENSITIVE FORAGING

One aspect of feeding that we have ignored so far is the *variability* associated with the rate of obtaining items of prey. In the language of statistics, this variance is referred to as *risk*—the term was first used in economics, where more variance implied a greater chance of loss (or gain). Using the word "risk" in foraging models is unfortunate, as this term is sometimes confused with risk in the sense of danger—one type of risk need not have anything to do with the other, and it is important to keep them separate in your thinking. When we speak of risk in this section, we are using it in the economic sense—increased variance in prey availability increases both the odds that an animal will find very little prey and the odds that it will find a bonanza of food.

Consider the following scenario: An animal can choose to forage for six hours in one of two patches. Further imagine that both patches have the same exact type of food item, and that animals know what to expect in each patch. In patch 1, each forager will always receive eight items. In patch 2, there is a 50 percent chance a forager will receive sixteen food items and a 50 percent it will get nothing. The mean number of food items that the foragers can expect in both patches is identical (eight), but the variance (risk) in food intake per hour is greater in patch 2 (Figure 10.11). Should our foragers take the differences in the variability into account when deciding between patches? This is the sort of question that **risk-sensitive optimal foraging models** address (Caraco, 1980; McNamara and Houston, 1992; Real and Caraco, 1986).

One key component to understanding risk-sensitive foraging is the hunger state of an animal. Thus, how hungry an animal is plays a part in how much it values a given item of food and affects how it assesses the variability in food. To see this, consider foragers who can be in one of three different hunger states. Forager 1 has a hunger state in which it values every new food item equally. Whether it is eating its first or fiftieth item, each item provides it with the same

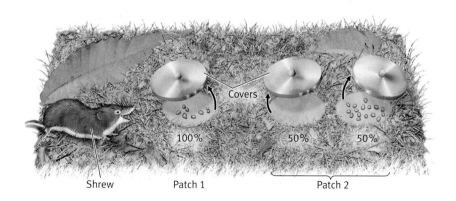

FIGURE 10.11. Risk-sensitive optimal foraging model. Imagine a shrew that must decide between a patch (1) that always yields eight pellets once the cover is removed and a patch (2) in which half the time there are no pellets and half the time there are sixteen pellets. Both patches have the same mean (eight), but the variance is greater in patch 2. If our forager takes variance into account, it is foraging in a risk-sensitive manner.

Covers

100%   50%   50%

Shrew   Patch 1   Patch 2

reward value. Forager 2 is fairly satiated, and although every additional item it takes in has some value, each additional item is worth less and less. Think about the value to you of a slice of cake after you have just had two ice cream sundaes. It might be worth something, but not what it would have been worth before consuming the sundaes. Forager 3 is starving, and every additional item it eats is worth more and more (to a limit), perhaps providing the difference between surviving or starving to death (Figure 10.12).

Risk-sensitive foraging models, though they can be mathematically complex, make a very straightforward, but powerful, prediction. Returning to our two patches, which have the same mean number of food items but different variances, risk-sensitive models predict that the hunger state of a forager will determine whether it prefers the patch with more or less variance. Our fairly satiated predators are predicted to be *risk-averse*—that is, they should choose to forage in patch 1, as that patch has less risk associated with it. On the flip side of the coin, our starving foragers should opt to be *risk-prone*, and select to forage in patch 2—the patch with the greater variance. All other foragers should be indifferent with respect to variance and should not show preference for one patch type or another.

To see why variance is favored in starving birds but avoided by relatively satiated birds, we need to cast the problem in terms of survival probabilities. For the forager who is not all that hungry, each additional piece of food isn't worth that much more, and so it should opt for a consistent food source, since sixteen pieces of food isn't worth all that much more than eight food items when the animal is stuffed. For our starving bird, eight pieces of food may not be enough to provide it with enough energy to survive the night, but sixteen food items may. In that case, it is worth taking the chance of getting no food at all (one possible outcome in our risky patch) in exchange for the chance of getting sixteen items. The reasoning here is that since eight food items, even if they appear with certainty, would not be enough to pull the starving

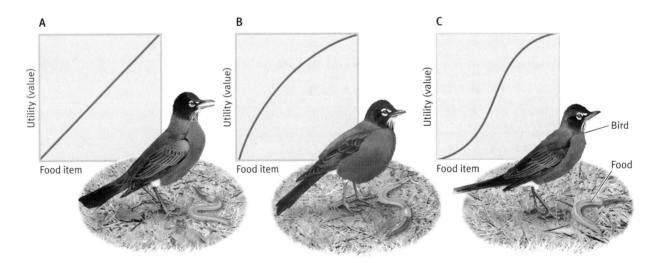

FIGURE 10.12. Utility of food. A forager may value each and every food item the same **(A)**, it may value each additional food item less and less **(B)**, or each additional food item more and more, as shown in the left part of the curve in **(C)**. The bird in **(A)** is predicted to be risk insensitive, the bird in **(B)** is predicted to be risk averse, and the bird in **(C)** is predicted to be risk prone.

forager through to the next foraging period, it should opt for the patch with more variance, where there is at least a chance it will receive enough food items to avoid starvation.

As with all the mathematical models we analyze, we are not suggesting that animals make the mental calculations that we just went through, but rather that natural selection favors any "rule-of-thumb" behavior that allows the animals to solve the problem at hand. In this case, the favored rule-of-thumb might be: "when starving, use patches of food that have high variances."

One of the first, and best, studies of risk-sensitive foraging was that of Thomas Caraco and his team in which they examined foraging behavior in yellow-eyed juncos (Caraco et al., 1980). Caraco and his colleagues presented juncos with two trays containing birdseed, and once a bird made the choice to go to one tray, the other was immediately removed (Figure 10.13). One tray had a "fixed" amount of food—for example, a fixed tray might always have five seeds—while the other tray had a "variable" amount of food—for example, no seeds half the time, and ten seeds half the time. Keep in mind that the variable tray had a mean number of seeds (five) equal to that on the fixed tray. Caraco and his team calculated the value of every new item of food both for hungry birds (who were said to be on a negative energy budget) and for birds that were meeting their daily food requirements (birds on a positive energy budget). Birds on a negative energy budget valued every additional food item much more than those on a positive energy budget (Figure 10.14).

When choosing between trays, risk-sensitive theory predicts that birds on a positive energy budget should choose the fixed trays, while very hungry birds should choose the variable trays. Caraco's juncos behaved in a fashion remarkably similar to that predicted from theory. Yellow-eyed junco foraging is indeed risk-sensitive, shifting between risk-averse foraging and risk-prone foraging according to energy budgets. Following the publication of this work, similar results on risk-sensitive foraging were uncovered in other birds, as well as in mammals and in invertebrates such as honeybees and crayfish. This broad taxonomic distribution of risk-sensitive foraging suggests that variance plays an important role in animal foraging behavior across many species.

FIGURE 10.13. Optimal juncos. Junco foraging behavior has been used to test numerous optimal foraging models. *(Photo credit: William Leaman/Alamy Images)*

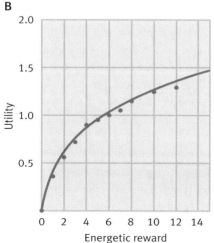

FIGURE 10.14. Utility functions and risk sensitivity. (A) Risk-prone juncos. The utility function for this junco indicates that each additional item the bird eats is worth more and more. Such a bird tends to be risk prone. **(B)** Risk-averse juncos. Here each additional item a junco receives is worth less and less. Juncos with this sort of utility function tend to be risk averse. *(From Caraco et al., 1980)*

Foraging and Group Life

For individuals that spend all or part of their lives in groups, many aspects of group life can impact both foraging behavior and foraging success. With that in mind, we will tackle the following questions in this section:

▶ What is the role of group size per se on animal foraging?
▶ What role does cooperation within groups play in foraging, and how can this be distinguished from the effect of group size?
▶ How does work on the "public information" available in some groups shed light on animal foraging?

GROUP SIZE

In many species that live in groups, increasing the foraging group size increases the amount of food each forager receives (Krause and Ruxton, 2002). This may be because more foragers flush out more prey, or because cooperative hunting creates a division of labor between different group members and increases the success rate of the cooperator. Below, we examine an example of each of these possibilities.

FORAGING IN BLUEGILLS. Consider foraging success in bluegill sunfish. These fish primarily eat small aquatic insects that live in dense vegetation (Figure 10.15). Such prey items need to be flushed from the vegetation, and success in flushing out prey may increase as a function of group size (Bertram, 1978; Mock, 1980; Morse, 1970). That is, while bluegill prey are quite difficult to catch in dense vegetation, increasing the size of foraging groups may force more prey out of the vegetation. While such prey may not be taken by the specific bluegill chasing them, they may be ingested by other bluegill group members, and cause an increase in the average number of prey obtained per group member. Gary Mittlebach examined this hypothesis by experimentally manipulating foraging group size of bluegills in a controlled laboratory setting (Mittlebach, 1984).

Mittlebach began his experimental work by placing 300 small aquatic prey (called amphipods) into a large aquarium containing juvenile bluegill sunfish. He examined the success of bluegills that were foraging alone, in pairs, and in groups (ranging from three to six bluegills). Mittlebach measured the number of prey captured per bluegill, and he uncovered a clear positive relationship between foraging group size and individual foraging success (Figure 10.16). It appears that the increased feeding rate per individual was due to two factors. First, more prey were flushed when group size rose. Second, prey clumped together, and so when one group member found amphipods, others swam over to this area, and then they often found food themselves (Figure 10.17).

While increased group size in bluegills does benefit each individual forager in its intake of food (its per capita foraging success), there is no evidence to suggest that bluegill foragers hunt in any coordinated fashion (see below for more on cooperative foraging). That is, the flushing effect is merely a byproduct of having more individuals searching for food. Furthermore, the manner by which bluegills increase foraging efficiency in larger groups (that is, by flushing) is only one means of increased foraging efficiency through group living. For example, in a number of species, increased group size reduces the amount of

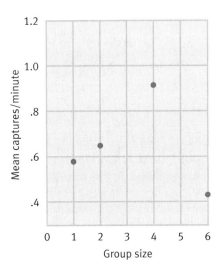

FIGURE 10.15. Bluegill foraging. Bluegill sunfish forage for small aquatic insects in dense vegetation. The bluegills' foraging patterns approximate those predicted by theory. *(Photo credit: U.S. Fish and Wildlife Service)*

FIGURE 10.16. Group size and foraging success. In bluegill sunfish, the mean rate of prey captured increases with group size until group size reaches about four individuals. *(Based on Mittlebach, 1984, p. 999)*

FIGURE 10.17. Bluegill group foraging. When bluegills forage in groups, they flush out more prey and attract other fish to the foraging site.

time that any given individual needs to devote to antipredator activities and this often, but not always, increases per capita foraging success (Caraco, 1979; Ens and Goss-Custard, 1984; Sullivan, 1984).

Though certainly not universal, the general relationship between group size and foraging success uncovered by Mittlebach has been found over and over in animal studies. For example, Scott Creel ran a meta-analysis on foraging success and group size in seven different species that hunt in groups (Creel, 2001). Overall, Creel found a strong positive relationship between foraging success and group size.

DISENTANGLING THE EFFECT OF GROUP SIZE AND COOPERATION ON FORAGING SUCCESS. Individuals may cooperate with one another when hunting in groups. For example, when wild dogs hunt down a prey item, it is a coordinated effort (see Chapter 2). Different members of the hunting pack play different roles in the hunt—flushing the prey, making the initial attack, disemboweling the prey, and so forth. In such cases, it is useful to separate out the effects of coordinated cooperation from that of group size per se. To see how animal behaviorists disentangle such effects, let us examine hunting behavior in chimps.

Cooperative hunting or the lack of it has been examined in chimp populations in (1) the Gombe Preserve in Tanzania (Boesch, 1994b; Busse, 1978; Lawick-Goodall, 1968; Telecki, 1973), (2) the Mahale Mountains in Tanzania (Nishida et al., 1983; Uehara et al., 1992), and (3) the Tai National Park in the Ivory Coast (Boesch, 2002; Boesch and Boesch, 1989). The most comprehensive studies of cooperative hunting among chimps are those of Christophe and Hedwige Boesch, who compared hunting patterns across the Gombe and Tai chimp populations. Major differences in hunting strategies emerged between these populations.

In Tai chimps, hunting success was positively correlated with group size in what is called a nonadditive fashion. That is, adding more hunters to a group did not simply increase the amount of food by a fixed amount for each new hunter added. Rather, with each new hunter, all group members received more additional food than they did when the last new hunter was added to the group (up to a limit). In addition to these group-size effects, Christophe Boesch found

FIGURE 10.18. Cooperative chimps.
While we often think of chimps as primarily vegetarian, they readily add meat, when it is available, to their diet. In the Tai Forest (Ivory Coast), chimps cooperate in both capturing and consuming prey. Once a prey is caught, subtle rules for food distribution are invoked. *(Photo credit: Christopher Boesch)*

clear evidence of cooperation in Tai chimp hunting behavior (Boesch, 1994a; Figure 10.18). Very complex, but subtle, social rules exist that regulate access to fresh kills, and assure hunters—that is, those who actually cooperate during the hunt—greater success than those who fail to join a hunt.

The situation was quite different with Gombe chimps—no correlation between group size and hunting success was found in chimps from this population. That is, no group-size effect was uncovered in the context of foraging. In addition, unlike in the Tai population, behavioral rules limiting a nonhunter's access to prey were absent, and such individuals received as much food as those who hunted cooperatively (Boesch, 1994a; Goodall, 1986). Part of the difference in hunting behavior in Tai and Gombe chimps may be due to the fact that the success rate for Gombe solo hunters was quite high compared with the individual success rate for chimps in the Tai population, obviating the need for cooperative hunting in the Gombe population.

GROUPS, PUBLIC INFORMATION, AND FORAGING

Tom Valone and his colleagues have suggested that another potential foraging-related benefit associated with group life is the acquisition of public information (Danchin et al., 2004; Valone, 1989; Valone and Templeton, 2002). The idea behind public information models is that a forager needs to be assessing a whole host of environmental variables—food availability, predators, and so on. One way to update such information is to use the actions of others as a cue to changes in environmental conditions. This public information differs from the sort of information acquired during social learning. In social learning, individuals learn something specific (a new behavior, the preference of others). In public information models, individuals simply use the actions of others as a means of assessing the condition of the environment, and as such, public information allows group members to reduce environmental uncertainty (Valone and Giraldeau, 1993). While public information models are general in nature and can apply to numerous environmental parameters, here we shall focus on how these models have been tested in the context of foraging behavior.

Solitary foragers can reduce environmental variability by acquiring knowledge about patches of food before arriving at a patch and/or by keeping track of how long they have been in a patch and how much they have eaten (Danchin et al., 2004). Foragers in a group, however, can acquire information in these same

FIGURE 10.19. Public information. Social foragers such as starlings have been used to test "public information" models of foraging behavior. Starlings in this public information experiment were tested using an array of food placed into cups. *(Photo credit: Jennifer Templeton)*

ways, but they also have access to public information. In particular, a forager in a group can use the foraging success of others as an estimate of patch quality. This public information should allow social foragers access to quicker and better estimates of the productivity of a patch of food than solitary foragers.

As a case in point, public information models predict that social foragers in poor patches should leave such patches earlier than solitary individuals would, since social foragers may use the failed foraging attempts of their groupmates as additional information about when they themselves should leave a patch of food. Jennifer Templeton and Luc-Alain Giraldeau tested this prediction by examining the use of public information by the starling (*Sturnus vulgaris*). Starlings in Templeton and Giraldeau's experiment fed at an artificial feeder that had thirty cups that were either empty or contained a few seeds (Templeton and Giraldeau, 1996; Figure 10.19). A given bird (B1) fed from such a feeder either alone or paired with a second bird (B2). Prior to being paired with B1 partners, B2 birds had either been given the chance to sample a few cups in this feeder, or to sample all such cups. Two results support the predictions of public information models. First, when tested on completely empty feeding patches, B1 birds left such patches earlier when paired with any B2 bird than when foraging alone. Even more importantly, B1 birds left patches earliest of all when paired with B2 birds that had complete information about the patches (as compared with those B2 birds with only partial information).

Natural Selection, Phylogeny, and Seed Caching

Here we will consider the phenomenal ability of some birds and mammals to remember where they have stored literally thousands of food items. Watching a squirrel find the nuts it has stored for winter all over your garden often inspires a sense of awe in the observer. And it isn't only squirrels; for example, many bird species in the families *Corvidae* and *Paridae* possess such uncanny abilities, with some species of birds caching tens of thousands of items per year, and others an astonishing hundreds of thousands of items each year (Balda and Kamil, 1992; Pravosudov and Clayton, 2002). How is that possible? How can an animal find scores of food items that are scattered across its environment, and often hidden over the course of months and months?

HIPPOCAMPAL SIZE AND CACHING ABILITY

To address foraging and spatial memory, Sue Healey and John Krebs examined hippocampal volume and food-storing abilities in seven species of corvid birds (Healey and Krebs, 1992). They chose to study the hippocampal region because in birds this area of the brain is known to be associated with food retrieval (Krebs et al., 1989; Sherry, 2006; Sherry and Vaccarino, 1989). Moreover, the corvids are an ideal group in which to examine the relationship between hippocampal volume and food storage in more detail, since so much variation in food-storing behavior exists within this group (Balda and Kamil, 1989; de Kort and Clayton, 2006; Emery, 2006; Goodwin, 1986). Some corvids store no food, while others rely on the food they have stored over the course of nine months.

Healey and Krebs studied two species—jackdaws (*Corvus monedula*) and Alpine choughs (*Pyrrhocorax graculus*)—that rarely if ever stored food; four species—rooks (*Corvus frugilegus*), European crows (*Corvis corone*), European magpies (*Pica pica*), and Asian red-billed blue magpies (*Cissa erythrorhyncha*)—in which food storing plays some role; and one species—the European jay (*Garrulus glandarius*)—in which not only does food storing play an important role, but the location of 6,000 to 11,000 seeds must be remembered for nine months. When food-storing behavior was examined in relation to hippocampal volume in these seven species, a strong positive relationship was uncovered (Figure 10.20). The more food-storing behavior seen in a species, the greater the hippocampal volume, strongly supporting the hypothesis that hippocampal volume is a critical variable in the evolution of spatial memory and foraging.

In addition to the comparative approach adopted by Healey and Krebs, animal behaviorists have also examined the relationship between hippocampal size and caching ability within a single species. For example, one might expect that, within a given species, individuals from populations where food resources are relatively scarce would be better at caching and recovering food and would possess a larger hippocampus than individuals from food-rich environments (Pravosudov and Grubb, 1997; Pravosudov et al., 2001). That is, natural selection should favor better caching and retrieval abilities when individuals live in harsh foraging environments, where caching and retrieval is at a premium, and selection should favor larger hippocampal areas and more hippocampal neurons in such individuals. Vladimir Pravosudov and Nicky Clayton tested this idea using black-capped chickadees (*Poecile atricapilla*) from two populations—Colorado (food rich) and Alaska (food poor) (Pravosudov and Clayton, 2002).

Pravosudov and Clayton captured fifteen chickadees from a site in Anchorage, Alaska, and twelve birds from a population near Windsor, Colorado, and transported them back to their laboratory at the University of California at Davis. Forty-five days after being brought into the lab, the birds were tested on their ability to retrieve seeds they had cached. When provided with seeds that could be cached, the birds from Alaska (food-scarce population) cached a greater percentage of seeds than the birds from Colorado (food-rich population).

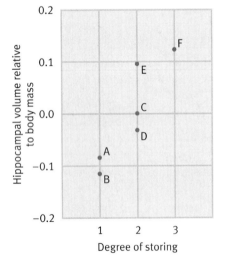

FIGURE 10.20. Foraging and brain size. The volume of the hippocampal region relative to body mass was positively correlated with the extent of food storing in six species of birds: (A) alpine chough, (B) jackdaw, (C) rook and crow combined, (D) red-billed blue magpie, (E) magpie, and (F) European jay. *(Based on Healey and Krebs, 1992)*

A

B

FIGURE 10.21. Population differences in food storing. **(A)** Mean number of sunflower seeds eaten and cached. Birds from both populations ate about the same number of seeds, but the birds from the resource-scarce environments (the Alaskan birds) cached significantly more seeds than the birds from the resource-rich environments (the Colorado birds). **(B)** Mean number of sites inspected. Note that it took the Alaskan birds fewer looks to find their caches, showing that they were more efficient at locating their caching sites than were the Colorado birds. *(Based on Pravosudov and Clayton, 2002, p. 519)*

Equally important, the Alaskan birds found more of their cached seeds than did the Colorado birds, and their searches were more efficient in that they made fewer errors (Figure 10.21).

In terms of hippocampal size, even though the birds from Alaska weighed less and were smaller than the Colorado birds, the hippocampal volumes of the Alaskan birds were greater and their hippocampuses contained more neurons than those of the Colorado birds. What's more, when Pravosudov and Clayton compared birds from Colorado and Alaska that were *not* given the chance to cache seeds, the same hippocampal differences were found, suggesting that the caching experience per se was not what gave Alaskan birds a larger hippocampus. Instead, the differences between birds from harsh and abundant food environments were the result of natural selection acting on hippocampal size. These differences fit nicely into an adaptationist framework, and much work in this area continues.

PHYLOGENY AND CACHING ABILITY

Another evolutionary approach to seed caching is to study this phenomenon from a phylogenetic perspective (de Kort and Clayton, 2006). In an attempt to understand the evolutionary history of caching behavior in corvids, Selvino de Kort and Nicky Clayton built a phylogeny of forty-six species from this family of birds. To do this, each species was categorized on its tendency to cache seeds. Based on a combination of published laboratory and field studies, each of the forty-six species was placed into one of three categories. Non-cachers were defined as species that virtually never cache food. Moderate cachers were those that cached food throughout the course of a year and cached many different types of food, but were never entirely dependent on cached food sources for survival. Finally, specialized cachers were defined as species in which individuals cached a large number of items, the cached items were typically one food type, and caching was seasonal (dependent on when the food item was available). In addition, specialized cachers often recovered their cached items after long periods of time had passed.

When the information on caching is analyzed, a phylogenetic analysis indicates that the ancestral state of caching in corvids is "moderate caching."

In other words, the ancestor species that gave rise to all corvids was a moderate cacher. This is critically important information. Many animal behaviorists initially argued that the ancestral state in corvids was non-caching. What that meant was that they assumed that evolution was moving some species on a trajectory from non-cacher to cacher. De Kort and Clayton's findings that the ancestral state was moderate caching suggest that some corvid species evolved into specialized cachers, while others lost the caching trait altogether. Indeed, de Kort and Clayton found evolution toward highly specialized cachers occurred independently at least twice, and perhaps as many as five times. Conversely, over evolutionary time, at least two species completely lost the ability to cache seeds, perhaps because the benefits of caching did not make up for the metabolic costs of maintaining a relatively large hippocampus (Attwell and Laughlin, 2001; Laughlin et al., 1998).

Learning and Foraging

While the studies described so far often involve animals learning something about their foraging environment, they were not designed as studies on foraging and learning per se. To even touch on the tip of the iceberg of studies done on learning and animal foraging would require a series of books. After all, these sorts of studies have been a mainstay in psychology over the last fifty years, and there have been thousands of studies examining learning in the context of foraging (Balda et al., 1998; Kamil et al., 1987; Kamil and Yoerg, 1982; Pietrewicz and Richards, 1985; Shettleworth, 1998; Stephens and Krebs, 1986; Yoerg, 1991). Here, we shall look at a tiny, but important, subsection of the work on foraging and learning by focusing on:

▶ Foraging, learning, and brain size in birds.
▶ Learning and planning for the future.

FORAGING, LEARNING, AND BRAIN SIZE IN BIRDS

A number of animal behaviorists have hypothesized a neurobiological link between forebrain size and learning abilities in animals (Byrne, 1993; Clutton-Brock and Harvey, 1980; Dunbar, 1992; Johnstone, 1982; Jolicoeur et al., 1984; Mace et al., 1981; Wyles et al., 1983). The premise underlying this link is as follows: Since the forebrain appears to be associated with behavioral plasticity—including learning—animals with larger forebrains should often be better learners. While this approach is susceptible to numerous potential biases, Louis Lefebvre and his colleagues used its basic principles to test for a relationship between "foraging innovations" and forebrain size in North American and British Isle bird groups (Lefebvre et al., 1997a, 1997b).

Lefebvre and his colleagues defined a "foraging innovation" as "either the ingestion of a new food type or the use of a new foraging technique." For our purposes here, we will focus on the latter types of innovations (which include some examples of social learning). The researchers used descriptions of birds mentioned in nine ornithology journals to gather data on 322 foraging innovations—126 in British Isle birds and 192 in North American birds

TABLE 10.1. Examples of foraging innovations in birds. Lefebvre and his colleagues gathered data on 322 foraging innovations, including those in this list. *(Based on Lefebvre et al., 1997b, pp. 552–553)*

SPECIES	INNOVATION
Cardinal (Florida subspecies)	Nipping off nectar-filled capsule on flower and eating it
Herring gull	Catching small rabbits and killing them by dropping them on rocks or drowning them
Ferruginous hawk	Attracted to gunshot, preys on human-killed prairie dog
Magpie	Digging up potatoes
Storm petrel	Feeding on decaying whale fat
Great skua	Scavenging on roadkill
House sparrow	Using automatic sensor to open bus station door
House sparrow	Systematic searching and entering of car radiator grilles for insects
Galápagos mockingbird	Pecking food from sea lion's mouth
Common crow	Using cars as nutcrackers for palm nuts
Osprey	Opening conch shells by dropping them on concrete-filled drum
Turnstone	Raiding gastric cavities of sea anemones
Red-winged + Brewer's blackbirds	Following tractor and eating frogs, voles, and insects flushed by it
Sparrowhawk	Drowning blackbird prey
Carrion crow	Landing on floating sheep corpse and feeding from it
Downy woodpecker	Using swaying caused by wind to catch meat hung from a branch

(Table 10.1). Innovations included behaviors ranging from herring gulls "catching small rabbits and killing them by dropping on rocks or drowning" to common crows "using cars as nutcrackers for palm nuts" (Grobecker and Pietsch, 1978; Young, 1987). Lefebvre's group then calculated how these innovations were distributed across different orders of birds, at the same time taking into account how common or rare a particular bird order was in Britain or North America.

With the data about foraging innovation in hand, Lefebvre's team obtained information about relative forebrain size in the bird species of interest (Holden and Sharrock, 1988; Portmann, 1947; Scott, 1987). In both North American and British Isle birds, relative forebrain size correlated with foraging innovation. Bird orders that contained individuals that possessed larger forebrains were more likely to have high incidences of foraging innovation (Figure 10.22).

Although many of the cases of foraging innovation were based on a single observation, the fact that a larger-scale analysis spanning 322 cases found a striking relationship between forebrain size and one measure of learning (foraging innovation) suggests that this is an important but relatively understudied area in ethology. In support of this, Lefebvre's group ran a similar analysis on Australasian birds and uncovered very similar results with respect to foraging innovation and forebrain size (Lefebvre et al., 1998).

Daniel Sol, Lefebvre, and their colleagues examined whether there is a fitness advantage associated with being a large-brained bird (Sol and Lefebvre, 2006; Sol et al., 2005a, 2005b, 2006, 2007). One long-held, but largely untested, hypothesis for the fitness advantage associated with large brains (relative to

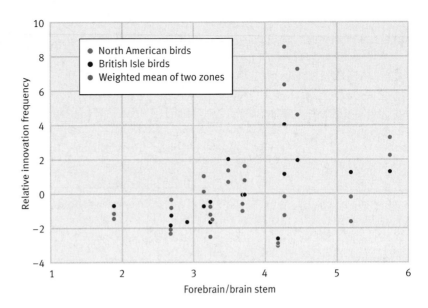

FIGURE 10.22. Brain size and foraging innovation in birds. In North American and British Isle birds, and in the weighted mean of North American and British samples, the relative frequency of foraging innovation is positively correlated with the ratio of forebrain mass to brain stem mass. *(Based on Lefebvre et al., 1997b)*

body size) was that large brains would be particularly helpful when a population was introduced into novel or altered environments, where innovation might be especially important (Allman, 1998; Reader, 2004; Reader and Laland, 2003). Sol and his colleagues put this hypothesis to the test by examining the 646 introductions (involving 196 species) in which humans had placed a population of birds in a novel environment, most often an island or a park outside its native range (Cassey et al., 2004; Sol et al., 2005a). The researchers collected data on brain size from 156 of the 196 species, and in the 40 remaining species in which there were no direct measures, they estimated brain size by using the brain size found in the closest phylogenetic relative for which data were available. Because larger-brained birds are generally bigger than smaller-brained birds, Sol and his team corrected for this potential bias by using brain size relative to body size as their key parameter.

As we discussed in Chapter 5, Sol and his team found a positive relationship between relative brain size and the birds' success in novel environments. What's more, after correcting for potential confounding factors, they found evidence that the success of large-brained species was, at least in part, due to their relatively high use of innovative new foraging techniques, which increased their rate of food intake (Figure 10.23). These findings suggest that there is a strong fitness component for relatively large brains and the innovative abilities associated with them.

PLANNING FOR THE FUTURE

Learning theory is fundamentally tied to the idea that current action is in part a function of prior experience. At the same time, it is also true that if animals could *plan* for the future based on prior experience, as we humans clearly do, there would be huge fitness benefits associated with such an ability. Research on this topic is scarce, however, because for a long time scientists argued that planning for the future was a uniquely human quality—indeed, it was posited that planning for the future was one of the most fundamental differences between humans and all other animals (Suddendorf and Corballis, 1997). Yet,

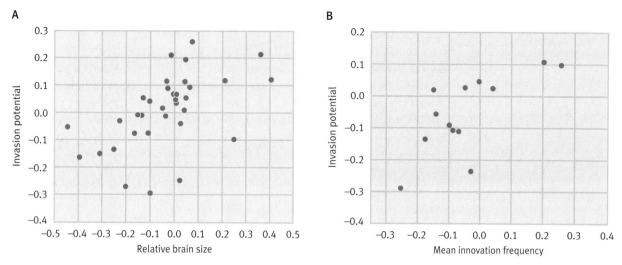

A

B

FIGURE 10.23. Brain size, innovation, and survival in birds. (A) The relationship between mean relative brain size and invasion potential (survival in a new environment) across avian families. **(B)** The relationship between mean foraging innovations and invasion potential across avian families. *(From Sol et al., 2005a)*

over time, it has become clear that animals are capable of other behaviors that we initially believed were uniquely human—for example, tool use—and so animal behaviorists have begun to test animals for their ability to plan for the future.

Both animal and human behaviorists posit that two requirements must be met to demonstrate planning for the future. First, the behavior must be novel, so that we can be certain that we are not seeing the manifestation of some innate action. For example, migration behavior, which has many underlying innate components, may appear "planned," but would not be considered such under our definition. Second, the behavior in question must not be tied to the current motivational state of the animal, but rather to the anticipated motivational state at some point in the future (Shettleworth, 2007; Suddendorf, 2006). Here, we will examine a recent study of the ability of western scrub jays (*Aphelocoma californica*) to modify their foraging behavior in an attempt to plan for the future (Figure 10. 24).

Western scrub jays are a model system for such experiments, as they display incredible feats of episodic memory—recollecting specific events or episodes—in that they cache and later uncover large amounts of food. In addition, these birds not only remember where they have stored items, but they remember who was watching them when they cached their food and in such cases will later dig up and rehide the food, presumably to protect their stored food from being stolen (Clayton and Dickinson, 1998; Dally et al., 2006). With such impressive cognitive abilities, the hypothesis that western scrub jays can also plan for the future seems worth testing, especially considering that studies in humans suggest that the same neurobiological processes involved in episodic memory are involved in planning for the future (Atance and Meltzoff, 2005; Okuda et al., 2003; Rosenbaum et al., 2005).

Caroline Raby and her team used a simple, but elegant, experimental procedure to examine whether western scrub jays could plan for the future (Raby et al., 2007). On alternate mornings over the course of six days, birds were exposed to one of two compartments—one compartment contained food

FIGURE 10.24. Western scrub jays and planning for the future. Researchers have examined whether western scrub jays plan into the future when making foraging decisions. *(Photo credit: David A. Northcott/Corbis)*

in the form of ground-up pine nuts, and the other compartment contained no food. On the evening before each test, the birds were not fed any food, and they were therefore hungry during their exposure to test compartments. After the six days of exposure to the two compartments, the birds were denied access to any food for two hours before dark, and then they were unexpectedly provided with a bowl of whole pine nuts—that is, food that could be cached. They were then allowed to move freely in the area with the whole pine nuts and could access both of the compartments they had been exposed to earlier. But now each of the compartments had a "caching tray" added to it, so the birds could cache food before it got dark, if they so chose.

Remarkably, Raby and her team found that jays cached more nuts in the compartment in which they had consistently received no food in the past, strongly suggesting that they were planning for the fact that, when next exposed to that compartment, there would be no food present unless they cached it there. In an ingenious follow-up experiment, Raby and her colleagues had birds learn that they would be fed peanuts in one compartment, but dog kibble in the other (jays like both these food types). When an experiment like the one described above was run, jays cached peanuts in the compartment associated with kibble, and kibble in the compartment associated with peanuts, suggesting they prefer a varied diet, and that they plan for such a diet accordingly. The extent that other animals can plan for the future remains a relatively unexplored question in ethology.

SOCIAL LEARNING AND FORAGING

In addition to learning per se, information about foraging can be culturally transmitted when individuals observe others to see how they find food and what they eat (recall the work on foraging and cultural transmission in rats in Chapter 1). To understand more about such social learning, we will consider social learning and foraging in pigeons. Like rats, pigeons (*Columbia livia*) are an ideal species in which to examine cultural transmission of feeding behavior (Figure 10.25). Being primarily scavengers feeding on human garbage, pigeons face the same dilemma faced by rats: Which new food items are safe, and which are

FIGURE 10.25. Urban foragers.
Pigeons are scavengers, coming across novel food items all the time. Such a species is ideal for studying foraging and cultural transmission.
(Photo credit: Blickwinkel/Alamy)

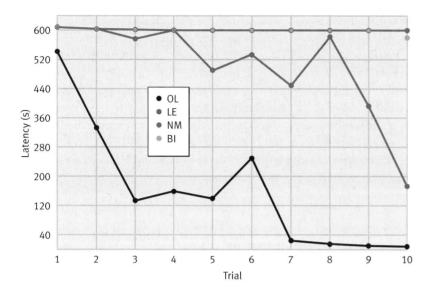

FIGURE 10.26. Social learning and foraging in pigeons. Pigeons in this experiment need to learn to pierce the red half of a paper covering a box of seeds. The graph shows average latency to eating for four groups: NM (no model) group—these birds were never exposed to a model; BI ("blind" imitation) group—these birds observed a model bird pierce a paper cover but never eat; LE (local enhancement) group—these birds observed a model bird eat through a hole in the paper made by the experimenters; and OL (observational learning) group—these birds saw a model bird pierce the paper and eat the seeds in the box. Pigeons in the NM and BI treatments never learned to feed in the experimental apparatus. The quickest learning occurred in the OL treatment. *(Based on Palameta and Lefebvre, 1985)*

dangerous? Louis Lefebvre and his colleagues Luc-Alain Giraldeau and Boris Palemeta have run an intriguing series of experiments that attest to the strength of cultural transmission in shaping diet in the pigeon. This work has focused on three related issues: (1) What type of information do pigeons transfer about food? (2) How does such information spread or fail to spread through a population of pigeons? (3) What factors favor the cultural transmission of information over alternative means of acquiring information?

Palemeta and Lefebvre set out to examine cultural transmission in a three-part experiment that used observer and demonstrator animals (Palameta and Lefebvre, 1985). The task that observer pigeons needed to master was piercing the red half of a half red/half black piece of paper covering a box. Under the paper was a bonanza of seeds for the lucky bird who made it that far.

An observer pigeon was placed in an arena with such a food box—with a half red/half black paper cover—and exposed to one of four scenarios. In the first group, birds saw no model on the other side of a clear partition. None of the pigeons in this group learned how to get at the hidden food, suggesting that this was indeed a difficult task to master through individual learning. In a second group, observers were shown a model that was eating from a hole in the paper. The hole was made by Palameta and Lefebvre, and as such, although observers did see a model eating, they did not see the model solve the hidden food "puzzle"—that is, they did not see the model pierce the red half of the cover. Once again, pigeons in this treatment failed to learn how to get food from the multicolored box. In the final two treatments of the experiment, birds either saw a model pierce the red side of the paper but get no food, or they saw a model both pierce the paper and eat. Although birds in both of these treatments learned to solve the food-finding dilemma, those in the latter treatment did so much faster (Figure 10.26), suggesting an important role for cultural transmission in the foraging behavior of pigeons.

There is an interesting twist to the pigeon story. In many animals that live in groups, there are two strategies for foraging that individuals can adopt: producing and scrounging. **Producers** find and procure food, while **scroungers** make their living parasitizing the food that producers have uncovered (Barnard, 1984; Giraldeau and Caraco, 2000). Layered onto the social learning and foraging story we have seen in pigeons, we find producers and scroungers in this species as well (Giraldeau and Lefebvre, 1986). And it is the unusual way that producing and scrounging interacts with social learning that makes the pigeon story particularly useful in furthering our understanding of cultural transmission and foraging.

Despite Palameta and Lefebvre's work demonstrating social learning in pigeons in cages, when birds are tested in groups, only a few birds seem to learn new feeding behaviors by observing others. This apparent paradox caused Giraldeau and Lefebvre to examine whether scrounging behavior somehow inhibited cultural transmission (Giraldeau and Lefebvre, 1987). To do so, they used a different set-up than the one described above (Figure 10.27).

In the new experimental protocol, flocks of pigeons were allowed to feed together. Forty-eight little test tubes were placed in a row and five of these tubes had food. Which five had food was unknown to the birds. To open a tube, an individual had to learn to peck at a stick in a rubber stopper at the top of the tube. When this task was done correctly, it caused the test tube to open and the contents to spread over the floor below. Once the food was out, any bird in the vicinity, not just the one that opened the tube, could eat it.

The results of this experiment were striking. As predicted based on earlier work, only two of the sixteen pigeons in their group learned to open tubes— that is, the flock was composed of two producers and fourteen scroungers. Two additional findings suggested to Giraldeau and Lefebvre that scrounging inhibited an individual from learning how to open tubes via observation. To begin with, scroungers followed producers and seemed more interested in *where* producers were, than in *what* producers did, to get food; the scroungers' attention was not directed at the actions taken by the producers to open the tubes. Second, by removing the two producers from the group, Giraldeau and

FIGURE 10.27. Producing and scrounging. When a group member finally opens a tube with food in it, the food spills on the floor and is accessible to all. In Giraldeau and Lefebvre's study using such a scenario, out of sixteen pigeons, only two learned to open tubes (these were the producers), while fourteen acted as scroungers. Labels show where millet was hidden, but the birds were not privy to this information.

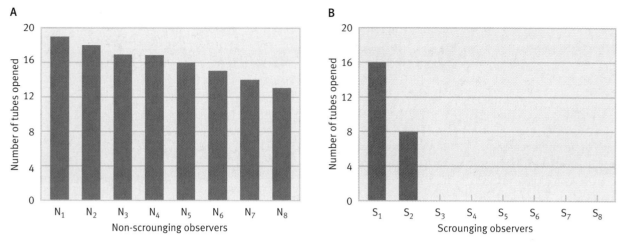

FIGURE 10.28. Scrounging prevents social learning. In an ingenious experiment, Giraldeau and Lefebvre trained two groups of pigeons. **(A)** One group of birds saw a model bird peck at a stick in a rubber stopper at the end of the tube. This provided food to the model. These birds learned to peck at the stick to obtain food after observing the model, and so they were considered non-scroungers. **(B)** In the second group of birds, when the model pecked at the stick, food was released, but to the observer. In this group, observers were scroungers. Scroungers fared much worse than non-scroungers when faced with the task of pecking at the stick. *(Based on Giraldeau and Lefebvre, 1987)*

Lefebvre were able to ascertain that scroungers not only didn't *display* the tube-opening trait, but they also didn't know how to open these tubes. That is to say, it was not as if scroungers could open the tubes, but opted not to; they truly never learned from observing the producers.

In order to get a firm handle on just how scrounging blocked cultural transmission of foraging skills, Giraldeau and Lefebvre ran a second set of controlled experiments. Here, they paired a single observer with a single demonstrator who already knew how to obtain food. If an observer had the chance to view a demonstrator open tubes and obtain food, over time the observer learned how to open tubes. That is, all birds were capable of learning the foraging task. In an ingenious manipulation, Giraldeau and Lefebvre then set up the experimental cages so that every time the demonstrator opened a tube, the food in that tube slid over to the observer's side of the cage. In these treatments, the observers rarely learned how to open the tubes themselves (Figure 10.28). Their scrounging on the food that was found by others interfered with the transmission of information about how to go about getting the food themselves.

Current work on foraging behavior continues in most of the areas we have covered in this chapter—prey choice, patch-leaving rules, risk sensitivity, group effects, planning for the future, the role of phylogeny in shaping behavior, as well as in the role that both individual and social learning play in making foraging decisions.

Now that we have spent a chapter on animal behavior and foraging, we are ready to examine what is, in a sense, the flip side of the foraging coin. In the next chapter, we shall examine antipredator behaviors, which often amount to strategies to avoid becoming a prey item.

INTERVIEW WITH

Dr. John Krebs

How did it come to be that someone whose father won a Nobel Prize for coming up with the Krebs cycle made his initial mark in science by studying animal behavior?

No single factor, but a concatenation of many events led me to a career in animal behavior. I came to zoology as a bird-watcher; as a high school pupil I spent two summers working in the laboratory of the famous ethologist, Konrad Lorenz; and as an undergraduate at Oxford, I was lucky enough to be taught by two giants of their generation, David Lack and Niko Tinbergen. Having said all this, my father dissuaded me from my first choice of a university course, namely archaeology, and I ended up as a zoologist, having failed to get in to study medicine! My Ph.D. at Oxford was unusual in that I studied population ecology in Niko Tinbergen's animal behavior group. This meant that right from the start I saw the linkages between ecology and behavior that led to the emergence of "behavioral ecology."

One of the most innovative aspects of your work on foraging in great tits was the use of a conveyer belt to present food to the birds. How did you come up with that idea? What did this allow you to do that otherwise would have been impossible?

Throughout my career I have been extraordinarily fortunate in the exceptional colleagues, students, and co-workers I have had. The "conveyor belt" was not my idea. A graduate student in the animal behavior group

at Oxford, Jon Erichsen, had devised it for psychophysical studies of reaction times in birds. Together we saw its potential for foraging studies. It would enable us to control encounter rates very accurately by having the prey move past the bird, rather than vice versa. I remember vividly posting to (no e-mail in those days) Ric Charnov

the first results from the conveyor belt. These showed that the inclusion or exclusion of the less profitable prey type depended exclusively on the encounter rate with the more profitable prey. The theory actually worked!

Psychologists have been studying the feeding behavior of animals for more than fifty years. Why the lag in ethological studies in this area? Why did they start up in earnest in the 1970s?

Ethologists had in fact been studying feeding behavior for many

years. The important concept of "search image" was well established, and there were many studies of the cues used by animals for detecting food, the development of feeding skills during the life of an individual, as well as of predator avoidance strategies, such as crypsis, mimicry, and warning colors. The new approach in the 1970s, known as "optimal foraging theory," resulted from a confluence of ideas from ethology, ecology, evolution, psychology, and economics. As so often happens when new ideas are beginning to crystallize, more than one person independently came to similar conclusions. The seeds of foraging theory were more or less independently sown by J. T. Emlen, R. H. MacArthur and E. R. Pianka, J. D. Goss-Custard, and G. A. Parker. The attraction of foraging theory for me at the time, and I think for many others, was the juxtaposition of a broad theoretical framework, testable predictions from mathematical models, and both field and laboratory data.

How do classical psychologists and ethologists differ in the way they study animal foraging?

Traditionally, psychologists studied the mechanisms of behavior in the laboratory whilst ethologists and behavioral ecologists studied function or adaptation in the field. In the last fifteen years, these boundaries have become blurred, to the benefit of both disciplines. For example, ethologists have adopted some of the experimental and theoretical tools of operant and classical conditioning as well as of cognitive psychology. Psychologists have increasingly taken on board the potential value of an evolutionary framework for understanding behavior.

Many optimal foraging models involve complex mathematics. Does that mean the animals have to know how to solve mathematical equations to forage efficiently?

Mathematical models of flight are complex, but birds do not need to be mathematicians in order to fly. Nor do they need to do sums in order to forage according to the predictions of optimal foraging models. Mathematics is the universal language used by a scientist to describe and analyze what goes on in nature. There is no implication that nature itself uses mathematics.

A number of foraging models focus on what are called "rules of thumb." Could you explain the basic idea here?

Traditional foraging models were concerned with the end result (or adaptive significance) of foraging—for example, maximizing energy intake, rather than about the mechanisms that control feeding behavior. The notion of "rules of thumb" is that the end result, analyzed in a foraging model, might be achieved by a mechanism that approximates the "right" answer. If, for example, you were trying to find the best textbook of animal behavior, the rule of thumb "read if it is by Dugatkin" might bring you close enough to the optimal solution to be virtually indistinguishable from a more complex search strategy. If students following a different rule of thumb did better in exams, over time, the "Dugatkin rule" would be replaced by

another rule that came closer to the optimal solution. In other words, rules of thumb are themselves subject to evolution by natural selection.

One potential critique of the foraging literature in ethology is that so many of the experiments undertaken are run in the laboratory and not in the field. In your estimation, how serious a problem is this?

If you are studying fundamental properties of animals—for example, decision-making rules—then they can be elucidated in the laboratory as well

> The attraction of foraging theory . . . was the juxtaposition of a broad theoretical framework, testable predictions from mathematical models, and both field and laboratory data.

as in the field. A potential danger is that in the laboratory you may end up finding out more about the properties of your apparatus and experimental set-up than about the animal! This is a criticism that has sometimes been leveled at earlier studies of "schedules of reinforcement" by operant psychologists. Probably the ideal approach is to use a combination of field and laboratory work. Laboratory work certainly has the advantage that it is possible to control the variables more precisely. For laboratory work, intelligent design of the experimental set-up will help to ensure that the essence of the natural situation is captured.

What's "the big question" to be tackled next in the study of animal foraging behavior?

Foraging theory, like any other branch of inquiry, will continue to evolve and change. I do not see a single "big question" on the horizon, but I see several potentially important ways in which the study of foraging behavior could develop. One of these is to apply ideas from foraging behavior to conservation. The pioneering work of J. D. Goss-Custard and W. J. Sutherland has shown how foraging models can be used to predict the effects of habitat loss and disturbance on threatened populations. The key has been to link the foraging of individuals to density-dependent influences on the population as a whole. Another area of recent, and likely continuing, growth consists of the links between behavioral economics, decision theory, and foraging behavior. This is a development of the links between animal psychology and foraging behavior that began about twenty years ago. New insights are flowing in both directions. More generally, I do not think we should regard "foraging behavior" as an ineluctable, distinct field of inquiry. The basic ideas may be reconfigured, remolded, and, reinvented so that the categories used to describe behavior today might seem outmoded in ten years' time.

Dr. John Krebs is a professor at Oxford University in England. Dr. Krebs's work on foraging behavior was seminal to the development of optimal foraging theory. Dr. Krebs (along with Dr. Nick Davies; see Chapter 7 interview) is the editor of Behavioural Ecology: An Evolutionary Approach, *4th ed. (Blackwell Science, 1997), the most well-read book in the field of behavioral ecology.*

SUMMARY

1. One way animals determine what sort of food to search for is through the development of a search image. The idea behind a search image is that when animals encounter a prey type more and more, they form some sort of representation of the prey, and that as this representation or image becomes more and more detailed with experience, the forager finds itself more successful at finding that type of prey.

2. Optimal foraging theory encompasses a class of models that predicts what and where animals should eat, as well as nutrient constraints and the effect of hunger state on risk-sensitive foraging.

3. Somewhat surprisingly, optimal foraging models predict that the encounter rate with the less profitable of two prey items does not affect whether that item should be added to the diet or not. Rather, a critical encounter rate with the *most* profitable item is what determines which prey items should be added to a diet.

4. The marginal value theorem predicts how long a forager should stay in a given patch, given that it can leave and travel to feed in more undisturbed patches. Moving between food patches, however, is assumed to entail some cost, including lost time foraging while traveling and the increased rate of predation while traveling.

5. In addition to *maximizing* their rate of energy intake, animals are constrained by a need to spend time foraging for specific nutrients that are essential for survival.

6. Hungry foragers should be risk prone, that is, willing to assume greater variance (risk) in food intake. Less hungry individuals tend to be more risk averse.

7. Foraging while in groups often, but not always, increases the foraging success of individuals (compared to solitary foraging). Benefits of group life include the ability to learn about various aspects of the foraging environment from observing others.

8. A phylogenetic analysis of caching in corvid birds suggests that "moderate caching" was the ancestral state of caching behavior in this group. This finding suggests that some corvid species evolved into specialized cachers, while others lost the caching trait altogether.

9. Animals often learn how and on what to forage; indeed work in this area has been a mainstay in the psychological literature for years. Learning sometimes manifests itself in foraging innovations; brain size often correlates with the frequency of such foraging innovations. In addition, some evidence now exists that some animals can use what they have learned to plan for the future.

DISCUSSION QUESTIONS

1. Read R. Pulliam's 1973 article "On the advantages of flocking," in the *Journal of Theoretical Biology* (vol. 38, pp. 419–422). Based on the article, outline the "many eyes" hypothesis, and discuss how it relates to foraging behavior.

2. Read E. L. Charnov's 1976 article, "Optimal foraging, the marginal value theorem," in *Theoretical and Population Biology* (vol. 9, pp. 129–136). How

might you modify the model to examine other behaviors displayed by animals?

3. Using Math Box 10.1 (see pp. 340–341) as a starting point, construct a foraging model with three prey types. Imagine that you already know that it pays for a forager to eat prey type 1 and prey type 2. What are the conditions under which it should add prey type 3?

4. Why do you suppose it took so long for ethologists and psychologists to recognize the larger literature on foraging behavior that exists in each other's field? What do you think were the biggest differences in the way foraging was studied in these two disciplines?

5. Using the graphs in Figure 10.7 (see p. 344) as a starting point, examine what happens to the time an animal should spend in the patch as a function of how profitable that patch is. This will involve changing the shape of the curve that describes food intake as a function of patch residence time and examining what this change does to optimal time in a patch.

6. How does the corvid phylogeny paper we discussed show that the adaptationist and phylogenetic approaches to studying brain size and caching can complement one another?

SUGGESTED READING

Belovsky, G. E. (1978). Diet optimization in a generalist herbivore: The moose. *Theoretical and Population Biology, 14,* 105–134. One of the first optimal foraging studies that incorporated specific food constraints (the need for salt).

Giraldeau, L. A., & Caraco, T. (2000). *Social foraging theory.* Princeton: Princeton University Press. A comprehensive overview of social foraging theory, with many empirical examples to lead the reader through the math.

Krebs, J. (1978). Optimal foraging: Decision rules for predators. In J. R. Krebs & N. B. Davies (Eds.), *Behavioural ecology: An evolutionary approach* (pp. 23–63). Oxford: Blackwell. A good overview of early work on foraging.

Raby, C. R., Alexis, D. M., Dickinson, A., & Clayton, N. S. (2007). Planning for the future by western scrub-jays. *Nature, 445,* 919–921. The first evidence that nonprimates can plan for future events in an adaptive manner.

Stephens, D., & Krebs, J. (1986). *Foraging theory.* Princeton: Princeton University Press. Regarded by most as the definitive book on foraging theory and animal behavior.

11

Antipredator Behavior

At the California field site where Richard Coss, Donald Owings, and their colleagues have been studying predator-prey interactions, gopher snakes (*Pituophis melanoleucus*) and their prey—ground squirrels (*Spermophilus beecheyi*)—have been present for approximately a million years. After such a long period of evolutionary time, and with snakes relying so heavily on squirrels as a main staple of their diet, natural selection has strongly selected for ground squirrels to be able to identify their predators and to respond to them with fine-tuned behaviors (Coss, 1991; Coss and Owings, 1985; Owings and Coss, 1977). For example, groups of squirrels will often mob, or converge on, a gopher snake, biting and harassing it until the snake is forced to leave the area (Owings and Coss, 1977). In addition, squirrel antipredator behavior includes throwing dirt, pebbles, and roots at putative predators, as well as emitting alarm calls that are specifically made when snakes, but not other predators, are present (Owings and Leger, 1980; Figure 11.1). But there is more to it than that. The squirrel's immune system has also evolved in concert with the antipredator behaviors mentioned above. To see this, let us look at some behavioral immunological work undertaken by Naomie Poran and Richard Coss.

Poran and Coss focused on maturing young California ground squirrels and examined both antipredator behavior and immunological defenses against snakes (Poran and Coss, 1990). With respect to the latter, they examined serum-to-venom binding levels—a measure of immunological defenses against snake bites—in ground squirrels (Biardi et al., 2000, 2005, 2006). To do this, Poran and Coss employed radioimmunoassays of serum-to-venom binding levels in squirrels at ages fourteen, twenty, forty-eight, and eighty days. At very young ages, pups have very low serum-to-venom binding levels, but this measure shoots up to almost adult levels some time between days fourteen and thirty. This occurs even when pups are not exposed to snakes during the experiment. Why is there a spike in serum-to-venom binding levels?

The answer is tied to the natural history of the squirrels. Squirrel pups don't emerge from their natal burrows until they are about forty days old (Linsdale, 1946). In their burrows, the pups are relatively safe from snake predation, at least compared to the threats they face when emerging from their burrows. But just prior to when the pups will emerge, when the threat of gopher snake predation will

FIGURE 11.1. Snakes and squirrels. (A) Ground squirrels recognize snakes as predators upon emergence from their burrow. **(B)** Confrontations with rattlesnakes are common, and **(C)** they sometimes lead a squirrel to throw dirt and roots at the snake (note the snake's head at the left) to defend itself. Arrows indicate the location of the snake in each photo. *(Photo credits: Richard Coss)*

increase dramatically, natural selection has favored a spike in serum-to-venom binding levels (Figure 11.2). Such a spike will help to protect young squirrels from snake bites when they emerge from their burrows (Figure 11.3).

There is one thing for certain about animal behavior: If an individual makes an error with respect to antipredator tactics, its future fitness may well be zero. This obvious, but striking, fact suggests that natural selection should operate very strongly on antipredator behavior and that, in addition, we might expect fine-tuned learning in this behavioral venue as well. Both because interactions between predators and their prey are often spectacular to observe, and because such interactions are so critical for understanding the process of natural selection, ethologists have a long history of studying antipredator behavior (Lind and Cresswell, 2005). Indeed, we have already touched on some cases of antipredator behavior in an earlier chapter—recall from Chapter 2 that among other things, guppies in areas of high predation live in larger groups than guppies from corresponding areas of low predation. Not only does the chance of being taken by a predator go down as group size increases, but large group size allows for more individuals to be vigilant for predators in the first place (the so-called "many eyes" hypothesis; Pulliam, 1973).

At the most fundamental level, there are essentially two forms of antipredator behaviors: those that help prey avoid detection by predators, and those that function once a prey encounters a predator. Here, we will try to place our proximate and ultimate perspectives of antipredator behavior within these two categories. Before proceeding, here are two caveats: (1) while these two categories encompass most antipredator behaviors, they are not meant to be exhaustive, and (2) only biotic (living) predators are considered in this chapter. Fire, for example, kills many animals, and there is evidence that reed frogs (*Hyperolius nitidulus*) respond to the sound of oncoming flames and flee (Grafe et al., 2002). We will not be considering such instances here.

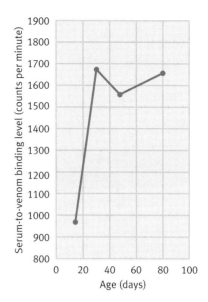

FIGURE 11.2. Immunology and predation. Ground squirrel pups emerge from their burrows at about forty days. Shortly before this, there is an increase in their immunological defenses (their serum-to-venom binding levels) against snakes. *(From Poran and Coss, 1990, p. 237)*

FIGURE 11.3. Danger at emergence. Ground squirrel pups often face serious predation threat on their first emergence from their burrow.

Avoiding Predators

If putative prey can avoid their predators in the first place, they can decrease not only the probability of being captured and eaten but also the costs associated with fleeing, fighting back against a predator, and so on (Ruxton et al., 2004). Below, we shall examine three ways that animals can avoid their predators: (1) blending into the environment, (2) being quiet, and (3) choosing a safe habitat.

BLENDING INTO THE ENVIRONMENT

Naturalists have long recognized that one way for animals to avoid predators is to blend into their environment and become **cryptic**—that is, hidden through camouflaging, making their detection by predators unlikely. This sort of background matching need not be behavioral per se. For example, in a classic natural history study, Francis Sumner found that populations of the mouse *Peromyscus polionotus* matched the background of the beaches on which they lived (Sumner, 1929a, 1929b). Here, individual mice were not behaving in any particular way that increased their crypsis. Instead, natural selection had acted so that "beach mouse" variants of *P. polionotus* had color patterns that matched their environment—in particular, "beach mice" displayed light skin pigmentation that better matched the sand upon which they lived, and pigmentation became darker in populations farther from the beach and closer to the inland areas. Indeed, a single amino acid mutation plays a major role in this example of crypsis (Hoekstra, 2006).

Animals can increase their ability to remain hidden from their prey by behaviorally changing color to match their environment. Cephalopods—which include octopuses, squids, cuttlefish, and nautiluses—are especially adept at quickly changing color to blend into their background, and in so doing, they decrease their chances of being attacked by a predator (Hanlon and Messenger, 1988; Packard, 1972). While most work on camouflage to stay hidden from predators has been conducted during the day or at sunset, Roger Hanlon and his team argued that a great deal of predation on cephalopods may occur at night, as many predators have sharp night vision.

Hanlon and his colleagues used a noninvasive light source—one that relied on a red filter—to observe the nocturnal behavior of the giant Australian cuttlefish (*Sepia apama*), and, in particular, to see whether the cuttlefish used camouflage at night, presumably to hide from predators with good night vision (fur seals, bottlenose dolphins, and some species of fish; Hanlon et al., 2007). The researchers found that cuttlefish were camouflaged in 71 of 83 (86 percent) nocturnal observations. This, of course, is probably an underestimation, because some cuttlefish may have matched the environment so well that the underwater camera employed may simply have missed them. More important than the raw numbers of how often crypsis was uncovered, Hanlon found that cuttlefish could match their background in one of three ways, and, rather remarkably, they could change their color and pattern to match their background in a matter of seconds (unfortunately, the neurobiology and endocrinology of this incredible ability to match their backgrounds is not well understood).

A   **B**   **C**

FIGURE 11.4. Cuttlefish camouflaging. **(A)** Cuttlefish using uniform color to camouflage itself against the rocks, **(B)** cuttlefish using a "mottled" camouflage pattern, with small dark splotches resembling the dark patches on rocks and sand, and **(C)** cuttlefish using a "disruptive" camouflage pattern, with large light and dark areas that enable it to blend in with the background. Arrows indicate where the cuttlefish are located. *(Photo credits: Roger Hanlon)*

The first kind of disguise consisted of a "uniform" camouflage pattern, in which cuttlefish adopted a single color for their skin—a color that matched their background (Figure 11.4). Although this form of camouflage was rare in Hanlon's observations, when it occurred, it often involved a cuttlefish mimicking rocks. The second kind of crypsis made up almost half of the instances of background matches that Hanlon's team uncovered and involved what are called "mottled camouflage" patterns. Here, the cuttlefish changed their appearance such that their skin had small dark and light splotches all over. The size and color of the splotches often mimicked the cuttlefish's background—for example, this patterning is often seen when the background is composed of small rocks and dark algae.

The final form of disguise employed by cuttlefish was "disruptive camouflage." This involved the cuttlefish changing color and pattern, and taking on large light and dark stripes. This had the effect of visually breaking up (disrupting) the animal's body, so it did not look like a cuttlefish. On some occasions, the stripes actually mimicked the pattern of the cuttlefish background, but this was often not the case.

All of these different forms of camouflage techniques support the notion that for large, soft-bodied creatures such as the giant cuttlefish, blending into the environment is an important antipredator behavior (Hanlon and Messenger, 1988).

BEING QUIET

In systems in which predators hone in on sounds made by their prey, one of the simplest things that an animal can do to avoid such predators is to be quiet (Ryan, 1985). With this in mind, Luke Remage-Healey and his colleagues examined the role of sound suppression in the antipredator repertoire of the Gulf toadfish (*Opsanus beta*) (Remage-Healey et al., 2006).

Gulf toadfish are a major food staple of adult bottlenose dolphins (*Tursiops truncatus*), making up 13 percent of the dolphin's diet (Barros, 1993). Prior work had shown that dolphins orient toward the "boatwhistle" sound produced by male toadfish during breeding season (Gannon et al., 2005). That is, dolphins are eavesdropping (see Chapter 14) on the sounds produced by toadfish to better

FIGURE 11.5. Gulf toadfish. Gulf toadfish are preyed upon by bottlenose dolphins. Dolphins orient toward the "boatwhistle" sound produced by male toadfish during the breeding season. *(Photo credit: Midge Marchaterre)*

orient toward their prey. Once a toadfish is located by eavesdropping, the dolphin locks onto this prey and tracks it. Given this, the question Remage-Healey and his colleagues addressed was whether the toadfish respond in kind, listening for sounds associated with bottlenose foraging behavior, and then reducing the boatwhistle sounds they produce (Figure 11.5).

Bottlenose dolphins produce a variety of different sounds, ranging from high-frequency whistles used in dolphin-to-dolphin social communication (not foraging), as well as two sounds that are particularly associated with foraging— "clicks" and low-frequency "pops" (Janik et al., 2006; Nowacek, 2005; Tyack and Clark, 2000). The pops are easiest for toadfish to hear, since this species hears most accurately in the low-frequency range, and so Remage-Healey and his team focused on these dolphin sounds.

The researchers captured toadfish during the breeding season, and they kept individual males in tanks until the breeding season ended. The males soon began to emit boatwhistle sounds, presumably to attract females. At that point, toadfish males were exposed to one of three sounds—the pops associated with dolphin foraging, the high-frequency whistles produced during dolphin social communication, and, as a control, the "snapping" sounds made by snapping shrimp. All sounds were broadcast using underwater speakers, and the activity of toadfish was recorded for the five minutes before sounds were emitted, the five minutes during which the experimental sounds were broadcast, and the five minutes after the sounds were played.

Remage-Healey found clear evidence of antipredator responses when the toadfish heard pop sounds. No differences were found in call rate between males before exposure to the experimental sounds (Figure 11.6). Males exposed to pop sounds, however, reduced their call rates by 50 percent. In addition, males exposed to the pop sounds maintained their reduced calling rate for the five minutes following exposure to pops—that is, they eavesdropped on their predators and reduced their activity in a way that made capture by a dolphin less likely. Males in the other treatments showed no changes in boatwhistle call rate when they heard the recorded sounds.

Remage-Healey and his team followed up their behavioral work on call rates and exposure to predators with a hormonal analysis that examined whether

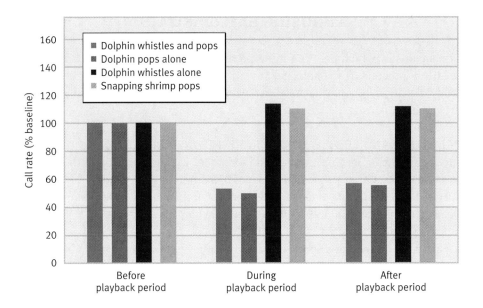

FIGURE 11.6. Gulf toadfish become silent. Gulf toadfish decrease their "boatwhistle" calls when they hear the sounds of bottlenose dolphins. They also continue to reduce their calling rate for a short while following exposure to dolphin pop sounds. *(From Remage-Healey et al., 2006)*

dolphin pops produce a stress response in the toadfish. After experimentally exposing the male toadfish to pops or snapping shrimp sounds, the researchers drew blood from the males, and they measured their cortisol levels. Males exposed to pops not only responded to the pops by reducing their own boatwhistle call, but they also showed higher levels of cortisol than males exposed to the sound of snapping shrimp.

Being quiet in the presence of predators is not unique to toadfish. A similar type of antipredator behavior is displayed by greater wax moths (*Galleria mellonella*) in response to their bat predators (Figure 11.7). Foraging bats emit echolocation pulses, and moths generally reduce their activity when they detect such pulses (Griffin, 1959; Jones et al., 2002; Jones and Holderied, 2007; Jones and Teeling, 2006). Female wax moths, however, face something of a dilemma, in that the temporal and spectral characteristics of bat echolocation pulses are very similar to the sounds produced by courting males.

Male courtship elicits a "wing fanning" behavior by females—a behavior that would make them a more obvious target for bat predators, who can hone in on vibrations associated with wing fanning. Females, then, must be acutely tuned in to the subtle differences between male moth sounds (which should elicit wing fanning) and bat echolocation sounds (which reduce female activity). To examine whether females were able to distinguish between the structurally similar sounds produced by male greater wax moths and bats, Gareth Jones and his colleagues used a playback experiment in which they exposed females to tapes of male great wax moth calls and bat echolocation calls (Jones et al., 2002). They found that females were indeed able to distinguish between these types of calls and responded appropriately—that is, fanning their wings when they heard male calls, but dramatically decreasing this behavior when they heard bat echolocation calls. In addition, females also distinguished between the pulses produced by bats that were searching for prey versus the pulses emitted by bats that were attacking a moth, with the latter producing a greater reduction in wing fanning by female moths.

FIGURE 11.7. Wax moths and predators. Foraging moths typically reduce their activity when bats' echolocation pulses are detected. Despite this, bats do capture some moths, as is about to happen here. *(Photo credit: Image courtesy of Wake Forest University)*

CHOOSING SAFE HABITATS

One means by which prey can avoid predators is by selecting habitats that are relatively predator free (Apfelbach et al., 2005). Here we will look at a case study that involves a phylogenetic perspective on habitat selection and predator avoidance in parrots.

PREDATION AND CHOICE OF NESTING SITES IN PARROTS.   As we learned in the "egg dumping" example discussed in Chapter 2, some birds build their nests in tree cavities. Other birds nest in cavities of a different kind—for example, some species build their nests in old termite mounds, and others, like the white-fronted bee-eaters we discussed in Chapter 8, build cavities into the sides of cliffs. From a phylogenetic perspective, some bird taxa contain both species that nest in tree cavities (TC nesters), and species that nest in other sorts of cavities (let's call them OC "other cavity" nesters). This raises a number of questions: Which of these behavioral states—nesting in tree cavities, or nesting in other sorts of cavities—is the ancestral state? In addition, once we know the ancestral state, what selective force is responsible for the evolution of the other (derived) behavioral state? And especially critical for a discussion of antipredator behavior, did predation drive the choice of nesting area so as to minimize encounters with predators?

Donald Brightsmith addressed these questions in parrot species from two different areas—Australia and the Amazon region. Brightsmith obtained molecular genetic-based phylogenies that contained DNA sequences from six Australian parrot species and dozens of species of Amazon parrots (Brightsmith, 2005; Ribas and Miyaki, 2004; Rowden, 1996; Russello and Amato, 2003). Brightsmith also collected published data on the nesting behavior (TC or OC) of as many of the species in the above-mentioned phylogenies that he could uncover. He then mapped the nesting data onto the phylogenies to examine ancestral and derived nesting behaviors. This analysis showed that the ancestral state was tree cavity nesting, and that nesting in other cavities had evolved independently many times in both Australian and Amazonian parrot species.

Returning to the role of avoiding predators and cavity nesting, Brightsmith used the data he had collected to address the following question: What selective forces were responsible for the evolutionary shift from tree cavity nesting to OC nesting? In particular, ecologists had suggested two possible selective forces driving OC nesting: (1) competition for tree cavity nests is typically quite intense, and so selection in some species may have favored nesting in other sorts of cavities (Beissinger, 1996; Martin, 1993; Monkkonen and Orell, 1997), and (2) predation on eggs and chicks is very high during the nesting period, and shifting from tree cavities to nesting in such places as old termite mounds or the face of cliffs may have decreased predation pressure (Lack, 1968). Predation and competition, of course, are not mutually exclusive, and so both forces may have affected the switch in nesting behavior.

To test for the effects of competition and predation on the shift in nesting behavior, Brightsmith reasoned as follows: Prior work had shown that, when released from competition, an increase in clutch size often occurred over evolutionary time. Having had limited opportunities to find nests in the evolutionary past should favor investing heavily in offspring production—that is, producing large clutches when the opportunity arises. No evidence for increased clutch size was found in OC nesters, providing no support for the competition hypothesis.

To examine whether predation was the key force selecting for the shift away from tree cavity nesting, Brightsmith turned to an idea first suggested by David Lack (Lack, 1968). Lack had hypothesized an inverse correlation between nest predation rate and the length of nesting period, and a large-scale study of 101 North American species found such a correlation (Martin, 1995). As such, Brightsmith hypothesized that if the shift away from tree cavities was due to predation pressure, then OC nesters should have longer nesting periods. And the data on both Amazonian and Australian parrot species do, in fact, show that those species that nest in cavities other than tree cavities have longer nesting periods.

With respect to the Amazonian parrots, Brightside estimates that almost all of the species that rely on cavities other than trees arose in the late Oligocene–early Miocene geological period, 20 to 30 million years ago (Miyaki et al., 1998). South American mammal communities were undergoing a large change at that time, with rapid increases in the number of nest predators, including both tree rats and primates from Africa (Poirier et al., 1994). These nest predators may have been responsible, in part, for the Amazonian parrots' evolutionary shift away from tree cavity nesting.

Brightside's work on OC and TC nesting demonstrates nicely how both phylogenetic and adaptationist approaches can be employed to address questions relating to antipredator behavior.

What to Do When Prey Encounter Predators

Despite the various means by which prey can avoid predators, encounters with such dangers are, over the lifetime of an organism, inevitable (Figure 11.8). In this section, we will examine how animals respond when they do encounter predators. Before we go into detail on specific behaviors, it is important to have an understanding of the sort of neuroendocrinological changes that occur when a predator is encountered. Consider, for example, work by David Smith and his colleagues on the proximate effect of predator odor on mice (Smith et al., 2006). Prior work had shown that

FIGURE 11.8. Encounter with a predator. A scavenging skua gull descends from the air in search of penguin eggs or unattended chicks, while these two gentoo penguins attempt to fend it off. *(Photo credit: Seth Resnick/science faction)*

the frontal cortex area of the brain regulates the effect of stressors on behavior in rodents and humans, and that this area of the brain may alter neurological and endocrinological responses to stressors, such as predators (Amat et al., 2005; Drevets, 2000; Osuch et al., 2000; Spencer et al., 2005). To examine this in more detail, Smith and his team exposed mice to two different stressors. One group of mice was exposed to the odor of a predator—in this case, the predator was a rat, and mice were exposed to bedding that had been soiled by rats. A second group of mice was exposed to a physical stress—these individuals were immobilized in a device with the wonderful name of a Universal Mouse Restrainer (UMR). A third group of control animals was exposed to neither predator odor nor the UMR.

To measure the neuroendocrinological responses to predator stress (as well as UMR stress), the investigators anesthetized the mice prior to the experiment and implanted into their brains a device that allowed the investigators to draw out a small amount of fluid from their prefrontal cortex. The researchers then took fluid samples from the prefrontal cortex of the experimental mice throughout the course of the experiments. Smith and his group found that both predator odor and the UMR increased the circulation of the neurotransmitters acetylcholine, serotonin, and dopamine within the frontal cortex, but that the increase was greatest in response to predator odor.

While it is always difficult to measure whether a predator induces anxiety in nonhumans, Smith and his team did find that when chlordiazepoxide (Librium®), a drug that reduces anxiety in humans, was administered to mice before exposure to the odor of predators, the increases in acetylcholine, serotonin, and dopamine described above disappeared. This suggests that predators may indeed cause anxiety in nonhumans.

Just being exposed to the odor of a predator caused a significant change in the neurological and endocrinological states of the brain in mice—a greater change, in fact, than when they were being physically restrained. Such neuro-endocrinological changes will, in turn, produce antipredator behavior such as reduced foraging, burying for safety, and so on (Campbell et al., 2003; Koolhaas et al., 1999).

While it is not possible to include all possible behaviors that prey use once they encounter a predator, here we shall examine the following five antipredator actions: (1) fleeing, (2) approaching a predator to obtain information, (3) feigning death, (4) signaling to the predator, and (5) attacking (see Chapter 8 for a discussion of another example of antipredator behavior—alarm calling).

FLEEING

The most common response of prey that have spotted a predator is to flee for safety (Lima and Dill, 1990; Lima, 1998; Stankowich and Blumstein, 2005; Ydenberg and Dill, 1986; Figure 11.9). This might involve a squirrel sprinting to its underground den, a bird flying into the trees for safety, a fish heading for cover in a coral reef or, as we shall see in a moment, an embryonic tadpole falling from a branch into the relative safety of the water.

A META-ANALYSIS OF FLIGHT INITIATION BEHAVIOR. Animal behaviorists have measured **flight initiation distance**—that is, how close a predator can approach before prey flee—in a wide variety of species. This is a fairly easy measure for researchers to obtain, both observationally and experimentally,

FIGURE 11.9. Fleeing. The most common response of prey that have spotted a predator is to flee for safety. *(Photo credits: Johnny Johnson/Image Bank; Tom Brakefield/Getty Images; Klaus Nigge/NGS Images; Gerry Ellis/Minden Pictures/Getty Images)*

in part because experimentalists can manipulate predator behavior by using trained animals or through the use of "model" predators (for example, a stuffed hawk flown over an area with pigeons).

Ted Stankowich and Dan Blumstein gathered published data from sixty-one studies of flight initiation in mammals, fish, birds, and reptiles. With this data in hand, Stankowich and Blumstein were able to undertake a meta-analysis across a wide variety of taxa, searching for patterns in flight initiation behavior (Stankowich and Blumstein, 2005). They reviewed studies to see how characteristics of the predator, the physical condition of the prey itself, the prey's environment, and the prey's prior experience with predators affected the prey's decision as to when to flee from a predator.

At the most general level, Stankowich and Blumstein found that animals that were far from some sort of refuge (their territory, for example) initiated fleeing from a predator sooner than animals closer to their refuge. In addition to the distance to safety, the researchers found that animals involved in foraging, mating, or fighting were slower to flee from predators than animals that were not currently involved in such behaviors. That is, when animals were distracted by other activities, they were less alert for predators. These sorts of trade-offs between antipredator behavior and foraging, mating, and so on, are well documented in the literature (Lima and Dill, 1990).

Stankowich and Blumstein found that the predator's size, speed, and the directness of its approach affected the prey's perception of risk. They

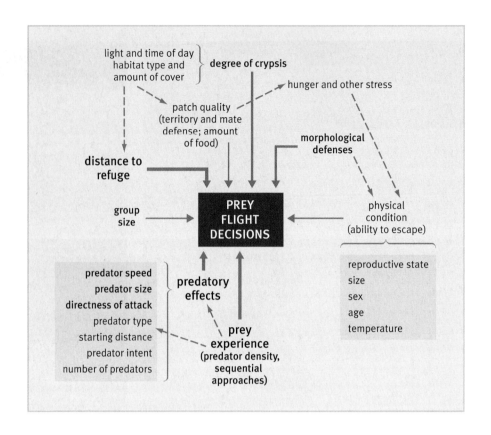

FIGURE 11.10. Flight initiation distance. A summary of the different factors that may influence when an animal decides to flee from a predator. Bolder and larger type and thicker arrows indicate more important factors—that is, there is more evidence for these factors influencing prey flight decisions than for the factors in lighter and smaller type. Dashed lines indicate factors that may have indirect effects on other factors. *(From Stankowich and Blumstein, 2005, p. 2630)*

also examined how morphological traits of the prey affected its behavioral decision of when to flee from a predator. They found that the presence of armor—spines, shells, and so on—reduced a prey's perception of risk. That is, at a given distance, armored animals were not as likely to flee from a predator as prey without armor. They also found that the prey's ability to camouflage itself (cryptic coloration) affected its flight decision. Other factors affecting its decision included the quality of the habitat and the physical condition of the prey (how hungry it was, its size and age, whether it was pregnant, whether it was defending young offspring), but more research is needed to investigate how important these factors are.

Stankowich and Blumstein found that experience and learning played a strong role in when prey initiated flight—prey typically flee at a greater distance as a function of experience with predators. For example, Larry Dill found that zebrafish that had experienced a predator fled at a greater distance from the predator than fish that had no experience with the predator (Dill, 1974). As a second, more practical example, published work suggests that animals flee humans at a greater distance during hunting season compared with during other times of the year (Fox and Madsen, 1997; Smits and Visser, 1993).

Across many diverse taxa, then, the behavioral decision of when to flee from a predator is affected by a suite of factors, but especially includes attributes of the predator (predatory effects), experience with the predator in question, the distance to safety, and the presence or absence of armor (Figure 11.10).

TREEFROG EMBRYOS AND SNAKES. While we tend to think of the anti-predator options available to embryos as limited, some research suggests that even embryos can, in a sense, flee from predation. As a case study of this phenomena, let us examine Karen Warkentin's work on red-eyed treefrogs

A   **B**

FIGURE 11.11. Predators that feed on treefrogs. Red-eyed treefrogs have numerous predators that specialize in feeding on their eggs. **(A)** Here a wasp forages on treefrog eggs. **(B)** Snakes are another dangerous predator on red-eyed treefrog eggs. *(Photo credits: Karen Warkentin)*

(*Agalychnis callidryas*) of Panama and their predators to see how natural selection can produce fleeing behavior on the part of embryos—a behavior that, in fact, lessens their risk of encountering predators (Warkentin, 2000).

Red-eyed treefrogs attach their eggs to the various types of vegetation that hang over water. As soon as eggs hatch, the tadpoles that emerge drop down into their aquatic habitat. Both the terrestrial habitat of the egg/embryo and the aquatic habitat of the tadpole have a set of dangerous, but different, predators that forage on treefrogs. If terrestrial predation from snakes and wasps is weak, eggs hatch late in the season (Warkentin, 1995, 1999; Figure 11.11). This serves two functions: First, it maximizes the time that the eggs/embryos are in a low-predator terrestrial habitat, and second, such late hatching allows the embryos to grow to a size that lowers the levels of fish predation once the eggs finally hatch and the tadpoles fall into the water.

Based on the results of some mathematical models, Warkentin predicted that treefrog eggs would hatch sooner if predation in the terrestrial environment increased. That is, natural selection should favor embryos that avoid terrestrial predators when such predators are at high frequencies (compared with the aquatic predators that feed on treefrogs; Warkentin, 2000). Both snakes and wasps are terrestrial predators on treefrog eggs—wasps feed on one egg at time, while snakes can eat entire clutches. When predation from snakes and wasps is high, it often pays to mature early and drop into the water, away from heavy terrestrial predation.

To test this idea, Warkentin marked 123 egg clutches of treefrog eggs. She found that less than half the eggs she kept track of survived to hatch, with the majority falling prey to wasp attacks. The question of interest then is whether the eggs that survived responded by hatching and having the emerging tadpoles "flee" by dropping to the water. Warkentin found that eggs in clutches that were not disturbed by predators often hatched at about six days. When comparing eggs from these undisturbed clutches to those clutches that had already suffered some predation by wasps, Warkentin found that hatching rates were dramatically different. Eggs hatched at a much quicker rate when their clutch had been the victim of some wasp predation, with most eggs from attacked clutches hatching at four or five days (as opposed to six) (Figure 11.12). Indeed,

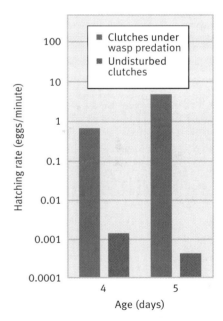

FIGURE 11.12. Wasp predation and development time. Red-eyed treefrogs respond to wasp predation by hatching early. Green bars represent hatching time of clutches that suffered some wasp predation, while orange bars indicate undisturbed clutches. Embryos are capable of hatching sometime during day 4. *(Based on Warkentin, 2000)*

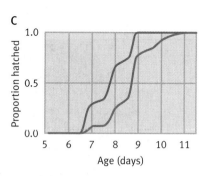

FIGURE 11.13. Snake predation and development time. Red-eyed treefrogs also respond to snake predation by hatching earlier than normal. Clutches attacked by the snake *Leptodeira septentrionalis* at **(A)** five days old and **(B)** six days old. **(C)** Clutches that were undisturbed by predation. *(Based on Warkentin, 1995)*

FIGURE 11.14. Sounds from red-eyed treefrog nests. Sounds recorded as waveform graphs at the nest of a red-eyed treefrog. **(A)** A *Leptophis* snake attacks and eats an entire clutch of eggs in a long sequence in which it bites clumps of eggs and then pulls back. **(B)** A segment of a *Leptodeira* snake attack in which the snake eats one or two eggs in a short series of bites. **(C)** A rainstorm. *(From Warkentin, 2005, p. 62)*

some embryos in clutches that were attacked ruptured their eggs, hatched, and dropped off branches immediately after such attacks. Remarkably similar results were found when examining the effect of snake predation on hatching rates (Figure 11.13).

Warkentin's work on predator avoidance raises an interesting question about proximate cues. What specific cues do the treefrog embryos use to determine when to shift from terrestrial to aquatic habitats? That is, we know that if the developing embryos survive an attack by snakes, survivors drop off branches into the water, but what specific cues are they honing in on? Warkentin hypothesized that the embryos may be using the vibrational cues associated with snake attacks as the proximate cue for when to switch from terrestrial habitats to aquatic ones.

To test her hypothesis, Warkentin released a snake into a cage and, using a device called an accelerometer, she recorded the vibrations associated with this predator. Because Warkentin hypothesized that the vibrations associated with snake attacks—and not just vibrations in general—were the key to a habitat shift away from predators, she also recorded a different vibrational cue. In this case, she recorded the vibrations associated with rainfall. She then played back vibrational recordings of two kinds of snake attacks and of a rainstorm to clutches of developing treefrog eggs (Figure 11.14). As predicted, the cues associated with snakes resulted in treefrogs that hatched earlier than treefrogs that had been played the recording with rainstorm cues (Warkentin, 2005; Warkentin et al., 2006, 2007).

APPROACHING PREDATORS

While prey often flee from their predators, surprisingly animals sometimes approach predators when they initially encounter them. Typically, this approach behavior allows prey to gather important information about putative predators, and hence reduces their chances of mortality. Approach behavior is often undertaken by healthy adults, but it is not limited to this group. This type of behavior has been extensively documented in vertebrates, particularly in fish, birds, and mammals, and it has been referred to in the literature as approach behavior, boldness, investigative behavior, or predator inspection behavior (Curio et al., 1978; Dugatkin and Godin, 1992; Pitcher et al., 1986). Here, we will examine two examples: approach behavior in gazelles and predator inspection behavior in minnows.

Among vertebrates, the dynamics of approach toward a potential predator are quite similar. Prey typically approach a potential predator from a distance in a tentative, jerky manner. The approach is characterized by a series of moves toward the predator interrupted by stationary pauses and sometimes alternating with moves away from the predator (Curio et al., 1983; Dugatkin, 1997a; Milinski, 1987; Pitcher et al., 1986). The approach may culminate in a number of possible outcomes along a continuum, ranging from the prey simply retreating, to rejoining a social group of conspecifics nearby, to an escalation in which prey actually attack the predator (see more on escalation below).

For this sort of antipredator approach behavior to evolve and to be maintained in a population, the average fitness benefits accrued must equal or exceed the associated average fitness costs. To investigate these costs and benefits, we turn to work on Thomson's gazelles.

THE COSTS AND BENEFITS OF THOMSON'S GAZELLES APPROACHING A PREDATOR. Using natural populations of Thomson's gazelles as her experimental subjects, Clare Fitzgibbon undertook one of the most thorough analyses of the costs and benefits of approach behavior (Fitzgibbon, 1994; Figure 11.15). In the Serengeti National Park (in Tanzania), gazelles live in groups that can vary from fairly small (< 10 individuals) to fairly large (> 500), and they interact with four main predators: lions, cheetahs, spotted hyenas, and wild dogs. While we will focus on the predators that gazelles in fact do approach (lions and cheetahs), it is interesting to note that gazelles rarely approach wild dogs and hyenas. This difference appears to be primarily due to the fact that cheetahs and lions rely on surprise and short, fast chases, while wild dogs and hyenas rely on stamina. Approaching the former group may be wise, while approaching the latter is often a surefire invitation to a hunt.

With respect to the benefits of approaching a predator, Fitzgibbon examined three possible scenarios:

A   **B**

FIGURE 11.15. Gazelle antipredator behavior. (A) Gazelles are constantly vigilant for potential predators. **(B)** Many different species, including the cheetah (pictured here chasing a gazelle) hunt gazelles. *(Photo credits: Gerald and Buff Corsi/Visuals Unlimited; Joe McDonald/Visuals Unlimited)*

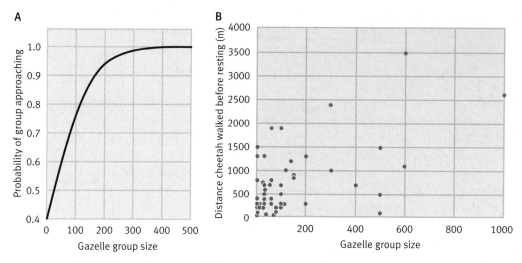

FIGURE 11.16. Approach behavior in gazelles. (A) The probability of approach behavior occurring in gazelles is a function of group size, as indicated by the logistic curve. **(B)** Cheetahs respond to gazelle approach behavior. The distance a cheetah moved away in response to gazelle approach behavior is a function of the gazelles' group size. *(Based on Fitzgibbon, 1994)*

> Approach behavior might decrease the current risk of predation.
> Approach behavior might allow gazelles to gather information about a potential threat.
> Approach behavior might serve to warn other group members of the potential danger associated with predators.

In the course of her two-year field study, Fitzgibbon found some evidence for benefit 1. In particular, she found that cheetahs responded to gazelle inspection behavior, which is most common and most pronounced in large gazelle groups (Figure 11.16A), by moving farther between rest periods and between hunting periods (Figure 11.16B). This in turn could cause cheetahs to leave a particular area sooner than normal as a result of gazelle approach behavior, leading to decreased rates of mortality among potential prey.

The cost of gazelle approach behavior is manifested primarily in terms of lost time/energy. Through detailed behavioral observations, researchers determined that gazelles actually spend approximately 4 percent of their waking hours involved in approach behavior. This 4 percent could otherwise be devoted to other activities (for example, foraging, mating, resting), and thus it represents a real "opportunity cost" to the animals. While this is not the detailed quantitative data on costs one would ideally like to have, the opportunity cost approach, especially when dealing with a behavior that takes up a real proportion of an animal's time, is a step in the right direction. And it may be the best animal behaviorists can do when working in the field on predator-prey systems involving large, long-lived mammals that are difficult to track over long distances. That said, Fitzgibbon's work on approach behavior represents one of the few cases in which the benefits and costs to approach behavior have been studied in the wild.

INTERPOPULATIONAL DIFFERENCES IN APPROACH BEHAVIOR IN MINNOWS.

Anne Magurran and her colleagues have examined antipredator behavior in two different populations of minnows (*Phoxinus phoxinus*). Minnows from the Dorset area of southern England and the Gwynedd area of northern Wales were chosen for study, as the Dorset population is under strong predation pressure from pike predators, while pike are absent from the Gwynedd population of minnows (and have apparently never colonized this area) (Magurran and Pitcher, 1987; Figure 11.17).

Both populations of minnows increased their group size when faced with predators in the laboratory, but the Dorset population tended to maintain larger groups. With respect to approaching predators, Dorset minnows engaged in predator inspection more often than did Gwynedd minnows, but they were also much more likely to stop inspecting if a conspecific was eaten by a pike (Figure 11.18). For our purposes here, we will focus on whether these discrepancies between the inspection behavior of the Dorset population, which co-evolved in the presence of pike, and the Gwynedd population, which did not, are a result of natural selection operating differently across these groups.

To address this question, adult minnows from Gwynedd and Dorset populations were captured in the wild, and their offspring were raised in the laboratory (Magurran, 1990). Four treatments were undertaken. In treatments 1 and 2, at two months of age, offspring from Gwynedd and Dorset minnows were exposed to a "model" pike predator (constructed from wood, but made to be a realistic representation of a predator) five times during development, and their antipredator behaviors were recorded. In treatments 3 and 4, rearing conditions were identical, except that no minnows in these treatments were exposed to the model predator.

When researchers compared the antipredator behavior of two-month-old fish exposed to predators, they found that young Dorset minnows differed from young Gwynedd minnows in the same manner uncovered in Magurran's earlier work (using wild fish). Dorset minnows inspected more often and tended to be found in larger groups, suggesting that natural selection has produced significant differences in antipredator behavior across these two

FIGURE 11.17. A population of minnows. Minnows from high-predation and low-predation areas respond very differently when confronted with a potential predator. For example, Gwynedd minnows (those from the low-predation site) totally ceased foraging and eating in the presence of a predator. In contrast, Dorset minnows (those from the high-predation site), who are used to foraging in the face of danger, curtailed their foraging activity, but not nearly to the extent of Gwynedd minnows. *(Photo credit: Melvin Grey)*

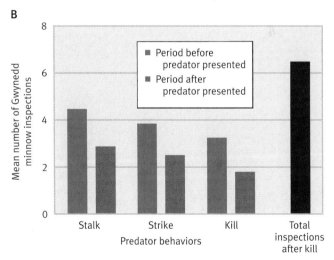

FIGURE 11.18. Inspection across populations. (A) Dorset minnows respond to pike behaviors (stalk, strike, kill another group member) by decreasing their predator inspection behavior, while **(B)** no statistically significant decrease in inspections occurs in the Gwynedd minnow population. *(Based on Magurran and Pitcher, 1987)*

FIGURE 11.19. Reaction to predators. (A) Population differences in inspection behavior were found when comparing two-month-old minnows, who had never before been exposed to a predator, from high-predation (Dorset) and low-predation (Gwynedd) sites. **(B)** Population differences in schooling behavior were also found in two-month-old inexperienced fish originating from high-predation (Dorset) and low-predation (Gwynedd) sites. *(Based on Magurran, 1990)*

populations (Figure 11.19). The story, however, is more complex, and hence it is more interesting.

After raising the minnows in the laboratory for a total of two years, Magurran examined the antipredator tactics of minnows in these four groups. The differences found in two-month-old Dorset and Gwynedd populations were also found in two-year-old fish, but experience also played a key role. That is, while all Dorset fish (experienced and inexperienced) inspected more and in larger groups than all Gwynedd minnows, there were also interesting between-population differences in the role that experience played in shaping antipredator behavior. In both populations, experienced adults inspected more often than inexperienced adults, but this difference was most pronounced in Dorset fish.

Natural selection seems to have operated in one, and perhaps two, ways on antipredator behavior in minnows. First, as a result of differences in predation pressure, Dorset and Gwynedd fish have genetically based differences in the antipredator tactics they employ. Second, it may be that selection has actually selected for stronger responses based on experience in the Dorset population of minnows from high-predation areas. As such, the minnow inspection experiment allows us to see how both the process of natural selection (across generations) and learning (within generations) can shape antipredator behavior.

FEIGNING DEATH

Faking, or feigning, death is an antipredator behavior seen across a spectrum of species. This behavior is expressed slightly across taxa, but because we shall focus on feigning death in insects, we shall adopt the definition most often applied to this group. Death feigning occurs in insects when, in response to a predator, an insect falls down and then remains frozen—that is, motionless (sometime referred to as tonic immobility) (Miyatake et al., 2004; Ruxton et al., 2004).

Tatsunori Ohno and Takahisa Miyatake have done extensive work on feigning death in the adzuki bean beetle (*Callosobruchus chinensis*) (Ohno and Miyatake, 2007). In this species, when a beetle is on a branch and a predator approaches, beetles can either fly away or feign death, but they cannot do both at the same time. Ohno and Miyatake hypothesized that a negative genetic correlation existed between the intensity of death feigning and the ability to fly—that is, they hypothesized that those beetles that feigned death for a long period of time would be poor flyers, and that those beetles that feigned death for shorter time periods would be especially good flyers.

Ohno and Miyatake first established two assays—one for feigning death and one for flying ability. For the former, they simply exposed beetles to danger and measured how long the beetles remained frozen, feigning death. For the assay on flying ability, they dropped a beetle through a hole into a cube-shaped apparatus that had a grid on its bottom. The researchers measured whether the beetle dropped straight down (poor flyer), or whether it flew away as it was falling and how far it flew (on a scale of 1–6). Once these assays were established, Ohno and Miyatake ran a classic artificial selection experiment with two treatments. In one treatment—the death-feigning (DF) treatment—a random sample of 100 flies was selected, and the researchers measured the duration of death feigning for each fly. In the second treatment, the researchers selected flies based on their flying abilities.

Two genetic "lines" were established within the DF treatment. In the "long duration" line, the fourteen individuals (seven males and seven females) that displayed the longest duration of death feigning were selected and allowed to breed with one another. In the "short duration line," the fourteen individuals (seven males and seven females) with the shortest duration of death feigning were selected and allowed to breed with one another. This was repeated for eight generations—that is, in each generation of the short duration line, the seven males and seven females with the shortest times for feigning death were selected. The same process of selection and breeding of the seven males and seven females with the longest times for feigning death occurred over eight generations of the long duration line.

Not surprisingly, eight generations of strong artificial selection on death feigning produced dramatic differences between the selected lines (Figure 11.20). Individuals in the long duration line showed death-feigning times that were about forty times as long as those in the short generation line. More critically, Ohno and Miyatake found a negative genetic correlation between death feigning and flying abilities. Individuals in the long duration line were very poor flyers, and, conversely, individuals in the short duration line were adept flyers. In other words, this experiment demonstrated a trade-off in terms of antipredator behavior—good flyers were poor at death feigning and poor flyers were good at feigning death—and this trade-off could be seen at the genetic level.

Ohno and Miyatake also ran a second artificial selection experiment. This time, they created two genetic lines—one in which the best flyers (BF) in every generation bred with one another, and a second in which the worst flyers (WF) bred with one another. Remarkably, the same negative genetic correlation found in the DF treatment was uncovered here. That is, after eight generations, the beetles in the BF were not only superb flyers, but they displayed very short death-feigning times. Conversely, the beetles in the WF treatment were very poor flyers, but they displayed death feigning for long periods of time.

Ohno and Miyatake's artificial selection experiments are an excellent example of how animal behaviorists can employ classic experimental protocols from genetics to better understand the trade-offs associated with different forms of antipredator behavior, as well as the genetics underlying this trade-off.

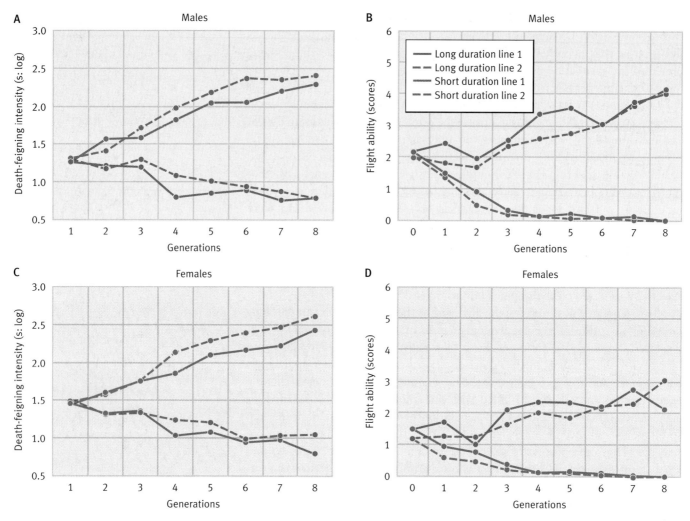

FIGURE 11.20. Selection for death feigning. Data from two replications (replicate 1 and replicate 2) of the long-duration and short-duration selection experiments on death feigning in the adzuki bean beetle. The death-feigning response is shown in males **(A)** and females **(C)**. The long duration lines are in green, and the short duration lines are in orange. There is a negative correlation with flying ability when selection is on death feigning (those who are good at feigning death are poor flyers; those who are poor at feigning death are good flyers) in males **(B)** and females **(D)**. Points on solid lines represent data from the first replicate; points on dashed lines represent data from the second replicate. *(From Ohno and Miyatake, 2007, p. 558)*

SIGNALING TO PREDATORS

Prey sometimes attempt to transmit signals to a predator regarding either the probability that they will be captured, or the consequences of such capture. For example, prey may transmit information to a predator, warning the predator about the dangers of contact, or that it has been sighted and will not succeed in capturing a prey, which may deter predator attack. These signals are often visual but they can also be auditory, as in the case of tiger moths that can produce warning sounds that cause bats to avoid them because they learn to associate the sounds with a noxious taste (Barber and Conner, 2007). Here we will consider two case studies of signaling: (1) warning coloration in monarch butterflies, and (2) tail flagging in ungulates.

WARNING COLORATION IN MONARCH BUTTERFLIES. As caterpillars, monarch butterflies (*Danaus plexippus*) ingest milkweed plants, which contain chemicals called cardiac glycosides. These chemicals, which are toxic to birds, do not harm the monarchs, and instead are sequestered by the butterflies—that is, they are stored in the tissue. When a naive bird predator eats a monarch, the toxins in the butterfly make the predator violently ill—temporarily (Figure 11.21). From that point forward, the color patterns of monarchs act as warning coloration for *that* predator who now avoids feeding upon monarchs. Such birds have learned to associate monarch color with illness.

It can be confusing to understand how natural selection acts on the prey to have the sort of warning coloration that we see in monarchs. If a naive predator must eat a monarch to learn how dangerous monarchs are, how could selection ever favor the monarch ingesting milkweeds and possessing a distinctive color pattern? That is, how could natural selection favor a trait in which the individual in possession of the trait must die for the predator to learn about the danger? There are a number of ways that this could occur, but here let us consider just one of these. The predator does not always kill the monarch before it senses the toxin (touching the monarch may be enough to alert the predator to the presence of the toxin). What this means is that the presence of the toxin and warning coloration may save the life even of a prey that is the victim of a naive predator's first encounter with a monarch.

TAIL FLAGGING AS A SIGNAL. Some animals send signals that may serve to notify a predator that it has been spotted. When the predator is an ambush hunter that relies on surprise, such a signal often causes it to move on and leave the area, and hence clearly benefits the prey. Even when predators aren't strictly ambush hunters, prey may still benefit by signaling predators if signals reduce the probability of capture. Consider tail flagging in ungulates, where individuals

A

B
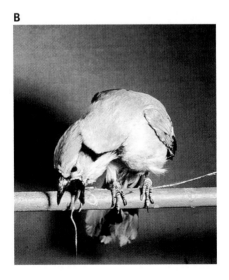

FIGURE 11.21. Monarch warning colors. (A) A bluejay holding the wing of a monarch butterfly that it is about to eat, and **(B)** a bluejay vomiting after eating a monarch butterfly. *(Photo credits: Lincoln Brower)*

FIGURE 11.22. Tail-raising event. In white-tailed deer, individuals often display a white patch while running from danger. At least a half dozen hypotheses have been put forth to explain the function of the patch. *(Photo credit: Gary Carter/ Visuals Unlimited)*

"flag" their tails after a predator has been sighted (Figure 11.22). Such flagging occurs as part of a sequence of antipredator behaviors, and often it involves an individual lifting its tail and "flashing" a conspicuous white rump patch. Flagging often, but not always, occurs when a predator is at a relatively safe distance from its potential prey (Hirth and McCullough, 1977).

In principle, tail flagging could serve many different functions. At various points in time, animal behaviorists have hypothesized that this behavior might: (1) warn conspecifics (both kin and nonkin) about the presence of a predator (Estes and Goddard, 1967), (2) "close ranks" and tighten group cohesion, which might make predation less likely (Kitchen, 1972; McCullough, 1969; Smith, 1991) and ensure group-related foraging and antipredator benefits in the future (Smith, 1986; Trivers, 1971), (3) signal to the predator that it has been sighted and should therefore abandon any attack (Caro, 1995a; Caro et al., 1995; Woodland et al., 1980), (4) entice the predator to attack from a greater distance, which is likely to result in an aborted attempt (Smythe, 1977), (5) cause other group members to engage in various antipredator activities, thereby confusing the predator, and making the flagger himself less likely to be the victim of an attack (Charnov and Krebs, 1975), or (6) serve as a sign for appeasing dominant group members, and only secondarily play a role in antipredator behavior (Guthrie, 1971).

Some evidence supports the hypothesis that tail flagging causes an increase in group cohesion (Bildstein, 1983; Hirth and McCullough, 1977; Smith, 1991), but here we will focus on the question of whether tail flagging is a signal to the predator. This "pursuit-deterrence" hypothesis about signals is supported by Tim Caro's work on white-tailed deer, as well as the work of other researchers (Bildstein, 1983; Caro, 1994b; Caro et al., 2004; Woodland et al., 1980). Caro and his colleagues found no evidence for a time cost to flagging—that is, flagging did not slow down prey—and no evidence that tail flagging was aimed at conspecifics in the context of cohesion. Rather, they showed that white-tailed deer that run fast flag their tails and are using this signal to communicate to the predator that an attack is unlikely to succeed because the fleeing deer will escape a pursuing predator. This sort of pursuit-deterrence signal is not limited to white-tailed deer or to tail flagging. For example, in a phylogenetic study involving 200 species and seventeen antipredator behaviors, Caro and his colleagues found that, in ungulates, snorting also serves as a signal to predators (Caro et al., 2004). This signal deters attack, presumably because snorting indicates the health and vigor of the signaler.

The monarch butterfly example and the work on tail flagging demonstrate how both morphological and behavioral traits work as signals that have an antipredatory function in nature. These signals warn predators against making attacks that will not succeed or that will have aversive consequences for the predator.

FIGHTING BACK

Although prey are typically physically smaller and weaker than their predators, that does not mean that they lack adaptations designed to help them fight back when their life is in danger. Here we will examine two such adaptations: chemical defense in beetles and mobbing behavior in birds.

CHEMICAL DEFENSE IN BEETLES. Thomas Eisner and his colleagues have demonstrated how bombardier beetles use chemical weapons to defend themselves against predators, including swarming ants, orb-weaving spiders, and toads (Dean, 1980a, 1980b; Eisner and Dean, 1976). In the bombardier beetle, *Stenaptinus insignis*, individuals blast potential predators with a highly noxious spray (Eisner and Aneshansley, 1982, 1999; Eisner et al., 2000). A beetle can discharge its acidic spray twenty times before depleting its supply of chemicals.

Production of *S. insignis*'s noxious spray is an act of engineering brilliance. These beetles have two glands, each of which has two separate compartments. The larger compartment in a gland is referred to as the reservoir, and it contains hydroquanines and hydrogen peroxide. The smaller compartment, called the reaction chamber, holds a variety of catalases and peroxidases. When they are threatened by a predator, bombardier beetles allow the contents of the two compartments to mix, causing a chemical reaction that produces an acidic spray composed of acidic and very noxious *p*-benzoquinones. The heat produced by this chemical reaction causes an audible pop, and the spray shoots out at a temperature of 100° C. Somehow, and it is not yet known how, the beetles themselves are not injured by their own noxious sprays, but predators are.

S. insignis does more than just produce an acidic spray that is released when a predator attacks. Using high-speed photography, Eisner and Daniel Aneshansley have shown that the beetles are quite adept at selectively aiming this spray at predators. That is, when they are attacked from the front, they fire the spray forward; when attacked from the rear, they fire the spray backward, and so on (Eisner and Aneshansley, 1999; Figure 11.23).

How did such a successful, but complicated, antipredator mechanism evolve? Eisner and his team are still working on that, but they have found a clue in the spray mechanism of the most phylogenetically ancient of the bombardier beetles, *Metrius contractus* (Eisner et al., 2000). Like other bombardier species, it has a reservoir that contains hydroquanines and hydrogen peroxide and a reaction chamber that holds a variety of catalases and peroxidases, suggesting that possession of these traits is an ancestral characteristic. Unlike other species, however, which often discharge their defensive spray as a jet, *M. contractus*'s spray is discharged as a fine mist. Again using high-speed photography, the researchers examined emission of this spray in more detail.

Eisner and his colleagues found that *M. contractus* emits its spray in a unique manner. When it is attacked from the rear, it produces a froth secretion, which builds up on the body of the beetle and wards off predators. When a beetle is attacked from the front, instead of spraying its attacker, it forces the chemical secretion it produces forward, along tracks on its forewings. Although it is not clear why, these mechanisms of discharging chemical weapons appear to lower the temperature of the disseminating chemicals from 100° C to approximately 55° C. This work on *M. contractus* suggests that spraying an extremely hot chemical secretion is a derived trait, whereas frothing and using the forewing tracks to disseminate a somewhat reduced heat spray represent the ancestral version of chemical defense in bombardiers.

Eisner and his team's work shows nicely how animal behaviorists (in this case, in conjunction with collaborators in chemistry) can: (1) study the function of a trait, (2) break down the complex anatomical and chemical underpinning of that same trait, and (3) use comparative studies to understand the evolution of behavior.

FIGURE 11.23. Bombardier defenses. When the bombardier beetle, *Stenaptinus insignis*, is threatened, it releases chemicals that ward off predators. This bombardier beetle is being attacked from the front, and so it is directing its chemical spray forward. *(Photo credit: Thomas Eisner)*

SOCIAL LEARNING AND MOBBING IN BLACKBIRDS. Chemical weapons are only one way prey can counterattack their predators. Blackbirds (*Turdus merula*), like many other bird species, undertake a form of attack called predator **mobbing** (Altmann, 1956; Sordahl, 1990). Once a flock of blackbirds spots a predator, they join together, fly toward the danger, and aggressively attempt to chase it away. Such group attacks often work well enough to force predators to leave the blackbirds' area.

Eberhard Curio and his colleagues examined whether young, predator-naive blackbirds learn what constitutes a predator by watching which species is mobbed, and classifying such a species as predators (Curio et al., 1978). In other words, is mobbing a form of cultural transmission that is useful in the context of antipredator activities? To examine this, Curio and his colleagues ran a fascinating laboratory experiment on mobbing.

In each trial of their experiment, Curio's team began with a "model" and "naive" bird, each in its own aviary. The experimental apparatus was designed so that each of the blackbirds could see another bird—a noisy friarbird (*Philemon corniculatus*). The friarbird was a species that neither the model nor the naive blackbird had seen before. Furthermore, it looked nothing like any known predator of blackbirds. The friarbird was presented in such a way that the naive blackbird saw the friarbird alone, but the model saw both a friarbird and, adjacent to it, a real predator of blackbirds—a little owl, *Athena noctua*. From the viewpoint of the naive subject, the little owl was out of sight. In other words, when the model mobbed the little owl, the naive individual saw it mobbing a friarbird.

Curio's team found that, once naive blackbirds had seen a model apparently mobbing a friarbird, the naive blackbirds themselves were much more likely to mob this odd new creature than if they had not been exposed to the model. The information about what constitutes a danger, then, was transmitted culturally. The researchers then took the experiment one step further and asked whether the (now not so naive) subject would act as a model for a new naive blackbird. And if that worked, how many times could they get a former naive blackbird to successfully act as a model? In other words, how long is the "cultural transmission chain" in blackbirds? The longer such chains are, the more powerful cultural transmission may be in spreading antipredator behaviors through a population. Though their sample was small, Curio and his colleagues found that the blackbird cultural transmission chain was at least six birds long. That is, after the initial model (bird 1) perceived friarbirds as being dangerous, a new model (bird 2) then saw bird 1 respond to friarbirds. If bird 2 then responded as if friarbirds were dangerous, a new model (bird 3) then observed bird 2 respond to the friarbird as a predator. This procedure went on until six different birds acted as if the friarbird were a predator, and then the "chain" was broken.

Curio's work on mobbing has implications not only for the study of antipredator behavior per se, but for conservation biology as well. In particular, many conservation "reintroduction" programs—in which animals raised in captivity are placed back into their natural habitat—fail. Researchers believe one critical reason for such failures is that animals need to learn about predators—sometimes by social learning—and that such opportunities are absent in captivity. A number of reintroduction studies using fish, marsupials, birds, and mammals have built on the work by Curio. In these studies, conservation biologists teach captive animals to learn what is dangerous and what isn't, and one part of the protocol involves watching trained animals respond to danger (Ferrari et al., 2006a, 2006b; McLean et al., 1996, 1999, 2000; Shier and Owings, 2006; Suboski, 1990; Suboski and Templeton, 1989).

Predation and Foraging Trade-offs

Ethologists who study antipredator tactics focus on "trade-offs" more than on any specific behavior. That is, when animals spend time engaged in antipredator activity, they could in principle, be doing something else— foraging, mating, resting, playing, and so forth (Lima and Dill, 1990; Figure 11.24). Or, rather than totally curtailing alternative behavior, antipredator behavior could be creating pressure to perform other behaviors in a different manner—for example, to forage in the vicinity of a refuge, to mate at times when predation is minimal, and so on. In either case, trade-offs between some other behavior and antipredator tactics are often a fact of life when it comes to animal behavior.

Foraging is one of the behaviors especially affected by predation. Predation pressure affects virtually every aspect of foraging—everything from when a forager begins feeding (Clarke, 1983; Lima, 1988a, 1988b), to when it resumes feeding after an interruption (De Laet, 1985; Hegner, 1985), where it feeds (Dill, 1983; Ekman and Askenmo, 1984; Lima, 1985; Schneider, 1984), what it eats (Dill and Fraser, 1984; Hay and Fuller, 1981; Lima and Valone, 1986) to how it handles its prey (Krebs, 1980; Valone and Lima, 1987). As an example, let us consider Steven Lima and Thomas Valone's work on predation and

FIGURE 11.24. Foraging-predation trade-off. When animals are being vigilant for predators, it is often at the cost of other activities. The starlings here can't be foraging for insects while they scan the sky for hawks.

INTERVIEW WITH

Dr. Anne Magurran

Why study antipredator behavior in animals? Are there unique aspects about this sort of behavior?

Predation risk is an uncompromising form of natural selection. An animal that is captured by a predator will be unable to reproduce, so any activity or response that increases an individual's chances of survival is favored. The study of antipredator behavior can therefore tell us a lot about the process of evolution. But it is not simply a matter of prey evolving skills that allow them to evade predators more effectively. Predators will also experience selection to improve their capture success rate. This is sometimes called an "arms race" since better defenses are countered by improved hunting tactics, which in turn will select for improved antipredator behavior. I particularly like Darwin's description of this co-evolutionary game: "Wonderful and admirable as most instincts are, yet they cannot be considered as absolutely perfect: there is a constant struggle going on throughout nature between the instinct of the one to escape its enemy and of the other to secure its prey."

Interpopulational comparisons have proved particularly useful in terms of understanding the evolution of antipredator behavior. Why is that?

I believe there are two main reasons why interpopulational comparisons have been so productive. First, when we compare populations we are, to a large extent, comparing like with like. An investigation of the antipredator behavior of,

say, blackbirds and robins could be confounded by all the other biological and ecological differences between the species. An intraspecies investigation, on the other hand, looks at groups of organisms that are broadly similar. It is a particularly powerful means of understanding the evolution of antipredator behavior

when the degree of predation risk is the single most important thing that differentiates populations. Moreover, if there are multiple populations experiencing each level of predation risk, then we can, by virtue of this replication, be even more confident that the variation in behavior that we observe is related to the activities of predators as opposed to some other variable (such as the history of the population or the temperature of the environment).

Trinidadian guppies, *Poecilia reticulata*, are a classic example of an interpopulational comparison. A number of rivers draining Trinidad's Northern Range have barrier waterfalls that have prevented

predators, though not guppies, from moving upstream. This means that the behavioral characteristics of guppy populations separated by very small distances, and exposed to similar ecological conditions, but differing in the types and numbers of predators that they coexist with, can be attributed to predation. It is also possible to perform simple manipulations in the wild, in which predators are added to, or removed from populations, to show that a shift in predation risk does indeed result in heritable change—i.e., evolution—of behavior.

The second reason why interpopulational differences are so illuminating is that changes in predation risk—and hence evolution—can be tracked over relatively short time scales. In guppies, for instance, a change in escape response is detectable within about 15 years of a shift in predation risk. I suspect that behavioral evolution occurs even more quickly than this in the guppy system—no one has looked carefully yet.

What is the most dramatic example of antipredator behavior that you know of?

There are many impressive antipredator behaviors and it is difficult to select a single example, but I think that the evasion tactics of schooling fish are particularly dramatic. Hundreds, or sometimes many thousands, of individuals engage in choreographed maneuvers, such as the flash expansion [in which tightly packed schools of fish "explode," and the fish swim off in all directions], that confuse and outwit their predators. Although it was originally thought that these seemingly cooperative tactics were for the "good of the species," we now know that they are underpinned by individual selection, and that the complex formations that emerge are based on simple decision rules. Unfortunately, this behavior offers little protection against modern fishing vessels since these are equipped with technology to locate and capture large shoals of fish.

Initially a great deal of work on predation focused on foraging/predation trade-offs. How would you summarize the findings from these studies?

One way of looking at this is in relation to what Richard Dawkins and John Krebs called the life-dinner principle. In other words, selection on an individual to remain alive is greater than the selection to find the next meal. So, all other things being equal, animals should invest more in predator avoidance than foraging. However, choices are rarely that simple. An individual that spent all its time in a refuge might avoid predators but would sooner or later die of starvation. This leads to a trade-off between the conflicting demands of foraging and predator avoidance. One resolution of this conflict is for an animal to select the habitat that allows it to minimize the risk of mortality (μ) while maximizing growth rate (g), typically by minimizing the ratio μ/g. Empirical studies—for example, experiments on creek chub, *Semotilus atromaculatus*, by Jim Gilliam and Doug Fraser—support these predictions. Of course, there is considerable variation, among individuals and species, in the trade-offs adopted. Sexually immature animals may place a higher priority on feeding so that they grow faster and reach the size class at which they are able to breed, whereas older ones may be more cautious to help ensure that they remain alive and continue to reproduce.

Your own work on predation pressure suggests that studying this phenomenon may have implications for understanding the process by which new species arise. Can you tell us a little about that?

Our work on guppies uncovered an interesting paradox. Population differences in antipredator behavior (as well as in life history and color pattern) arise over relatively short time periods (typically 10 to 100 generations). Reproductive isolation, in contrast, is slow to emerge and seems to take in excess of a million years to become established. When we looked at its evolution in detail, we found that some post-mating isolation has arisen among populations that have been separated for long periods of time. It occurs in the form of gametic isolation (the reduced ability of foreign sperm to compete with native sperm) and as a reduction in hybrid viability. However, there is little evidence for pre-mating isolation, even among long separated populations. In part this is because of female choice. Although females prefer certain male color patterns, particularly orange spots, they do not seem to discriminate against males from genetically divergent populations. Males show less discrimination of mating partner than females and use sneaky matings as well as consensual courtship to obtain copulations. Sneaky matings occur at a higher rate in populations that co-occur with predators, and are often directed at females preoccupied by predation avoidance.

Where do you see the study of predation and animal behavior heading over the next years?

Genomic techniques have revolutionized much of biology but have only recently been employed by researchers in animal behavior. This is partly because the emphasis has been on laboratory strains and inbred lines of model species, whose activity patterns tell us very little about natural behavior in the wild. In addition, behavior is shaped by subtle interactions between genes and the environment so it is more challenging to study than other "hardwired" traits. However, it seems likely that genomic tools will soon be used to answer ecologically meaningful questions—for example, to shed light on the mechanistic basis of population differences in antipredator behavior.

A second topic that seems bound to attract more attention is climate change and its effect on predator-prey interactions. Species ranges are altering rapidly, so that more and more species are encountering novel predators—or prey. It's already clear that the introduction of exotic predators can have far-reaching, and often negative consequences for the native fauna. I think there will be increasing interest in the behavioral component of invasion, particularly where species of economic importance, or conservation priority, are involved.

Dr. Anne Magurran is a professor at the University of Saint Andrews (Scotland). Dr. Magurran's work, using both guppies and minnows, has helped ethologists better understand the interaction of ecology, evolution, and behavior. She is the author of Measuring Biological Diversity *(Oxford University Press, 2004) and* Evolutionary Ecology: The Trinidadian Guppy *(Oxford University Press, 2005).*

FIGURE 11.25. Squirrel balancing act. (A) When squirrels forage in open fields, they need to balance the risk of predation (a function of distance to cover) against the benefits associated with various food items. Here a squirrel is foraging at a feeding station like that used in Steve Lima's work. **(B)** A squirrel in Lima's study heads for cover with a food item (part of a cookie) in its mouth. *(Photo credits: Steven Lima)*

foraging in the gray squirrel (*Sciurus carolinensis*) (Lima and Valone, 1986; Figure 11.25).

Early work by Lima had demonstrated that squirrels alter their foraging choices as a result of predation pressure from redtailed hawks (*Buteo jamaicensis*) (Lima, 1985). Squirrels who could either eat their food items where they found such items or carry the food to cover were more likely to carry items to an area of safe cover, particularly as the distance to safe cover decreased. That is, the closer the refuge from predation, the more likely they would use such a shelter when foraging; when it was a quick run to reach safety, squirrels generally chose to do so. Furthermore, squirrels were much more likely to carry larger (rather than smaller) items to safe areas before continuing to forage.

Lima and Valone followed up the above study with one in which they presented squirrels with two types of food—a large chunk of cookie (associated with long handling times) or a small chunk of cookie (associated with short handling times). Cookie chunks, rather than nuts, were used to avoid the confounding variable of food storage, as nuts are often buried, but cookies are always eaten. A combination of large and small items was placed either close (8 m) to an area of cover or farther from safety (16 m).

In order to make sense of Lima and Valone's results, we need two critical pieces of information. First, the profitability of small food items was greater than the profitability of large food items (see Chapter 10). Thus, in the absence of predation, we would expect that squirrels would always take any small food item that they encountered. Second, the total handling time associated with larger food items was great enough that, using optimal foraging theory, Lima reasoned that larger items should be brought to cover, where it is safe, before being eaten, particularly when the distance to cover was not great. This was not the case for smaller items. Lima and Valone reasoned that, if faced with predation, squirrels might sometimes pass up the smaller, more profitable food items, and continue to search for larger morsels to bring back to cover. This, in fact, is just what the squirrels did. Smaller items were indeed rejected in favor of larger items that needed to be brought back to cover. In other words, predation pressure redefined which food items should be taken and which should be passed up.

In this chapter, we have reviewed three ways that prey avoid detection by predators (blending into the environment, being quiet, and choosing a safe habitat), and five ways that prey react once they encounter a predator (fleeing, approaching a predator to obtain information, feigning death, signaling to the predator, and attacking the predator). In our investigation into both predator avoidance and the behaviors displayed when predators are encountered, we have seen how ultimate explanations (dealing with natural selection and phylogeny) and proximate explanations (neurobiological, endocrinological, and molecular genetic) help us better understand antipredator behavior.

SUMMARY

1. Because predation is a matter of life and death, natural selection should, and does, act strongly on antipredator behaviors.
2. There are essentially two forms of antipredator behaviors: those that help prey avoid detection by predators, and those that function once a prey encounters a predator. These two categories encompass most antipredator behaviors, but they are not meant to be exhaustive.
3. Studies using tools from genetics, neurobiology, endocrinology, and chemistry have helped animal behaviorists better understand proximate factors associated with antipredator behavior.
4. Predation pressure not only has an effect on how an animal behaves, but it can also have a dramatic effect on such life-history variables as development time—for example, when eggs will hatch.
5. If prey can avoid their predators in the first place, they can not only decrease the probability of being captured and eaten, but they can also reduce the costs associated with fleeing, fighting back against a predator, and so on. Three ways that animals avoid their predators are: (a) blending into the environment, (b) being quiet, and (c) choosing a safe habitat.
6. Despite the varied means by which prey can avoid predators, encounters with such danger are, over the lifetime of an organism, inevitable. Five types of behaviors that prey use once a predator has been encountered are: (a) fleeing, (b) approaching a predator to obtain information, (c) feigning death, (d) signaling to the predator, and (e) attacking.
7. Comparing a single species in populations with and without a particular predator is a powerful means for studying how selection operates on antipredator behaviors.
8. When there is predation pressure, animals are likely to alter their behavior, especially their foraging behavior, to avoid capture by predators.

DISCUSSION QUESTIONS

1. Pick your animal of choice, and sketch what a normal time budget (how much time it spends feeding, sleeping, mating, and so on) might look like for this animal. Now, besides the direct time spent looking for predators,

examine how predation might directly or indirectly affect all the behaviors on your time budget.

2. Some prey, particularly birds, actually mob their predators and harass them until the predators leave. List some of the costs and benefits associated with such mobbing, and construct a hypothesis for what sorts of environments might favor mobbing.

3. Abrahams and Pratt (2000) used a thyroid hormone to manipulate growth rates of the fathead minnow (*Pimephales promelas*) in the study described in their paper, "Hormonal manipulations of growth rate and its influence on predator avoidance: Foraging trade-offs" in Volume 78 (pp. 121–127) of the *Canadian Journal of Zoology*. Thyroid treatment stunted growth rates, and the researchers found that such stunted individuals were less likely to risk exposure to predators to gain access to food. Why might that be? Is it possible to construct an argument that would predict the exact opposite of what was found? Also, what does this study tell you about the relationship between proximate and ultimate factors shaping antipredator behavior?

4. In addition to the three ways we discussed that animals avoid predators, can you think of any other predator avoidance behaviors? How do they work? Why do they work?

5. A number of studies have found that laboratory raised animals can learn what constitutes danger by watching other animals respond to potential predators. How might such cultural transmission be employed by those interested in wildlife reintroduction programs?

SUGGESTED READING

Caro, T. M., Graham, C. M., Stoner, C. J., & Vargas, J. K. (2004). Adaptive significance of antipredator behaviour in artiodactyls. *Animal Behaviour, 67,* 205–228. A systematic study of the antipredator behavior in one group of large African mammals.

Kerfoot, W. C., & Sih, A. (Eds.) (1987). *Predation: Direct and indirect impacts on aquatic communities.* Hanover, NH: University Press of New England. This book looks at the ecological and behavioral implications of predation in aquatic communities.

Lima, S. L. (1998). Stress and decision making under the risk of predation: Recent developments from behavioral, reproductive, and ecological perspectives. *Advances in the Study of Behavior, 27,* 215–290. A very nice review of decision making in the context of antipredator activities, with a particular emphasis on the effects of stress.

Lind, J., & Cresswell, W. (2005). Determining the fitness consequences of antipredation behavior. *Behavioral Ecology, 16,* 945–956. A review of antipredator behavior from an ultimate perspective, with a focus on measuring complex antipredator behavior in relation to estimates of reproductive success.

Maren, S. (2001). Neurobiology of Pavlovian fear conditioning. *Annual Review of Neuroscience, 24,* 897–931. A review of antipredator behavior and fear from a psychological and neurobiological perspective.

Ruxton, G., Sherrat, T., & Speed, M. (2004). *Avoiding attack: The evolutionary ecology of crypsis, warning signals and mimicry.* Oxford: Oxford University Press. A comprehensive review of the evolution of antipredator behaviors that allow prey to avoid attack by predators.

Stankowich, T., & Blumstein, D. T. (2005). Fear in animals: A meta-analysis and review of risk assessment. *Proceedings of the Royal Society, B–Biological Sciences,* 272, 2627–2634. A concise overview of factors that affect antipredator behavior.

12

Communication

Life for vervet monkeys living in the Amboseli National Park in southern Kenya is not easy. Leopards hide in the bushes and pounce on passing vervets. Crowned eagles swoop from the sky and pick off vervets, and snakes are also a very real threat (Cheney and Seyfarth, 1990). Faced with such dangers, it is not all that surprising that vervets communicate information about predators to one another. But they do this in a remarkable fashion. Vervets don't just give an "alarm call" when a predator is sighted; they emit specific alarm calls for specific types of danger—that is, they communicate detailed information about danger to one another (Figure 12.1). Moreover, this sort of complex alarm calling has also been found in other primates such as chimpanzees and tamarins (Crockford and Boesch, 2003; Kirchhof and Hammerschmidt, 2006).

When an eagle is spotted, vervets emit a "cough" call. When other vervets hear the cough call, they look into the air or hide in the bushes, where they are safe from avian threat. In other words, vervets respond in an adaptive fashion when they hear an eagle alarm call. If a leopard is spotted, a "barking" alarm call is given, and vervets respond by heading up trees, where their agility makes them relatively safe from leopard attacks. That is, rather than respond to the leopard alarm call by looking up or hiding in the bushes—both of which would likely get the animal killed—they respond adaptively by heading for safety in the trees. And finally, when a python or cobra is sighted, vervets emit a "chutter" call. Since snakes often hunt vervets by hiding in the tall grass, a chutter call gets other vervets to stand and scan the grass around them for snakes.

Many other examples of animal communication—albeit not as dramatic as the communication among vervets as described above—have been documented in the ethological literature. When we see a chimp bare its canine teeth at another chimp, we, and any chimps in the vicinity, know that trouble is brewing. When female songbirds hear a male sing a certain song, breeding season has begun. In this chapter, we will address both "how" and "why" questions about animal communication systems.

A   **B**   **C**

FIGURE 12.1. Vervet alarm calls. Vervets give different alarm calls depending on what type of predator has been sighted. **(A)** Here we see vervets standing up after hearing a "chutter" alarm call indicating that a snake (approaching from the bottom left of the photo) has been spotted. When a leopard **(B)** is detected, vervets will give a "barking" alarm call and **(C)** climb up trees for safety. *(Photo credit: Anthrofoto; Ian Jones/Alamy)*

We will analyze **communication**—defined as the transfer of information from a signaler to a receiver—to help us better understand animal behavior. There is another, somewhat different, reason that some people study animal communication—namely, to understand how humans can communicate with animals. For example, people may study animal communication in order to better interact with their pets or domesticated livestock. Here, however, we are not interested in animal-human communication, except in terms of how it helps us better understand the evolution of animal communication.

There are a number of reasons not to focus on animal-human communication per se. First, this sort of communication likely only evolved with respect to a small number of species—dogs, cats, horses, and other species that humans have had as pets or livestock for thousands of years. Communication between these species and humans has evolved because only these species have been subject to intense artificial selection. Second, animal-human communications are notoriously difficult to study, primarily because it is very hard to know exactly what is being communicated from the animal side. A classic example of the sort of problems that arise here can be seen in the famous case of a horse named "Clever Hans" (Pfungst, 1911; Sebeok and Rosenthal, 1981).

Around the turn of the twentieth century, a schoolmaster named William von Osten gained fame because of the apparently prodigious ability of his horse, Hans. Hans was seemingly able to do mathematical puzzles, identify music, and answer questions regarding European history. He did this, of course, not by actually speaking, but by using his hoof to count out the right answer to a math problem, or shaking his head "yes" or "no" to a verbal query.

When the Prussian Academy of Science put Hans to the test in a controlled environment, they found something interesting. Hans could only give the right answer when someone in the room knew the right answer. If two people each gave Hans part of a question, but each was ignorant of what the other told Hans, the horse *never* got the correct answer. The reason was that Hans was indeed clever, but not in the way people thought.

Hans's cleverness, it turns out, was that he could pick up on very subtle body cues and facial cues that investigators in the room (unconsciously) emitted while they provided correct and incorrect answers for Hans to select from (Figure 12.2). So, for example, if the problem was "what is 10 + 10," Hans was able to pick up on subtle cues people emitted when he was approaching 20 hoofbeats on the floor. The cautionary lesson here is that human-animal communication can

* Translation: What is ten plus ten?

FIGURE 12.2. Clever Hans. Clever Hans, the horse, was thought capable of incredible mental feats. In fact, Clever Hans was picking up very subtle cues from the individual who asked him a question (and consequently knew the answer to that question).

be subtle and extremely difficult to pin down. Of course, the fact that something is difficult to study is no reason not to study it, but this, in conjunction with the first caveat about the evolutionary history of animal-human communication, leads me to focus on evolved animal communication systems.

We will begin our discussion of animal behavior and communication by addressing a fundamental question about communication—is it honest? That is, are individuals using communication to accurately convey information, or do they use communication to manipulate others? More specifically, we will examine a conceptual framework that will help us predict when communication is expected to be honest, and when it is not. Subsequent to this, and at the heart of the chapter, we will analyze communication systems in terms of the problems they were designed to solve. Communication is inherently social—that is, it involves more than a single individual. Animals communicate to convey information that is necessary to solve some problem, and we will organize the chapters around this functional, problem-solving approach to communication.

As we address these issues, it is important to recognize that the literature on animal communication is quite large, and so, while we will discuss some important conceptual questions in this chapter, we are touching on only the tip of the iceberg here. Using the approach just outlined, we will examine communication as it relates to problems associated with foraging, mating, and predation.

Communication and Honesty

If we adopt the definition of communication given above—the transfer of information from a signaler to a receiver—then an evolutionary approach to this topic immediately raises the question of honesty. That is, regardless of the problem a communication network is in place to solve, we can ask whether theory suggests that signalers should be honest in the information they convey, or whether they should attempt to deceive recipients (Dawkins and Krebs, 1978). Consider the following analogy of communication from Richard Dawkins and John Krebs:

> When an animal seeks to manipulate an inanimate object, it has only one recourse—physical power. A dung beetle can move a ball of dung only by forcibly pushing it. But when the object it seeks to manipulate is itself another live animal there is an alternative way. It can exploit the senses and muscles of the animal it is trying to control . . . which are themselves designed to preserve the genes of that other animal. A male cricket does not physically roll a female along the ground and into his burrow. He sits and sings, and the female comes to him under her own power. (Dawkins and Krebs, 1978, p. 282)

Dawkins and Krebs view communication not so much as the exchange of information between a signaler and a receiver, but as an attempt by the signaler to manipulate the recipient. They recognize that sometimes what is in the best interest of the signaler is also in the best interest of the recipient. They argue, however, that this need not be the case, but that when it is, it's usually just an incidental byproduct of what happens to be good for the signaler (see below for some exceptions). When what is good for the signaler is not good for the recipient, natural selection will favor signalers that send signals in whatever way that best increases the fitness of the signaler, even if that means manipulating recipients. The recipient is then selected for the ability to unscramble what is honest and what isn't, so it can act in ways that maximize its own fitness. In this light, Krebs and Dawkins refer to recipients as "mind readers." This view leads Krebs and Dawkins to speak of an "arms race" between signaler and recipient, in which the signaler is selected to better manipulate the receiver, who then is selected to better filter out only that information that benefits it, and so on (Krebs and Dawkins, 1984).

This is quite a different view from what Dawkins and Krebs refer to as "the classic ethological approach" of communication (Marler, 1968; W. J. Smith, 1968, 1977; Tinbergen, 1964). Implicit in the classic approach is that both parties usually benefit from the information exchange, and thus there is little selection pressure for either to be deceitful. In the classic ethological view, the signaler and receiver are "on the same page," and selection is thought to favor the most economical way to share information.

Krebs and Dawkins recognize that the sort of cooperative signaling that plays so prominent a role in the classic ethological approach may in fact be occurring in some systems, particularly those involving kin or reciprocal exchanges (see Chapters 8 and 9). They offer an ingenious way to distinguish between those systems in which there is an arms race between manipulators and mind readers, and those in which cooperation dominates.

Krebs and Dawkins argue that when communication is of the manipulator/mind-reader type, the signals employed should be exaggerated, as one might expect from a salesman attempting to convince a prospective buyer that his product is the top of the line. When cooperative signaling, however, is in play, Krebs and Dawkins hypothesize that natural selection should favor less exaggerated signals—what they refer to as "conspirational whispers." This is because signaling often involves some costs (for example, energy costs or drawing attention from predators), and so natural selection should favor minimizing these costs during conspirational whispers and hence reducing the conspicuousness of the communication itself (De Backer and Gurven, 2006; Johnstone, 1998; Noble, 1999). For example, take the case of ptarmigans (*Lagopus mutus*). Both male and female rock ptarmigans are a stark white against the snow of winter. Once spring arrives, females molt quickly, while males stay white, and as such the males are very conspicuous against the dark brown background (Figure 12.3). Such conspicuousness attracts females, but it also attracts predators. As the breeding season progresses, rather than molting, males soil their plumage to become less conspicuous (Montgomerie et al., 2001). In other words, males communicate information to females via coloration, but when the period during which communication is useful comes to an end, they shut down the communication system in a cost-efficient manner—by soiling their white plumage.

While formal mathematical models of the "conspirational whispers" versus conspicuous display hypotheses have shown that this dichotomy oversimplifies communication systems a bit, it is nonetheless a very useful heuristic tool. There is, however, another means besides cooperative signaling by which we might expect communication to be honest. Even within the manipulator/mind-reader view of communication, honesty might evolve if the signals being sent are either impossible, or at the very least, difficult to fake. To see how this might work, imagine that females produce more offspring when they are mating with larger males. All males, even small ones, would be selected to produce signals

FIGURE 12.3. Color and communication. During the breeding season, male ptarmigans remain white to attract females, but this also makes them vulnerable to predators. As the breeding season comes to an end, the male ptarmigans soil their plumage to make themselves less conspicuous to predators. *(Photo credit: Robert Montgomerie)*

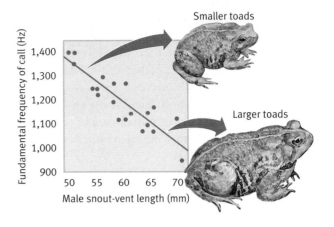

FIGURE 12.4. Toad size and croaks. Female toads *(Bufo bufo)* use the frequency of males' calls to gauge their potential mate's size. The relationship between a male's size (as indicated by his snout-vent length) and the frequency of his call is strong, suggesting that call frequency is an honest indicator of size, and hence of fighting ability. *(Based on Davies and Halliday, 1978)*

that made a female believe they were large. But selection should favor females paying attention only to those cues that are in fact true indicators of large size. As such, we should end up with a system in which females pay heed only to cues that can't be faked—that is, honest cues. This appears to be the case in toads, in whom deep croaks can only be produced by large males because of the design of their vocal system. Since male toads can't fake deep croaks, female toads can use croaks as one major cue in choosing among males (Davies and Halliday, 1978; Figure 12.4).

Amotz Zahavi has suggested that honesty is also possible when traits are not impossible, but merely very costly, to fake (Grafen, 1990a, 1990b; Zahavi, 1975, 1977, 2003; Zahavi and Zahavi, 1997). Under Zahavi's handicap principle, if a trait is costly to produce, it may be adopted as an honest signal, because only those individuals who can pay the cost will typically adopt the signal in question. For example, imagine that females are using the length of a male's energy-costly song as a cue for the amount of resources he is able to garner. While a male that is not particularly good at garnering resources could potentially use virtually all of his resources to sing, and thus could give the female a false impression of his resource-garnering skills, most of the time only the males that are genuinely good at gathering resources would be able to afford to sing, as singing is an energy-costly activity. Hence, honest communication may be an outcome even when deception is possible in principle, as long as deception is very costly in nature (Adams and Mesterton-Gibbons, 1995; Johnstone, 1995, 1998; Mesterton-Gibbons and Adams, 1998; Zahavi and Zahavi, 1997).

Communication Solves Problems

As mentioned earlier, communication systems evolve to solve problems that animals encounter in their natural environments. Here we will examine communication in terms of the problems associated with foraging, predation, and mating. In so doing, we will examine the costs and benefits of communication, the phylogenetic history of communication systems, the role of learning and social learning in shaping communication, and the underlying proximate basis for communication.

PROBLEM: HOW TO COORDINATE GROUP FORAGING

When animals forage in social groups, they face coordination problems. For example, when new food sources are found, how can that information be transferred to other group members if such transfer is beneficial to the signaler (Dornhaus et al., 2006; Galef and Giraldeau, 2001; Stevens and Gilby, 2004; Thierry et al., 1995)? We begin our discussion of foraging problems and communication by examining food calling in swallows. We then continue to explore the role of communication in foraging by describing the famous "waggle dance" that honeybees use to convey information about the location of food, and by discussing the intricate communication system underlying foraging in leaf-cutter ants.

FOOD CALLS IN BIRDS. Colonial breeding cliff swallows (*Petrochelidon pyrrhonota*) live in nests that serve as "information centers" (Brown, 1986; Ward and Zahavi, 1973). For some time, researchers believed that individuals living in nests only received "passive" information. That is, it was thought that group members simply observed their nestmates and followed them to potential resources. While this sort of system does allow for group foraging, it is not as efficient a solution to coordinating group behavior as an active form of communication about foraging sources—for example, *recruiting* foragers.

The idea that individuals are recruited to food sites was first suggested by Charles Brown and his colleagues (Brown et al., 1991). Using both playback experiments (playing tape-recorded bird calls) and provisioning experiments (putting food out to entice birds), Brown and his team found that cliff swallows gave off "squeak" calls, which alerted conspecifics that a new food patch— often a swarm of insects—had been found (Table 12.1). These calls served the specific function of facilitating group foraging, as squeak calls were emitted

TABLE 12.1. Squeak calls attract others. The mean number of birds and squeak calls heard two minutes before and two minutes after insects were flushed by foraging birds. For each two-minute period there were significantly more birds after insects were flushed than before, and there were significantly more squeak calls that were heard after the insects were flushed than before. *(From Brown et al., 1991, p. 559)*

PERIOD	MEAN NO. OF BIRDS		MEAN NO. OF CALLS/ BIRD/2 MINUTES		NO. OF TRIALS (*N*)
	BEFORE	AFTER	BEFORE	AFTER	
8 May 1990	37.8	240.3	0.062	0.267	11
9 May 1990	9.5	20.5	0.000	0.137	4
24 May 1990 A.M.	9.7	22.7	0.000	0.100	6
24 May 1990 P.M.	30.8	88.7	0.053	0.171	9
27 May 1990	7.9	45.4	0.031	0.133	7
29 May 1990	8.8	54.8	0.000	0.098	5
30 May 1990	8.5	38.5	0.033	0.109	2
15 June 1990	25.9	102.1	0.032	0.134	7

FIGURE 12.5. Raven yells. Under certain conditions, ravens emit a loud "yell" upon uncovering a new food source. Such yells attract other birds. *(Photo credit: Bernd Heinrich)*

FIGURE 12.6. Yellers are hungry. In ravens, "yelling" is often associated with foraging—in particular, calling others to a food bonanza. Immature ravens yell progressively more as a function of hunger. *(Based on Heinrich and Marzluff, 1991)*

only in the context of recruiting others to a food site—calls did not appear to be used in any other context.

In terms of the costs and benefits of this form of foraging-based communication, those recruited certainly obtain a resource—food. So, it is clearly in the interests of possible recruits to respond to squeak calls. Recruiters also obtain benefits from calling, however, because the increased group size that results from recruiting makes it more likely that one group member will find and track the insect swarm, and thus provide further foraging opportunities (Brown, 1988; Brown et al., 1991). This tracking behavior may be especially critical, as individual swallows must often return to the colony to provision young, and hence they would likely have great trouble relocating an insect swarm without the help of others.

Swallows are not the only birds that emit food calls. When ravens—who are scavengers that can often survive for days if they uncover a large food patch—find a new food source, they often emit a very loud "yell" that attracts other ravens to the caller's newly discovered bounty (Figure 12.5).

Bernd Heinrich and John Marzluff have addressed both proximate and ultimate questions associated with communication and foraging in common ravens (*Corvus corax*; Heinrich, 1988a, 1988b; Heinrich and Marzluff, 1991). On the proximate end, it appears that yelling is, in part, a response to hunger level, as hungry birds call more often than satiated birds (Figure 12.6). In terms of the costs and benefits of calling, it appears that yelling by juvenile ravens attracts other juvenile ravens to a food resource in order to overpower resident adult ravens and increase the yeller's fitness. Most of the juvenile ravens are unrelated "vagrants," and the only way an immature vagrant who comes upon a food source that is being defended by an adult territorial male can gain access to this source is to yell (Parker et al., 1994). Yelling attracts others, who together with the yeller can overpower those originally found at the food source (Heinrich and Marzluff, 1991).

Ravens also communicate about food when they roost together at night, and this form of communication appears to involve some type of learning (Marzluff et al., 1996). While many populations of ravens roost at the same spot for years, Marzluff and his team studied juvenile ravens in the forested mountains of Maine, where individuals form roosts near a newly discovered food source—a large animal carcass. They found that such roosts are very mobile (the ravens move where new prey has been discovered). Marzluff's team hypothesized that these mobile roosts served as "information centers" that provided roostmates with the chance to share information about prey that they had discovered when away from the roost.

Marzluff and his colleagues ran a series of experiments to test their ideas on communication at evening roosts. Information on naturally occurring mobile roosts suggests that a roost is comprised of both knowledgeable individuals—who know about nearby prey—and naive individuals who do not. And yet, when birds leave the roost in the morning, they all tend to go in the same direction, suggesting that they have communicated with one another, and that one or a few knowledgeable individuals lead the way. In one experiment, Marzluff's team captured ravens and denied them information about the prey environment. When these individuals were released and joined a roost, they tended to follow, rather than lead, other birds out of the roost in the morning.

Marzluff and his team ran a second experiment in which they again captured ravens, but this time they brought the captured birds to a location where there was a new prey item that the researchers themselves had placed into the environment. This information was unavailable to birds that were not captured, as they were not brought to the location of the new food source. When captured birds were released and joined roosts, they tended to be the individuals who led other roostmates out of the roost and to the newly discovered prey item (Figure 12.7). That is, birds that had learned the location of prey acted as leaders. Indeed, Marzluff found that the same individual would act as a leader when it learned the location of new prey, and as a follower when it was denied information that others in the nest knew. While it is not clear exactly how information about who is a knowledgeable forager and who is not is spread at the roost, Marzluff and his team noted that, prior to departure from the roost in the morning, a great deal of "honking" sounds were emitted by the ravens. Whether knowledgeable birds were more likely to emit such sounds remains to be tested.

Paola Laiolo and Antonio Rolando used a phylogenetic approach to study the evolution of vocalizations in genus *Corvus* (which includes crows, rooks, and ravens). They focused on the "caw" call that is often emitted in long-distance communication, including food calling. This call has numerous characteristics—frequency, amplitude, and so on—that can be analyzed with spectrographic techniques. Laiolo and Rolando studied the caw calls of twenty-eight corvid species—species that came from all over the planet, and included representatives of all three major geographic "stocks" of corvids (Laiolo and Rolando, 2003).

By analyzing phylogenetic relationships, Laiolo and Rolando found that *within* each of the three stocks—the "American," "Palearctic-African," and "Oriental-Australian"—there were significant differences in spectral and temporal components of caw calls. There are a number of possible reasons for variation in calls within different stocks of corvids. Variability in caw calls, for example, is consistent with the idea that vocalizations, and the communication that arises from them, may have been involved in the speciation process in this group of birds by providing a mechanism for individuals to recognize members of their own species.

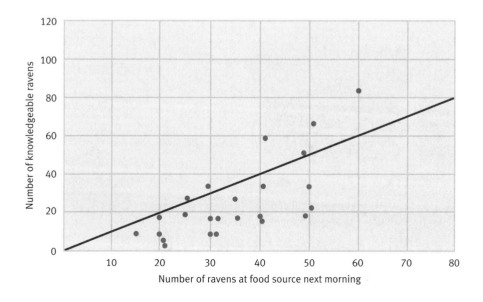

FIGURE 12.7. Raven recruitment. The line denotes when the number of ravens that knew of the prey source equals the number of ravens at the prey source the next day. Points *below* the line indicate recruitment to the food source. Green points indicate statistically significant recruitment. Orange points indicate that recruitment was not statistically significant. *(Based on Marzluff et al., 1996, p. 99)*

FIGURE 12.8. Bee foraging.
Honeybee foraging involves a complex communication system, including waggle dances. This dance, along with other informational cues, gives bees in a hive information about the relative position of newly found food sources. *(Photo credit: Leroy Simon/Visuals Unlimited)*

HONEYBEES AND THE WAGGLE DANCE. Food collecting in honeybees often involves thousands of workers covering large areas of ground, at least from a honeybee's perspective (Visscher and Seeley, 1982; Figure 12.8). Such a system poses enormous logistical problems for honeybees: How do they keep track of the changing distribution of resources (nectar, pollen) through time? How are they able to monitor the needs of their genetic relatives in the colony? Yet, for our purposes, we shall focus on an overarching problem: How do foragers communicate information about any food they uncover to other members of their hive? The answer, in part, lies in the now famous **waggle dance** of the honeybee.

The waggle dance of the honeybee was first studied experimentally by Karl von Frisch (von Frisch, 1967). Thomas Seeley eloquently describes the waggle dance as:

> a unique form of behavior in which a bee, deep inside her colony's nest, performs a miniaturized reenactment of her recent journey to a patch of flowers. Bees following these dances learn the distance, direction and odors of these flowers and can translate this information into a flight to specified flowers. Thus the waggle dance is a truly symbolic message, one which is separated in space and time from both the actions on which it is based and the behaviors it will guide. (Seeley, 1985, pp. 84–85)

The waggle dance has an almost mystical quality to it (Munz, 2005). Fortunately, it is possible to maintain that air of the amazing while at the same time studying this behavior in detail as ethologists have now been doing for more than half a century (Seeley, 1985). To see this, imagine that a worker bee has just returned from a bountiful cluster of flowers that are approximately 1500 meters from her nest, and that these flowers are located 40 degrees to the right of an imaginary straight line running between the worker's nest and the sun (Figure 12.9). How is our worker supposed to communicate this vitally important information to others in the hive?

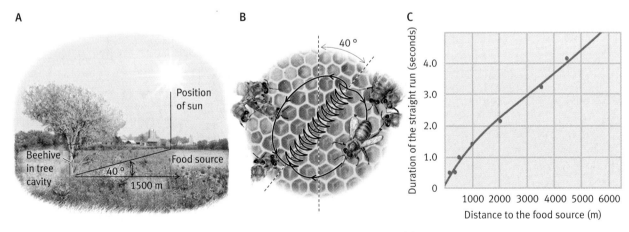

FIGURE 12.9. Honeybee waggle dances. (A) Imagine a patch of flowers that is 1500 meters from a hive, at an angle 40 degrees to the right of the sun. **(B)** When a forager returns, the bee dances in a figure eight pattern. In this case, the angle between a bee's "straight run" (up and down a comb in the hive) and a vertical line is 40 degrees. **(C)** The length of the straight run portion of the dance translates into distance from the hive to the food source. *(Based on Seeley, 1985)*

Upon returning to the nest, our worker bee would quickly start "dancing" up and down a vertical honeycomb within the hive; her sisters would try to keep up with her, making as much physical contact as possible with both our forager and each other in the process. While dancing vigorously (by waggling her abdomen), our worker would be conveying crucial information to her relatives in the hive. For example, her dance would provide topographical information (north, east, south, west, northwest, and so on) for finding the food source from which she had just returned. When compared to a straight up-and-down run along a comb, the angle at which our forager danced would describe the position of the food source of interest in relation to the hive and to the sun. Further, the longer the bee danced—in a part of the waggle dance known as the "straight line"—the farther away the bounty. In fact, every extra 75 milliseconds of dancing would translate into the resource being about an additional 100 meters from the hive. The more precise the information conveyed in the waggle dance, the greater the ability of other bees to find the food source, the more food brought back to the hive, and consequently the greater the inclusive fitness of the forager, since a hive is composed of individuals that are closely related to one another.

The honeybee waggle dance has been the subject of intense interest in ethology, and hence much work has been done on the genetics, endocrinology, and development of this fascinating behavior. For example, Ross Crozier and his colleagues studied the genetics of the honeybee dance by examining the point at which bees shift from other types of dances to the waggle dance (Johnson et al., 2002). When resources are close to the hive, honeybee foragers tend to use what is called a round dance. When the resources are at greater distances, bees switch to a sickle dance, and when food is very far from a hive, foragers use the waggle dance (Figure 12.10).

Crozier and his team ran a series of experiments in which they mated individuals from populations of bees that differed in terms of when they shifted from using the round dance to the sickle dance, and finally when they shifted from the sickle dance to the waggle dance. For example, in one population that the researchers studied, bees transitioned from the round to the sickle dance when food was more than 20 meters from the hive, and they shifted from the sickle dance to the waggle dance when food was 60 meters or more from the hive. The results of the genetic crosses undertaken by Crozier and his

FIGURE 12.10. Different honeybee dances. The three different honeybee dances: **(A)** round dance, **(B)** sickle dance, and **(C)** waggle dance. Each bee at its initial starting point is shown in full color, and the same bee is shown in gray as it moves along the path of its dance. *(Based on Johnson et al., 2002, p. 171)*

colleagues suggest that the transition across dance types is under the control of a single gene (Johnson et al., 2002). A single gene, then, can help us understand much about the waggle dance and its importance in foraging and honeybee communication.

The honeybee waggle dance has also been examined from a developmental perspective. On this front, Jurgen Tautz and his colleagues studied how hive temperature during development affected the waggle dance behavior of bees (Tautz et al., 2003). Tautz's team raised bees in one of three temperatures (all of which were in the normal temperature range within a hive): 32°C, 34.5°C, or 36°C. When bees in these treatments matured, they were individually marked and placed into "foster" hives. When the experimental bees in these hives matured into foragers, they were trained by Tautz and his colleagues to feed at an artificial food source placed 200 meters from the hives; the researchers observed differences in the waggle dance behavior in bees raised at different temperatures.

Bees from the 32°C treatment were less likely to use the waggle dance when they returned to the hive than were bees from either of the other treatments—60 percent of foragers from the 32°C treatment waggle danced versus 90 percent of foragers from the 34.5°C and 36°C treatments (this difference, however, was not statistically significant because of the large amount of variance found within treatments). In addition, bees from the 32°C treatment made significantly fewer "circuits" (trips around the figure eight in the waggle dance) than bees from the 36°C treatment (Figure 12.11).

Tautz and his colleagues found that bees raised in the 36°C treatment fared much better in individual learning tasks than did bees raised in the other treatments. These results suggest that differences in temperature during early development can have important effects for both individual bees and the hive as a whole. When bees were raised in colder temperatures, they were both poor learners and less adept at communicating important foraging-related information to other members of their hive. Because the food that foragers bring into a hive is eventually transferred into energy that keeps the hive temperature high, a dangerous feedback loop is put into play here—lower temperatures lead to bees that are both poor foragers and poor communicators, which in turn leads to less energy for the hive and hence to lower hive temperatures, which then leads to even worse foragers, and so on.

CHEMICAL AND VIBRATIONAL COMMUNICATION IN FORAGING ANTS. Like honeybees, ants often forage in huge groups and cover relatively large areas during their foraging bouts. And like honeybees, ants face the problem of how to communicate foraging-related information to those in their nest. Ants tend to solve this communication problem by using chemical markers and sound production through vibrations (stridulation) (Billen and Morgan, 1997; Holldobler and Wilson, 1990; Vander Meer et al., 1997; Wilson, 1971). Here we begin by examining chemical communication in the leaf-cutting ants of the genus *Atta* and then proceed to study vibrational communication in this same species (Holldobler and Roces, 2001).

Ants in the genus *Atta* are one of the dominant life-forms in the neotropics, consuming more vegetation than any other group in that ecosystem. Remarkably, leaf-cutters subsist entirely on the fungus they grow on leaves and on the sap produced by the plants whose leaves they harvest (Littledyke and Cherrett, 1976). Leaf-cutters live in nests containing hundreds of thousands of workers (plus a

FIGURE 12.11. Number of dance circuits. The number of "figure eight" circuits in a waggle dance when bees were raised at a temperature of 36°C or 32°C. *(Based on Tautz et al., 2003, p. 7345)*

single queen) and have evolved an elaborate, caste-based system for obtaining the leaves on which they subsist. Leaves must first be cut, then carried to the nest, ground up, chewed and treated with enzymes, placed into the "fungus garden," and subsequently cultivated. Bert Holldobler and E. O. Wilson liken the system to an assembly line where different castes handle different tasks (Holldobler and Wilson, 1990; Wilson, 1980a, 1980b; Wilson and Holldobler, 2005a, 2005b).

From a proximate perspective, when it comes to long-distance foraging communication in leaf-cutters, two chemicals are particularly important in *Atta* species—methyl 4-methylpyrrole-2-carboxylate and 3-ethyl-2,5methylpyrazine (Morgan, 1984). These substances are produced in the poison gland of leaf-cutter ants and are used to recruit fellow workers to foraging sites that are relatively long distances from their nest. Recruitment pheromones are incredibly powerful:

> . . . the discoverers of methyl 4-methylpyrrole-2-carboxylate . . . estimated that one milligram of this substance (roughly the quantity in a single colony), if laid out with maximal efficiency, would be enough to lead a column of ants three times around the earth. (Holldobler and Roces, 2001, p. 94)

Recruitment pheromones, which fade slowly, are placed along the trails leading to trees where leaves are being harvested. These pheromones are also deposited along branches and twigs, bringing recruited foragers very close to the leaves they need to harvest. When leaf-cutters are in the vicinity of the leaves, they rely on a second mode of communication—stridulation—to determine the precise leaves on which to work.

When *Atta* workers are cutting leaves, the process seems systematic. Sections of leaves are not randomly cut throughout a tree (or even a branch), but rather certain leaves are cut and cut until there is virtually nothing left (Figure 12.12). From an ultimate perspective, Holldobler and Roces hypothesized that *Atta* workers were cutting the most desirable leaves, where desirability might be measured in terms of maximizing leaf tenderness or minimizing the amount of dangerous secondary plant compounds present (Holldobler and Roces, 2001). They further hypothesized that because *Atta* workers appeared to raise and lower their gasters in a manner similar to the way they created stridulatory vibrations, the ants were actually using vibrational cues to recruit other workers to the best leaves in the vicinity, which increased the amount of high-quality food brought back to the nest (Markl, 1968).

To begin their work on vibrational communication, Holldobler and Roces used noninvasive laser Doppler vibrometry to test whether workers in *Atta cephalotes* stridulate while they are cutting leaves. Indeed, workers were stridulating while they were cutting the leaves, and the vibrations were being sent along the length of a leaf in a long series of vibrational "chirps" (Figure 12.13). Next, the researchers offered workers leaves that differed in toughness (tough or tender). In addition, in a follow-up experiment, tough and tender leaves were both dipped in sugar water and offered to ants. The results were clear-cut. While only 40 percent of the ants stridulated when cutting tough leaves (with no sugar water), the number increased to 70 percent when the leaves were tender (with no sugar water), and to almost 100 percent when either type of leaf was dipped in sugar water (Roces et al., 1993). Ants, then, clearly stridulate while cutting leaves, and they vary this behavior, depending upon the value of the leaf in question.

FIGURE 12.12. Devastating leaf-cutters. Leaf-cutter ants can ravage foliage in their path. The ants don't attack all the leaves, however, but instead they often strip some leaves to the stalk (for example, those that are most tender or have fewer secondary compounds present), while leaving other leaves untouched. *(Photo credit: Bert Holldobler)*

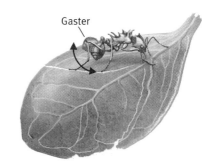

Gaster

FIGURE 12.13. Stridulating communication. A schematic of a leaf-cutter ant cutting a leaf and stridulating its gaster up and down. *(Based on Holldobler and Roces, 2001)*

FIGURE 12.14. Minim workers hitchhiking on a leaf. The stridulating signals emitted by leaf-cutters are used in numerous contexts. One such venue is between leaf-cutters and "minimum" workers (minims), who use these signals to eventually hitch rides on cut leaves that are carried on leaf-cutters' backs. *(Photo credit: Bert Holldobler)*

These two experiments, although powerful, do not demonstrate that ant workers are recruited by stridulation. To test for the potential recruiting nature of stridulatory communication, Holldobler and Roces hooked one leaf to a vibrator and used a similar ("silent") leaf as a control (Holldobler and Roces, 2001). When given the choice to cut either of the leaves, ant workers clearly preferred the vibrating leaf, demonstrating that these cues were not only produced by workers, but they were used to recruit workers. Further, through an ingenious set of experiments, the researchers were able to demonstrate that communicating to other workers was the primary function of stridulation (Roces and Holldobler, 1996). Moreover, stridulation was also found to serve another role in communication. In *A. cephalotes*, a small-sized caste, called minim workers, exists. These minim workers cannot cut leaves, but they are often found hitchhiking rides on leaves on the backs of leaf-cutters. Minims protect these other leaf-cutting workers from attack by parasitic flies, and so it is certainly beneficial for leaf-cutting ants to have minims find them (Eibesfeldt and Eible-Eibesfeldt, 1967; Feener and Moss, 1990). Hitchhiking minims apparently use the vibrational cues created by stridulating leaf-cutting nestmates to locate the leaf-cutters (Roces and Holldobler, 1995; Figure 12.14).

PROBLEM: HOW TO FIND AND SECURE A MATE

Animals often solve problems associated with mate choice by some form of communication. In this section, we will examine the role of (1) vocal communication (birdsong), and (2) tactile communication (ripples by insects that live in water), as they relate to problems that animals encounter as a result of both intrasexual and intersexual selection.

BIRDSONG. Some forms of animal communication are more pleasing to humans than others. Go to your local music store and you are bound to find dozens of CDs of birdsong. In addition to its practical, sedative effects on human listeners, birdsong has been studied by naturalists, ethologists, behavioral ecologists, comparative psychologists, and evolutionary biologists for hundreds of years. Indeed, few communication systems in vertebrates have been studied to the extent of birdsong (Beecher and Brenowitz, 2005; Catchpole and Slater, 1995; Clayton, 2004; Hauser and Konishi, 1999; Podos et al., 2004; Slater, 2003; Thorpe, 1961; Todt and Naguib, 2000).

While birdsong has many functions—colony formation, flocking, foraging, and so on (Kroodsma and Byers, 1991)—here we will focus on its role in problems relating to sexual selection. In particular, we will examine how and why birdsong is used to attract and secure mates. We will begin with two studies that address ultimate questions regarding the fitness consequences of birdsong and the phylogeny of birdsong, and then we will examine the proximate underpinnings of birdsong (for an in-depth case study of social learning and birdsong, see the discussion in Chapter 6 of Freeberg's work on cultural transmission in the cowbird).

In most species of songbirds, males don't just learn a single song, they learn *many* different songs. For example, the song sparrow (*Melospiza melodia*) sings about ten different songs, the western marsh wren (*Cistothorus palustris*) sings more than a hundred songs, and the brown thrasher (*Toxostoma rufum*) sings an incredible thousand different songs (Beecher and Brenowitz, 2005). Ethologists have hypothesized that females may use a male's song repertoire to choose mates if the repertoire size indicates such things as a male's age and/or genetic quality (Hosoi et al., 2005; MacDougal-Shackleton, 1997).

Aki Hosoi, Stephen Rothstein, and Adrian O'Loghlen examined the role of repertoire size in the mating success of male brown-headed cowbirds (*Molothrus ater*). Male cowbirds possess between two to eight different perched songs (songs sung from a perch, generally near the ground, rather than in flight), which they sing to attract females during the mating season. Earlier studies indicated a correlation between the size of the perched song repertoire and mating success, but no work had specifically examined whether female mate choice was affected by song repertoire in cowbirds (O'Loghlen, 1995; O'Loghlen and Rothstein, 1993, 1995, 2002). To fill in the gap in understanding and examine whether male repertoire size had an effect on female mate choice, Hosoi and her colleagues captured female cowbirds from two populations in California—one from Santa Barbara and one from Ventura—and brought them into an experimental aviary (Hosoi et al., 2005). The researchers then subcutaneously implanted the captured females with the hormone estradiol to increase the probability that they would respond to male song during experimental manipulations.

Hosoi and her team exposed each female in the experiment to five different song treatments—a *single* perched song sung three times in succession by a male Santa Barbara cowbird (treatment 1; smaller repertoire) or by a male Ventura cowbird (treatment 2; smaller repertoire), three *different* perched songs sung in quick succession by a male Santa Barbara cowbird (treatment 3; larger repertoire) or by a male Ventura cowbird (treatment 4; larger repertoire), and a control in which females were exposed to the song of males from a different species (song sparrow). The length of time that a female displayed ritualized "copulation-solicitation displays" (CSDs) to different songs was recorded and used as a measure of female choice.

Not surprisingly, female cowbirds displayed longer CSDs when they heard cowbird versus song sparrow songs, regardless of how many songs were sung. If we just consider the four treatments involving male cowbird song, females show a marked increase in CSD times when exposed to males with larger song repertoires (Figure 12.15). When females were exposed to males from their own

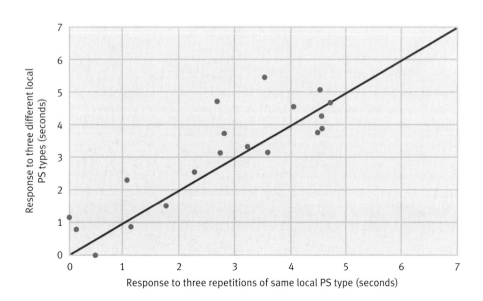

FIGURE 12.15. Same vs. different songs. Female cowbirds had longer copulation-solicitation displays (CSDs) when they were exposed to three different songs than to the same song played three times. Each point represents the CSDs of one female. The diagonal represents points where females respond in the same manner to three different songs and three repetitions of the same song. Most points are above the diagonal, indicating a stronger response to larger song repertoires. *(From Hosoi et al., 2005, p. 89)*

population, they preferred larger song repertoires on thirteen of nineteen trials. Moreover, females exposed to male cowbirds from a different population also preferred males with larger song repertoires. Larger song repertoire, then, has clear fitness effects and provides males with one solution to the problem of attracting a mate.

Phylogenetic studies of birdsong also point to the importance of sexual selection in the evolution of birdsong (Brenowitz, 1997; Price and Lanyon, 2002a, 2002b, 2004a, 2004b). Many phylogenetic studies of sexual selection look at a single trait—for example, feather length—to see whether this trait varies in ways that one would predict from the ecology of the species. This approach is more difficult to use when song is the trait of interest, as numerous studies show that the many components of song—repertoire size, amplitude, frequency, and so on—can vary across groups. So, to obtain an accurate assessment, phylogenetic analysis of birdsong and sexual selection needs to incorporate many measures of song—frequency, rate of pauses, maximum note length, and so forth (Price and Lanyon, 2004a). And, in particular, if researchers are interested in sexual selection and communication, it is especially useful for them to analyze components of song that are costly to produce, and hence hard to fake.

Recognizing the inherent complexity of birdsong, Jordan Price and Scott Lanyon mapped six components of birdsong onto a molecular phylogeny of seventeen species of blackbirds (Price and Lanyon, 2004a). Price and Lanyon's work focused on caciques and oropendolas—two groups of New World blackbirds from Argentina and Mexico. The caciques and oropendolas are well suited for analysis involving sexual selection and song, as tremendous variations in mating systems exist in these groups. Some species are monogamous (recall that this means individuals have one mate during a breeding season; see Chapter 7), while others are polygynous (recall that this means that the males have more than one mate per season; see Chapter 7). In addition, some species of caciques and oropendolas are sexually monomorphic (males and females are the same size), while others are sexually dimorphic (males are much larger than females). This variance is critical, as much work suggests that sexual selection operates more strongly in polygynous mating systems and in systems that are sexually dimorphic (Figure 12.16).

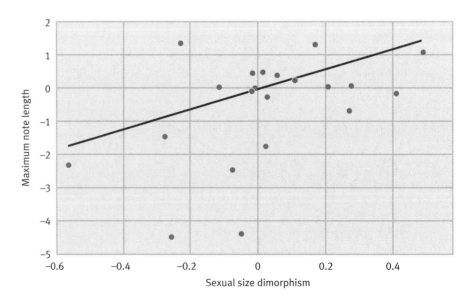

FIGURE 12.16. Sex differences and songs. Across seventeen species of blackbirds, the maximum note length of songs increased as the size difference between males and females increased. *(From Price and Lanyon, 2004a, p. 490)*

Price and Lanyon's phylogenetic analysis can get complicated. Nonetheless, for our purposes, what is most critical is that they uncovered multiple lines of evidence that evolutionary changes in song were most often associated with sexually dimorphic species, where sexual selection was likely strongest. For example, in one oropendola species, *Psarocolius oseryi*, in which males were much larger than females, phylogenetic analysis found changes in three components of song. More generally, in the phylogenetic tree that Price and Larson constructed, in eight of the ten branches that showed clear changes in song components, males were at least 15 percent larger than females. Thus, when sexual selection is powerful, and there is strong competition for access to females, natural selection acts strongly on the many components that make up male song.

In addition to the evolutionary literature on birdsong, there has also been a tremendous amount of work addressing birdsong from a proximate perspective. Part of this work centers on something of a riddle. As we have seen, birdsong is incredibly diverse in terms of structure, pattern, tempo, frequency, and repertoire size. At the same time, however, the vocal organ used in birds, the syrinx, varies little between different species in this group. How is it possible that morphological (structural) invariance in the syrinx can translate into great diversity in birdsong?

To address this question, we begin by recognizing that the avian syrinx has two compartments—left and right—and that the two sides of a bird's brain can control these compartments independently (Suthers, 1997; Suthers et al., 2004; Suthers and Zollinger, 2004; Table 12.2). This one piece of information sets the stage for moving from *invariance* in the structure of the syrinx to *variance* in the

TABLE 12.2. The different ways to sing. The costs and benefits of different song lateralization patterns. *(Based on Suthers, 1999)*

SONG LATERALIZATION PATTERN	SPECIES	ADVANTAGES	DISADVANTAGES
Independent bilateral phonation	Brown thrasher and gray catbird	Two independent voices increase spectral and phonetic complexity.	Expensive in use of air supply. Best suited for a low syllable repetition rate.
Unilateral dominance	Waterslager canary	Conserves air, favoring shorter minibreaths and longer phrases. Separation of phonatory and inspiratory motor patterns to opposite sides of syrinx. Both of these may facilitate higher syllable repetition rates.	Use of one voice limits frequency range and certain kinds of spectral and temporal complexity. Minibreath may be smaller than tracheal deadspace.
Alternating lateralization	Brown-headed cowbird	Enhances spectral contrast between notes. Efficient use of air supply. Extended frequency range for overall song.	Two-voice complexity limited to note overlap.
Sequential lateralization	Northern cardinal	Extended frequency range. Conserves air supply.	Lacks spectral complexity of two voices.

song output. That is, although the syrinx varies little in structure, its *parts* can be manipulated to create new permutations that may give rise to new sounds (Suthers, 1999).

Over a hundred years ago, theorists suggested that two different sides of the syrinx contribute differentially to the frequency component of birdsong. But stronger evidence of this phenomenon did not arise until 1968 (Greenewalt, 1968; Stein, 1968). Independence of the two sides of the syrinx allows songbirds to switch off one side at any time. This, in turn, facilitates variation in song production in that it permits some species to:

▶ operate both sides of the syrinx independently throughout their song without one side being dominant, as in brown thrashers (*Toxostoma rufum*) and gray catbirds (*Dumetella carolinensis*) (Suthers et al., 1994, 1996; Suthers and Hartley, 1990).

▶ have one side of the syrinx dominate song generation, as in canaries (*Serinus canaria*) (Nottebohm and Nottebohm, 1976).

▶ alternate which side of the syrinx dominates during a song, as in brown-headed cowbirds (*Molothrus ater*) (Allan and Suthers, 1994).

▶ have one side of the syrinx dominate for certain frequencies, and the other side dominate for the remainder of the frequencies used in a song (sequential lateralization), as in the northern cardinal (*Cardinalis cardinalis*) (Suthers, 1997; Suthers and Goller, 1996).

The respiratory muscles that supply air to the syrinx can also be employed to achieve the variance in song output across oscine birds. Varying the respiratory muscles can have dramatic effects on the structure and timing of birdsong. So, again, the syrinx itself is invariant, but variation around other anatomical structures can produce variation in the output of birdsong.

These sorts of proximate analyses help us to better understand the construction of communication systems that are designed to address problems that arise during sexual selection in songbirds.

RIPPLE COMMUNICATION AND MATE CHOICE IN AQUATIC INSECTS. Vocal signaling, as in birdsong, is only one way for animals to communicate about mating-related issues. Indeed, animals communicate information relevant for mate choice and sexual selection in many different ways—vocally, visually, chemically, and so on. In 1972, Stim Wilcox discovered a new form of communication—ripple communication—in water striders, insects that live in freshwater lakes, ponds, streams, and small rivers. This form of communication has now been demonstrated in numerous species of water striders, and it has also been found in giant water bugs (Bottger, 1974; Kraus, 1989; R. L. Smith, 1979).

In water striders, ripples are usually produced by an up-and-down movement of the legs, with both right and left legs in synchrony and in constant contact with the water surface (Wilcox, 1995). The water striders produce different patterns of ripples (waves with different amplitudes and frequencies) for different kinds of behaviors, including signals for calling mates, courtship, copulation, postcopulation, sex discrimination, mate guarding, spacing, territoriality, and food defense. Such signals can range from 0.2 second during the courtship behavior of the water strider, *Rhagadotarsus anomalus* (Wilcox, 1972), up to 30 seconds in other water strider species (Polhemus, 1990). Here we will touch on what is known of ripple communication and courtship.

A

B

C

FIGURE 12.17. Ripple communication by water striders. **(A)** The concentric circles of these ripples in a pond are part of the communication used by the water strider, *R. kraepelini*. **(B)** A closeup of the male water strider *(R. kraepelini)* and the ripples he is making to communicate with other water striders. **(C)** An experimental set-up to study ripple communication, in which an *A. remigis* female is making a signal via a magnet glued to her leg. In nature, female water striders don't emit such signals. *(Photo credits: Stim Wilcox)*

Ripple production appears to have significant benefits associated with it. In *R. anomalus*, males produce ripple signals that can travel more than 60 cm, and females find such ripple signals very attractive. Wilcox undertook a series of ingenious playback experiments that demonstrated that females from as far away as 60 cm were attracted to mating ripple signals—ripples that are quite different from those produced by aggressive males (Wilcox, 1972; Figure 12.17). Females would often grasp males and even begin to oviposit (lay eggs) in response to playbacks of calling signals. In addition, Wilcox speculates that ripple calls designed to attract mates also serve as a means for species identification, as *R. anomalus* are often found in the same streams and ponds as other water striders (Polhemus and Karunaratne, 1993).

Ripple signals are also employed by giant water bugs in the context of mating (Bottger, 1974; Kraus, 1989; R. L. Smith, 1979). While performing courtship displays, giant male water bugs pump up and down with their legs, thereby creating ripples, which attract female water bugs. The roots of such pumping behavior may lie in the motion that giant water bugs use to aerate eggs (which are laid on their backs) (R. L. Smith, 1979).

PROBLEM: HOW TO WARN OTHERS ABOUT PREDATORS

As we saw in the opening to this chapter, communication can be used to warn conspecifics about predators. Animals that live in social groups often derive benefits from keeping group size above some minimum level, in order, for example, to forage efficiently. In addition, the probability that any given individual will be attacked by a predator often decreases as group size increases (see Chapter 11), yielding another benefit from group living. Predation obviously decreases group size, and so animals often must solve a problem: how, when, and why to communicate to other group members that a predator is in the vicinity.

FIGURE 12.18. Protecting a mate. While downy woodpeckers don't give alarm calls when they are paired with same-sex partners, they emit such alarm calls when they are paired with a member of the opposite sex. *(Photo credit: E. R. Degginger/Color-Pic, Inc.)*

WOODPECKER AND CHICKADEE ALARM CALLS. In Chapter 8, we saw the powerful role that genetic kinship plays in shaping alarm calls, and hence communication. Recall that in Belding's ground squirrels, alarm calls are primarily driven by the degree of relatedness between caller and recipient. Yet, protecting genetic kin is not the only function associated with communication via alarm calls. For example, Kimberly Sullivan found that in both downy woodpeckers (*Picoides pubescens*) and black-capped chickadees (*Parus atricapillus*), individual alarm calls are emitted to protect *mates*, but not other individuals (Figure 12.18). This form of alarm call communication has been termed "mate investment."

During the winters of 1979–1981, Sullivan observed mixed-species flocks of birds in the Great Swamp National Wildlife Refuge in New Jersey. During her observations, she recorded alarm calls given by downy woodpeckers and black-capped chickadees to three naturally occurring predators—sharp-shinned hawks (*Accipiter straitus*), Cooper's hawks (*Accipiter cooperii*), and American kestrels (*Falco sparverius*). In addition, Sullivan examined alarm calls in response to (stuffed) models of these predators. These models were "flown" over a group of birds on a pulley that ran down a wire between two trees. Sullivan found that downy woodpeckers never gave alarm calls when they were foraging alone (0/46—that is, there were 0 alarm calls in 46 instances of solo foraging), when in a flock with no other woodpeckers (0/23), or when with a same-sex downy woodpecker (0/6). The situation was very different, however, when downy woodpeckers were in the presence of a woodpecker of the opposite sex. In seven of nine such instances, they emitted alarm calls (Sullivan, 1985). Three of these calls were made by females and four by males, suggesting that both sexes use this form of communication to attract opposite-sex partners.

Sullivan found no evidence that either black-capped chickadees or tufted titmice used alarm calls to attract mates. But other researchers have found evidence that black-capped chickadees do preferentially give alarm calls in the presence of potential mates (Ficken et al., 1980; Witkin and Ficken, 1979). This "mate investment" form of communication may account for alarm calls in other birds as well (Curio and Regelmann, 1985; East, 1981; Hogstad, 1995; Krams et al., 2006; Leopold, 1977; Morton, 1977).

DEVELOPMENT, LEARNING, AND ALARM CALL COMMUNICATION IN MEERKATS. In species in which parental care is present and lengthy, natural selection will often favor development pathways in which young individuals learn what communicative signals mean from adults (Platzen and Magrath, 2005). This should be especially true when signals are complex, as in the alarm calls of vervets. Indeed, the evidence suggests that young vervets do learn about alarm calls from older individuals (Seyfarth and Cheney, 1986). Meerkats also experience prolonged parental care and learn complex alarms calls for terrestrial and avian predators.

Meerkat pups spend the first three weeks of their lives underground, and then they emerge and join groups of juveniles (meerkats that are six to twelve months old) and adults. Once above ground, pups are subject to intense predation pressure from avian and terrestrial predators. Linda Hollen and Marta Manser examined the development of the response to alarm calls in maturing meerkat pups (Hollen and Manser, 2006). They studied eleven groups of free-ranging meerkats in the Kalahari Desert, and they used a combination of observation of meerkat encounters with predators in natural settings and experimental mani-

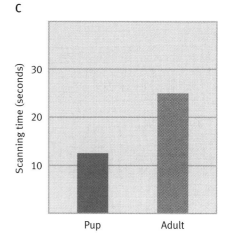

FIGURE 12.19. Age differences in reaction to alarm calls. In meerkats, a pup's response to alarm calls was not as strong as the response seen in adults: **(A)** time until reaction after hearing playback of alarm call (adults react to predators more quickly than do pups), **(B)** duration of response to playback of alarm call, and **(C)** length of time spent "scanning" the environment for predators after hearing predator alarm call. Adults remain vigilant and continue to watch out for predators longer than do pups. *(Based on Hollen and Manser, 2006, p. 1350)*

pulation through playback experiments in which meerkats were exposed to recorded alarm calls.

Behavior observation indicates that, compared to adults, pups were *initially* more likely to respond to alarm calls in the presence of less dangerous or nondangerous predators, and they were more likely to ignore alarm calls emitted in the presence of dangerous predators. Other evidence also suggests that pups don't react as appropriately to alarm calls as adults. For example, after hearing an alarm call, pups often moved to shelter when they observed adults only briefly look up and scan for aerial predators. And even when pups displayed antipredator behaviors similar to those of adults, as when the pups looked up after they observed adults move to shelter, they reacted more slowly than did adults (Figure 12.19). As time passed, however, pups began to display more adult-like, adaptive, responses to alarm calls. Thus, pups appear to learn about alarm calls and predators from adults.

From a social learning perspective, two things about meerkat alarm calling and development are worth noting. First, female pups (and juveniles) exhibited adult-like responses to alarm calls more quickly than did males, and this apparently had a significant impact on fitness, as female pups suffered less mortality than did males (Russell et al., 2002). Second, throughout development, females remained closer to adults than did males. Together these results suggest that meerkat pups may learn the appropriate response to alarm calls from adult models, and that female pups are more adept at this than are male pups.

ALARM CALLS AS DECEPTIVE COMMUNICATION. Because alarm calls are a powerful form of communication—failure to listen might lead to death—natural selection should favor paying close attention to such calls. Nonetheless, these same selection pressures set up the possibility of using alarm calls in a deceptive manner. In Chapter 11, we mentioned that using alarm calls in a deceptive manner is probably the exception rather than the rule. That being said, there is, in fact, some evidence that deceptive use of these calls exists in a number of species.

Cheney and Seyfarth suggest that vervets sometimes use deceptive predator alarm calls during some intergroup encounters—encounters that can lead to serious aggression between group members (Cheney and Seyfarth, 1990). Occasionally, male vervets give an alarm call when encountering a new troop, even though no predator is in the vicinity. It is unlikely that these predator alarm calls are mistakes, as vervets are quite sophisticated when it comes to such calls, and their behavior seems to indicate that they know when a predator is around and when it isn't (see Chapter 11 and opening section of this chapter). An additional reason that ethologists doubt that such calls are given in error is that the response to alarm calls may provide alarm callers with a benefit: when these calls are emitted, all vervets head for cover, and so a potentially dangerous intergroup encounter is avoided and the alarm caller does not have to fight, at least for the moment.

In the 264 intergroup interactions that Cheney and Seyfarth observed, males gave false alarm calls regarding the presence of leopards about 2 percent of the time. Moreover, it was almost always a low-ranking male—an individual near the bottom of a dominance hierarchy who thus stood the most to lose from aggressive intergroup interactions—who gave the call. On the other hand, vervets don't have the whole deception package that, say, people might have at their disposal. For example, on a number of occasions, one vervet named Kitui emitted an alarm call when an interloper from another group was near his troop. Cheney and Seyfarth described what happened next:

> As if to convince his rival of the full import of his calls, Kitui twice left his own tree, walked across the open plain, and entered a tree adjacent to the interloper's, alarm calling all the while. Kitui acted as if he got only half the story right; he knew that his alarm calls had caused others to believe there was a leopard nearby, but he did not seem to realize that other aspects of his behavior should be consistent with his calls. To leave his tree and to walk toward the other male simply betrayed his own lack of belief in the leopard. (Cheney and Seyfarth, 1990, p. 215)

Deceptive alarm calls are not unique to primates and have been found in at least three studies on birds (Møller, 1988, 1990; Munn, 1986). In one such species—the barn swallow—males may emit false alarm calls when they see their mate engaging in an extrapair copulation that may result in the mate having an offspring by another male (see Chapter 7; Møller, 1990). Anders Møller hypothesized that these alarm calls break up extrapair matings, as a male swallow that is attempting an extrapair mating with the alarm caller's mate should take flight when the call is emitted. To test this idea, when males were away from their nests, Møller chased their mate away from the nest as well. This was done both during the period when extrapair copulations were most likely (during egg laying) and when such pairings were least likely (during egg incubation periods). When females were absent during egg laying, the males who returned to their nests almost always gave false alarm calls, which might serve to disrupt any extrapair copulation that their mate was undertaking. In the same situation, during periods when extrapair copulations were unlikely,

A

Territory
1 male

Returning territory 1 male
sees no female and
emits "false" alarm call

B

Territory
2 male

Territory 1 female

Extrapair copulation by
territory 1 female and
territory 2 male interrupted

C

100

75

50

25

0

% males giving alarm calls

■ Solitary
breeding
swallows

■ Colonial
breeding
swallows

Nest building   Egg laying   Incubation

Time in breeding cycle

FIGURE 12.20. Dishonest alarm calls in swallows? (A) Male barn swallows often give false alarm calls when their fertile mates leave the nest vicinity. **(B)** These false alarm calls sometimes disrupt extrapair copulations (EPCs). **(C)** Møller hypothesized that male swallows would give false alarm calls when they were at the greatest risk of EPCs to disrupt the EPCs. To test this, Møller removed a female from the nest at different stages in the breeding cycle for both solitary breeding swallows and colonial breeding swallows. Solitary breeding males almost never emitted alarm calls when their mate was temporarily gone. Colonial breeding males emitted false alarm calls during the period in which EPCs were most likely (during egg laying). *(Based on Møller, 1990)*

males almost never emitted alarm calls (Figure 12.20). Thus, male swallows who emitted false alarm calls during possible periods of extrapair copulations were tapping into an evolved response to the real threat that predators pose, co-opting this form of communication and, in the course of such deception, making alarms calls a less reliable signal.

When signals, such as alarm calls, become less reliable, natural selection should favor paying less and less attention to them. This raises the question of whether animals who receive inaccurate information from a signaler respond by eventually ignoring the signaler. James Hare and Brent Atkins experimentally examined this question in Richardson's ground squirrels (*Spermophilus richardsonii*; Figure 12.21). Hare and Atkins placed juvenile ground squirrels into one

FIGURE 12.21. Alarm calls in Richardson's squirrels. Over time, when predator alarm calls are unreliable, juvenile squirrels began to ignore such false alarm cues. *(Photo credit: John Cancalosi/naturepl.com)*

INTERVIEW WITH

Dr. Rufus Johnstone

What do ethologists mean when they speak of communication? How did you come to study this phenomenon?

Different people have defined communication in different ways. I would say, though, that it entails the use of specialized structures or behaviors (signals) by one individual to modify the behavior of others. The key feature of this definition is the emphasis on specialized signals, by which I mean traits that have been favored by natural selection specifically because of their influence on the behavior of receivers. There are plenty of cues that can provide receivers with useful information, but have not been selected for that reason. Consider, for instance, a field mouse that rustles the grass as it moves and draws the attention of a predator such as an owl. The rustling noise provides the predator with a cue to the prey's location, but selection has not favored noisy mice for this reason—quite the reverse! So I would not see this as a true instance of communication, nor the rustling as a true signal. By contrast, when a peacock displays its train or a nightingale sings, their behavior has been favored by selection because of the responses it elicits from others.

Animal signals are so striking and so diverse, one can't help being fascinated by them. Just think of a bowerbird's elaborately decorated bower, or the complex song of a humpback whale, or take a look at the gape of a parrot finch chick—what could possibly have driven the evolution of such an extreme display? But more than any individual example,

what most appealed to me about the study of communication was the idea that there might be unifying principles of signal evolution underlying this great diversity of different displays.

What is meant by honest communication? When do animal behaviorists expect to find this type of communication, and when don't they?

Again, different people use the word "honesty" in different senses. In everyday speech, it usually carries "intentional" connotations. That is, an honest individual is one who bears no intent to deceive, but rather means to convey reliable, truthful information. In this sense, however, the concept of honesty is inapplicable to many animals (though not perhaps to all), who lack any awareness of the responses their signals may evoke (or the meanings they may convey). Nevertheless, biologists often speak of honest and dishonest signals—one

might, for instance, describe the aposematic coloration (bright warning colors) of a palatable hoverfly that mimics a wasp as dishonest. This is not to imply that the hoverfly is engaged in intentional deceit. Rather, a dishonest signal in this sense is one that elicits a response that is beneficial to the signaler, but detrimental to the receiver. In this case, the hoverfly obviously benefits when its bright colors deter a predator, but the predator loses out because it has foregone a potentially palatable meal. Conversely, an honest signal is one that elicits responses that are beneficial for the receiver as well as for the signaler. The aposematic coloration of the wasp model, for instance, unlike that of the hoverfly, is honest—the wasp gains if its black and yellow stripes deter attack, but so too do the predators that avoid it.

When do we expect to find honest communication? To begin with, if there is no evolutionary conflict of interest between signaler and receiver, then there should be no selection for deceitful signals, because what benefits the receiver also benefits the signaler. This is typically the case when we consider communication between close relatives. A nice example is the waggle dance of the honeybee. When a worker returns to the hive with food, the waggle dance she performs conveys information to her fellow workers about the direction and distance of the food source. There is no evolutionary incentive for deceit here, because the worker benefits by recruiting others to the food; all share the same evolutionary interest in the productivity of the colony.

What about communication between individuals with conflicting interests? Even here, we might expect that honest communication is the norm. The reason is that in the long run, selection will favor receivers that ignore a consistently dishonest signal, and that attend only to signals which provide reliable information at least some of the time. Moreover, signals which are costly to produce or maintain are likely to provide such information, because it only pays signalers to employ them if they are of high quality or in great need—this is Zahavi's handicap principle. Of course, there are plenty of examples of dishonesty, but deceitful signalers must typically exploit some underlying system of reliable communication— and dishonesty cannot be too frequent or too costly to receivers if the system is to persist.

How does an ethologist build a mathematical model of something as complex as communication?

Constructing a model always involves a lot of simplification. This is not necessarily a bad thing—in fact, a model that is too detailed and complex is often rather unhelpful, because it is likely to be applicable only to one specific system, and it may be very difficult to understand the results it yields. The best models are those that strike a good balance between generality and specificity. The difficulty lies in identifying which factors to include, and which you can omit. In modeling communication, a distinction is often made between efficacy and strategy. The details of signal design have an important influence on the ease with which receivers can detect and identify a signal (its efficacy), but strategic issues of honesty and reliability

depend principally on the costs of signal production, the benefits of eliciting certain responses, and the fitness consequences of those responses for the receiver. So many strategic models ignore the details of signal form and focus solely on costs and benefits. This approach has generated many insights, although in the long run, I suspect it will be necessary to integrate both efficacy and strategy in a more comprehensive analysis.

Do you think communication is more important in some behavioral venues (for example, foraging, aggression, cooperation) than others? If so, why?

I think that communication plays an important role in almost every behavioral interaction. In any social context, individuals are likely to benefit from information about those with whom they interact—their nature, identity, motivation, and physiological state may all be relevant. So we would expect animals to attend to behavioral and morphological cues that provide such information. But whenever receivers do attend to a cue, selection will favor those individuals who tend to elicit the most beneficial responses—leading to the elaboration of cues into true signals. In fact, many behaviors that are not obviously displays may be modified in this way. When a parent bird, for instance, brings food to the nest, it is engaging in parental care. But this behavior may also indicate to its mate that the offspring are hungry, or that the focal parent is a good provider, encouraging the mate to work harder or deterring it from seeking an alternative partner. Indeed, it may be that frequent feeding is partly driven by the need to impress the mate, rather than simply to supply the young. So cooperation over offspring care might entail communication, even if there are no

obvious display behaviors involved. In general, I think it is very difficult to fully understand the evolution of social foraging, aggression, cooperation, or any other type of interaction without thinking about the information that an individual's actions convey to others in this way— and in that sense, communication is always important.

Do you think of human communication via language as fundamentally different from all other forms of communication?

Human language is certainly exceptional. I don't think all of its striking features are individually unique to our species. Other animals, for instance, employ apparently arbitrary signals to convey information about the external world—the usual example is the alarm calling of vervet monkeys, who make distinct vocalizations to alert others to the presence of leopards, eagles, and snakes. Similarly, other species can produce varied signals by combining distinct display elements in different ways—songbirds provide a good example. But there is no animal signaling system even remotely comparable to human language in complexity, flexibility, and scope of reference. What's more, from a strategic perspective talk is cheap; honesty among humans is not maintained by the costs of faking an exaggerated display, but by social sanctions. This is very different from the costly signals with which ethologists are often concerned.

Dr. Rufus Johnstone is a professor at the University of Cambridge (England). Dr. Johnstone's game theory models of animal behavior have shed light on many questions surrounding the evolution of communication.

of two treatments. In one treatment, juveniles heard a recorded alarm call and then saw a predator (a stuffed badger). They then heard the same alarm call, which was paired with the presentation of the predator nine more times (for a total of ten presentations). In a second treatment, ground squirrels again heard an alarm call, but subsequently they did not see a predator. In this treatment, the same alarm call was repeated ten times but not followed by presentation of a predator. Individuals in the second group were receiving unreliable—that is, false—alarm calls (Hare and Atkins, 2001).

Hare and Atkins examined how long the squirrels remained vigilant (vigilance duration) and the extent to which juvenile squirrels in the two treatment conditions turned in the direction from which an alarm call emanated (postural change). No differences across the two groups were found in their response to the first alarm call, which was to be expected, as the squirrels had no knowledge beforehand as to which alarm calls would be reliable and which would not. Even after hearing five alarm calls, no differences in vigilance duration were found across the two treatment groups, although there was a difference in postural change, with squirrels that had heard unreliable calls less likely to look in the direction of the call than were squirrels that had heard reliable calls. After hearing the alarm call ten times, differences in vigilance duration between the two groups of squirrels emerged. Squirrels in the group in which the alarm was paired with a reliable caller (who accurately alerted them to the presence of a predator) responded to alarm calls in a typical manner—by remaining vigilant and looking in the direction of the call. Squirrels in the other treatment—in which the information they had been receiving was inaccurate—essentially ignored the alarm calls, and they were unlikely to look in the direction from which the calls emanated (Figure 12.22). Given enough

FIGURE 12.22. **Responses to reliable and unreliable alarm calls.** Postural change (elevation of the head in the direction of the perceived threat) was virtually the same in response to all alarm calls by reliable callers (green bars). There was less postural change in response to unreliable alarm callers (orange bars) by the fifth unreliable alarm call, and much less postural change by the tenth unreliable alarm call. *(From Hare and Atkins, 2001, p. 110)*

information, then, Richardson's ground squirrels can distinguish between real and false alarm calls.

The transfer of information from a signaler to a receiver—communication— is a fundamental component to many aspects of animal behavior. In this chapter, we have seen when we expect communication to be honest, and when it might be deceptive. We have also examined the specific sorts of problems that communication may help solve—how to coordinate group foraging, how to find a mate, and how to alert others to the presence of a predator. In the course of reviewing communication, we have examined both the costs and benefits of communication, the phylogeny of communication systems, the role of learning, and the underlying proximate basis for communication.

SUMMARY

1. Communication is most often defined as the transfer of information from a signaler to a receiver.
2. A question that consistently rises to the surface when studying communication is whether it is "honest." One framework to study this question begins by assuming that the exchange of information between signaler and receiver is an attempt by the signaler to *manipulate* the recipient. Recipients are then selected to be good "mind readers."
3. Zahavi's handicap principle hypothesizes that honest signaling can evolve when traits are very costly to fake.
4. Communication systems are designed to solve problems that animals encounter in their natural environments.
5. When animals forage in social groups, they face coordination problems. When new food sources are found, that information must be transferred to other group members. Communication systems that solve the problem of recruiting others to food, including "squeak calls" by swallows, the waggle dance by honeybees, and chemical markers and stridulation by leaf-cutter ants, have been favored by natural selection.
6. Animals use communication to attract mates. For example, male birds use birdsong to attract females during the mating season, and male water striders use ripple communication to signal their location to female water striders.
7. Animals use communication to warn others in their family or group about predators. They teach their young to be alert to alarm calls about the approach of predators. But deceptive communication, such as fake alarm calls, has also been uncovered in primates and birds, suggesting that animals may adopt communication tactics designed to trick others in a manner beneficial to the deceiver.
8. Work on the costs and benefits of communication, the phylogenetic history of communication systems, the role of learning and social learning in shaping communication, and the underlying proximate basis for communication is providing ethologists with a much improved picture of signaler-receiver dynamics.

DISCUSSION QUESTIONS

1. Bacteria often release chemicals that affect other bacteria in their vicinity. Would you consider this communication? If so, why? If not, would you consider the chemical trails that ants use to direct one another to a food source communication? How does that differ from the bacteria case, if at all?

2. One problem examining whether a communication system more resembles exaggerations or "conspirational whispers" is that it is difficult to know how to define those terms for any given animal social system. How might you overcome this problem? Consider using a comparative study involving many species.

3. Imagine you are studying a group of amphibian species that vary in their habitats, some living in dense, murky water, and others living in very clear ponds. What kind of communication problems exist in each environment? What sorts of differences in communication systems would you expect to see across such species?

4. Suppose you are studying a heretofore unexamined species of primates. During your observations, you note that individuals are often throwing heavy rocks against trees, causing a large "booming" sound. You speculate that individuals are communicating to one another using this technique. How might you go about testing this hypothesis?

5. How has research on birdsong provided insight into both proximate and ultimate questions regarding communication?

SUGGESTED READING

Beecher, M. D., & Brenowitz, E. A. (2005). Functional aspects of song learning in songbirds. *Trends in Ecology & Evolution, 20,* 143–149. A review that touches on many aspects of birdsong.

Bradbury, J. W., & Vehrencamp, S. (1998). *Animal communication.* New York: Oxford University Press. A well-done overview of animal communication systems.

Cheney, D. L., & Seyfarth, R. M. (1990). *How monkeys see the world.* Chicago: University of Chicago Press. A wonderful look into how vervet monkeys perceive the world. Contains what is probably the best discussion of work on animal deception.

Dawkins, R., & Krebs, J. R. (1978). Animal signals: Information for manipulation? In J. R. Krebs & N. B. Davies, *Behavioural ecology* (pp. 282–315). Oxford: Blackwell. Also Krebs, J. R., & Dawkins, R. (1984). Animal signals: Mind reading and manipulation? In J. R. Krebs & N. B. Davies, *Behavioural ecology* (pp. 380–401). Oxford: Blackwell. A pair of book chapters that nicely outline the question of manipulation and mind reading.

Hauser, M. (1997). *The evolution of communication.* Cambridge, MA: MIT Press. Also Hauser, M., & Konishi, M. (Eds.) (1999). *The design of animal communication.* Cambridge, MA: MIT Press. A pair of books that synthesize biological and psychological perspectives on communication.

McGregor, P. (Ed.) (2005). *Animal communication networks*. Cambridge: Cambridge University Press. An edited volume that focuses on the transfer of information in social groups (networks).

Zahavi, A. (1997). *The handicap principle*. New York: Oxford University Press. A book-length treatment on the evolution of traits that are hard to fake, including traits related to communication.

13

Habitat Selection, Territoriality, and Migration

Virtually every aspect of an animal's behavior is affected by where it lives. This is true for animals that take up residence in a single place, as well as for those that move from place to place. From an ethological perspective, habitat choice is interesting, not only because the habitat of an animal affects its behavior (for example, what sorts of antipredator strategies will be successful, what types of foraging behaviors will yield the most food, what mating opportunities will be available, and so on), but also because the behavior of an animal affects its choice of habitat. For mobile animals, individuals can decide where to live, and in that sense they have some control over the ecological and evolutionary forces operating upon them.

To better understand the relationship between animal behavior and habitat choice, let's walk through a hypothetical scenario. Imagine a male bird that lives near a large marsh (Figure 13.1). Where should he spend his time during the remainder of the day? To answer that, our bird must balance many factors. If it is the mating season, one question would be: Where are the females? Females may prefer the safety of the reeds, so perhaps our male should go there. The reed area, however, may be home to organisms that parasitize this bird species. That is, there are both costs and benefits to staying in the reeds. Even if the reeds do not have parasites, courting a mate is energetically expensive, and it may be that prey are not found in the reeds, but over the marsh water, and so there might be reason to spend time over the marsh first. On the other hand, predators may also prefer the area over the marsh, and so, as with the reed area, there are costs as well as benefits to spending time over the marsh. The decision-making process is complicated, as it now includes mates, food, and

FIGURE 13.1. Habitat choice. Imagine a red-winged blackbird deciding where to form a territory. All sorts of factors—mates, temperature, predators—play a role in the decision making. Another factor in habitat choice is the availability of prey, such as the presence of dragonflies (not drawn to scale) shown flying above the marsh.

predators. Other factors, too, may play a role in determining where our bird goes. Temperature will vary both across the day and across the marsh, and this may affect where the bird spends time. The point of all this being that the choices faced by animals are complex and multidimensional.

Let's imagine that in deciding where to spend his time, our bird ends up flying between the reeds and the marsh water but does not spend that much time in any one area and does not stop others from using any of those areas. In such a case, we might speak of those areas being his **home range**. In other species, it might be that individuals are **nomads**, constantly wandering and never returning to the same place with any regularity.

Now suppose that our bird flies between the reeds and the marsh area but that he regularly returns to a particular area in the central part of the reeds, and actively tries to keep intruders outside of this area. Now we can speak of this bird as having a **territory**—an area occupied and defended by the bird. It might be that while our bird frequents the central marsh area as his home range, he only keeps intruders out of half of that area. In that case, his home range would be twice as big as his territory.

Some species stay in the same territory and home range for long periods of time. Naturally, what constitutes a long period of time will vary dramatically across species, but as an extreme example, some long-lived birds, such as Florida scrub jays, can maintain the same territory for years upon years and pass that territory down to their offspring (Woolfenden and Fitzpatrick, 1978, 1984).

Animal behaviorists have made considerable progress in understanding habitat choice and territoriality. In some cases, abiotic (nonliving) factors dominate habitat choice; in other cases, biotic (living) factors do. The abiotic factors that affect habitat choice include heat, availability of water, wind, refuge from danger, availability of specific nutrients, and so on. The biotic factors affecting habitat selection may include the location of mates, food, predators, and parasites. We will examine some of these in more depth in the remainder of the chapter.

Ethologists have gone far beyond simply creating a laundry list of variables that affect habitat choice. Far more interesting are the studies that delve into how such variables interact in determining habitat selection and territoriality. Researchers are also explicitly incorporating learning into habitat selection and finding fascinating new trends that may pave the way for future work in this area.

Even animals with defined home ranges and territories, however, can make dramatic shifts in the habitats in which they live; that is, they can periodically move long distances—from one region to another—through **migration**. The most dramatic examples of this are the large-scale migrations that are common in insects, reptiles, mammals, and birds. Let's imagine that we continue studying our bird, who wanders about his home range and defends his territory. Six months after watching our subject, we note that he actually leaves the marsh we have been studying and spends the next half year 2,000 miles south of where we first saw him. At the end of these six months, our bird returns back to the central reed area of the marsh and starts back where he began. In this case, we have home ranges and territories mixed in with large-scale migration. We might, in fact, get any number of permutations here. It may be that 2,000 miles south, our subject has another home range or territory or neither.

Animal behavior researchers have moved well beyond simply observing and recording migration. This is not meant to denigrate the labor-intensive work still under way documenting monumental migrations like those of the monarch butterflies, but only to suggest there is a lot more migration work these days that focuses on hypothesis testing per se. For example, we now have a much better handle on the physiology and resultant behavioral changes associated with switching from a "nonmigratory" to a "migratory" mode, as well as the costs and benefits of migration. What seemed impossible to study experimentally a generation ago is now commonplace in the study of migration.

Having introduced habitat selection, territoriality, and migration, we will take the rest of the chapter to examine the following topics in more depth:

- models of habitat choice and territoriality,
- territoriality and learning,
- family dynamics and territoriality,
- migration and navigation,
- migratory "restlessness,"
- parasites and migration,
- phylogeny and migration.

Models of Habitat Choice

Before examining territoriality per se, we will first explore a more general phenomena, that of habitat choice. While territoriality implies the defense of a set area, **habitat choice models** simply examine how animals distribute themselves in space and time with respect to some resource in their environment (Bateson, 1990; Brown and Rosenzweig, 1985; Kacelnik et al., 1992; Kennedy and Gray, 1993; Morris, 1994; Rosenzweig, 1981, 1985, 1990, 1991). The resource might be food items, mates, refuge from predators, and so on. Ecologists have examined how animals distribute themselves into different habitats—that is, where they end up living. What makes the work in ethology different from earlier work in ecology is that ethologists specifically focus on the role of behavioral decision making (how they choose where to live) and how that affects the distribution of animals in time and space.

THE IDEAL FREE DISTRIBUTION MODEL AND HABITAT CHOICE

Work in natural history has long suggested that animals seem to distribute themselves in relation to the distribution of resources. If two habitats differed in terms of the amount of food available, and one habitat had more food than the other, more animals tended to be found where there was more food. In a sense, this finding confirms our intuition, but animal behaviorists wanted to understand why this was such a common finding. What's more, they were interested in what behavioral rules animals use to distribute themselves between habitats. The **ideal free distribution (IFD)** model was developed to address these sorts of issues (Brown, 1969; Fretwell, 1972; Fretwell and Lucas, 1970; Orians, 1969; Parker and Stuart, 1976).

To see how the ideal free distribution model works, consider the case where individuals choose between only two habitats, which we will call H1 and H2, and these habitats have resources R1 and R2, respectively. For example, we might be looking at two patches that serve as possible habitats: one habitat (H1) provides five food units/minute (R1), and the other habitat (H2) provides animals with three food units/minute (R2). Imagine that we are studying a population that has N individuals, that individuals can move freely from habitat 1 to habitat 2, and that moving between food patches has no costs associated with it. How many individuals should end up in habitat H1 and how many in habitat H2?

The ideal free distribution model predicts that the equilibrium distribution of individuals into patches should be that distribution at which, if any individual moved to the patch she was not in, she would suffer a reduced payoff. That is, at the ideal free distribution equilibrium, any individual that moved from H1 to H2, or vice versa, would obtain fewer resources as a result of her move. Mathematically, it can be shown that this translates into individuals settling in habitats in proportion to the resources available in that patch. The equilibrium proportion of individuals in H1 and H2 should be reached when $R_1/N_1 = R_2/N_2$—that is, when the per capita intake rate of individuals in both patches is equal. This solution—$R_1/N_1 = R_2/N_2$—is also known as the resource matching rule, as the distribution of individuals at equilibrium matches the distribution of resources across patches.

THE IFD MODEL AND FORAGING SUCCESS

The IFD model has been applied to cases in which the resource driving habitat choice ranges from availability of mates to safe refuge from predators (Hoglund et al., 1998; Parker and Stuart, 1976). Here we will focus on two studies where the critical resource is food, and in particular we will address: (1) whether animals distribute themselves as the matching resource rule predicts, and (2) at such a distribution, whether all individuals receive about the same amount of food, as predicted by the IFD model.

The first direct test of IFD models of foraging was conducted by Manfred Milinski (Milinski, 1979). In an elegantly simple experiment, Milinski had six stickleback fish in a tank. The tank had two feeders that distributed food—water fleas (*Daphnia magna*)—at opposite ends of a tank. The foraging behavior of six sticklebacks was then observed in two treatments. In one treatment, water fleas were released from the two feeders in a 5:1 ratio (five times as much food at one feeder than the other); in the second treatment, the ratio of water fleas released from the feeders was 2:1. Milinski found that, after some initial sampling, the fish in both treatments distributed themselves under feeders in a ratio similar to the resource matching rule (Figure 13.2). For example, in the treatment in which five times more food was available at one feeder, five of the six fish were found at that feeder. While Milinski's work was the first experimental work demonstrating the resource matching rule, it was not designed to examine the feeding success of each individual, and hence could not determine whether individual foraging success was approximately equal across the two feeding patches. To examine that prediction of the IFD model, we turn to David Harper's work on habitat choice in mallard ducks.

FIGURE 13.2. Ideal free fish.
(A) When sticklebacks are presented with two foraging patches that produce food at a 5:1 ratio (5 water fleas being dropped into the tank from the left feeder versus 1 water flea being dropped into the tank from the right feeder), they distribute themselves in accordance with predictions from the ideal free distribution model. **(B)** Using this setup with sticklebacks foraging from two feeders on opposite sides of an aquarium, Milinski tested the ideal free distribution model for a 5:1 profitability ratio and then for a 2:1 ratio. The arrow on the left indicates the start of feeding; the arrow on the right indicates the point at which the profitabilities of the more and less profitable patches were reversed. For a 5:1 profitability ratio, the green points indicate the number of fish in the less profitable patch, and the green line shows the predicted number of fish at the less profitable patch. For the 2:1 profitability ratio, the orange points indicate the number of fish in the less profitable patch, and the orange lines show the predicted number of fish in the less profitable patch. *(Based on Milinski, 1979)*

Using individually recognizable mallards (*Anas platyrhynchos*) living in a pond at Cambridge University, Harper ran an IFD experiment similar to that of Milinski (Harper, 1982). Harper had two observers who were stationed 20 meters apart throw pre-cut, pre-weighed pieces of food (bread) into the pond. The observers acted both as data takers *and* as the food stations themselves. Harper varied the profitability of a patch by varying either the number of pieces of food added to that patch or the weight of each piece (Figure 13.3).

When equal amounts of food were thrown into patches by both observers, ducks quickly distributed themselves in a 1:1 ratio (Figure 13.4). In addition, as predicted by the IFD model, when one patch had twice as much bread as the other, the ducks distributed themselves in a 2:1 ratio.

During trials of his experiment, Harper noticed that some ducks seemed to be very aggressive and tended to receive a disproportionate amount of food within the patches. What this meant was that, although individuals distributed

A **B**

FIGURE 13.3. Ducks feeding at a pond. (A) One of the first controlled experiments on the ideal free distribution model involved ducks feeding at a pond. **(B)** To test the ideal free distribution model, food was thrown into a pond from two locations, and the distribution of ducks to each feeding station was recorded. *(Photo credit: Marc Epstein/ Visuals Unlimited)*

themselves across food patches in a manner similar to the resource matching rule, all individuals were *not* receiving the same amount of food across patches, and as such, the ducks' behavior might be better represented by a modified IFD model that takes into account such aggression (Parker and Sutherland, 1986; Sutherland, 1983; Sutherland and Parker, 1985).

Territoriality

With a general understanding of habitat choice via the IFD model, we can move on to examine territoriality—the occupation and defense of particular areas within a habitat. Territories can provide their owners with exclusive access to food, mates, and safe haven from predators, and are typically vigorously defended from intruders. Such defense can be costly, both in terms of time and energy, representing a cost of territoriality.

Most of our discussion of territoriality will focus on territories that contain either a single individual or a family. But it is important to recognize that territories are sometimes defended by groups of unrelated individuals. This sort of group territoriality can often result in dramatic between-group interactions, in which groups attempt to enlarge their own territory by taking over another group's territory. For example, consider the "between-group raiding" that is occasionally seen in natural populations of chimps. Between-group interactions often appear to be "war-like," and in fact resemble the raiding behavior that is common among many tribes of humans (Boehm, 1992). During raids, all-male chimpanzee "patrol groups" travel into areas that border their territorial boundaries (Bygott, 1979; Goodall, 1986; Nishida, 1979). In contrast to excursions for food, in which foraging chimps often emit vocalizations, chimps in patrols move in a wary fashion and remain silent (Goodall, 1986). These raids often involve the killing of a small number of members of the raided group, and the capture of females. Occasionally raiding parties from two groups will meet one another.

FIGURE 13.4. Ideal free ducks? The two foraging patches created when two individuals threw bread into a pond from different locations had equal profitability. The dashed line represents the predicted number of ducks at site 1. *(Based on Harper, 1982)*

In such instances, rather than engaging in extremely violent interactions, both groups engage in hostile vocalizations and then withdraw (Goodall, 1986). Despite the fact that all-out warfare does not emerge when two raiding parties meet, raiding can, in the long run, amount to the slow extinction of one group. For example, raiding behavior in the Mahale Mountains of Tanzania led in part to a larger group eradicating a smaller group of chimps (Nishida et al., 1985; see also Goodall, 1986, for evidence of this at Gombe).

TERRITORIALITY AND LEARNING

While most models of territoriality assume that animals are capable of assessing various characteristics about a potential territory—how much food is in the area, how safe the area may be from predators—they do not explicitly consider how learning affects the establishment and maintenance of a territory. Such learning-based models, however, have been constructed, and below we examine two models that examine how learning affects decisions regarding both the acquisition and subsequent maintenance of territories.

TERRITORIALITY AND LEARNING DURING SETTLEMENT. Territoriality in juvenile *Anolis aeneus* lizards has been the subject of an in-depth analysis by Judy Stamps (Stamps, 2001). These lizards form territories early in life, and Stamps was interested in, among many other things, where and how juveniles decided to stake out a territory (Figure 13.5). Because much of the work on territoriality has centered on the distribution of food resources, Stamps's initial inclination was to test for the importance of food availability in structuring territoriality in *A. aeneus*. Yet, despite numerous experiments manipulating food availability, she did not uncover a clear-cut effect of food availability on territory formation. Rather, in subsequent experiments, Stamps found that safety from predators and suitable temperature appeared to be the most important attributes of a desirable territory. But *how* do juvenile lizards determine which territories are suitable with respect to temperature and predation pressure? More specifically,

A

B

FIGURE 13.5. Territorial lizards. (A) Juvenile *Anolis aeneus* are very territorial, and their territory formation has been studied in the context of habitat choice and learning. **(B)** *Anolis aeneus* stake out territories in areas such as those depicted here. *(Photo credits: Judy Stamps)*

FIGURE 13.6. Conspecific cueing and territorial lizards. (A) Focal juveniles not only spent more time on experimental (E) versus control (C) homesites, but they also arrived at experimental homesites more quickly. **(B)** Juvenile lizards were drawn to experimentally manipulated homesites (E) over control (C) homesites. Control territories remained empty prior to the focal's choice, while experimental territories had formerly contained a territorial juvenile. *(Based on Stamps, 1987a)*

given that these factors affect what areas lizards choose as territories, do lizards *learn* what areas are best from their interactions with other lizards (Stamps and Krishnan, 1999, 2001)?

From earlier work, Stamps had noticed that juvenile *A. aeneus* were interested in what other lizards were doing, and she hypothesized that they might be determining territory quality as a result of their interactions with conspecifics. In other words, if another individual has already determined a territory is safe and has temperatures that will not cause overheating, then it probably is safe and probably will not cause overheating. This sort of decision-making process, in which individuals use the choices of others to determine the quality of a potential territory, has been called "conspecific cueing."

Stamps tested the conspecific cueing hypothesis by examining whether a territory that had been occupied by an owner sometime in the past but was currently vacant would be viewed as attractive to other lizards (Stamps, 1987a). In this experiment, a juvenile would be allowed to observe two very similar territories, one that was currently occupied and one that was vacant. When given the choice between these two areas, with the territory owner now removed, juveniles showed a strong preference for the previously inhabited area (Figure 13.6). Furthermore, juveniles who had not observed the territories during the initial part of the experiment but were given a choice between these territories displayed no preference for the previously occupied territory, suggesting a strong visual component to conspecific cueing in *A. aeneus* (Stamps, 1987b).

TERRITORY OWNERS AND SATELLITES

As we have seen, territory ownership often requires constant vigilance against both predators and conspecific intruders who might attempt to make that territory their own. This relationship between vigilance and territoriality can be

FIGURE 13.7. Territorial wagtails.
Economic models of territorial ownership, and the acceptance of intruders, have been put to the test in pied wagtails. *(Photo credit: Charles McRae/Visuals Unlimited)*

complex. Here we will examine this complexity by addressing whether the costs and benefits of territory defense are ever such that it is in a territory holder's interest to allow other individuals to share its territory, at least temporarily.

OWNERS, SATELLITES, AND TERRITORY DEFENSE IN PIED WAGTAILS. From the perspective of a territory holder, intruders onto a territory need not always be a liability. To see why, let's examine the economics of territoriality in pied wagtail birds (*Motacilla alba*; Figure 13.7). During the winter season, pied wagtails defend riverside territories, where they forage on insects that have washed up onto riverbanks (Davies, 1976; Figure 13.8). This food source is "renewable" in the sense that, even after insects are consumed, more insects eventually will wash up on shore. What this means is that if a pied wagtail can time its movement within a territory correctly, it can deplete the insects in one part of its territory, proceed to search other parts of its territory for food, and by the time it returns to the original section again, find more insect prey there for it to consume.

Nick Davies and Alasdair Houston tracked the movement and foraging activity of a population of pied wagtails on a riverbank along the Thames River, near Oxford, England, and found that these birds systematically searched their territories and timed their movements such that they did not return to an area on which they had foraged until sufficient time had elapsed for a new crop of insect prey to wash up onto the banks (Davies and Houston, 1981).

While on their winter territories, pied wagtails must often deal with territorial intruders (Davies and Houston, 1981). Under certain conditions, intruders are tolerated, at which point ethologists refer to them as satellites. Under other conditions, intruders are aggressively chased off a territory. Davies and Houston wanted to know what determines when intruders are allowed onto a territory as satellites and when they are not.

To understand how territory owners make such decisions, we need to recognize that a territory is worth more to a pied wagtail owner than to an intruder, because intruders do not know which areas in a territory have recently been cropped (and so have few prey), but owners do. If an owner permits an intruder to stay, it loses some foraging-related benefits, but it will also gain the satellite's assistance in territory defense against other intruders (Table 13.1). Having a satellite around makes a territory owner's residence a bit safer, but not quite as profitable in terms of food.

A

B

FIGURE 13.8. Pied wagtails and food search. Pied wagtails systemically search for food on their territories along riverbanks. **(A)** A single bird can complete a circuit of the riverbank in 40 minutes and gets all the food it finds. **(B)** When a territory is shared by two birds, however, the circuit is divided up as well, and so each bird primarily gets the food that it finds in its 20 minutes of walking the riverbank. *(Based on Davies and Houston, 1984)*

TABLE 13.1. Owners and satellites. Pied wagtails form winter foraging territories along a river. Owners often allow "satellite" individuals to forage on such territories. Some territorial defense is provided by the satellites. *(Based on Davies and Houston, 1981)*

| | NUMBER OF DEFENSES BY | | PERCENT DEFENSES |
TERRITORY	OWNER	SATELLITE	BY SATELLITE
1	13	5	27.8
2	2	1	33.3
4	8	2	20.0
5	6	6	50.0
7	44	22	33.3
8	8	7	46.7
9	13	15	53.6
Total	94	58	38.1

Davies and Houston built a mathematical model to predict when owners would allow satellites on their territories and when they would not. In general, their model predicts that when the benefits of having a satellite on a territory outweigh the costs, satellites will be allowed on the territory. And, indeed, this seems to be what happens. For example, on days when food availability was particularly high, territory owners tolerated satellites; otherwise, they evicted such intruders. This is a particularly interesting case of conditional cooperation because it suggests that the costs and benefits of byproduct mutualism (see Chapter 9) can vary depending on territory-holding status. Would-be satellites, who have no foraging territories of their own, always face a harsh environment with respect to food allocation, and they are willing to pay the costs of territory defense in order to have access to food on territories. When food becomes sparse for owners, however, they do not allow intruders in. So, intruders are always willing to undertake cooperative territory defense in exchange for food, but the costs and benefits of byproduct mutualism do not always select for owners to permit this cooperative act (Brown, 1982).

HOW TO KEEP A TERRITORY IN THE FAMILY

For more than thirty years, Glen Woolfenden, J. Fitzpatrick, and their colleagues have been studying Florida scrub jays at the Archibold Biological Station (Woolfenden and FitzPatrick, 1990). Unlike closely related species in the western United States in which the young disperse from their natal territories before their first birthday, Florida scrub jays have an elaborate system of helpers-at-the-nest (see Chapters 3 and 8), resulting in an interesting territorial inheritance system, in which territory ownership is passed down across generations, leading

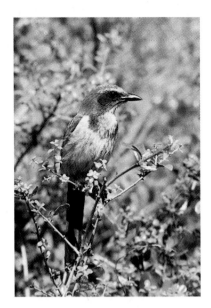

FIGURE 13.9. Scrub jays and territories. In Florida scrub jays, territories are "inherited" across generations, leading to the establishment of "family dynasties." Territory size is increased through a process called budding. *(Photo credit: Charlie Heidecker/ Visuals Unlimited)*

to "family dynasties" (Fitzpatrick and Woolfenden, 1984, 1988; Quinn et al., 1999; Woolfenden and FitzPatrick, 1990; Figure 13.9).

Each Florida scrub jay territory is initially occupied by a monogamous pair of birds. In addition, territories contain up to six helpers-at-the-nest and all individuals, including helpers, defend the territory. When territories are formed, they may be relatively small. But, as family size increases, so does territory size (up to a point). The way this typically occurs is through a process known as territorial budding (Woolfenden and Fitzpatrick, 1978). At about two and a half years of age, a male scrub jay, with the help of his family members, will expand the boundaries of family territory and actively defend this new area (the "budded" territory) as his own. While there are some aggressive interactions between the male who has acquired this budded territory and the family members in adjacent territories, these are rare compared to the aggressive acts between such a male and any nonfamily members that border his territory.

The budding procedure serves to increase a family's total territory size, provides a male with his own smaller territory, and essentially creates a form of inheritance. This inheritance system, with larger families outcompeting smaller families, may lead to very large territorial family dynasties.

CONFLICT WITHIN FAMILY TERRITORIES

Because they are genetically related, family members that share a territory usually do not differ in terms of what constitutes the best behavioral decisions affecting all group members. But this is not always the case. Under certain conditions, family members on a territory may differ on decisions about when a territory member—let's call it individual X—should leave a territory and breed on its own. For example, it may be in individual X's best interest to leave its natal territory and breed at time 1, while it may be in the best interest of other family members on the territory for X to remain at home, not to breed, and to help family members at time 1. Conversely, it may be in X's interest not to breed, but in the interests of other family members for X to breed on its own territory. In fact, there is a burgeoning literature on **optimal skew theory**, which studies the distribution of breeding within a group and whether there will be cooperation or conflict over reproductive activities (see Chapter 8). For a good example of conflicting interests in terms of breeding, we turn to Steve Emlen's work on parent-offspring conflict over breeding opportunities in white-fronted bee-eaters (*Merops bullockoides*) (Emlen and Wrege, 1992).

Like the young in many communally breeding bird species, young male white-fronted bee-eaters often remain on their natal territory and aid their relatives, usually their parents, in raising young (typically their siblings). When breeding opportunities for young males are rare, no conflict exists between young males and their parents—it is in the best of interest of all parties for the young male to remain at home and help his parents. The situation gets more complex when breeding opportunities away from the natal nest are more readily available to such a young male. Under these conditions, it may be in the best interest of a young male to breed on his own, but in the best interest of this male's parents for him to remain at home and help raise his siblings. This leads to conflict between offspring and parent.

To understand this conflict of interest, consider the following: Pairs of mates without helpers raise on average 0.51 offspring per clutch. Every helper a pair has at its service adds approximately 0.47 offspring. Keeping in mind that young males who breed for the first time will rarely have a helper of their own, let's start with the perspective of a young male's parents. If their son attempts to breed, he will, on average, produce 0.51 offspring. But, if instead, he helps them, he will add, on average, 0.47 offspring to their next clutch. Since the young male's parents are twice as related to their own offspring ($r = 0.5$) as they are to grand-offspring ($r = 0.25$)—that is, the offspring that their son would have produced had he not helped but instead gone off to find a territory and a mate—the parents will have an incentive to keep their son around to help. Therefore, ethologists predict that parents will try to block any attempt on the young male's part to leave.

The genetic accounting is different from the young male's perspective. Because he is equally related ($r = 0.5$) to his own offspring and to his siblings (individuals he would assist if he were to help his parents), there is no incentive for such a male to resist his parents' attempt to suppress his breeding. Hence, parental suppression of offspring breeding is met with little resistance on the part of their son. This interpretation is bolstered by the fact that when a breeding pair tries to suppress the reproductive efforts of more distant kin, or even nonkin, their actions are met with much stiffer resistance than when they attempt to suppress the reproduction of their own offspring.

Migration

While we often think of choosing a habitat as leading to a sedentary lifestyle, it need not always be the case. For animals that migrate, particularly those that migrate long distances, choice of the appropriate habitat throughout a year may require vast amounts of energy to be spent on traveling. Consider this eloquent summary of bird migration:

> Twice each year, billions of birds, entire species, swarm across the globe, traveling thousands of miles as they follow the sun to populate regions that are habitable for only part of the year. The spatial scope of these migrations exceeds all other biological phenomena. So fantastic are they that ancient civilizations devised a host of myths to explain the periodic appearance and disappearance of such vast numbers of animals. Those apocryphal stories were concocted in part because what we know to be true seemed then so completely beyond the pale. It seemed more likely that swallows buried themselves in the mud at the bottom of ponds than that they flew all the way from Europe to Africa and back twice each year. But the truth turned out to be more amazing than the myth. (Able, 1999, p. vii)

And migration is not limited to birds. From wildebeests swarming across the African plains to monarch butterflies heading by the tens of millions to Mexico each year, migration is seen across many different groups of animals, and is certainly one of the most spectacular of all animal behaviors. In some species, annual migration is obligatory, occurring like clockwork; in other species, it occurs only when conditions become poor (in what is called irruptive migration); in still other cases, only a portion of a population will migrate, while the rest stays put (Able, 1999). No matter where a species falls on this migration

FIGURE 13.10. Animal migration. In some species of birds and mammals, massive yearly migrations take place. Here we see migration in **(A)** geese and **(B)** gnu. *(Photo credits: William J. Weber/Visuals Unlimited; Joe McDonald/Visuals Unlimited)*

continuum, questions abound—how do they know where to go, when to go, how to go, how to prepare (Able, 1999; Alerstam, 1990; Baker, 1978; Gauthreaux, 1980; Heape, 1931; Ramenofsky and Wingfield, 2007; Salewsk and Bruderer, 2007; Wiltschko and Wiltschko, 2003; Figure 13.10)?

MIGRATION AND NAVIGATION

To migrate long distances, animals must navigate through the environment. That is, they must use cues to assess where they are in relation to where they are heading. As we are about to see, these cues can come in many forms—the position of the sun, the position of the stars, various landmarks on the ground, the odor of a stream, and so on—but one way or another, migrating animals must determine if they are heading where they want to go, and if not, how they can get back on track.

MIGRATION AND THE SUN COMPASS. Both because the sun is such a large, prominent object in the sky, and because it provides information about direction, ethologists have long speculated that migrating animals use the sun to help them navigate. Here we shall examine exactly how monarch butterflies use the sun to guide them on their journeys.

Few natural spectacles are as magnificent as seeing tens of millions of monarch butterflies (*Danaus plexippus*) migrating each year from North America to the mountain ranges of central Mexico. During their annual migration, the air is so thick with monarch butterflies that branches of trees have been known to collapse from the weight of too many butterflies (Figure 13.11). Monarch butterflies traverse up to 6,000 miles on their migratory trip, and they almost always navigate successfully without getting lost, even on their first migration.

As they travel south, monarch butterflies use the position of the sun in relation to the time of day to help them navigate (Mouritsen and Frost, 2002; Perez et al., 1997). To examine the role of solar navigation in this species, Sandra Perez and her colleagues ran a classic "clock-shift" experiment (Perez et al., 1997). The basic idea in such studies is to experimentally manipulate

FIGURE 13.11. Monarch migration.
Migration of monarch butterflies can involve tens of millions of individuals. Here we see a tree covered in monarchs. *(Photo credit: Fritz Polking/ Visuals Unlimited)*

the amount of daylight and darkness animals are exposed to such that they experience a light-dark cycle that is different from the normal cycle at that time of year. For example, more hours of daylight are typically experienced in the summer than in the winter, but clock-shift experiments allow an experimenter to take an animal during the winter and expose it (in the laboratory) to the light-dark cycle it typically experiences in the summer. This manipulation of its biological clock tricks the animal into acting as if it were summer.

At the start of the experiment, Perez and her team raised one group of monarch butterflies in a laboratory and slowly shifted the butterflies' body clocks back six hours—when the real time, for example, was noon, the clock-shifted monarchs acted as if it were six hours later. The researchers also kept a second group of butterflies in the laboratory, but these butterflies' body clocks were not shifted; they were the control group. During the period of autumn migration south, Perez and her team released individual monarch butterflies that they had raised in the laboratory. They then watched these individual butterflies and noted their position by using handheld compasses. The control butterflies headed south, just as wild populations of monarch butterflies typically do in the autumn migration (Figure 13.12). The clock-shifted butterflies, however, flew almost due west, which is just where Perez and her team expected them to fly if they were using a sun compass to help them navigate during their migration. That is, the six-hour clock shift caused the butterflies to misinterpret the

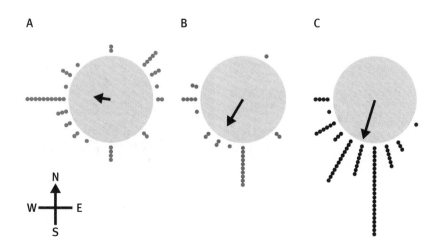

FIGURE 13.12. Clock-shifted monarch butterflies and navigation. The diagrams show the mean body position of monarch butterflies during the first five minutes of autumn migration. **(A)** Clock-shifted birds fly west, **(B)** laboratory raised butterflies, who were raised on a normal light-dark cycle for autumn, fly south, and **(C)** butterflies from natural populations fly south. *(From Perez et al., 1997, p. 29)*

FIGURE 13.13. Insect flight simulator. A flight simulator for monarchs was constructed in the laboratory, and a butterfly was tethered to this device. The pipe at the bottom of the simulator directed a constant flow of air up toward the butterfly so that it could fly; a video camera was connected to the bottom of the simulator (so that the researchers could see when the butterfly was flying, gliding, or stopping; the four images show the images from four flight simulators); an encoder (recording the butterfly's direction) was attached to the butterfly from the top of the simulator and was connected to a computer that kept a timed record of all the butterfly's movements. With this setup, researchers could track the direction the butterfly was orienting toward and whether it was actively flying or gliding. *(From Mouritsen and Frost, 2002, p. 10163)*

FIGURE 13.14. Bunting migration. **(A)** Indigo buntings can use the stars as a navigation tool. **(B)** Planetarium in which indigo buntings in funnel-shaped cages were shown the stars. *(Photo credits: Maslowski/ Visuals Unlimited; Cornell University)*

information that the sun was conveying about direction and to fly west, rather than south.

Henrik Mouritsen and Barrie Frost examined in even greater detail monarch butterflies' use of a sun compass to navigate. They built a miniature flight simulator (Figure 13.13) that allowed them to follow the orientation of a tethered monarch butterfly for much longer than the five-minute time frame in the Perez experiment (Mouritsen and Frost, 2002). Using this flight simulation device and the clock-shift protocol we discussed above, Mouritsen and Frost confirmed the use of the sun compass during monarch butterfly migration.

INDIGO BUNTINGS AND NAVIGATING BY THE STARS. The vast majority of passerine birds migrate almost exclusively at night (Able, 1999). What cues might such birds use when traveling after the sun has set? One of the earliest and best-known studies of how migrating individuals use the stars to guide them was undertaken by Stephen Emlen. Building on prior ethological work by Kramer and Sauer, Emlen undertook an ingenious set of experiments involving indigo buntings (*Passerina cyanea*), a nocturnal migratory species that travels 2,000 miles each winter from the northeastern United States to the Bahamas, Mexico, and Panama (Emlen, 1967, 1970, 1975; Figure 13.14).

Emlen began by creating funnel-shaped test cages for buntings, at the bottom of which he placed an ink pad. The cages were constructed such that each time a bunting tried to fly out, the location of its footprint was marked by ink, and so its orientation pattern was easily recorded (Figure 13.15). When these cages were placed under a star-lit sky, the buntings clearly oriented their attempts in the direction they would normally migrate—toward the south in September and October, and toward the north in April and May. In addition, these patterns all but disappeared on cloudy nights when stars were not visible, suggesting a strong role for some sort of star-based navigation system.

Emlen repeated his experiments inside a planetarium, where he could control what the birds saw in a simulated night-time sky. Results were very similar to those obtained in the field, but Emlen was now able to artificially

A

B

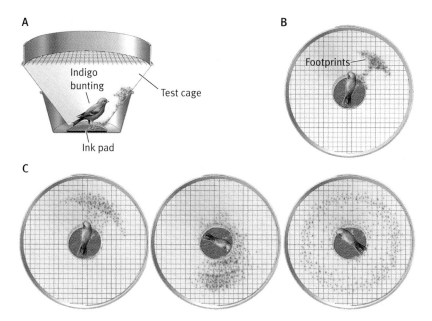

FIGURE 13.15. Migration and orientation. (A) A cross-sectional view and **(B)** a top view of the circular test cage used by Emlen in his orientation/migration work in indigo buntings. The funnel portion of the cage was made of white blotting paper, with an ink pad at the bottom. The entire apparatus was placed in an outdoor cage. The migration tendencies of the buntings were recorded as the bird tried to hop out of the funnel. **(C)** Each time the bunting hopped in one direction, it appeared as black footprints on the blotting paper. The left footprint records show a bunting during spring (when it orients north), the middle footprint records show a bunting during fall (when it orients south), and the right footprint records show a bunting on nights when the stars are obscured (and it hops randomly with respect to direction). *(Based on Emlen, 1975)*

shift the position of the North Star. In response to this manipulation, buntings shifted to the "new south" or "new north" (depending on the season). Emlen was able to further demonstrate that buntings appear to use the geometric patterns of stars in northern skies as one guide on their long journey.

There are numerous constellations that fall within 35 degrees of the North Star, and buntings appear to be able to cue in on more than one of these constellations. Removal of one star from the normal pattern does *not* throw the birds off track, as they apparently fall back to relying on the stellar information that remains. Emlen sums it up nicely by noting that "since birds frequently migrate on nights when there is variable cloud cover, such redundancy is obviously adaptive."

THE EARTH'S MAGNETIC FIELD AND ANIMAL MIGRATION. The hypothesis that the earth's magnetic field might affect animal navigation and migration has been in the behavioral literature for more than a century, but the first experimental work on this idea was not undertaken until the late 1960s and early 1970s, when it was found that magnets glued to the back of pigeons disoriented birds navigating across a fifteen- to thirty-mile route (Keeton, 1971; Wiltschko, 1968; Wiltschko and Wiltschko, 1995, 2003).

FIGURE 13.16. Magnetic fields and bobolinks. Research has examined whether bobolinks use the magnetic field of the earth to help guide them on their annual migration, which involves a 12,400-mile round-trip. *(Photo credit: Jim Fenton/pbase)*

Evidence that the magnetic field of the earth is important in migration has been found in a wide diversity of animals, including birds, amphibians, reptiles, and insects (Freake et al., 2006). To see how magnetic fields can affect navigation and migration, let's examine the behavior of the bobolink (or rice bird; *Dolichonyx oryzivorus*), which has one of the longest round-trip annual migrations of any animal—12,400 miles. These birds spend the summer months in the northern United States and Canada and then undertake a migration to South America (primarily Brazil, Paraguay, and Argentina) before they return to the Northern Hemisphere (Figure 13.16). Do they use the magnetic field of the earth to help guide them on this incredible journey?

To answer that question, Robert Beason and Joan Nichols examined the "headings"—the direction to which the birds oriented—at the time of their fall migration to South America (Beason and Nichols, 1984). They did this by bringing birds into a planetarium and projecting the star patterns that were appropriate for the autumn sky in the Northern Hemisphere. In other words, the birds were given correct visual cues with respect to migration, and in response they oriented south (toward South America). Beason and Nichols could also use equipment in the planetarium to manipulate the magnetic polarity that the birds experienced. When the visual cues and the magnetic polarity provided the same information—the northern sky was associated with magnetic north—the birds again oriented in the correct southern direction.

The most critical treatment in the Beason and Nichols experiment was the one in which the visual cues were correct, but the magnetic polarity was reversed—that is, when the appropriate star pattern for autumn in the north was displayed, but the magnetic field was reversed so that the visual cues suggested south was in one direction and the magnetic cues indicated south was in the opposite direction. In this treatment, the birds headed toward the magnetic south, indicating that magnetic cues were critical in the annual round-trip migration.

How are the bobolinks able to sense changes in magnetic polarity? To address this question, when their experiment was complete, Beason and Nichols autopsied the bobolinks, focusing on the head area of the birds. They found high levels of an iron-rich, magnetically sensitive substance, most likely magnetite, in the bobolinks. In particular, this magnetically sensitive substance was consistently found around the olfactory nerves and the bristles that project into the nasal cavity, as well as in the tissue between the nasal cavity and the eyes. While it is not clear precisely how the birds use magnetite to make navigational decisions, the presence of magnetite strengthens the claim that magnetic orientation is important in bobolink migratory behavior (Freake et al., 2006; Lohmann and Johnsen, 2000).

THE HERITABILITY OF MIGRATORY RESTLESSNESS

Given the broad and varied consequences that migration has on an individual's fitness, it is not that surprising that evolutionary biologists and ethologists have examined the possibility that some aspects of migratory behavior are heritable. For example, using an array of different techniques, Peter Berthold compared the onset of migratory activity between laboratory and wild birds in eighteen different species (Berthold, 1990). He found a strong correlation between onset of migratory activity in both groups of birds, suggesting that the timing of departure for migration may be under genetic control. Such studies cannot, however, directly measure heritability. To do this, Francisco Pulido and his colleagues (including Berthold) designed a selection experiment on autumn migration behavior, choosing the German blackcap bird (*Sylvia atricapilla*) as the species they would study (Pulido et al., 2001).

Pulido and his team brought blackcaps in from the field and measured their migratory restlessness ("zugunruhe") during the autumn migratory season. During migratory restlessness, caged birds in the laboratory show intense movement and activity (including wing-flapping behavior) in their cages; normally, the birds would be migrating during the evenings in the autumn, and this is replaced in the laboratory by extreme activity. Pulido and his team defined the onset of such restlessness as the first night on which a bird was active during at least five thirty-minute periods.

In 1994, the researchers collected forty blackcaps from the field and brought them back to the lab. The ten birds with the latest dates for migratory restlessness were selected and allowed to mate. They produced a total of twenty-six offspring, and from that group four breeding pairs with late-onset migratory restlessness were again allowed to breed, producing fourteen second-generation birds in a line selected for late migratory activity. Somewhat remarkably in only two generations, migratory restlessness was delayed for an average of 7.65 days (Figure 13.17), with Pulido and his co-workers calculating a heritability of 0.72 for the onset of this behavior. In conjunction with the other findings, this suggests that variance in migratory patterns may indeed be due to genetic variance in migratory behavior rather than to some sort of phenotypically plastic response on the part of birds.

FIGURE 13.17. The heritability of migratory activity. In each generation, German blackcap birds with the latest onset of migratory activity were chosen to breed. In just two generations, the onset of migratory activity was set back more than a week. The y-axis here measures a statistical term known as "residuals," rather than the actual change in absolute days until migration. *(Based on Pulido et al., 2001)*

MIGRATION AND DEFENSE AGAINST PARASITES

The energy expended during long migration can reduce immune responsiveness, making animals more susceptible to disease (Hoffman-Goetz and Pedersen, 1994; Leffler, 1993). In addition, long-distance migrants also face new parasites and diseases upon arrival at their migratory end point. That is, while nonmigratory birds must combat parasites in one environment, migratory birds face that challenge in two very different environments, and they are thus combating a more diverse array of potential parasites. Anders Møller and Johannes Erritzøe hypothesized that migratory birds should therefore invest more heavily in immune function compared to related resident relatives (Møller and Erritzøe, 1998).

Møller and Erritzøe tested their hypothesis by comparing the size of immune defense organs in pairs of bird species. One member of each pair was from a migratory species and the other pair member was from a closely related species that was nonmigratory. The immune defense organs that were compared were the spleen and a lymphoid organ called the bursa of Fabricus. The researchers assumed that a larger size in either of these defense organs would provide better immunological resistance to parasites (John, 1994; Toivanen and Toivanen, 1987). Møller and Erritzøe found that, in nine of ten pairwise comparisons, the bursa of Fabricus was larger in birds from the migratory species, while in nine of thirteen pairwise comparisons, the spleen was larger in birds from the migratory species.

Are there other variables besides the tendency to migrate or not that might explain differences in the size of immune defense organs when comparing the pairs of bird species that Møller and Erritzøe tested? The authors themselves note that differences in sexual selection pressure, mating systems, and the pattern of nest use and reuse are also known to affect investment in immune defenses (Møller and Erritzøe, 1996). As such, they reanalyzed their data, using only pairs of species that were known not to differ on any variable (besides migratory tendencies) that might affect the size of immune defense organs. While this comparison lowered their sample size to six pairwise comparisons for both the bursa of Fabricus and the spleen, their initial findings remained unchanged, suggesting an important relationship between migratory habits and the immune system.

PHYLOGENY AND MIGRATORY BEHAVIOR

Migratory behavior has also been studied in a phylogenetic context (Outlaw and Voelker, 2006; Outlaw et al., 2003; Zink, 2002). Diana Outlaw and Gary Voelker, for example, have examined migratory behavior in the avian family Motacillidae, which includes such species as the pied wagtail (*Motacilla alba*), the golden pipit (*Tmetothylacus tenellus*), and the yellow-throated longclaw (*Macronyx croceus*) (Figure 13.18). In particular, one of the hypotheses they set out to examine was the "evolutionary precursor" model of migration. This hypothesis posits that migration will be associated with species that live in open or edge habitats (so-called nonbuffered areas) rather than species that live in forests (buffered areas) (Chesser and Levey, 1998; Levey and Stiles, 1992). The underlying logic here is that open and edge habitats exhibit much greater seasonal variation in

A B   C

FIGURE 13.18. Migratory behavior in Motacillidae birds. Migratory behavior has also been studied in a phylogenetic context in the avian family Motacillidae, which includes such species as **(A)** the pied wagtail (*Motacilla alba*), **(B)** the golden pipit (*Tmetothylacus tenellus*), and **(C)** the yellow-throated longclaw (*Macronyx croceus*). *(Photo credits: David Chapman/Alamy; Tina Manley/Animals/Alamy; Arco Images GmbH/Alamy)*

food resources than do forest habitats, and that this variation might select for migration in the birds that occupy such open and edge habitats.

To test the evolutionary precursor model in a phylogenetic context, Outlaw and Voelker categorized the migratory behavior of forty-nine species in the Motacillidae family as either "migratory" or "sedentary," and their habitat as either open/edge or forest. Using an already published molecular genetic phylogeny of Motacillidae, they found that there was no association between habitat in terms of open/edge versus forest—that is, species that were associated with open/edge habitats were no more likely to migrate than were species that lived in the forest.

Outlaw and Voelker's phylogenetic analysis found that the ancestral state of migration in Motacillidae was "sedentary" and that the ancestral habitat was open/edge. Migratory behavior then evolved independently in many species in Motacillidae, but these species were just as likely to live in the forest as in open/ edge habitats. Outlaw and Voelker's analysis did, however, find one ecological variable that was associated with migration. Species that lived at higher altitudes were much more likely to migrate than species that lived at lower altitudes. Overall, their analysis found numerous independent evolutionary transitions from sedentary to migratory and that these transitions were most likely in species that lived at high latitudes.

Habitat choice, including the choice of territories, plays an important role in the life of many animals. In this chapter, we have examined numerous aspects of such choices, including models of habitat choice and territoriality, the manner in which learning affects choice of territory, and family dynamics and territoriality. One specific aspect of habitat choice that has been the subject

INTERVIEW WITH

Dr. Judy Stamps

Of all the systems you could have chosen to study territoriality, how did you end up working with small lizards?

I originally began studying social behavior in lizards because of a comment made by my professor in an undergraduate animal behavior class. He suggested that lizards might be a good choice for studying stereotyped behavior patterns (displays) because many lizards use stereotyped behavior—headbobbing patterns—to communicate with each other. So, I began by studying the displays of male *Anolis* lizards in captivity. After several years of studying lizards in the laboratory, I became curious about their behavior under natural conditions, and made a preliminary field trip to their native habitat, in the West Indies, to observe their behavior there. This first trip not only convinced me that these lizards were doing some pretty interesting things in nature, but also that the place they were doing them (the West Indian island of Grenada) had obvious attractions of its own. So, my first fieldwork focused on the social behavior of adult lizards in the West Indies.

While observing adults in the field, I noticed that tiny hatchlings exhibited many of the same behavior patterns as adults, including headbob displays, chasing, fighting, and the defense of territories. In addition, since territory size typically scales with body size, hatchlings that weighed only 2 grams had commensurately small territories, on the order of only 0.5 square meter in size. As a result, it was possible to study an entire "neighborhood"

of territories in a small area in the field and to manipulate structural features of habitats under natural conditions to determine the features that free-living juveniles preferred in their territories. After several months of playing around with juvenile lizards, it was obvious that they were much more amenable to both laboratory

and field studies of territorial behavior than adults, and from that point on, I focused on the juveniles.

You've modeled territoriality in terms of learning. What spurred you to take on this approach?

Many hours spent observing juveniles in the field convinced me that I needed to consider the role of learning in territorial behavior. For instance, it was quite apparent that a juvenile who entered a neighborhood for the first time had no idea where any of the territory boundaries were, and that it only became aware of their locations as a result of being chased

from one territory to the next by the residents. Similarly, two juveniles of similar size meeting for the first time engaged in an extended, strenuous fight, involving lengthy exchanges of a wide array of headbob patterns, and culminating in physical combat, in which the two parties grabbed one another by the jaws, and then banged one another against the perch. It seemed that this "knock down, drag out" fight made a strong impression on both combatants, because when they encountered each other again the next morning, both seemed reluctant to venture near that opponent, and instead they began to exchange headbob displays from adjacent perches, across an intervening "no-man's-land" that eventually became the border between their two territories. Other observations indicated that if an individual was summarily attacked the first time it ventured into a novel area, it almost never returned to that area. In contrast, if an individual received a comparable attack in an area it had used for an extended period of time, its first response was to flee, but typically it returned to the area within an hour or so, and persisted in using its familiar area in the face of repeated attacks by its opponent. These and other observations suggested that salient experiences, both positive (a snooze on a familiar, comfortable perch with a full stomach) and negative (being attacked by an opponent), had important effects on the subsequent social and spatial behavior of these animals.

Inspection of the psychology literature revealed that scientists studying the effects of positive and aversive stimuli on space use had already described very general behavioral phenomena that could account for the behavior of these lizards. For instance, rodents who receive aversive stimuli (e.g., electric shock) as soon as they first venture into an unfamiliar area are unlikely to return to that area, whereas comparable individuals who receive the same stimulus in an area in which they have previously been rewarded are much more likely to return to that area. Translated into territorial terms, these studies suggested that territorial animals may be behaving like little psychologists, delivering punishment to one another in an attempt to dissuade members of their own species from using a particular area.

Does being bigger usually mean you are guaranteed a good territory? If not, what else plays a role in territory acquisition?

In some situations, large body size can be helpful in acquiring a good territory, because if two individuals are competing for an area that is novel to both of them, and if one is larger than the other, the larger one is capable of delivering more punishment to its opponent during aggressive interactions than vice versa. However, size is not everything, because individuals who are already in possession of an area typically retain possession of that area, even when competing with larger opponents, a phenomenon called the "prior residency advantage." The prior residency advantage may be attributable to the fact that a resident knows more about an area than does a newcomer, as a result of which the resident is likely to fight more vigorously for that area, and persistently return to that area even after losing one or more fights to a larger newcomer.

Regardless of the reason, the prior residency advantage means that animals can acquire space by being the first to settle in an area, rather than by being bigger than their opponents. This means that in many species, the ability to find newly vacant territories, and the ability to settle in them before anyone else finds them, plays an important role in territory acquisition. Thus, the prior residency advantage may explain why some birds establish territories weeks

> A resident knows more about an area than does a newcomer, as a result of which the resident is likely to fight more vigorously for that area, and persistently return to that area even after losing one or more fights to a larger newcomer.

or months in advance of the time that the territory will be needed for reproduction: the early bird gets the territory.

Are there any general patterns in territoriality that emerge when you look across taxa?

There are a number of general patterns that occur in territorial species from a wide range of taxa. I have already mentioned the prior

residency advantage, which occurs in virtually all territorial animals. Another generalization is that individuals in territorial species exhibit site tenacity, meaning that a given individual tends to remain in the same area for an extended period of time. Site tenacity is observed in all territorial species, but the reverse is not the case (e.g., all species with site tenacity do not defend areas in which they live). The basic elements of territorial behavior (stay in an area and use aggressive behavior to discourage other individuals from remaining in or returning to that area) are exhibited by a very large array of species, ranging from sea anemones to primates, but taxa with a long evolutionary history of territoriality typically add certain refinements to this basic pattern. For instance, territory owners in birds, mammals, frogs, lizards, and insects may produce songs, olfactory signals, conspicuous visual displays, or other conspicuous signals using other sensory modalities. These broadcast signals indicate to other inhabitants of the area that the territory is occupied, as well as providing additional information about the sex, condition, and (sometimes) identity of the territory owner. Territory owners in species with a long evolutionary history of territoriality are also likely to be able to recognize different categories of conspecifics, and tailor their aggressive behavior accordingly.

Dr. Judy Stamps is a professor at the University of California at Davis. Her long-term work on lizards and territoriality has produced fundamentally new ideas on both territoriality and the role of learning in territory formation.

of much work in ethology is migratory behavior. Here we have reviewed work on migration and navigation, migratory "restlessness," parasites and migration, and phylogeny and migration. An ethological overview of these topics provides a scientific context for the pure majesty of animal migrations that can cover round-trips of more than 12,000 miles each year.

SUMMARY

1. Both biotic and abiotic factors affect habitat choice in animals. Abiotic factors include, but are not limited to, heat, availability of water, wind, "cover" from danger, and the availability of specific nutrients, while biotic factors encompass the location of potential mates, food, predators, and parasites.

2. Territories provide exclusive access to food, mates, and safe haven from predators, and are defended from intruders. Defense can be costly, both in terms of time and energy, and it represents a cost of territoriality.

3. The ideal free distribution model is a simple, but powerful, predictor of habitat choice as a function of resource distribution. This model predicts that the equilibrium distribution of individuals into patches (or habitats) should be that distribution at which, if any individual moved to a patch (or habitat) it was not in, it would suffer a reduced payoff.

4. Animals can learn about territory quality through a process known as conspecific cueing, wherein they judge the suitability of a territory by whether it previously was occupied by an owner sometime in the past.

5. Ethologists studying migration focus not only on the obvious costs (for example, the energy needed for travel) and benefits (breeding in a warmer climate) of migration, but also on more subtle factors such as the immunological costs of being a migrant, the various cues that migrants use to locate their breeding and nonbreeding grounds, and the interaction between genetic and environmental factors in shaping migratory behavior.

6. Phylogenetic studies of migration have tested the "evolutionary precursor" model of migration, which posits that migration will be associated with species that live in open or edge habitats (so-called nonbuffered areas) rather than species that live in forests (buffered areas).

DISCUSSION QUESTIONS

1. Make a general list of the costs and benefits of territoriality. Using that list, determine what sort of environments would generally favor the formation of long-term territories.

2. The ideal free distribution model predicts that animals will distribute themselves among patches in proportion to resources. What sort of cognitive abilities, if any, does this assume on the part of animals? Would bacteria potentially distribute themselves in accordance with the predictions of IFD models?

3. Suppose that young individuals watch older conspecifics choose their territories and subsequently use such information in their habitat-choice decisions about valuable resources. Outline one scenario by which such observational learning could increase competition for prime habitat sites, and one in which it would decrease competition for such sites.

4. Consider Møller and Erritzøe's work on immune defense organs and migration behavior. Can you make any predictions regarding how a migrating species might fare against local parasites (in both its habitats) as compared to resident species? What is the logic underlying your hypothesis?

SUGGESTED READING

Able, K. P. (1999). *Gatherings of angels: Migrating birds and their ecology.* Ithaca, NY: Comstock Books. A wonderful, easy-to-read book on migration in birds.

Brown, J. L. (1969). Territorial behavior and population regulation in birds. *Wilson Bulletin, 81,* 293–329. A classic paper that examines the effects of territoriality on population dynamics.

Freake, M. J., Muheim, R., & Phillips, J. B. (2006). Magnetic maps in animals: A theory comes of age? *Quarterly Review of Biology, 81,* 327–347. A current review on the role of magnetic fields and migration in animals.

Milinski, M., & Parker, G. (1991). Competition for resources. In J. R. Krebs & N. B. Davies (Eds.), *Behavioural ecology: An evolutionary approach* (pp. 137–168). Oxford: Blackwell. A nice overview of all variations of the ideal free distribution model.

Stamps, J. (2001). Learning from lizards. In L. A. Dugatkin (Ed.), M*odel systems in behavioral ecology* (pp. 149–168). Princeton: Princeton University Press. A review of learning and territory establishment.

14

Aggression

457

One of the most vivid of all the popular depictions of animal behavior is two rams facing one another, putting their heads down, charging, and butting horns. During the mating season, this sort of fighting behavior is common, and winners are more likely to mate with females. But aggression between members of the same species is not restricted to this sort of dramatic display, nor is it always associated with immediate access to mating opportunities. Animals fight over obtaining food, securing space (territories, home ranges), and providing safety for their family members.

As we have seen throughout the book, when valuable resources such as space, food, and mates are at stake, animals can be aggressive—that is, they fight or threaten to fight. Aggression has been studied in relatively solitary species, in which individuals fight when they occasionally interact at a territory boundary, as well as in species that live in social groups year-round. When aggression occurs in group-living species, and individuals interact with each other many times, we can measure **dominance hierarchies** (rank orderings of the individuals) in such groups. In the simplest case of group living—when animals live in groups of three—we might have individual 1 winning the majority of its fights with individuals 2 and 3, individual 2 winning the majority of its fights with individual 3, and individual 3 losing the majority of its fights with individuals 1 and 2. In that case, individual 1 would be the top-ranked or alpha (α) member of the hierarchy, individual 2 would be the second ranked or beta (β) member, and individual 3 would be the third ranked or gamma (γ) member of the hierarchy. Where an individual places in a dominance hierarchy has both proximate and ultimate implications. Individuals at the top of hierarchies often have access to more food, more mating opportunities, and safer territories than individuals at the lower end of hierarchies. At the proximate level, we will see that androgen and glucocorticoid levels differ between individuals that hold different ranks in a hierarchy.

Ethologists and naturalists have long been fascinated with animal aggression, and the literature in this area is huge, going back to at least the time of Darwin (Archer, 1988; Drummond, 2006; Huntingford and Turner, 1987; Mock and Parker, 1997). For example, Thomas Henry Huxley, one of the leading intellectual figures of the nineteenth century and Darwin's most vociferous defender, argued that interactions in the animal world resulted in a bloodbath. Huxley thought that aggression, often extreme aggression, was the norm for everyday interactions among animals, and he made his claim in no uncertain terms:

> From the point of view of the moralist, the animal world is on about the same level as the gladiator's show. The creatures are fairly well treated, and set to fight; whereby the strongest, the swiftest and the cunningest live to fight another day. The spectator has no need to turn his thumb down, as no quarter is given . . . the weakest and the stupidest went to the wall, while the toughest and the shrewdest, those who were best fitted to cope with their circumstances, but not the best in any other way, survived. Life was a continuous free fight, and beyond the limited and temporary relations of the family, the Hobbesian war of each against all was the normal state of existence. (Huxley, 1888, p. 163)

In contrast, Russian Prince Peter Kropotkin, a well-respected naturalist, whose book *Mutual Aid* is regarded as a classic early work on behavior, looked around and saw a world that seemed almost antithetical to that of Huxley's:

. . . in all these scenes of animal life which crossed before my eyes, I saw mutual aid and mutual support carried on to an extent which made me suspect in it a feature of the greatest importance for the maintenance of life, the preservation of each species and its further evolution. (Kropotkin, 1902, p. 18)

The point of presenting the Huxley and Kropotkin quotes is not to determine whether animals are aggressive or not. To some extent and under certain circumstances, toned-down versions of both views capture aspects of animal behavior at different times and under different conditions. At present, rather than asking whether animals engage in aggression or cooperation, ethologists are interested in the costs and benefits that favor animals in a population fighting or not fighting with one another, cooperating or not cooperating with each other in different situations. It is also important to note that cooperation and aggression are not the flip sides of a coin—individuals in groups often cooperate with each other in order to compete, often aggressively, with individuals in other groups (Dugatkin, 1997a; Gadagkar, 1997). Aggression is part and parcel of even the most cooperative of units—the social insect group. In wasps, for example, while cooperation is common within hives, when "foreign" individuals from other hives try to enter a nest, wasp guards often respond with vigorous and sometimes deadly defensive behaviors (Gamboa et al., 1986; Figure 14.1).

Rather than attempting to summarize the large literature on aggression, we will focus on: (1) some proximate mechanisms of aggression, (2) models of aggression, including the hawk-dove game, the sequential assessment model, and the war of attrition model, and (3) the implications of experience, particularly social experience, on aggressive interactions and hierarchy formation, including the effects of winning and losing in one aggressive interaction on subsequent interactions, and the effects of observing or being observed on aggressive bouts. Let us begin with a brief discussion of the "fight or flight" response, which we first discussed in Chapter 3, and tie this response more directly to proximate mechanisms of animal aggression.

FIGURE 14.1. Intruder aggression.
When a wasp (left) approaches a nest, guards at the nest determine whether it's a hive mate or an intruder. Intruders are aggressively repelled.

Fight or Flight?

In the "fight or flight" response, a surge in adrenaline and norepinephrine produces a quick increase in blood sugar, which, along with oxygen, is delivered to strategic areas such as the brain, skeletal muscles, and heart. "Nonessential" systems, such as digestive and reproductive systems, are often temporarily shut down at this point. This response most often occurs when prey must decide to fight off a predator or flee. The same sort of response—albeit not as dramatic—occurs when animals encounter aggressive individuals from their own populations. An individual can choose to fight or flee from a potential antagonistic opponent.

We can think about the decision as to whether or not to fight against conspecifics at a number of different levels. From an ultimate perspective, this decision revolves around the costs and benefits of aggression. When the benefits of victory, on average, outweigh the costs of fighting, ethologists predict that animals will fight; otherwise, they will not. From a proximate perspective, we can ask questions about immediate causation and aggression. And, as in the case of responding to predators, when animals opt to fight or flee from others in their own population, ethologists focus on the endocrinological underpinnings of such behavior, often uncovering similar hormonal responses across different species. Dominant individuals typically display increased androgen levels—for example, increased testosterone—and are more likely to fight than flee. Likewise, winners of fights tend to have their circulating levels of androgens increase—that is, the relationship between androgen level and aggression cuts both ways. Subordinates, who are more likely than dominants to flee than fight, usually lose aggressive interactions in which they are involved. Subordinates tend to have higher circulating levels of glucocorticoid "stress" hormones (for example, cortisol or corticosterone) than dominants when going into fights, and even higher levels when a fight is over. But it is not always the case that subordinates and losers are the only individuals that display high levels of circulating stress hormones. For example, dominant individuals defending territories often must expend a large amount of energy fending off competitors and predators, and this can lead to high glucocorticoid levels. Similarly, alpha individuals in a hierarchy are often challenged by many subordinates in their group, and this too can lead to increases in glucocorticoid levels.

If fighting is costly, then once it is clear that an animal is losing a fight, it will often be beneficial for it to signal subordination, and hence reduce future costs (Enquist and Leimar, 1990; Geist, 1974a; Hurd, 1997). It may inhibit its aggressive behaviors, refraining from charging, biting, or rapidly approaching the dominant fish. In addition, it may communicate its subordinate status via color change. Color change may be a particularly good communication vehicle in aggressive contests, where color may be linked to "badges of status," and hence color change can quickly indicate an individual's relative rank in a hierarchy and whether it will engage in aggressive behaviors (Rohwer, 1982; Roper, 1986).

Because fish have tight hormonal and neuronal control over the expansion of pigment cells, they are particularly adept at quick color change over short time periods and have been the subject of numerous experiments on color change and aggression (Baerends et al., 1986; Barlow, 1963; Guthrie and Muntz, 1993; Hulscher-Emeis, 1992). For example, researchers have studied Atlantic salmon (*Salmo salar*), a species in which aggression is most often associated with territorial defense. Males pair up during fights and undertake a series of behaviors, including circling, charging, and biting. Losers—who display increased levels of cortisol—often swim close to the surface to avoid future aggressive interactions with individuals that have defeated them. In terms of communicating relative status in a dominance hierarchy, and hence minimizing costly encounters, in Atlantic salmon, dominant males develop dark vertical eye bands and subordinate individuals develop darker body color (Keenleyside and Yamamoto, 1962; Figure 14.2).

Two caveats before we move to the next section. First, many hormones, not just androgens and glucocorticoids, affect decisions about whether or not to fight. Second, while androgens and glucocorticoids tend to play the same role in aggression and submission across many species, this is not necessarily the case for all chemical messengers associated with aggression and submission. To see this point more clearly, let us briefly examine the role of the neurotransmitter serotonin in aggressive behavior.

Most researchers agree that serotonin plays an important role in animal aggression. That role, however, appears to differ across animal systems. In mammals, low serotonin levels are often linked with high levels of aggression but lower social status (Coccaro, 1992; Raleigh et al., 1991; Sheard, 1983). The situation can be complex, however, as the effect of serotonin (and its chemical precursors) may depend on whether animals were raised in social or asocial environments and on what specific type of aggressive behavior is being studied (Balaban et al., 1996; Raleigh and McGuire, 1991).

In fish, as opposed to mammals, enhanced serotonergic function is seen in more subordinate individuals, leading to reduced fighting behavior (Clotfelter et al., 2007; Winberg et al., 1992, 1997). For example, Svante Winberg and his colleagues studied brain serotonergic activity and hierarchy formation in Arctic charr (*Salvelinus alpinus*). In phase 1 of their work they constructed four groups, each consisting of four fish. They then determined the dominance hierarchy of the four fish in each group. After a stable hierarchy had formed in each group, groups were disbanded. In phase 2, Winberg and his team placed all four top-ranked males in one group, all four second-ranked males in a second group, all four third-ranked males in a third group, and all four bottom-ranked males in a

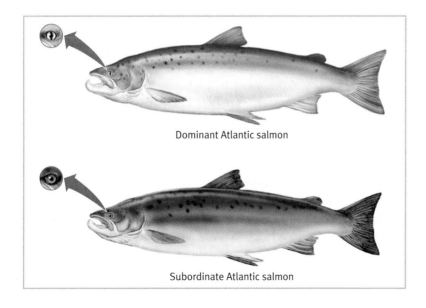

Dominant Atlantic salmon

Subordinate Atlantic salmon

FIGURE 14.2. Color as a signal. In Atlantic salmon, subordinate individuals often assume a much darker body color. Dominants' body color remains light, but they develop dark vertical eye bands.

FIGURE 14.3. Serotonin and aggression. A small individual was made subordinate by being matched against an individual that was 30 percent larger than it was. When serotonin was continuously infused into subordinates (red bar), their aggressive levels surged. Subordinates returned to their pre-infusion levels within 30 minutes after serotonin infusions were turned off. **(A)** The intensity of the aggression over time, and **(B)** the duration of the aggression. *(Based on Huber et al., 1997)*

fourth group. Correlating serotonin and serotonin-related chemicals with social status, they found that fish that were subordinate in phase 2 showed higher serotonergic activity. The subordinate fish were known to curtail their aggressive activity, presumably to avoid aggressive interactions with dominant fish. The researchers suggested that the stress experienced by the subordinate fish in relation to the dominant fish increased the subordinates' serotonergic activity, which in turn inhibited the neural circuitry associated with aggression.

A different picture emerges when we look at the relationship between serotonin, aggression, and social status in crustaceans (Edwards and Spitzer, 2006; Huber et al., 1997; Kravitz, 1988; Panksepp et al., 2003; Yeh et al., 1997). In crustaceans, increased serotonergic function leads to enhanced aggression and high social status. Take the case of lobsters. When lobsters are paired up in fights, they generally escalate their aggressive behaviors through a series of ritualized combats (Huber and Kravitz, 1995). Once an individual loses a fight, however, it avoids aggressive interactions for days. But losers can be made more aggressive if they are given injections of serotonin (Huber et al., 1997; Figure 14.3). Furthermore, if fluoxetine (Prozac), an inhibitor of serotonin, is injected into the lobster at the same time as serotonin, this effect disappears, suggesting a strong role for serotonin in lobster aggression.

While serotonin appears to play an important role in aggression across this wide spectrum—crustaceans, fish, and mammals—the neuroendocrinological effect of serotonin differs dramatically across these groups.

Game Theory Models of Aggression

As we discussed in Chapter 9, game theory models are built to examine behavioral evolution when the fitness of an individual depends on both its own behavior and on the behavior of others, as in the case of fighting behavior. If, for example, an individual is willing to fight for a contested resource, its fitness is going to depend on whether its opponent opts to fight or simply to flee, and so we can model fighting using game theory.

Evolutionary game theorists have built a suite of models that examine the evolution of fighting behavior (Riechert, 1998). Here we will focus on the three most well-developed game theory models of aggression—the hawk-dove game, the war of attrition model, and the sequential assessment model. All three of these game theory models share certain attributes. For example, a cost to fighting is assumed in hawk-dove, war of attrition, and sequential assessment models. Such a cost can take many different forms, ranging from opportunity costs—the cost associated with not doing something else—to the cost of physical injury, up to and including mortality costs (Enquist and Leimar, 1990).

All game theory models must have some sort of variable that represents the value of the resource being contested. In some cases, the value of a resource will be fairly easy to calculate. When two individuals, for example, are contesting an item of food, the value of the resource will be straightforward to calculate. In other cases, such as a male's access to reproductively active females, resource value can be much more difficult to calculate. As we shall see in a moment, the

A   B

FIGURE 14.4. Deciding to fight. (A) One of the many resources animals will fight over is food, as shown here by these vultures that are fighting over a carcass. **(B)** Males also fight over females. Here, male elephant seals are fighting over access to reproductively active females. *(Photo credits: Tom Vezo; Jeff Mondragon/mondragonphoto.com)*

value of a resource affects not only an animal's decision to fight, but how long and/or how hard it is willing to fight (Figure 14.4).

Two individuals contesting a resource may not assign the same value to that resource. For example, imagine that two animals—one of whom is starving, and the other of whom is hungry, but not starving—are contesting a ten-pound prey item that has just been discovered. While ten pounds of meat is ten pounds of meat, it may be *valued* differently by putative fighters. To a starving animal, ten pounds of food might make the difference between life and death, while to a less hungry animal the value of that ten pounds of meat might be much lower. In that case, we might see our starving animal fight harder for the food than its opponent (Figure 14.5). As another example, consider the value of territory to a potential intruder and to a territory holder. Above and beyond the fact that the territory holder might be on a territory because it is a good fighter to begin

FIGURE 14.5. Value estimation. When two animals contest a resource, the hungrier animal may fight harder or longer to obtain it. If one of these cats is hungrier than the other, it may be willing to risk more to obtain the remains of the fish.

TABLE 14.1. Resource value and fighting. The value that an individual animal assigns to some resource affects how long contests last and to what extent they escalate. *(Based on Riechert, 1998)*

RESOURCE	CONTEST DURATION	LEVEL OF ESCALATION
Duration of food deprivation		
▸ Crayfish		increases
▸ Domestic cat		increases
Limited mating opportunities		
▸ Marine isopod crustacean		increases
▸ Bowl-and-doily spider	increases	
▸ Dungfly	increases	
▸ Red-spotted newt	increases	
▸ Red deer	increases	
Limited food/site availability		
▸ Funnel-web spider	increases	increases
▸ Digger wasp	increases	
▸ Iguana		increases
▸ Fulmar		increases
▸ Bald eagle		increases

with, it may well be that a territory holder will value a contested area (that is, its territory) more because it has already invested time and energy in learning where the resources in such a territory are located (Kokko et al., 2006; Table 14.1). These sorts of asymmetries in value have been documented many times in the ethological literature (Barnard and Brown, 1984; Ewald, 1985; Verrell, 1986).

Let us now examine some specific evolutionary game theory models in a bit more detail.

THE HAWK-DOVE GAME

The earliest and most well-known game theory model of the evolution of aggression is the **hawk-dove game** (Maynard Smith, 1982; Maynard Smith and Price, 1973). John Maynard Smith and George Price's paper introducing the hawk-dove game is regarded as a watershed event in theoretical ethology, as it introduced game theory to animal behaviorists. Prior to the description of this game, only a few papers discussed how game theory might be used to address evolutionary issues, particularly behavioral evolution (Hamilton, 1967; Lewontin, 1961; Trivers, 1971).

Given the impact of the hawk-dove game on ethologists, it is remarkable how simple (yet brilliant) a game this really is. Imagine that individuals can adopt one of two behavioral strategies when contesting some resource: (1)

hawk—wherein a player will escalate and continue to escalate until either it is injured or its opponent cedes the resource, or (2) dove—wherein a player displays as if it will escalate, but retreats and cedes the resource if its opponent escalates (this strategy was originally labeled "mouse").

If we let V = the value of the contested resource, and C = the cost of fighting, we can create a payoff matrix for the hawk-dove game (Table 14.2). In this matrix, we see that if a hawk interacts with a dove, the hawk receives the entire value of the resource (V), while the dove receives nothing. To understand the two remaining payoffs—the hawk-hawk and the dove-dove payoffs, we need to be aware of two assumptions underlying the payoff matrix. First, we are assuming that if two doves encounter one another, on average, they receive half the value of the resource (for example, they split a food item in half). Second, when two hawks interact and fight, we are assuming that only the loser pays the cost of fighting (for example, the cost of being injured). This means that hawks have a 50 percent chance of obtaining the resource (V/2) and a 50 percent chance of being injured and not receiving the resource (C/2), and so their total expected payoff from an interaction with another hawk is equal to (V − C)/2.

When calculating the evolutionarily stable strategy (see Chapter 9) to this game, the ESS depends on whether the value of the resource or the cost of fighting is greater. If V > C, then hawk is an ESS, as the hawk/hawk payoff, (V − C)/2, is positive, and hence greater than the payoff dove obtains when it meets hawk (0). Dove, however, is not an ESS, as the dove/dove payoff (V/2) is less than the payoff hawk obtains when it meets dove (V). Hence, when V > C, hawk is the only ESS. This makes sense, since V > C implies that the cost of fighting, paid only by hawks, is low compared to the prize that awaits the winner of any contest (V), and as a result, hawks do well. The situation is a bit more complicated when the cost of fighting is greater than the value of the resource. Now, neither hawk nor dove is an ESS. But it can be shown that

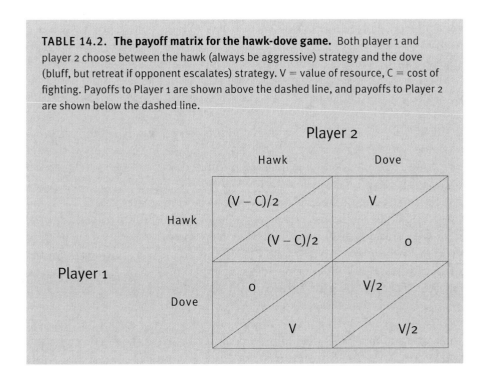

TABLE 14.2. The payoff matrix for the hawk-dove game. Both player 1 and player 2 choose between the hawk (always be aggressive) strategy and the dove (bluff, but retreat if opponent escalates) strategy. V = value of resource, C = cost of fighting. Payoffs to Player 1 are shown above the dashed line, and payoffs to Player 2 are shown below the dashed line.

MATH BOX 14.1

The Hawk-Dove Game

Let's look at the case of the hawk-dove game, when C > V, in a bit more detail.

If C > V, then hawk is not an ESS, as hawk's payoff against other hawks, (V–C)/2, is now negative, while dove's payoff against hawk is 0. Using the same calculations as we did for the case of V > C, we can see that dove is not an ESS either.

To see if some combination of hawks and doves is an ESS, let p = the frequency of hawks, and 1–p be the frequency of doves. Hawk's payoff is then:

$$p(V-C)/2 + (1-p) V \qquad (1)$$

where the first term is hawk's payoff against other hawks and the second is hawk's payoff against dove.

Dove's payoff can be calculated as:

$$p(0) + (1-p)V/2 \qquad (2)$$

where the first term is dove's payoff against hawk and the second term is dove's payoff against other doves.

When (1) = (2), the fitness of hawks is equal to the fitness of doves, and we then have our equilibrial frequency of hawks and doves. A little algebra shows that this occurs when p = V/C.

some mixture of hawks and doves is an evolutionarily stable strategy in this case (Math Box 14.1).

There are more complicated varieties of the hawk-dove game than the one we examined above (Mesterton-Gibbons and Adams, 1998; Riechert, 1998). One interesting version of this game adds in two new strategies called bourgeois and antibourgeois. The bourgeois strategy instructs an individual to play hawk if it is a territory holder, but to play dove if it does not own a territory. The antibourgeois strategy instructs players to do just the opposite—play dove if you are a territory holder, and hawk if you are not. Below we will look at the use of the bourgeois strategy (in butterflies) and the antibourgeois strategy (in spiders).

BOURGEOIS BUTTERFLIES. In the speckled wood butterfly (*Pararge aegeria*), territories are not set in space. That is, rather than having a territory with a set place in three dimensions, a male has a territory that is an open patch defined by well-lit areas that emerge when the sun breaks through the clouds. When a male comes upon an empty well-lit patch, he immediately occupies it and secures a mating advantage, compared to males not in sunlit territories.

When a male speckled wood butterfly comes upon a territory that has another male in it, the contest is settled as follows: resident wins, intruder retreats. In fact, there is very little aggression at all when males come upon occupied territories, perhaps because a prolonged fight over a short-lived resource, such as a sun patch, is not worth the costs. Rather, once a male is aware that a territory is occupied, he simply leaves (Figure 14.6). What makes the "resident wins" rule so dramatic is that an individual need only be the resident of a sun patch for a few seconds to secure victory over an intruder. To see this, let us

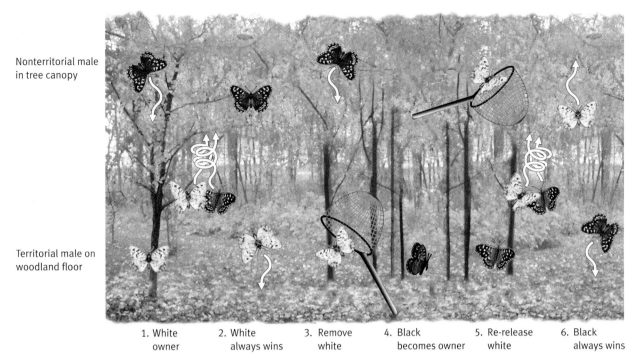

Nonterritorial male
in tree canopy

Territorial male on
woodland floor

1. White   2. White   3. Remove   4. Black   5. Re-release   6. Black
   owner   always wins   white   becomes owner   white   always wins

FIGURE 14.6. Conventional rules. The set-up for Davies's experiments on territory
ownership and contest rules in the speckled wood butterfly *(Pararge aegeria). (Based on
Dawkins and Krebs, 1978, p. 299)*

examine a study by Nick Davies. In Davies's work, a male (let's call him M1)
was experimentally made a territory owner (Davies, 1978). M1 then always
defeated M2, an intruder male. Yet, if M1 was removed from his territory and
M2 then occupied it, even if M2 was resident for only a short period of time,
M1 would now defer to M2 when he was reintroduced into his original sun
patch. The only escalated contests occurred when two males both acted as if
they were the rightful owner of a sun patch. This happens naturally when two
butterflies come to a sun patch at about the same time but do not notice the
other individual for some period (this can also be simulated experimentally). In
such cases, real fights can and do occur between the speckled wood butterfly
males (for an alternative view, see Kemp and Wiklund, 2004).

ANTIBOURGEOIS MEXICAN SPIDERS. The only well-documented instance
of the use of the antibourgeois strategy is during territory establishment and
home range defense in a small, territorial Mexican spider, *Oecobius civitas*
(Burgess, 1976). These spiders establish their territories under rocks, and when
an intruder approaches a territory, the territory holder flees rather than fighting.
The former territory holder then searches for a new territory, and if he comes
upon such a prize, the territory owner presently *there* vacates. This produces
a potentially long, bizarre series of events in which a territory owner leaves,
then challenges a spider in possession of another territory, causing that territory
owner to leave, and so on.

Given that in most species, territory holders win fights with an intruder,
how can ethologists explain such a seemingly strange cascade of events in
O. civitas? What factors might be responsible for the antibourgeois strategy
evolving in these Mexican spiders (Hodge and Uetz, 1995; Komers, 1989)?

FIGURE 14.7. Reverse bourgeois strategy. In *Oecobius civitas*, territory holders relinquish their territories when challenged by an intruder. This can have cascading effects throughout a cluster of *O. civitas* territories. *(Based on Mesterton-Gibbons and Adams, 1998)*

The answer can be understood in terms of the costs and benefits of fighting for territories, the number of available territories, and the cost of moving between territories. Imagine that the cost of fighting is relatively high, numerous territories are available, and movement between territories is not particularly dangerous. Under such circumstances, fleeing a territory when an intruder challenges—that is, playing the antibourgeois strategy—may in fact be the most profitable option available to individuals (Mesterton-Gibbons, 1992; Mesterton-Gibbons and Adams, 1998). These ecological and behavioral conditions (high cost of fights, many vacant territories) appear to describe the situation well for *O. civitas* (Figure 14.7).

THE WAR OF ATTRITION MODEL

Some potentially aggressive interactions are settled by animals displaying aggressively to one another, but not actually fighting, with the victor being the individual that displays the longest. In order to examine this scenario, the **war of attrition model** was developed by theoreticians (Bishop et al., 1978; Hammerstein and Parker, 1982; Maynard Smith, 1974; Maynard Smith and Parker, 1976; Parker, 1974a; Uehara et al., 2007).

The war of attrition model of fighting behavior has three important underlying assumptions: (1) individuals can choose to display aggressively for any duration of time, (2) display behavior is costly—the longer the display, the more energy expended, and (3) there are no clear cues such as size, territory possession, and so forth, that contestants can use to settle a contest (Riechert,

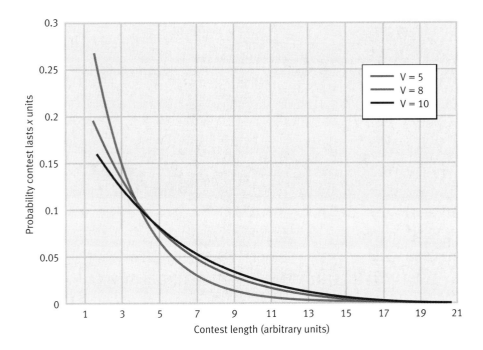

FIGURE 14.8. **The war of attrition model and fighting.** In this model, the probability that a contest will last a certain length of time is a function of the value (V) of the resource.

1998). If we again let V = the value of the resource being contested, and we now define x as the length of a contest involving displays, it can be shown that, at the ESS, the probability that a contest lasts x units of time is equal to $(2/V)e^{-2x/v}$ (Parker and Thompson, 1980). That is, rather than predicting a set time for aggressive display, the war of attrition model predicts that animals will choose randomly from a specific exponential distribution of contest lengths defined by the probability function $(2/V)e^{-2x/v}$ (Figure 14.8). All contest lengths from this ESS probability function—that is, any choice of display time from this function—lead to equal fitness gains to individuals.

This predicted distribution of contest lengths matches certain display durations in nature (Broom and Ruxton, 2003; Crowley et al., 1988; Field et al., 1998; Parker and Thompson, 1980; Stoewe et al., 2006). For example, recall the dungflies we discussed in Chapter 7. Females arrive at fresh dung pats to lay eggs, and males aggregate at such pats for access to females. The question, in terms of the war of attrition model, is how long should a male stay at a given pat? If he stays too long, he will encounter fewer and fewer females with time. If he leaves too quickly, he will pay the cost of moving, and may miss the opportunity to mate with females at the patch he left.

Using detailed measurements of the costs and benefits of dungfly mating, Parker and Thompson found that males' "stay times" (the time they remained at a patch) were exponentially distributed, as predicted from a war of attrition model (Parker and Thompson, 1980). When Parker calculated the mean time to find and move to a new patch from the dungfly fieldwork, he found that it was approximately four minutes (Curtsinger, 1986; Parker and Maynard Smith, 1987). When the travel time between patches is about four minutes, in accordance with the predictions of the war of attrition model, the stay times observed in the dungflies translate into approximately equal fitness for all males (Figure 14.9).

FIGURE 14.9. War of attrition over females. Male dungflies appear to engage in wars of attrition when determining how long to stay on a dung pat where females may alight. Assuming it takes four minutes to move from patch to patch, male mating success appears equal for a wide range of "stay times." *(From Maynard Smith, 1982, p. 31)*

THE SEQUENTIAL ASSESSMENT MODEL

A third game theoretical model of aggression, developed by Magnus Enquist and Olof Leimar, is called the **sequential assessment model** (Enquist and Leimar, 1983, 1987, 1990; Enquist et al., 1990; Leimar and Enquist, 1984). They created the sequential assessment model of aggression because they felt that other models did not realistically analyze how animals fought. Enquist and his colleagues argue:

> … the hawk-dove game, the war of attrition and similar games are not based on realistic behavioural mechanisms, i.e., mechanisms that produce sequences of behaviour patterns as a result of internal and external stimulation. This means that much of the behavioural diversity found in fighting behaviour, like the use of different behavioural elements, cannot be analyzed with such models. (Enquist et al., 1990, p. 1)

What separates the sequential assessment game from other models of aggression is that it is designed to analyze fights in which individuals continually assess one another in a series of "bouts." Let us examine how this model works, what predictions it makes, and what experimental evidence is available to test its basic predictions.

In the sequential assessment model, individuals assess their opponent's fighting abilities. Assessing an opponent's fighting ability, Enquist and his colleagues argue, is analogous to a process of statistical sampling (Enquist et al., 1990). A single sample (for example, a single assessment of fighting ability) introduces significant random error. The more sampling (assessment) one does, the lower the error rate, and hence the more confident one can be in whatever is being estimated; in our case, the opponent's fighting ability. After some period of sampling, one individual will determine that its odds of winning a fight are so low that it should end any further aggressive interaction with its opponent.

The sequential assessment game examines contests in which the level of aggression varies from relatively mild to very dangerous. At the evolutionarily stable solution to the sequential assessment game, the following type of scenario is predicted: Individuals should begin with the least dangerous type of aggressive behavior (let's call it behavior A), and "sample" each other with respect to behavior A for some period of time. Soon, however, all the information about an opponent with respect to A will be garnered. At that point, the next most dangerous behavior (B) should be the dominant action among protagonists. Again, at some point, information about an opponent and behavior B will reach saturation; that is, the animal will now have gathered as much useful information as it can gather about behavior B. Depending on the behavioral repertoire of the animals in question, more and more dangerous behaviors will be tacked onto the sequence. Because gauging your probability of winning a fight is most difficult when your fighting ability is similar to your opponent's fighting ability, the sequential assessment model predicts that the more evenly matched opponents should engage in the more dangerous behaviors.

Studies testing various predictions of the sequential assessment game have produced mixed results. Most studies find partial support of the model's basic predictions (Brick, 1999; DiMarco and Hanlon, 1997; Hack, 1997; Jennions and Backwell, 1996; Jensen and Yngvesson, 1998; Koops and Grant, 1993; McMann, 1993; Molina-Borja et al., 1998; Smith et al., 1994). Other studies more definitively support the great majority of the basic predictions of the sequential assessment game (Leimar et al., 1991). One such study examined contest behavior in the fish *Nannacara anomala*.

SEQUENTIAL ASSESSMENT IN *NANNACARA ANOMALA*. *Nannacara anomala* is an ideal species in which to test the sequential assessment model (Figure 14.10). Males form hierarchies, and aggressive interactions in males of this species range from "changing color" (least dangerous) and "approaching" through "tail beating," biting and mouth wrestling, up to "circling," which is the most dangerous of the aggressive activities, wherein fish repeatedly attempt to bite each other while they swim in a circular pattern (Figure 14.11).

Enquist and his collaborators staged pairwise interactions among male fish to test predictions of the sequential assessment game (Enquist et al., 1990). All trials were videotaped so as to allow a detailed analysis of subtle behavioral changes through time. Overall, interactions between aggressive males matched the predictions of the sequential assessment model very well.

One of the most elementary predictions of the sequential assessment model is that the more evenly matched the opponents are, the longer the fights and the more phases a fight should go through. In *N. anomala*, as in many fish, individuals are able to assess weight asymmetries (Enquist et al., 1987), and weight differences appear to have a very large effect on contest outcome, with heavier fish more likely to emerge from a contest victorious. In accordance with the predictions of the sequential assessment model, fights do indeed take longer when fish are more closely matched for weight than they do when large asymmetries exist.

FIGURE 14.10. Fighting fish.
Nannacara anomala has proven to be an ideal species for testing various predictions derived from the sequential assessment game. *(Photo credit: Magnus Enquist)*

FIGURE 14.11. Sequential assessment.
Much work on the sequential assessment model has been done in the fish *Nannacara anomala*. Here two individuals are engaged in a "mouth wrestle." *(Based on Enquist et al., 1990)*

The sequential assessment model also predicts that when numerous behaviors are used in aggressive contests, they should be used in approximately the same order across all fights. That is, while some fights are predicted to last longer and contain more elements than others, the order in which new aggressive behaviors appear in a fight should be similar in all contests, and hence shorter contests should simply have fewer types of behavior. Again, the behavior of *N. anomala* matches the model's prediction quite nicely. Males typically begin aggressive interactions with some sort of visual assessment, progress to tail beating, and then to biting and mouth wrestling, and occasionally to circling. How many acts in this sequence are played out depends on differences in an opponent's weight, but as predicted by the sequential assessment model, the order in which these acts are displayed tends to be the same, regardless of weight differences.

Winner, Loser, Bystander, and Audience Effects

Prior experience with an opponent can provide important information that can be used during future potentially aggressive interactions. If animal 1 has recently defeated animal 2, then animal 1 may decide to be more aggressive during the next interaction between these two individuals, and animal 2 may decide to be less aggressive. Indeed, experience with other individuals can be indirect, but still important. Suppose that animal 3 has recently seen animal 4 lose a fight to animal 5. If animals 3 and 4 interact at some point in the future, animal 3 may be more aggressive after seeing animal 4 lose his contest with animal 5. That is, observation, as well as direct interaction, provides information that may affect aggressive interactions. Ethologists have also found that being observed can affect the behavior displayed during, and the outcome of, aggressive interactions. Here we will examine the effect of direct and indirect experience by focusing on what are referred to as winner effects, loser effects, bystander effects, and audience effects.

WINNER AND LOSER EFFECTS

In sports, individual athletes, as well as teams, go on "winning streaks" and "losing streaks"—that is, winning itself sometimes begets more winning, and losing begets more losing. A similar set of phenomena exists in the animal behavior literature on aggression, wherein winning a fight increases the probability of future wins—so-called **winner effects**—and losing an aggressive interaction increases the probability of losing future fights—so-called **loser effects** (Hsu et al., 2005; Landau, 1951a, 1951b; Rutte et al., 2006).

Winner and loser effects are usually defined as an increased probability of winning at time T, based on victories at times T-1, T-2, and so on, and an increased probability of losing at time T, based on losing at times T-1, T-2, and so on, respectively. Although loser effects are more common than winner effects, both have been documented many times (Chase et al., 1994).

Generally speaking, at the proximate level, loser effects are coupled with increased circulating levels of glucocorticoid stress hormones. Increased glucocorticoids are sometimes also seen in winners, but winners usually, but not always, return to baseline hormone levels much faster than losers. Losers tend to have suppressed levels of testosterone, and winners tend to have increased levels, but the precise effects of testosterone on winning are less understood (Hsu et al., 2005). To get a better flavor for the behavioral dynamics of winner and loser effects, as well as some of the proximate underpinnings of these effects, let us examine some case studies in birds, fish, and snakes.

WINNER AND LOSER EFFECTS IN BLUE-FOOTED BOOBIES. In our discussion of sibling rivalry in Chapter 8, we learned that aggressive interactions sometimes occur between siblings at a nest (Mock and Parker, 1997). In a long-term study of nestmate aggression, Hugh Drummond and his colleagues have been investigating such aggressive behaviors during nestmate hierarchy formation in blue-footed boobies (*Sula nebouxii*) (Benavides and Drummond, 2007; Drummond, 2006; Drummond and Canales, 1998; Drummond and Osorno, 1992; Gonzalez-Voyer et al., 2007; Figure 14.12). Drummond's earlier work on the role of experience in shaping hierarchy formation found that if older chicks were aggressive and dominant early on, and younger chicks were submissive and subordinate, the older chicks would later be able to defeat the younger chicks even if the younger chicks were considerably larger than the older chicks (Drummond and Osorno, 1992). While this work clearly hints at the possibility of winner and loser effects in blue-footed boobies, it is not possible to definitively say whether loser effects (in younger chicks), winner effects (in older chicks), or both played a role in establishing hierarchies in this species.

In order to experimentally uncouple winner and loser effects, Drummond and Canales followed up the study mentioned above by pitting each dominant and subordinate individual against *inexperienced individuals* (Benavides and Drummond, 2007; Drummond and Canales, 1998). In their experimental protocol, in any given trial, only one of the animals had prior experience, and it was possible to examine winner and loser effects in isolation from one another. Specifically, Drummond and Canales predicted that when initially subordinate animals were pitted against inexperienced individuals (neutrals),

FIGURE 14.12. Blue-footed boobies. For blue-footed booby chicks involved in aggression, both winner and loser effects are in play. Winner effects, however, are much shorter lived. *(Photo credit: Hugh Drummond)*

A

B

FIGURE 14.13. Winning and losing booby chicks. (A) When subordinate chicks (green curve) who have experienced many losses are paired against neutral singleton chicks (red curve), they display very little aggressive behavior. **(B)** When dominant chicks (orange curve) who have recently won many aggressive interactions are paired against neutral chicks (red curve), they are very aggressive. The pattern begins to dissipate after four hours. *(Based on Drummond and Canales, 1998, p. 1672)*

the subordinate bird would have a decreased probability of winning aggressive bouts—to be conservative, they pitted subordinates against inexperienced partners that were slightly smaller (thus *increasing* a subordinate's chance of victory). The researchers also had initially dominant individuals interact with inexperienced partners (neutrals) and predicted that the dominant individual would have an increased probability of winning future aggressive interactions. Again, to be conservative, they pitted dominant individuals against slightly larger inexperienced individuals (*decreasing* the dominant bird's probability of victory).

Drummond and Canales uncovered strong winner and loser effects early on (at about four hours) in their experiment. At this stage of development, subordinates were much less aggressive than were their inexperienced pairmates, and dominants were much more aggressive than their pairmates (Figure 14.13). The winner effect waned with the passage of time, but the loser effect stayed intact throughout the ten days of observation. As such, young blue-footed boobies learned to accept the subordinate role (Drummond and Canales, 1998).

WINNER AND LOSER EFFECTS IN *RIVULUS MARMORATUS*. More controlled experimental studies of winner and loser effects have been undertaken in fish than in any other group. Why this is the case is hard to know for certain, but in all likelihood it is related to the fact that (1) aggression is common in fish, (2) aggression in fish is easily quantified in controlled laboratory settings, and (3) the endocrinology of aggression in fish has been well documented in numerous species.

Yuying Hsu and Larry Wolf have examined winner and loser effects in the hermaphroditic fish, *Rivulus marmoratus* (Hsu and Wolf, 1999, 2001). They examined not only the effect of wins and losses on the next aggressive interaction in which an individual was involved, but also the effect of wins and losses that had occurred two moves back in time (penultimate wins and losses).

Hsu and her team subjected fish to a number of different combinations of wins (W), losses (L), or "neutral" (N, no win, no loss) events (Table 14.3). The wins and losses an experimental fish received before it was tested were controlled by the researchers. This was accomplished by using a group of fish that were not used as experimental subjects in the winner/loser trials. These fish were allowed to fight, and the individual that defeated all others was used to fight with the experimental fish, defeat them, and thus create an experimental fish that began trials with a loss. A similar approach was used to create experimental winners—these fish had been paired with another fish that had been defeated by many others.

By comparing fish in the WW versus LW and LL versus WL treatments, (see caption of Table 14.3), Hsu and Wolf were able to document the first experimental evidence that the penultimate (next to last) aggressive interaction a fish experiences also affects its current probability of winning or losing (Hsu and Wolf, 1999). To see this, let us focus on the penultimate interactions and their implications for winner effects. Here, fish experiencing WW are significantly more likely to win a fight than fish experiencing LW. If the penultimate interaction had no effect on current aggressive interactions, one would expect no such difference across the WW versus LW treatments. Comparing numerous other treatments, Hsu and Wolf were able to demonstrate that, while penultimate interactions were important, their impact on winning or losing a current interaction was not as

TABLE 14.3. **Penultimate and ultimate contests.** Hsu and Wolf examined many combinations of winner and loser effects on contest outcomes through time. WW = win at time T-1, win at Time T; LL = loss at time T-1, loss at time T; WL = win at time T-1, loss at time T; NN = "neutral," no loss, no win. Outcomes of (1) and (2) directly measured the effects of penultimate winner and loser experiences. Outcomes of (3) measured the importance of penultimate versus ultimate experience on the probability of winning. Outcomes of (4) showed the difference between LL-WL and LN-WL, measuring immediate loser effects. Outcomes of (5) showed the difference between LW-WL and LN-WL, measuring immediate winner effects. Finally, outcomes at (6) showed the difference between WW-LW and NN-LW, measuring the effects of penultimate and ultimate winning experiences. *(From Hsu and Wolf, 1999)*

			(6)		
		(4)			
			(5)		
Opponent 1	WW	LL	LW	LN	NN
Opponent 2	LW	WL	WL	WL	LW
	(1)	(2)	(3)		

powerful as the outcome of the interaction immediately preceding the interaction underway. In addition, unlike many other species, *Rivulus marmoratus* showed no asymmetry in winner and loser effects—that is, the loser effect was not stronger than the winner effect, nor vice versa.

WINNER AND LOSER EFFECTS IN COPPERHEAD SNAKES. Gordon Schuett has examined both the behavioral dynamics and endocrinological correlates of winner and loser effects in copperhead snakes (*Agkistrodon contortrix*) (Schuett, 1997; Schuett and Gillingham, 1989). Because male-male aggression has a significant impact on mating success, Schuett examined whether winner and loser effects had an impact on aggression and mating success.

The experimental protocol involved a trial arena that housed a female in the center and one male at each end. Schuett used males that had had no aggressive interactions for six to twelve months prior to his study, and he pitted two males that differed in size by approximately 10 percent. In all thirty-two trials, the larger male emerged as dominant and gained reproductive access to the female.

Ten winners and ten losers from the "size" contests described above were chosen, and each was matched against a same-sized male copperhead that had no prior experience. Schuett found that prior winners were not more likely to win again, nor were they more likely to win than their opponents who had no experience to obtain access to a female. That is, no winner effects were uncovered in copperhead males. A loser effect, however, was uncovered—losers were more likely to lose again and to cede access to reproductively active females to other males. In an interesting twist, Schuett then examined how individuals who had now lost twice (in the initial "size contests" and then in loser effect treatments) fared against opponents who had no experience and who were about 10 percent smaller. Would the loser effect outweigh the positive size advantage that the

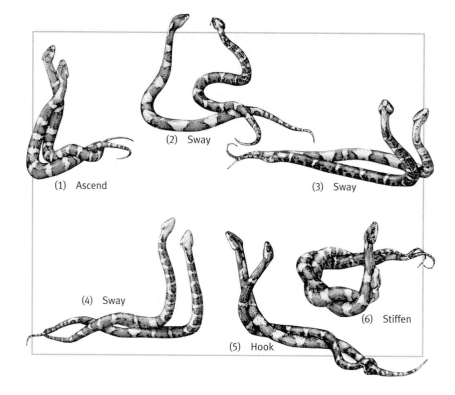

FIGURE 14.14. Winner and loser snakes. In copperhead snakes, losses can have a significant effect on future contest outcome. Snake fights in *Agkistrodon contortrix* include such aggressive behaviors as: (1) ascend, (2) ventrad-to-ventrad sway, (3) laterad-to-laterad sway, (4) ventrad-to-dorsad sway, (5) hook, and (6) stiffen. *(Based on Schuett and Gillingham, 1989, p. 248)*

(1) Ascend
(2) Sway
(3) Sway
(4) Sway
(5) Hook
(6) Stiffen

losers possessed, or vice versa? Results were crystal clear and pointed to the strength of the loser effect in copperheads—two-time losers lost all contests with smaller opponents (Figure 14.14).

Besides the behavioral work, Schuett and his colleagues also studied endocrinology and aggression in copperheads by examining hormonal correlates to the loser effect (Schuett et al., 1996; Schuett and Grober, 2000). Researchers allowed pairs of males to fight when a female was present. The snakes were kept together until one male was judged dominant to the other, at which point the individuals were separated and a blood sample was collected for hormonal analysis. In addition to this treatment, two controls were run; in the first, a lone male in his home cage was used, while in the second, a single male and a female were placed in the arena. The researchers took radioimmunoassays of plasma corticosterone in winners, losers, and both classes of control males, and they found that plasma corticosterone was significantly greater in losers than in winners or controls (Figure 14.15).

Increased levels of corticosterone produced dramatic effects in terms of both fighting and courting behavior in male copperheads. Not only do males who lose fights, and consequently have raised corticosterone levels, act subordinate, and rarely, if ever, challenge other males, they almost never court any females that are in the vicinity of where they fought.

Experimental work in a number of other species suggests that the stress-related hormones, such as glucocorticoids, often inhibit learning and/or memory (de Kloet et al.,1999, 2002; de Quervain, 2006; de Quervain et al., 1998, 2000; Lemaire et al., 2000; Sapolsky et al., 2000). Whether winners and losers differ in their ability to learn as a function of hormonal changes that occur as a result of fights is a fascinating, but unexplored question.

FIGURE 14.15. Hormones, winning, and losing. Losers show increased levels of plasma corticosterone compared to controls. No such change was found in winners. *(Based on Schuett et al., 1996)*

MATHEMATICAL MODELS OF WINNER AND LOSER EFFECTS. In addition to empirical work on winner and loser effects, there are a number of mathematical models that examine the implications of winner and loser effects on the formation of animal hierarchies (Beacham, 2003; Bonabeau et al., 1996, 1999; Dugatkin, 1997b; Landau, 1951a, 1951b; Mesterton-Gibbons, 1999).

You should recall from the beginning of the chapter that a dominance hierarchy is usually defined as a rank ordering of individuals in a group based on their aggressive interactions with each other. For example, if individual A wins the majority of fights with B, C, and D, then A is the top-ranked (or alpha) individual in a hierarchy. If B beats C and D, C beats D, and D beats no one, then a linear hierarchy exists (A > B > C > D) and that hierarchy is said to be transitive, in that if A defeats B and B defeats C, then A defeats C as well.

Part of the interest in hierarchy formation no doubt arises from the difficulty in understanding why an animal would ever "accept" a role other than that of alpha individual in a group (Allee, 1951; Dugatkin, 1995; Reeve and Ratnieks, 1993; Vehrencamp, 1983). Initial work on the impact of winner and loser effects on hierarchy formation was undertaken by H. G. Landau over fifty years ago (Landau, 1951a, 1951b). Landau was troubled that when he modeled hierarchy formation mathematically, he found that the linear, transitive hierarchies often found in nature did not seem to emerge from his mathematical work—work in which he only considered inherent differences in fighting abilities across individuals. So Landau added winner and loser effects to his models to examine if linear, transitive hierarchies then emerged. And such hierarchies did emerge from Landau's more complex models.

Despite the importance and impact of Landau's papers on research in the area of dominance hierarchies, a number of critical questions surrounding winner and loser effects and how they interact remained unanswered more than forty years after the original papers were published. In particular, Landau did not examine winner and loser effects independently, but he only considered the effect on hierarchy formation when both were present. Furthermore, Landau did not take into consideration the fact that animals assess each other's fighting ability, technically referred to as **resource holding power (RHP)**. Is it possible that when RHP is assessed, winner effects can have different implications for hierarchy formation than loser effects?

To address these questions, Dugatkin developed a simple computer simulation that independently examined winner and loser effects when individuals assessed each other's fighting abilities and could choose to fight or flee (Dugatkin, 1997b). The most salient result of these models is that the type of hierarchy predicted depends critically on whether winner effects exist alone, loser effects exist alone, or some combination of these forces are acting in a system.

Winner effects alone produce hierarchies in which the rank of individuals all the way from top rank (α) to bottom rank can be unambiguously assigned. Loser effects alone produce hierarchies in which a clear α individual exists, but the relationship among other group members remains murky. The difference between the hierarchies generated by the winner effect and by the loser effect appears to be that winner effects create a situation in which pairs of individuals primarily interact by fighting, which makes assigning position in the hierarchy fairly straightforward. Conversely, loser effects quickly produce individuals that are not going to be aggressive because of their low estimate of their own fighting ability after a few losses. Hence, with loser effects, most interactions will end in

TABLE 14.4. Winning, losing, and hierarchy formation.

TABLE 14.4. Winning, losing, and hierarchy formation. When winner effects alone are at play (green box), a clear linear hierarchy exists, with the position of each individual clearly delineated. When loser effects alone are at play (orange box), only the alpha individual is clear. Loser effects tend to outweigh winner effects (red box). *(Based on Dugatkin, 1997b, p. 585)*

Winner Effect

Loser Effect = 0, Winner Effect = 0:
No winner or loser effects in play here.

Loser Effect = 0, Winner Effect = 0.1:

	A	B	C	D
A	—	146	136	140
B	8	—	8	172
C	21	170	—	168
D	6	18	7	—

Loser Effect = 0, Winner Effect = 0.2:

	A	B	C	D
A	—	146	172	160
B	6	—	168	158
C	7	9	—	167
D	2	2	3	—

Loser Effect = 0.1, Winner Effect = 0:

	A	B	C	D
A	—	0	0	0
B	171	—	171	163
C	0	0	—	0
D	0	0	0	—

Loser Effect = 0.1, Winner Effect = 0.1:

	A	B	C	D
A	—	161	195	156
B	0	—	2	0
C	0	0	—	0
D	10	159	153	—

Loser Effect = 0.1, Winner Effect = 0.2:

	A	B	C	D
A	—	177	173	157
B	0	—	0	0
C	0	0	—	0
D	0	0	0	—

Loser Effect = 0.2, Winner Effect = 0:

	A	B	C	D
A	—	156	168	174
B	0	—	3	3
C	0	0	—	0
D	0	0	0	—

Loser Effect = 0.2, Winner Effect = 0.1:

	A	B	C	D
A	—	156	178	149
B	0	—	0	0
C	0	0	—	0
D	0	0	1	—

Loser Effect = 0.2, Winner Effect = 0.2:

	A	B	C	D
A	—	1	1	0
B	0	—	0	0
C	157	173	—	148
D	1	3	0	—

neither individual opting to fight, making it difficult to assign relative ranks to most individuals in a hierarchy (Table 14.4).

BYSTANDER EFFECTS

When the observer of an aggressive interaction between two other individuals changes its assessment of the fighting abilities of those it has observed, the **bystander effect**—sometimes called the "eavesdropper effect"—is in operation. Through observing, bystanders learn beforehand something about the opponents they may face one day in the future (Coultier et al., 1996; Johnsson and Akerman, 1998; Oliveira et al., 1998). Verbal models and computer simulations have found that bystander effects can have important consequences on hierarchy formation (Chase, 1974, 1982, 1985; Dugatkin, 2001b). Experimental work has found bystander effects in birds, mammals, and fish (McGregor, 2005).

Bystander effects have been examined in the green swordtail fish (*Xiphophorus helleri*), a species in which males establish linear dominance hierarchies where rank-order fights and/or attack-retreat sequences are common (Beaugrand and Zayan, 1985; Franck et al., 1998). In these experiments, eavesdroppers first observe aggressive interactions and extract information from watching those who are fighting. The eavesdroppers are then tested in later aggressive interactions with those they had previously observed.

To experimentally examine the bystander effect, Earley and Dugatkin had eavesdroppers on one side of an experimental tank and a pair of swordtails who were involved in aggressive interactions on the other side. In one treatment, the eavesdropper could observe the pair of fish through a one-way mirror (mirror treatment) in which he could see the fish who were fighting but they could not see him and so would not be affected by the eavesdropper's presence. In the other treatment, the eavesdropper could not see the pair because of an opaque partition placed into the tank (opaque treatment) (Earley and Dugatkin, 2002, 2005). After this observation period, the eavesdropper was pitted against either the winner of the observed fight or the loser of the observed fight. The opaque partition treatment served as a control for winner and loser effects. Since the eavesdropper could not observe the interaction between pairs of individuals in the opaque partition treatment, the dynamics of the subsequent interaction between the eavesdropper and the winner, or between the eavesdropper and the loser, were the result of winner and loser effects, respectively. In contrast, both bystander effects and winner and loser effects could affect contests between the eavesdropper and winners and losers in the one-way mirror treatment. This means that when we compare the dynamics of contests involving eavesdroppers in the opaque treatment (where there are only winner and loser effects) and the one-way mirror treatment (where there are winner, loser, and bystander effects), we are able to experimentally determine the contribution of bystander effects.

Eavesdroppers that observed a contest in the one-way mirror treatment were much more likely to try and avoid the winner of that contest than were fish in the opaque treatment (Figure 14.16). That is, eavesdropping per se affected future interactions with winners. In addition, eavesdroppers avoided observed winners regardless of how badly they had defeated their prior opponent. The results were quite different when eavesdroppers interacted with losers. In general, eavesdroppers responded in a similar way to all losers, regardless of whether they had witnessed the losers' defeat. But if we break down the data on losers by how badly they lost fights, there is one piece of evidence that suggests that eavesdroppers deal differently with losers because they have observed them lose. Results indicate that in the one-way mirror treatment (observed contests), eavesdroppers were less likely to initiate aggressive behavior and win against (1) losers that had persisted in their fights, or (2) losers that had escalated their aggressive actions, than they were to initiate aggression against losers that had

FIGURE 14.16 Eavesdroppers, winners, and losers. Eavesdroppers could either observe aggressive interactions between a pair of other fish (one-way mirror treatment; green bars) or such interactions were blocked from view by an opaque partition (opaque treatment; orange bars). When eavesdroppers were then paired against winners of the previous contests, those who had observed the previous contests were less likely to **(A)** initiate interactions, and **(B)** escalate aggressive interactions. Those who were paired with the losers of the previous contest were more likely to initiate aggressive contests, whether or not they had been able to observe the previous contests, and less likely to escalate contests. That is, the difference between orange and green bars for losers was not statistically significant. *(Based on Earley and Dugatkin, 2005, p. 90)*

A

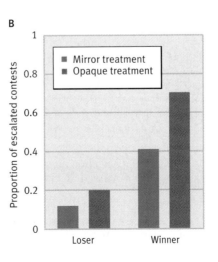

B

Dr. Karen Hollis

As a psychologist, what drew you to the study of animal aggression?

I first became interested in aggression as a graduate student working with *Betta splendens*, a territorial freshwater fish native to Southeast Asia. Although my project addressed a question of underlying learning processes, not aggression per se, it afforded me a serendipitous observation of aggressive behavior, one that provided the raw material for years of subsequent research. My project required me to transport each *Betta* male in its home tank to another room where it would have the opportunity to display to a rival. After a few days of this procedure, I noticed that when I approached the shelf on which the males were located and reached for a particular male's tank, it became quite agitated. After a few more days, each male that I selected began to display—at me. And at eye level that display looked quite ferocious! I recognized that some features of my appearance obviously had become a learned cue for the subsequent interaction with a territorial rival. At that time, associative learning in *B. splendens* was pretty well established (even if the experimenter-as-signal was a little unconventional). However, what was even more interesting to me was the realization that this kind of learning could be a wonderfully adaptive mechanism, providing a territory owner with a definitive competitive edge: Confronting a potential usurper with a full-blown aggressive display could be a very effective aggressive strategy for a territory owner. A few

years later, as a postdoctoral student at Oxford, I had the opportunity to conduct those experiments with blue gouramis, *Trichogaster trichopterus*, and, as the data showed pretty convincingly, the best defense is, indeed, a good offense.

What do animals usually fight over? Do they display different types of aggression depending upon what the fight is about?

No matter what the situation— from nest-mate aggression and sibling rivalry to parent-offspring conflict and territorial behavior—aggression is all about resources. Moreover, as behavioral ecologists have demonstrated quite convincingly across a variety of taxa, particular forms of aggressive behavior emerge under particular selection pressures. For example, aggressive behavior in the context of resource-defense polygyny is a mating strategy in which individuals of one sex, typically

males, defend a resource that is in short supply, critical for females, and defendable, both in terms of the reliability of its location and its quality. That resource—and, thus, what males fight over—could be anything that meets these criteria. Many species of freshwater fish, including my own study species, blue gouramis, defend a location where aspects of the habitat, such as the temperature and pH of the water, are favorable for the development of eggs and fry. Territorial lizards defend spots safe from predators. Some birds defend shady spots, necessary for the development of eggs. And, of course, many animals, from territorial male bumblebees and green frogs to sunbirds and burrowing owls, defend food sites.

Aggression also appears in another mating strategy, called harem defense, in which a few males defend a group of females directly, rather than a needed resource. Harem defense polygyny is characteristic of grizzly bears, red deer, and elephant seals. Because the benefits of winning are tied more directly to reproductive success whenever males are defending access to reproductively active females than when they are defending only the resources to which females are drawn, and because only a few males, namely those powerful enough to mount this kind of defense, are able to reproduce, the aggressive behavior differs enormously. Males are much more aggressive, and injuries are potentially more lethal, wherever harems are concerned. So, yes, aggressive behavior differs dramatically, depending on what the fight is about, as predicted by evolutionary theory.

How flexible are the aggressive strategies employed by animals? What role does learning play in aggressive behavior?

Many of the learning phenomena studied by animal learning psychologists map nicely onto naturally occurring aggressive behavior and, thus, demonstrate the flexibility of—and modulating influence on—aggression. For example, the "dear enemy effect"— where two adjoining territory holders form a temporary alliance to fight intruders that are threats to both of them—obviously depends upon habituation. Habituation is the progressive decrease in responsiveness resulting from repeated presentation of a stimulus. Although some instances of attenuated responsiveness are merely the result of sensory adaptation or muscular fatigue, true habituation is a phenomenon of neural memory: The response to repeated sensory stimulation is chocked off somewhere in the brain—or nerve net—of the animal. Aggression between territorial neighbors, which is initially both intense and frequent, gradually wanes to a point of sporadic and relatively mild aggressive interactions. Yet, while neighbors spare one another from their territorial aggression, producing dear enemies, newcomers face its full measure. Laboratory experiments on habituated aggression have reproduced successfully the basic components of the dear enemy effect. That is, the habituated response is stimulus-specific: Neighbors, and only neighbors, no longer elicit aggressive behavior. Moreover, habituation itself is neither permanent nor ephemeral, lasting just long enough to handle the time intervals observed in natural settings.

Other examples abound. Many species of territorial fish are capable of recognizing their competitors, even when they do not belong to the same species; fish of other species whose ecological requirements overlap with the territory holder are driven away while noncompetitive species are permitted to remain within the territory. In short, individuals not only learn which species to attack, but also make fine discriminations between different species of the same genera.

Finally, in the same way that animals can use signals to determine when or where an aggressor might appear and, thus, focus their aggression in cost-effective ways, inhibitory learning—the ability to learn that a cue predicts the absence of a particular event for some period of time—provides a mechanism to avoid useless energy expenditure at times when, or places where, rivals are less likely to occur. For example, territory owners often exhibit "spontaneous" aggressive displays, favoring particular locations—locations, as the research shows, where they have encountered rivals in the past—and ignoring places where rivals have not appeared and, thus, are unlikely to pose a threat.

What do you predict will be the next major breakthrough in the study of animal aggression?

To me, science is like a very large construction project, with different teams of professionals arriving on site at particular points to contribute their special expertise, then making way for the next group, and so on. Only, in the case of science, the project never really ends. Not only does the edifice get renovated over and over again, but also those teams of experts return with new and improved technology. In the study of aggression, behavioral ecologists have laid an extensive and solid foundation of intra- and interspecific behavioral similarities and differences, all of which reflect particular selection pressures. It's now time for geneticists to step on site with their array of exciting new tools.

In particular, I predict that genomic analyses will allow us to explore the vast expanse of questions that lie between genes and the expression of aggressive behavior. Concerning intraspecific differences, what does an ESS look like from a genetic perspective? What are the genetic and developmental differences that separate individuals that become harem defenders from those that are forced to adopt surreptitious strategies to obtain copulations? Single nucleotide polymorphisms (SNPs), locations on the genome where individuals differ by just one chemical compound, already have been implicated in the aggressive threat behavior of monkeys, making this approach a very promising one for addressing individual differences in aggression. At the interspecific level, to what extent do the genomes differ between closely related species that express different types of male-male competition? Conversely, to what extent might the aggressive behavior of convergent species possess similar genetic mechanisms? In short, I predict not only that geneticists and molecular biologists will add a completely new wing to the edifice that is our science of animal behavior, but also that the connectors between these and other groups of behavioral scientists will get easier and easier to traverse.

Dr. Karen Hollis is a professor at Mount Holyoke College. Her work on animal learning and Pavlovian conditioning represents a classic example of how researchers can integrate biological and psychological approaches to animal behavior.

FIGURE 14.17. Eavesdropping and testosterone. In *Oreochromis mossambicus*, the level of testosterone increases after eavesdropping on a fight. *(Photo credit: Johnny Jensen/Image Quest Marine)*

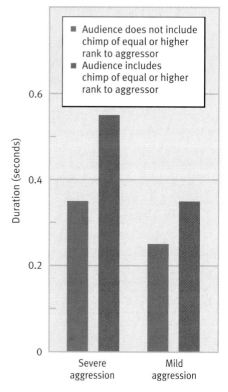

FIGURE 14.18. Audience effects in chimpanzees. Chimpanzees that were victims in severe aggressive interactions emitted distinctive screams. Significantly longer screams were emitted when fights were watched by an audience that included a chimp of equal or higher rank to the aggressor (orange bars) than when the audience did not contain such an individual (green bars). No significant difference was found in the case when victims were involved in mildly aggressive interactions. *(Based on Slocombe and Zuberbuhler, 2007)*

retreated immediately in the observed contests. This was not the case for the opaque treatment, suggesting the presence of subtle bystander effects when the eavesdroppers are interacting with losers.

Ethologists are also beginning to understand the underlying proximate mechanisms associated with bystander effects. In the cichlid fish *Oreochromis mossambicus*, for example, when eavesdropping males watch a fight between a pair of other males, their androgen levels rise (Figure 14.17). In particular, Rui Oliveira and his team measured the levels of testosterone in the urine of eavesdroppers before they saw a fight and after they observed a fight, and they found a significant increase in testosterone levels (Oliveira et al., 1998, 2001, 2002, 2005). This increase in testosterone may have better prepared the eavesdropper for future aggressive interactions by indirectly affecting attention, learning, and memory in ways that might prove adaptive to observers. For example, this increase in testosterone may be adaptive for the eavesdropper if the winner of the observed fight subsequently attacks others, including the eavesdropper, in the immediate vicinity.

AUDIENCE EFFECTS

Not only do bystanders change their estimation of the fighting ability of those they observe, but individuals involved in aggressive interactions change their behavior if they are watched. This latter phenomenon is referred to as the **audience effect** (Doutrelant et al., 2001; Evans and Marler, 1994; McGregor and Peake, 2000). A particularly interesting example of audience effects has been found in the context of aggression and "recruitment screams" in chimpanzees.

Wild chimpanzees are known to emit screams during pairwise aggressive interactions. The screams of those winning a fight are very different from those losing a fight, and it is possible for researchers to categorize screams as "aggressor screams" and "victim screams" (Slocombe and Zuberbuhler, 2005). Victim screams may, in part, function to entice support from observers—for example, a scream by a victim may entice an observer to intercede and break up the fight. Kate Slocombe and Klaus Zuberbuhler examined this possibility in a population of wild chimpanzees in the Budongo Forest of Uganda (Slocombe and Zuberbuhler, 2007).

Slocombe and Zuberbuhler began their work by categorizing pairwise aggressive interactions between chimps as either mildly or severely aggressive. From their observations, they were able to gather data on eighty-four screaming bouts, and they found evidence suggesting a cognitively complex form of audience effects. When they compared the screams of victims in mildly aggressive interactions, no differences were found whether or not there was an audience. When interactions involved severe aggression, however, victim screams were sometimes much longer and more intense when there was an audience present (compared to when there was no audience). But this audience effect was only seen when at least one of the audience members held a rank in the hierarchy that was equal to or above the rank of the aggressor (Figure 14.18). This screaming strategy was successful, as victims who emitted longer and more intense screams were able to entice support from observers, who would proceed to intervene and break up fights.

The proximate and ultimate underpinnings of aggression continue to be a subject of active research in ethology. Work in this area combines experiments and observations on fighting behavior and, in group-living species, dominance hierarchy formation. The three most well-examined models for the evolution of aggression are the hawk-dove game, the war of attrition model, and the sequential assessment model, and these models have been tested in everything from insects to birds, fish, and mammals. A growing area of interest in work on aggression focuses on winner, loser, bystander, and audience effects. Understanding how these four effects operate may provide animal behaviorists with a more comprehensive understanding of dominance hierarchies in nature.

SUMMARY

1. Individuals from very different species tend to fight over the same resources (space, mates, and food), but this does not translate into similar proximate mechanisms being involved in all aggression.

2. In mammals, low serotonin levels are often linked with high levels of aggression, but lower social status. In fish, enhanced serotonergic function is seen in more subordinate individuals, leading to reduced fighting behavior. In crustaceans, increased serotonergic function leads to enhanced aggression and high social status.

3. Ethologists and evolutionary game theorists have built a series of models that examine the evolution of fighting behavior. The three most well-developed game theory models of aggression are the hawk-dove game, the war of attrition model, and the sequential assessment model. In all three of these game theory models, a *cost to fighting* is assumed.

4. There are many varieties of the hawk-dove game. One version adds two new strategies: bourgeois and antibourgeois. The bourgeois strategy instructs an individual to play hawk if it is a territory holder and dove if does not own a territory. The antibourgeois strategy codes for the opposite—play dove if you are a territory holder and hawk if you are not.

5. The war of attrition model was created to examine aggression when the choice available to individuals is more continuous—for example, "fight for *x* seconds, then stop." Rather than getting a set time for fighting, the war of attrition model predicts an ESS distribution of contest lengths.

6. In the sequential assessment model, individuals constantly assess and update their assessment of their opponents' fighting skills. Assessing one's opponent is analogous to statistical sampling. A single sample (assessment) introduces significant random error; the more sampling (assessment) one does, the lower the error rate and hence the more confident one can be in whatever is being estimated.

7. Winner and loser effects are usually defined as an increased probability of winning at time T, based on victories at times T-1, T-2, and so on, and an increased probability of losing at time T, based on losing at times T-1, T-2, and so on.

8. Bystander effects occur when the observer of an aggressive interaction between two other individuals changes its assessment of the fighting abilities of those it has observed. Not only do bystanders change their estimation

of the fighting ability of those they observe, but individuals involved in aggressive interactions change their behavior *if they are watched*. This latter phenomenon is referred to as the audience effect.

DISCUSSION QUESTIONS

1. In 1990, Enquist and Leimer published a paper, "The evolution of fatal fighting" in *Animal Behaviour* (vol. 39, pp. 1–9). Based on reading their paper, as well as your own thoughts on the costs and benefits of extreme aggression, when do you think fighting to the death might be likely to evolve?

2. The classic hawk-dove game we examined in this chapter assumes that losers pay a cost (C) that is not paid by winners. In the matrix below, we are assuming that both hawks in a fight pay a cost.

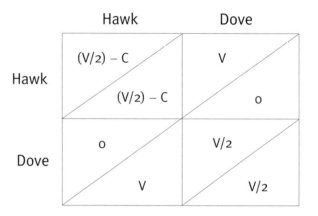

	Hawk	Dove
Hawk	(V/2) – C / (V/2) – C	V / 0
Dove	0 / V	V/2 / V/2

   For the case of both V > C and V < C, calculate the ESS for this new game.

3. A number of studies have suggested that loser effects are both more common and more dramatic than winner effects. Construct a hypothesis as to why this might be. How could you test your hypothesis?

4. If stress-related hormones such as cortisol often inhibit learning and/or memory, how might that compound the difficulties subordinate fish face in trying to raise their rank in hierarchies?

SUGGESTED READING

Archer, J. (1988). *The behavioural biology of aggression*. Cambridge: Cambridge University Press. A short book that provides an overview of biological and psychological approaches to animal aggression.

Edwards, D. H., & Spitzer, N. (2006). Social dominance and serotonin receptor genes in crayfish. *Current Topics in Developmental Biology, 74*, 177–199. A detailed analysis of serotonin and aggression in crayfish.

Hsu, Y., Earley, R. L., & Wolf, L. (2005). Modulation of aggressive behavior by fighting experience: Mechanisms and contest outcomes. *Biological Reviews, 80,* 1–42. A very nice review of both proximate and ultimate perspectives on winner and loser effects.

Maynard Smith, J., & Price, G. (1973). The logic of animal conflict. *Nature, 246,* 15–18. The classic paper introducing ethologists to mathematical models (game theory) of aggression.

Riechert, S. (1998). Game theory and animal contests. In L. A. Dugatkin & H. K. Reeve (Eds.), *Game theory and animal behavior* (pp. 64–93). New York: Oxford University Press. A review chapter on game theory and animal behavior.

15

Play

Give a kitten a ball of yarn or throw a new squeeze toy on the floor for your puppy and watch what happens. Kittens and puppies appear to play with these objects. Take two puppies and put them in the same room, and again it looks like they are playing—this time with each other. Pet owners will swear to you that their animals play—indeed, pet play stories are legendary and numerous.

As we will see in this chapter, play can take many forms. Evidence from ethology suggests that, while not all species engage in play, it is common, particularly among young individuals. Young animals gently wrestle with each other, toss, kick, and push objects they find in their environment, chase one another for no apparent reason, jump, climb up and down trees over and over, and practice hunting prey that aren't present.

While play is probably more common in big-brained vertebrates (such as primates) than in other species, it is not limited to this group (Figure 15.1). Take the case of Pigface, an animal at the Washington Zoo. Pigface would play with whatever new objects (brown balls, orange balls, hoops, and so on) that zookeepers added to his otherwise bland environment (Burghardt, 1998). Pigface approached the new objects, followed them, pushed them around, and so on—he played with them.

Two things make Pigface's story particularly interesting. First, Pigface isn't a dog or a chimp; he's a turtle. Second, play had a profound effect on Pigface's health. Before objects were introduced into his environment, Pigface was in the habit of clawing his own limbs and neck, causing infection and fungal growth. Once the play objects were introduced, this self-destructive behavior dissipated to a great extent. That is, once the bland environment Pigface once lived in was livened up with potential play items, he chose to play rather than self-mutilate.

Nonetheless, play remains a contentious subject in the ethological literature (Burghardt, 2005). Why? One possible explanation is that pet owners' and zookeepers' stories are usually anecdotal at best, and huge exaggerations at worst. Ethologists tend to focus on topics that can be studied experimentally, and, whenever possible, in a controlled manner. But play simply has not been examined experimentally until very recently.

A second possible reason that play behavior was (and is) relatively understudied is that animal behaviorists tend to study behaviors that appear to have an

A

B

FIGURE 15.1. Play. Play behavior in **(A)** sea lions, and **(B)** polar bears. *(Photo credits: Marty Snyderman/Visuals Unlimited; Jeff Vanuga/Corbis)*

evolutionary function. When it comes to play, function is sometimes very hard to determine, and hence there is a tendency to shy away from work in this area. A third, related reason for the relative lack of controlled studies of play is tied to theory. Robert Fagan and others have argued that a lack of concrete *theory* for the function of play can explain why play research lagged behind other areas of interest in ethology (Fagen, 1981). But recently, a theoretical underpinning for play behavior has begun to emerge, and we will examine this more throughout the chapter (Bekoff and Byers, 1998; Burghardt, 2005).

The situation with respect to the study of play has undoubtedly improved (somewhat) since 1975, when E. O. Wilson wrote that "no behavioral concept has proved more ill-defined, elusive, controversial and even unfashionable than play" (Wilson, 1975). There is now a sizable literature on many aspects of animal play, which seeks to answer various proximate and ultimate questions dealing with play behavior (Bekoff and Byers, 1998; Bruner et al., 1976; Burghardt, 2005; Fagen, 1981; Power, 2000; Symons, 1978). In this chapter, we will examine:

- how play is defined,
- the different types of play behavior (object, locomotor, and social play) and their purported functions,
- the endocrinological and neurobiological bases of play,
- the phylogeny of play.

Defining Play

Throughout this book, whenever possible, we have relied on definitions that already exist in the ethological literature, and these definitions often match the everyday meaning of the subject we are tackling. Since everyone knows what "foraging" means, for example, when we discuss how animals obtain food, we usually don't run into much in the way of definitional problems. The same holds true for subjects like "parental care" and "antipredator activities" as well as a whole host of other behaviors. Definitional issues, however, do become something of a concern when it comes to play. Indeed, some of the reluctance of ethologists to study play centers on the notion that play is some amorphous, fuzzy behavior that defies definition.

In the animal behavioral literature there are numerous definitions of **play**. The most widely cited of these definitions is that of Marc Bekoff and John Byers, who propose the following:

> Play is all motor activity performed postnatally that appears to be purposeless, in which motor patterns from other contexts may often be used in modified forms and altered temporal sequencing. If the activity is directed toward another living being it is called social play. (Bekoff and Byers, 1981, pp. 300–301)

This definition clearly centers on the structure of play rather than its function. One problem with it is that behaviors such as repetitive pacing (pacing back and forth for long periods of time in what appears to be a purposeless manner) meets the above definition, but no one would argue that this is really play behavior (Bekoff and Allen, 1998). In addition, it is not only extremely difficult to determine when a behavior is "purposeless," but behaviors that are apparently purposeless may be so for three very different reasons (Heinrich and Smokler, 1998): (1) observers may simply fail to decipher what the immediate benefit of the play behavior is, (2) the purpose and potential benefit may not be accrued until long after play has occurred (Fagen and Fagen, 2004), and (3) the benefits may be multiple and confounding. The situation is actually more complex, because the Bekoff and Byers's definition does not claim that play is purposeless, only that it appears to be so (Heinrich and Smokler, 1998).

So where does that leave us with respect to a definition of play? It seems that those who study play have adopted a definition similar to the United States Supreme Court's definition of pornography—"we can't say exactly what it is, but we know it when we see it." This is not quite as bad a state of affairs as it may seem. For example, in an edited volume on play behavior in animals, many of the authors adopt this view of play. They argue that since experimental work on play lags behind controlled work in other areas of animal behavior, it is best to take a "wait and see" approach, wherein observers study play in many species. The hope is that such work will eventually uncover certain commonalities in play behavior, and that such commonalities will then be used to construct a definition.

Types and Functions of Play

Ethologists generally speak of three different types of play—object, locomotor, and social play. We will examine each of these, and in so doing, attempt not only to provide examples of what constitutes each type of play but also to examine the function of each of the three types of play.

OBJECT PLAY

Object play refers to play that centers on the use of inanimate objects such as sticks, rocks, leaves, feathers, fruit, and human-provided objects, and the pushing, throwing, tearing, or manipulating of such objects (Hall, 1998). A wonderful example of object play has been documented in a chimpanzee population living in the Mahale Mountains of Tanzania. Researchers examining videotapes of the chimps in this population found a behavior they labeled "leaf-pile pulling" (Figure 15.2). As groups of chimps move down the slope of a mountain, an individual will sometimes stop and walk backwards, pulling handfuls of leaves along with him as he proceeds, making quite a racket along the way. Then, the chimp stops and either walks or somersaults through the pile of the leaves that he created (Nishida and Wallauer, 2003).

Object play has been documented in animals in a wide array of taxa, and is particularly well-studied in captive populations—such as zoo animals—where "toys" are given to animals to provide them with new items in an otherwise relatively constant environment. Object play has been distinguished from object exploration, with play often following exploration (Hutt, 1966; Wood-Gush and Vestergaard, 1991; Figure 15.3). Animals undertaking object exploration appear to be examining what an object is, while object play appears to have the animal addressing the question "what can I do with this object?" (Hutt, 1970; Power, 2000).

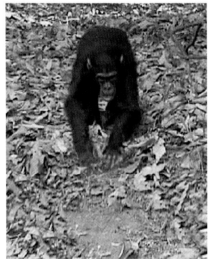

FIGURE 15.2. Leaf play in chimpanzees. Chimpanzees living in the Mahale Mountains of Tanzania play in what is called "leaf-pile pulling." As they go down the slope of a mountain, individuals sometimes walk backwards, pulling handfuls of leaves and then stopping and either walking or somersaulting through the pile of leaves. The top photo shows the chimp as he starts to gather a pile of leaves, and the bottom photo shows the same chimp as his leaf pile accumulates. *(Photo credits: Toshi Nishida)*

FIGURE 15.3. Play or exploration?
Here a cheetah cub comes upon a novel object: a can. Exploring the can appears designed to address the "what is it?" question, while play appears designed to tackle the "what can I do with this object?" question.

OBJECT PLAY IN JUVENILE RAVENS. Young animals often have more "free time" than adults to engage in object play (Burghardt, 1988). From a functional perspective, object play in young animals is often associated with some aspect of practice where an animal learns something that will benefit it either in the short or long term—for example, young predators may use object play to practice hunting (Beck, 1980; Fagen, 1981; Martin and Caro, 1985; Smith, 1982).

In his delightful and thought-provoking book *Mind of the Raven*, Bernd Heinrich describes how play occupies a raven's time more than one might predict from a general survey of the avian behavioral literature (Heinrich, 1999; Figure 15.4). For example, young ravens play with virtually every new kind of object they encounter—leaves, twigs, pebbles, bottle caps, seashells, glass fragments, and inedible berries (Heinrich and Bugnyar, 2007; Heinrich and Smokler, 1998). Heinrich, who has studied these birds for thousands of hours, writes of young birds' obsessive drive to contact and manipulate any objects they encounter (Heinrich and Smokler, 1998).

Object play in young ravens sets the stage for what individuals fear, or don't fear, when they mature (Heinrich, 1988a; Heinrich et al., 1996). Adult ravens still manipulate objects after they mature. Yet, compared with how they react to items they played with when they were younger, they treat items they have never encountered before—including potential food sources—with great trepidation. To demonstrate the potential fitness benefit of object play, Heinrich ran an experiment involving both observation and manipulation.

FIGURE 15.4. Hanging around. Various "hanging games" Heinrich observed in ravens. *(Based on Heinrich, 1999, p. 289)*

TABLE 15.1. Raven play. Young ravens play with almost any new item they encounter. Below are the forty-four novel items that Heinrich added to the raven's environment classified according to their conspicuousness and whether or not they were organic. *(Based on Heinrich, 1995)*

ORGANIC INCONSPICUOUS	ORGANIC CONSPICUOUS	INORGANIC CONSPICUOUS
Tenebrio larvae*	Small green apples	Seashell fragments
Squash stems	*Raja* egg cases	Bottle caps
Fucus seaweed bladders	*Ovalipes* crab shells	Red glass chips
Promethea (empty) cocooons	Pistachio (closed) nuts	Beach pebbles
Caddisfly *(Ephemeroptera)**	*Libinia* crab shells	Cigarette butts
Tenebrio adults*	*Busycon* egg cases	White glass chips
Leather chips	Mushrooms	Buttons
Spongomorpha seaweed	*Emerita* crabs*	Glass vials
Wood burls	*Ovalipes* crab claws	
Leaf rolls	*Papilio* butterfly wings	
Onion flower buds	Sparrow eggs*	
Dry beans	Wild strawberries *(Fragaria)**	
Brown birch cones	Red checkerberries *(Gaultheria)*	
Silver maple samaras	Carrot slices	
Red maple samaras	Green *(Ribes)* gooseberries	
Red spruce cones	Wild raspberries *(Rubus)**	
Green birch cones	Blueberries *(Vaccinium)**	
	Red bunchberries *(Cornus)*	
	Soft maize kernels*	

Edible items.

Heinrich examined object play in four young juvenile ravens raised by experimenters in a controlled, but relatively natural, forest environment in Maine (Heinrich, 1995). Young ravens were observed in thirty-minute sessions for more than thirty days. During the first ten observation periods, Heinrich noted all the naturally occurring objects the birds encountered. Nine hundred and eighty naturally occurring items that fell into ninety-five different categories were encountered by the young birds during their first ten trials, and such encounters often involved some combination of exploration and play.

After the first ten trials, Heinrich then added forty-four "novel" items—objects the ravens had never seen before—to the birds' environment and observed the manner in which juveniles interacted with these new objects (Table 15.1). He found that exploration and play were directed at novel items. Novelty, per se, rather than other characteristics such as shininess, palatability, or conspicuousness, explained which items they chose. Yet, while they did not choose items based on their palatability, they quickly treated inedible items as background material (that is, they did not handle these items much after their initial encounters with them) and edible novel items as their preferred foods. This suggests that juvenile play and exploration in ravens has the important benefit of enabling the juvenile ravens to identify new food sources. Ravens are scavengers (as well as predators), and in a world where many objects may be food, play and curiosity in ravens seem to be selected as a means to decipher what counts as food and what doesn't (Heinrich, 1999; Heinrich and Bugnyar, 2007).

OBJECT PLAY IN YOUNG CHEETAHS. Tim Caro examined play in cheetah cubs in the Serengeti National Park in Tanzania for three years (Caro, 1995b; Figure 15.5). He observed cubs for more than 2,600 hours and documented many cases of object, social, and locomotor play (Table 15.2). In particular,

TABLE 15.2. Types of cheetah play. Young cheetahs benefit from a wide variety of play activities in nature. *(From Caro, 1995b, p. 335)*

TYPE OF PLAY	BEHAVIOR PATTERNS*	RECIPIENT
Locomotor play	Bounding gait Rushing around	No recipient
Contact social play	Patting Biting Kicking Grasping	Any family member
Object play	Patting Biting Kicking Carrying	Object
Noncontact social play	Stalking[†] Crouching[†] Chasing Fleeing Rearing up	Any family member

*Definitions: bounding gait: slow run with stiff legs causing a rocking motion; rushing around: short sprint often including turns; pat: slap or touch with forepaw; bite: close jaws on animal or object; kick: strike with hindfeet; grasp: hold with forepaws or forelegs; carry: move with object in mouth; stalk: slow approach with body held low; crouch: stationary posture with body low and belly often on ground; chase: run after another animal; flee: run away from another animal; rear up: forelegs off the ground; sniff: place nose close to object.
[†]Crouches and stalks that continued from one cub's focal minute to the next were scored just once.

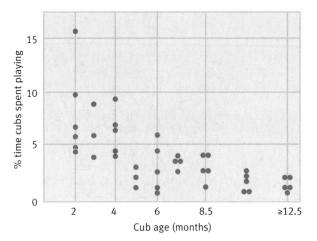

FIGURE 15.6. Play in younger and older juvenile cheetahs. In cheetahs, play progressively disappears with age. *(From Caro, 1995b)*

Caro was interested in the role of each type of play in shaping how cheetahs would learn to capture prey and what the costs associated with each type of play might be.

Given that cheetahs spend a considerable amount of time playing as cubs (Figure 15.6), Caro examined the possible costs associated with juvenile play. Estimating the cost of any behavior, particularly a behavior as complex and difficult to measure as play, is never an easy task, but a number of studies, involving various species, indicate that under certain conditions play may be very costly (Arnold and Trillmich, 1985; Berger, 1980; Douglas-Hamilton and Douglas-Hamilton, 1975; Harcourt, 1991; Lawick-Goodall, 1968). As an extreme case, while play accounted for just over 6 percent of young fur seals' time, twenty-two of the twenty-six pups that were killed over the course of long-term observations were engaged in some sort of play at the time they were killed (Harcourt, 1991).

To estimate the potential costs of play in young cheetahs, Caro measured both the distance that a cub rushed around or chased during play, and the distance cubs moved from their mothers during object, motor, and social play. The former was an attempt to measure energetic costs of play for the young cheetah cubs, while the latter was an estimate of predation or general injury costs associated with play (the farther the cub was from its mother, the greater was its risk of being harmed either during play or by a predator such as a lion or a spotted hyena).

Caro's data suggest that cheetah play—including object play such as patting, biting, kicking, and carrying—is a very low-cost activity. To begin with, while it turned out to be nearly impossible to measure the direct energy costs of play, cubs were never seriously injured during play. In addition, while young cheetah cubs that were involved in play were slightly farther from their mothers than cubs not playing, in all cases the cubs' mothers were so close that their cubs were not under any serious predation threat. Costs of play in juvenile cheetahs may still exist, but Caro's study was about as comprehensive as one can get under difficult field conditions, and if such costs do exist, they are in all likelihood minor.

In terms of benefits, increased play led cubs to display increased rates of patting, grasping, and biting live prey that their mother had just released. Such predatory-like behavior on the part of the cubs should, in all likelihood, make them more successful hunters when they mature.

LOCOMOTOR PLAY

In this section, we will consider one type of **locomotor play**, which is technically referred to as locomotor-rotational play (Power, 2000). One description of this type of play is as follows:

> The single most frequent and phylogenetically widespread locomotor act of play must surely be a leap upward. . . . Hops, springs, bounces and bucks are variations on the basic vertical leap. . . . Animals may somersault, roll, flip forward or backward, spin, whirl, pirouette, make handstands, chase their tails, rear and kick up their heels. . . . Often a vertical leap is decorated with body-twists, rear-kicks or head shakes. These acrobatics can be spectacular. (Fagen, 1981, pp. 287–291)

Two major hypotheses have been put forth to explain the function of locomotor play in animals and humans. The first is that locomotor play provides both exercise and training for specific motor skills needed later in life (Byers, 1984, 1998). A second potential benefit is that locomotor play provides animals with a better understanding of "the lay of the land"—that is, where things are in relation to one another—and this may provide immediate benefits (Power, 2000; Stamps, 1995; Symons, 1978). Here we will focus on the exercise-related benefits.

Locomotor play has been studied primarily in rodents, primates, and ungulates, and it includes such actions as leaps, jumps, twists, shakes, whirls, and somersaults (Figure 15.7). In an attempt to quantify the possible fitness

A

B

FIGURE 15.7. Pronghorn play.
Pronghorns undertake various forms of locomotor play, including **(A)** "high-speed running," **(B)** "fast turns," and **(C)** "stots" (jumping with all four legs simultaneously off the ground, like the pronghorn in the bottom left corner of the photo). *(Photo credits: John Byers)*

C

TABLE 15.3. Physiological effects of elevated motor activity. In examining the potential benefits of locomotor play, Byers and Walker listed nineteen benefits that might be associated with elevated motor activity. *(Based on Byers and Walker, 1995)*

SPECIFIC EFFECT	PRESUMED BENEFIT TO FITNESS	EFFECT AVAILABLE TO JUVENILES?	EFFECT PERMANENT?	EFFECT AVAILABLE TO ADULTS?
Increase in VO₂ max*	Greater endurance	Yes	No	Yes
Decrease in heart rate during exercise	Greater endurance	Yes	No	Yes
Decrease in blood lactate level during exercise	Greater endurance	Yes	No	Yes
Increased heart weight : body weight ratio	Greater endurance	Yes	No	Yes
Increased myoglobin	Greater endurance	Yes	No	Yes
Greater numbers and size of skeletal muscle mitochondria	Greater endurance	Yes	No	Yes
Increased muscle glycogen and triglyceride stores	Greater endurance	Yes	No	Yes
Greater capacity to oxidize fat	Greater endurance	Yes	No	Yes
Greater slow-twitch fiber area	Greater endurance	Yes	No	Yes
Greater total blood volume	Greater endurance	Yes	No	Yes
Greater muscle capillary density	Greater endurance	Yes	No	Yes
Greater maximal ventilation rate	Greater endurance	Yes	No	Yes
Increased maximal muscle blood flow	Greater endurance	Yes	No	Yes
Bone remodeling	Increased strength	Yes	No	Yes
Fast-twitch fiber hypertrophy	Increased strength	Yes	No	Yes
Increased recruitment of motor units	Increased strength	Yes	No	Yes
Modification of cortical areas involved in movement	Increased motor skill/ energetic economy of movement	Yes	No	Yes
Modification of muscle fiber type differentiation	Increased motor skill/ energetic economy of movement	Yes	Probably	Unlikely
Modification of cerebellar synapse distribution	Increased motor skill/ energetic economy of movement	Yes	Yes	Diminished

*VO₂ max measures maximum oxygen reuptake.

consequences of locomotor play, John Byers and Curt Walker reviewed a list of nineteen potential anatomical and physiological benefits associated with exercise and physical training (Byers and Walker, 1995; Table 15.3). They went through their list of putative benefits and began by searching for benefits that were available to individuals as juveniles, but not as adults, but that were long-lasting in their effects. Only two of the nineteen possible benefits met their criteria.

One hypothesized benefit associated with locomotor play is an increase in the creation of synapses in the cerebellum (technically referred to as cerebellar synaptogenesis). The cerebellum plays a critical role in limb coordination, movement, postural changes, eye-limb coordination, and many other aspects of movement in mammals (Byers and Walker, 1995; Thatch et al., 1992). During development, more cerebellar synapses are created than are used in later life, and some of these synapses may be pruned as a function of experience (Brown et al., 1991; Greenough and Juraska, 1979; Jacobson, 1991; Purves and Lichtman, 1980; Pysh and Weiss, 1979).

Researchers have asked how play behavior maps onto cerebellar synapse formation and elimination. With respect to motor play in juvenile mice, the fit is quite good (Figure 15.8A). Mice start playing at about fifteen days of age and peak in their locomotor play activities at nineteen to twenty-five days, and this ontogeny (development) of play corresponds with a peak in cerebellar synaptogenesis. The same general pattern is found when examining locomotor and social play in rats (Figure 15.8B) and social play in cats (Figure 15.8C). A second major developmental change—the differentiation of muscle fibers that will be important for use in foraging and antipredator behaviors also maps nicely onto the development of play (Close, 1972; Edgerton, 1978; Roy et al., 1988).

It is important to realize that this sort of work is correlational. As Byers and Walker note in their study, we do not know if an increase in locomotor play causes an increase in cerebellar synaptogenesis or if an increase in cerebellar synaptogenesis leads to an increase in locomotor play. Future work is needed to infer causation.

FIGURE 15.8. Play and brain development.
Cerebellar synaptogenesis (green curve) is plotted along the ontogeny of play (orange curve) in **(A)** mice, **(B)** rats, and **(C)** cats. *(Based on Byers and Walker, 1995)*

Social play—that is, playing with others—is the most well-studied type of play. Three functions of social play have been proposed (Thompson, 1996): (1) Social play may lead to the forging of long-lasting social bonds (Carpenter, 1934). For example, among immature chimps in the Arnhem Zoo (in the Netherlands) male-male social play is especially common (Mendozagranados and Sommer, 1995). A possible benefit of male-male social play sessions is to provide young males with coalition partners that may be important in their adult life (de Waal, 1992; see Chapter 9). (2) Like other forms of play, social play may provide much-needed physical skills, such as those relating to fighting, hunting, and mating. (3) Social play may aid in the development of cognitive skills (Bekoff, 2000, 2004, 2007). Let us examine the last two of these benefits of social play in a bit more detail.

SOCIAL PLAY AND BIGHORN SHEEP. In bighorn sheep (*Ovis canadensis*), as in many ungulates, males compete aggressively for females (Geist, 1966, 1974a), and male reproductive variance is much higher than that of females—only a few males win many aggressive contests and hence mate, while almost all females have mating opportunities. Joel Berger reasoned that if males and females differ in the degree to which aggression shapes their adult interactions, then such differences may manifest themselves much earlier, perhaps as early as lamb social play interactions (Berger, 1980).

Berger studied juvenile social play in two populations of bighorn sheep, one in the sloping grassy hills of British Columbia and one in the Colorado Desert (Figure 15.9). In line with his prediction, Berger found that males engaged in much more contact play than female lambs. This contact play may help males prepare for the battles that will play a large factor in their struggle for reproductive success in later life.

Three other interesting results emerged from the bighorn sheep study. First, social "contact" play (butting, pushing, and so on) was often preceded by "rotational" movements that appeared to serve as a signal that contact was part of a play sequence (see below for more on play signals). Second, it turns out that social play behavior in bighorn sheep does not begin at a certain age per se; rather it starts after young individuals have associated with each other for a certain amount of time. Young who stayed by the side of their mothers began contact play at later ages than did lambs that associated with other lambs from an early

A   B

FIGURE 15.9. Bighorn play. Juvenile bighorn sheep who (**A**) stayed close to their mothers for extended periods of time play less often than (**B**) other juveniles.

age. Finally, Berger also found differences in the frequency of play across his two populations. In both populations, lambs were involved in play at very early ages, but play tapered off much more quickly in the desert population than in the grassy slope population. One possible explanation for this difference is that young sheep in the desert were more energetically stressed. The data suggest otherwise, however, as lambs in the desert actually receive more milk from their mothers than lambs in the grassy hill population (Berger, 1979). Instead, it appears that desert lambs often bump into cactus while playing, and the consequent pain they suffer acts as a negative reinforcement for social play (Berger, 1980).

SOCIAL PLAY AND COGNITION. One cognitively related benefit of social play revolves around the idea of "self-assessment." Here, animals use social play as a means to monitor their developmental progress as compared to others. For example, in infant sable antelope (*Hippotragus niger*), individuals prefer same-age play partners. While this preference could be due to numerous factors, Kaci Thompson has hypothesized that it is primarily a function of infants attempting to choose play partners that provide them with a reasonable comparison from which to gauge their own development (Thompson, 1996; Figure 15.10).

With respect to cognition and social play, one question that ethologists have addressed is how do animals, especially young animals, know that they are engaged in play (Bekoff, 2000, 2004, 2007)? And even more to the point, how do they communicate this information to each other? Since many of the behavior patterns seen during play are also common in other contexts—hunting, mating, dangerous aggressive contests—how do animals know they are playing and not involved in the real activity? Bekoff has proposed three possible solutions to this important, but often overlooked, question (Bekoff, 2000).

One way that animals may distinguish play from related activities is that the order and frequency of behavioral components of play is often quite different from that of the "real" activity (Hill and Bekoff, 1977). That is, when play behavior is compared with the adult functional behavior that it resembles, behavioral patterns during play are often exaggerated and misplaced. If young animals are able to distinguish these exaggerations and misorderings of behavioral patterns by, for example, observing adults that are not involved in play, a relatively simple explanation exists for how animals know they are playing.

A

B

FIGURE 15.10. Antelope play. Young sable antelope like this pair often engage in play, particularly with same-age partners. *(Photo credits: Kaci Thompson)*

A B

FIGURE 15.11. Play markers. (A) Play signals override canine aggression. The dog on the right growls, while the dog on the left "paws." Pawing is a play signal that can turn a potentially dangerous encounter into a playful one. **(B)** Play bows are also often used as signals that the bowing individual wants to play. The dog in this photo is play bowing to another individual. *(Photo credits: Marc Bekoff)*

A second, somewhat related, means by which animals may be able to distinguish play from other activities is by the placement of **play markers** (Bekoff, 1977, 1995; Berger, 1980). These are also known as "play signals" and can serve both to initiate play and to indicate the desire to continue playing and to warn adults that the young are playing and not in danger of injury. In canids, for example, biting and shaking are usually performed during dangerous activities such as fighting and predation. Yet, biting and shaking are also play behaviors of young canids. Bekoff found that play markers such as a "bow" would precede biting and rapid side-to-side shaking of the head to indicate that they were not dangerous behaviors (Bekoff, 1995; Figure 15.11). The bow would communicate that this action should be viewed in a new context—that of play. Another play marker might be a particular kind of vocalization—for example, chirping in a rat, whistling in a mongoose, panting in a wolf or a chimpanzee—before or during a play interaction. Or there might be a distinctive smell that indicated that the animals were engaged in play.

Play markers have also been found in primates such as the lowland gorilla (Palagi et al., 2007). Juvenile lowland gorillas play with each other often, and play ranges from what Elisabetta Palagi and her colleagues call "gentle play" to "rough play." Palagi's team discovered that when juvenile gorillas—particularly males—were involved with rough play, the play was often preceded by a facial gesture they call the "play face" (Figure 15.12). This facial gesture, which is not seen in other contexts, includes slightly lowered eyebrows and an open mouth. In addition to using this facial gesture during rough play, juvenile gorillas also displayed it when a play session was in a place that made escape (leaving) difficult—another context in which it may be important to signal to others that "what is about to occur is play."

Yet another way by which young animals may be able to distinguish play from related behaviors is by **role reversal**, or **self-handicapping**, on the part of any older playmates they may have. In role reversal and self-handicapping, older individuals either allow subordinate younger animals to act as if they are dominant during play or the older animals perform some act (for example, an

FIGURE 15.12. Play face in gorillas.
Preceding bouts of aggressive play, juvenile gorillas use a facial gesture called a "play face," which appears to signal that "what is about to occur is play." *(Photo credit: William H. Calvin)*

aggressive act) at a level clearly below that of which they are capable. Either of these provides younger playmates with the opportunity to recognize that they are involved in a play encounter.

The obvious follow-up question to "how do animals know they are engaged in play?" is "even when you know it's playtime, why play fairly?" One likely answer is that "cheating" at play—for example, hurting a partner during social play by inflicting damaging bites or swipes of a paw—probably does net an individual many real benefits. But cheating may lead others to ostracize an individual at social playtime. If the benefits of social play are great enough (Figure 15.13), such ostracism could have a significant negative impact on a cheater.

FIGURE 15.13. The benefits of play. Bekoff has hypothesized that young animals learn to cooperate during play (left) and that this might have benefits later in life, when cooperation is necessary—for example, when adult lions are hunting a wildebeest (right).

FIGURE 15.14. Role reversal. In play fighting between older and younger juvenile squirrel monkeys, role reversal sometimes occurs, wherein an older, larger playmate will allow a younger, smaller playmate to act as if he is dominant and to obtain the superior position when they wrestle.

PLAY FIGHTING AND COGNITIVE TRAINING IN SQUIRREL MONKEYS. Squirrel monkeys (*Saimiri sciureus*) are a model species for studying play fighting in both the lab and the field (Baldwin, 1969, 1971; Biben, 1986; Dumond, 1968). Play begins at age five weeks old, when infants start interacting with each other while still on their mothers' backs. Young of each sex prefer playing with same-sex partners, and one fascinating aspect of play fighting in young squirrel monkeys is the important position that role reversal plays, particularly in male-male play bouts (Biben, 1986; Figure 15.14).

As in young human children, young male squirrel monkeys prefer to play with others lower in dominance rank (Biben, 1986; Boulton, 1991; Humphreys and Smith, 1987). Nonetheless, while their preference may be to play with those who are subordinate to them, squirrel monkeys often do accept a dominant play partner. But why would subordinate individuals play with someone who is dominant to them (Altmann, 1962)? The answer appears to be that individuals that are clearly dominant *outside* the context of play often allow subordinates to take on the dominant role when it comes to play—that is, they engage in role reversal, wherein the subordinate does not defer to the dominant individual as he would outside the play situation, thus providing normally subordinate individuals with an incentive for playing. Somewhat surprisingly, role reversal breaks down in between-sex play. Males, who are typically dominant to females, do not engage in role reversal when playing with females.

Why are dominant males so quick to engage in role reversal when play fighting with same-sex partners? Part of the answer is that role reversal during play does not appear to influence the dominant/subordinate relationship *outside* of play. So, the cost of role reversal is probably minimal. Yet, why bother with role reversal in the first place? The answer is that without role reversal, few play partners would be available since subordinates would not be willing to play with dominants, and so any benefits associated with play would be hard to come by.

What might such benefits be for young male squirrel monkeys? One benefit might be that play fighting trains males for true aggressive behavior later in life. Yet, the direct evidence for such benefits later in life are absent in squirrel monkeys—it is not as if those who play more win more fights later in life or those who win play fights win real fights. Instead, Maxeen Biben offers three possible benefits to play fighting in squirrel monkeys (Biben, 1998):

1. Behavioral flexibility: since play involves little in the way of costs to squirrel monkeys, it may be an ideal means for individuals to learn how to be behaviorally flexible. This may be particularly relevant with respect to role reversal in squirrel monkey male play fights.
2. Gauging the intentions of others: real fighting in adult squirrel monkey life can be very dangerous. Play fighting might provide males with training in gauging the intentions of others in adult life.
3. Experience in both the subordinate and dominant roles: males that end up as dominant in adult life must "work their way up" a dominance hierarchy. As they do, they will lose as well as win many encounters. Play fighting may teach males how to act both as a subordinate and as a dominant—roles they will encounter throughout life (again, this is particularly relevant to the role reversal aspect of male play fighting in squirrel monkeys).

Which, if any, of these possible benefits drives play in the squirrel monkey system remains to be tested.

A GENERAL THEORY FOR THE FUNCTION OF PLAY

Marek Spinka and his colleagues have hypothesized that the main function of play is to allow animals to develop the physical and psychological skills to handle unexpected events in which they experience a loss of control. Specifically, they propose that "play functions to increase the versatility of movements used to recover from sudden shocks such as loss of balance and falling over, and to enhance the ability of animals to cope emotionally with unexpected stressful situations" (Spinka et al., 2001, p. 141). So, for example, the loss of control and balance associated with being chased by predators or losing an aggressive interaction may be dealt with more effectively if play allows animals to prepare for such events.

Spinka and his collaborators list twenty-four predictions that emerge from their hypothesis. Here we will touch on a number of these predictions and the evidence available to judge them. At the most general level, Spinka and his colleagues predict that the amount of play experienced will affect an animal's ability to handle unexpected events. While this prediction has not been directly tested, some correlational work in both humans and nonhumans supports it. In rats, for example, individuals deprived of social play often react more negatively to unexpected stimuli than those not deprived of play (Potegal and Einon, 1989). In humans, measures of rough-and-tumble play are sometimes correlated with scores on social problem-solving tests (Pellegrini, 1995; Saunders et al., 1999).

A second prediction that emerges from Spinka and his colleagues' hypothesis is that self-handicapping, where dominant animals allow subordinates to defeat them during play fights, should be ubiquitous in species that play. Self-handicapping is thought to be an excellent means for preparing for the unexpected, as individuals put themselves in a position very different from that in which they normally find themselves. Evidence from many species supports the presence of self-handicapping in species that exhibit play.

During play, the brain must deal with sensory inputs that are different from the sensory inputs from other behaviors and with problems that must be solved by what Spinka and his group call "kinematic improvisation and emotional flexibility." As such, they predict that play should have measurable effects on an animal's somatosensory, motor, and emotion centers. In support of this prediction, rats that have been deprived of social play have long-term changes in opioid receptors, and they have permanently altered levels of dopamine and other neurotransmitters, all of which are important components of the stress response seen in these animals (Paul et al., 2005; Spinka et al., 2001; van den Berg et al., 1999).

One of the more obvious predictions from Spinka's general theory of play is that locomotor play should be most common in species that live in the most variable environments. If locomotor play allows one to experience loss of locomotor control, this effect might be most beneficial in environments that change most rapidly. More generally speaking, individuals who engage in play should be more prepared for the unexpected, which is more likely to occur where there is environmental change. Unfortunately, there is currently very little evidence available to test this particular prediction.

Endocrinological and Neurobiological Bases of Play

With one exception (the work on synapses and locomotor play), so far we have focused our analysis on ultimate questions about play behavior. In this section, we will take a more proximate perspective on play, by focusing on the endocrinological and neurobiological bases of play in rats and squirrels.

PLAY FIGHTING IN YOUNG MALE RODENTS

Male rats fight with one another from early on in development. While such fights among adult males can be dangerous and can have significant effects on male reproductive success, aggression among younger rodents, including rats, often takes the form of a much less dangerous form of play fighting (Figure 15.15). This type of social play may prepare rats for the "real" fights they will engage in as adults—and the stress that will arise from such fights. Here we will examine some work on the endocrinology and neurobiology of play fighting behavior in young male rodents.

Work on the endocrinology of play has focused on testosterone because this hormone has long been linked to male aggression (Nelson, 2005). As we have seen in earlier chapters, when examining the relationship between testosterone and aggression, it can often be difficult to assign cause and effect. For example, suppose you hypothesize that young male rats with high levels of testosterone are more likely to win play fights than males with lower levels of testosterone. If you took testosterone measures after a fight and found that males with higher levels of testosterone won more aggressive encounters than their losing counterparts, you would not be able distinguish cause and effect—winning may be a result of high levels of testosterone, or high testosterone levels may be a result of winning. Even if you had been able to measure testosterone levels in males before they fought, and victors had high levels of pre-fight testosterone, determining cause and effect would still be difficult, as some other factor might have caused an increase in both testosterone and the probability of victory—

FIGURE 15.15. Play fighting in rodents. (A) Djungarian hamsters (*Phodopus campbelli*); **(B)** Fat sand jirds (*Psammomys obesus*); **(C** and **D)** Syrian golden hamsters (*Mesocricetus auratus*).

that is, testosterone level per se may not have caused an increased probability of winning play fights.

To see how experimental work can distinguish between cause and effect with respect to hormones and play fighting, let us examine the work of Serge Pellis and his colleagues on play fighting and testosterone in rats (Pellis et al., 1992a; Pellis, 2002). Play fighting in rodents typically involves attack and defense of the nape area around the neck, and males engage in this sort of activity significantly more often than do females. Early work suggested that sex differences in play fighting were related to testosterone levels, as males that were castrated at birth reduced their play fighting to levels typically seen in juvenile females, and young females whose levels of testosterone were experimentally increased were involved in more play fights (Beatty et al., 1981; Olioff and Stewart, 1978).

Pellis and his team injected neonatal male rats with either testosterone propionate (TP) or an oil substance (as a control) (Pellis et al., 1992a). This enabled them to experimentally examine the effect of testosterone levels on play fighting. The researchers compared play fighting of TP- and oil-treated rats between days thirty and thirty-six, and subsequent to that, they observed true fighting when the males reached adulthood. Pellis and his team found that the rate of initiating playful attacks was significantly greater for TP-treated rats.

Evelyn Field, Pellis, and their colleagues next examined whether it was the presence of testosterone or the transformation of testosterone into other substances that affected play fighting in rats. To do this, they worked with a unique strain of rats, called the *tfm* strain (Field et al., 2006). Male *tfm* rats have testes that secrete normal levels of testosterone, but they lack the testosterone receptor gene and their appearance is feminized (Purvis et al., 1977; Yarbrough et al., 1990). Because they lack the testosterone receptor gene, the typical process in which some testosterone is transformed into estrogen by the aromatase enzyme in the liver does not occur in male *tfm* rats (McCarthy, 1994; Olesen et al., 2005; Olsen and Whalen, 1982). Pellis and his team reasoned that work with *tfm* males would allow them to determine whether it was the presence of testosterone or the transformation of testosterone into estrogen that was most important in the development of male play fighting. Their results suggest that both the production of testosterone and its transformation (technically called aromatization) to estrogen are important in the development of play fighting in males, with some components of play fighting being more tightly tied to the former, and other components being linked more closely to the latter (Field et al., 2006).

Ethologists have also examined the neurobiology and neurochemistry of play. Broadly speaking, neuroethologists use one of two techniques to study play behavior. In the first, neurotransmitters are targeted to examine their role in play (inhibition, stimulation, and so on), and in the second, the actual neural pathways involved with a particular form of play are targeted, either by making surgical lesions or by some pharmacological means that "lights up" a neural pathway. Both of these techniques have proved useful in studying the biochemistry of play fighting in rats (Siviy, 1998).

With respect to examining neurotransmitters and their role in social play, researchers often systemically administer a compound that either blocks or enhances a particular neurotransmitter. If they do this with enough neurotransmitters, a broad picture of the neurochemistry of play emerges. For example, three neurotransmitter systems—those involved with dopamine, norepinephrine, and serotonin—seem to be involved in rat play fighting. Dopamine inhibitors typically reduce play (Beatty et al., 1984; Holloway and Thor, 1985; Niesink and Van Ree, 1989). Rather than looking at dopamine in terms of increasing or decreasing play activities, however, a number of researchers have argued that dopamine's most important function may be to invigorate or "prime" an animal to prepare for play (Blackburn et al., 1992; Salamone, 1994; Siviy, 1998).

Rats can be trained to anticipate play, and hence it is possible to directly examine whether anticipation of play is concurrent with any changes in dopamine levels (Humphreys and Einon, 1981; Normansell and Panksepp, 1990). Stephen Siviy constructed an experimental apparatus that consisted of two chambers connected by a tube, and he counted the number of times that rats crossed the tube each day (Siviy, 1998; Figure 15.16). Two groups of rats were tested. Those in the "play group" were allowed to play with another rat in the experimental apparatus for five minutes each day. Those in the control group had five minutes in the apparatus, but no other individual was present, and hence no social play occurred. Rats in the play treatment crossed back and forth in the tube *before*

FIGURE 15.16. Rat city. This experimental apparatus served as a "play city" for Siviy's work on rats, play, and neurotransmitters. *(Photo credit: Steven Siviy)*

their partner was placed in the experimental apparatus much more than did rats in the control condition at the same point in time.

One interpretation of the Siviy experiment is that rats in the play treatment anticipated the opportunity for play and searched it out, hence the increased number of crossings. To further examine this possibility, half the rats were given a dopamine inhibitor drug. These rats reduced their tunnel crossings significantly, but their play behavior, once a partner was present, remained level, providing support for the notion that dopamine acts to increase the anticipation of play (Figure 15.17). Dopamine may also be involved in the increase in the "chirping" sound that is often heard during rat play but not at other times (Panksepp, 2005; Panksepp and Burgdorf, 2003). By neurochemically stimulating dopamine receptors in the rat brain, researchers have increased the rate of chirping, and behavioral geneticists have even bred strains of rats that chirp excessively during play (Burgdorf et al., 2005).

A second general question addressed in the neurobiological literature on play fighting in rats is: What neural pathway(s) underlie play? One technique used in searching for neural pathways is lesioning various areas of the brain and testing for the effect of such a lesion on play. While this technique has had some limited success (Panksepp et al., 1984; Pellis et al., 1992b, 1993; Siviy, 1998; Siviy and Panksepp, 1985, 1987), more recent work suggests that modern biochemical tools may provide an even greater window into the neurobiology of play, enabling us to identify areas of the brain that are involved as well as the genes that are active and the changes that are occurring in the neurons. For example, early work had shown that lesions to the parafascicular area (PFA) of a rat's brain reduces play fighting (Siviy and Panksepp, 1985, 1987). Siviy followed up this work using biochemical and immunohistological tools to better understand whether a neural pathway underlying play could be identified in the PFA (Siviy, 1998). He hypothesized that if the PFA was critical to play behavior, then cells in this portion of the rat brain should be very active during play. This activity can be measured by quantifying the amount of a protein product (associated with the *c-fos* gene) that is found in the PFA.

Siviy found that rats that had just been involved in play (and then were sacrificed for brain extraction) had much higher neural activity in the PFA than did control rats. Somewhat surprisingly, however, this increased neural activity was not limited to the PFA, but rather it was found in other areas of the brain (in the cortex and hypothalamus) as well. As such, play seemed to require the use of much of a rat's brain, not just its PFA.

FIGURE 15.17. Anticipating play. Mean number of tunnel crossings in Siviy's rats. Rats in the "play" treatment were given a five-minute opportunity to play with a same-age partner in a "play city" right before the test. Control animals had no such opportunity. *(Based on Siviy, 1998, p. 229)*

The neurobiological approach to play outlined above has some implications for understanding the evolution of social play. Siviy raises two interesting hypotheses for the functions of play that emerge from the neurobiological work that he and many others have undertaken (Siviy, 1998). First, play may serve as a mechanism for coping with stress throughout development. This hypothesis is generated from the finding that the same neurochemicals that are involved in play behavior (dopamine, norepinephrine, and serotonin) are also critical in animal stress responses (Goldstein et al., 1996). Second, the neural circuit work described earlier supports the hypothesis that play may facilitate learning and creativity (Piaget, 1951). That is, while the lack of a precise neural circuit for play may frustrate some researchers, since learning and creativity appear to be driven by general brain activity levels, this finding suggests a large potential benefit associated with play. In fact, it turns out that the transcription of the *c-fos* gene that Siviy studied appears to be an important component of the molecular machinery associated with learning (Kaczmarek, 1993; Morgan and Curran, 1991; Siviy, 1998).

BASIS OF SEXUAL PLAY IN YOUNG BELDING'S GROUND SQUIRRELS

In natural populations of Belding's ground squirrels (*Spermophilus beldingi*), males initiate much more sexual play than do females, but no differences in play behavior are evident across the sexes with respect to play fighting (Figure 15.18). Sexual play in this species involves young assuming the positions and behaviors associated with copulation.

In order to better understand the proximate basis for this difference in sexual play, Scott Nunes and his colleagues treated one group of newborn females with testosterone (in an oil capsule) and a second control group with a capsule that contained only water (Nunes et al., 1999). In both treatments, total play behavior was highest near weaning and gradually decreased during postweaning time. Females in the testosterone treatment displayed a significantly increased frequency of sexual play behavior. In fact, testosterone-treated females displayed sexual behavior at almost the level displayed by same-age males.

In addition to examining proximate underpinnings to play via hormonal manipulation, Nunes and his team manipulated the food available to young squirrels to test whether what they had eaten affected their play behavior. In a "provisioned" treatment, pregnant females and their newborns had their diets supplemented with a high-fat/high-energy nutrient (peanut butter), while controls received no such supplement. The provisioning treatment had a significant effect on juvenile play behavior. In the provisioned groups, rates of play increased, while no change in play was uncovered in the nonprovisioned groups (Figure 15.19).

FIGURE 15.18. Squirrel play. Belding's ground squirrels exhibit social play. Social play often resembles adult copulation and fighting. *(Photo credit: Scott Nunes)*

A Phylogenetic Approach to Play

As is the case whenever possible, ethologists wish to understand the role that phylogeny plays in the expression of a given behavior in animals. To even undertake a phylogenetic analysis of behavior, the behavior in question must

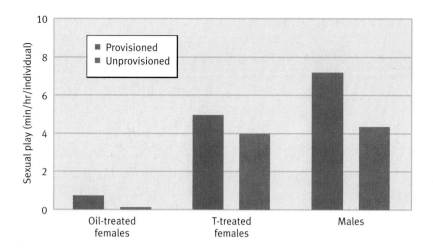

FIGURE 15.19. Testosterone, play, and food. In juvenile Belding's ground squirrels, males typically display much higher levels of sexual play than do females. Females in the testosterone treatment (T-treated females) increase sexual play. For both young males and females, provisioning (supplementing the diet with a high-fat/high-energy nutrient) increased rates of sexual play. *(Based on Nunes et al., 1999)*

have been the subject of investigation in many closely related species. Social play behavior in rodents meets that criteria.

Social play has been investigated in detail in muroid rodents. Within this family of rodents—a family whose phylogeny is well established—a wide range in the complexity of play has been observed (Jansa and Weksler, 2004; Pellis and Iwaniuk, 1999). Serge Pellis and Andrew Iwaniuk examined this range of complexity in a phylogenetic context and tested whether species with relatively complex play share a common ancestor(s), and whether species with simpler play repertoires share a different common ancestor that displayed simpler forms of play. In other words, is the variation we see today the result of a few ancestral forms of rodents differing in their play complexity and passing such differences down to the species that evolved from them?

To begin their analysis, Pellis and Iwaniuk developed a composite score for play "complexity" for each of the thirteen muroid rodent species they examined. These composite scores were based on seven different measurements of play seen in rodents—where higher scores indicate greater play complexity. Values for this complexity measure varied from 0 in *Pseudomys shortridgei* to 0.94 in *Rattus norvegicus*. Using a phylogenetic analysis program, the researchers tested whether similarities in complexity scores could be a function of phylogeny in the sense that complexity scores mapped well onto the phylogenetic relationship between the species they studied (Maddison and Maddison, 1992; Pellis and Iwaniuk, 1999). None of the aspects of play fighting that were examined could be explained by phylogenetic relationships, in that closely related species of rodents were no more likely to share similar play complexity scores than were species that were much more distantly related.

Pellis and Iwaniuk hypothesized that the ancestral state of play in muroids was moderately complex. From this state of moderate complexity, species independently evolved either more complex or less complex play-fighting repertoires. This hypothesis remains to be tested, but if it is correct, it will re-shape the way play evolution is conceptualized. Now, not only must we explain what selection forces acted to make play more complex, but how natural selection can favor less complex play as well. Pellis and Iwaniuk's hypothesis forces us to test whether both complex and simple play are adaptive in their own right.

While play behavior remains an under-explored area in ethology, recent work has helped us to better understand object, locomotor, and social play

INTERVIEW WITH

Dr. Bernd Heinrich

Were you ever worried that people wouldn't take the idea of play in ravens seriously? Was that part of the reason you documented the phenomenon so meticulously?

I suppose most people do not associate play with birds. For the most part, they think of play as a human activity, or an activity of one of the higher mammals. But I can't say I was worried about what anyone might think. I was interested in ravens, and play seemed like a very important aspect of their lives that gave me a window to see them and understand them better.

Isn't play a waste of an animal's time?

Play is traditionally defined by the fact that it does not have an immediate visible payback. The emphasis here is on immediate and visible. For example, young ravens play with (peck, manipulate) all sorts of objects that are new to them. Anyone watching only that would conclude this activity is a waste of time, unless they realized that the birds thereby get to sample and hence learn about almost all available potential food items in whatever environment they might live. By approaching predators cautiously, and jumping back and advancing again, they learn almost precisely what they can risk in a later feeding situation when scrounging food from the same predator. So play is no waste of time at all. In proximate terms it is fun. In ultimate terms it is investing in the future, especially an uncertain one

requiring flexibility of response that can't be predetermined.

What does an investigator have to see before he can feel comfortable calling an activity play?

I don't feel totally comfortable calling any activity play, any more than I feel totally comfortable characterizing any activity as demonstrating intelligence. There are so many gradations and angles. I think that the more precisely we try to define "it," the less we may see, because play like intelligence is an emergent property that is likely revealed as something "extra" above its components. It's a little bit like the analogy of putting an elephant under the microscope to try to see it more precisely. Play includes and grades into all sorts of activities with no discrete boundaries. Take just one activity—bathing. The ravens

that I study bathe obsessively in the first few months of their lives after they leave the nest. They jump into water whenever they get the chance, vocalize with many comfort sounds, and thrash till they are soaked, come out, preen and dry off, and do "it" again and again. This is long before, and greatly in excess of, any potentially useful function such as cleaning themselves; for example, dirtying the feathers does not affect the bathing frequency. As the birds get older they bathe more infrequently (but show no apparent behaviorally better or more practiced response), but even if they did they probably still do it because it is an enjoyable experience for them. However, watching them bathe then, one is not likely to mistake it for the "pure" play of the youngsters anymore. Play is supposedly practice for future benefits, but even in the young a few days out of the nest the activity already seems "perfect." Nevertheless, I doubt that anyone watching the young would not agree that their activity in a washbasin is not the purest of fun. I have no hesitation calling it playful. Is it play? I'm not sure. Nor am I sure that it matters.

What's the most unexpected thing you've learned from your work on play in ravens?

I think the most unexpected thing I learned was that the raven's attraction to shiny things, such as coins or rings, etc., has less to do with conspicuousness but more with variety. These items are rare to them, and hence when we see the birds play with them it is because they have not yet learned that they are useless.

Do you think play exists outside birds, mammals, and the occasional reptile?

I could envision play only being important for long-lived animals who may experience a diversity of situations. If they are short-lived and/or face a constantly uniform environment, then specific programming would be better. Thus, I do not expect play in insects.

How important is it to study play behavior in the field versus in the laboratory?

If it doesn't occur in the laboratory, then that does not mean it does not exist in the field. So I'd start with the field. However, some details are best observed under controlled conditions. That is, both field and lab have unique deficiencies, and both also have unique possibilities. It depends on what one wants to find out, but generally one complements the other.

Is it possible to experimentally examine whether animals enjoy playing?

No. First, what do we mean by "enjoy"? When we run a marathon, we could equally well say it is an extremely painful experience, or a very satisfying one. We could stick electrodes in the pain and pleasure center and add up discharges and define play by a number. Even if we could for one species, we could not transfer that equation to another.

> So play is no waste of time at all. In proximate terms it is fun. In ultimate terms it is investing in the future, especially an uncertain one requiring flexibility of response that can't be predetermined.

I personally think we can't avoid some subjectivity, and I doubt that our understanding of animals is greatly reduced because of it.

Do you think our constantly improving understanding of the brain will send play researchers down new paths?

Unfortunately I'm not well-informed on the frontiers of brain research. Of course, we are all aware that through medical research we've now identified brain regions in humans (and possibly other mammals) that are associated with sensation, emotions, sensory and motor processing, etc. It is conceivable that by NMI or some other method we can detect the location of neural activity associated with unambiguous play, and then see if we can also detect the same activity in the same area during some other activity that we also perceive as play. But, even if we might find a correlation, we would still be no closer to knowing what it *is*.

Dr. Bernd Heinrich is a professor at the University of Vermont. His long-term work on raven behavior, as discussed in his book Mind of the Raven *(HarperCollins, 1999), is a wonderful example of how to test hypotheses on everything from foraging to cognition in the wild.*

from both proximate and ultimate perspectives. A combination of work on costs, benefits, and functions of different kinds of play has elucidated the way that natural selection has acted on play behavior, while phylogenetic analyses are shedding light on the role of common descent in shaping play. Work from developmental biology and neurobiology—particularly the neurobiology of brain areas associated with complex cognition—is also beginning to help ethologists better understand the proximate underpinnings of play behavior.

SUMMARY

1. The most widely accepted definition of play is "all motor activity performed postnatally that appears to be purposeless, in which motor patterns from other contexts may often be used in modified forms and altered temporal sequencing. If the activity is directed toward another living being, it is called social play." Yet this definition is not without its problems, including determining when a behavior is purposeless.

2. Ethologists studying play behavior generally speak of three different types of play: object, locomotor, and social play.

3. From a functional perspective, object play in young animals tends to be associated with some aspect of "practice" that will benefit the animal either in the short or long term and is tied to learning.

4. One hypothesis for the function of locomotor play in animals and humans is that it provides both general exercise and trains specific motor skills needed later in life.

5. With respect to social play, three functional hypotheses are: forging long-lasting social bonds; sharpening physical skills, such as those relating to fighting, hunting, and mating; and aiding in the development of cognitive skills.

6. Spinka and his colleagues have hypothesized that play allows animals to develop the physical and psychological skills to handle unexpected events in which they experience a loss of control. From this, they generate twenty-four specific predictions regarding animal and human play.

7. Neuroethologists often use two techniques to study play behavior. In the first, certain neurotransmitters are targeted and either inhibited or stimulated to examine their role in play. In the second, the actual neural pathways involved with a particular form of play are targeted and studied making surgical lesions or using some pharmacological means to "light up" a neural pathway to determine what brain areas are affected, what gene products are involved, and what changes are occurring in neurons.

8. Play has been studied extensively across many species of rodents. With such data available, a phylogenetic analysis of play is possible.

DISCUSSION QUESTIONS

1. Based on what you have learned in this chapter, try to construct a definition of play. After you have done so, answer the following questions: Does your definition cover all cases of play? Does it cover behaviors that you don't consider to be play?

2. In the interview, Bernd Heinrich argues that we can never know whether play is enjoyable to nonhumans. Can you construct an argument that it is, at least in principle, possible to know the answer to this question? If so, what would your argument be? If not, can you give other reasons besides those covered by Heinrich that explain why you believe we can't know whether animals enjoy play?

3. Recall from the start of the chapter Gordon Burghardt's work with play in turtles. How could this sort of study help in the design of animal habitats in zoos?

4. Think about play in young children. Does reading a book for pleasure count as play? Does watching a movie or television show or playing a video game count as play? If they are considered play, how might these activities fit into Spinka's hypotheses about play?

5. Some researchers have suggested that play facilitates "creativity." After constructing your own definition of creativity, how would you test this hypothesis? Can you construct tests that measure both the behavioral and neurobiological/endocrinological correlates of play as they relate to creativity?

SUGGESTED READING

Bekoff, M., & Byers, J. (Eds.) (1998). *Animal play: Evolutionary, comparative and ecological perspectives*. Cambridge: Cambridge University Press. An excellent overview of the ecology and evolution of play.

Burghardt, G. (2005). *The genesis of animal play: Testing the limits*. Cambridge, MA: MIT Press. The most current book on ethology and play.

Heinrich, B. (1999). *Mind of the raven*. New York: HarperCollins. A beautifully written account of the complexities of raven life, including a nice section on raven play.

Pellegrini, A. D., Dupuis, D., & Smith, P. K. (2007). Play in evolution and development. *Developmental Review, 27*, 261–276. An up-to-date review on various aspects of the ontogeny of play.

Spinka, M., Newberry, R., & Bekoff, M. (2001). Mammalian play: Training for the unexpected. *Quarterly Review of Biology, 76*, 141–168. A review that attempts to integrate all aspects of play under one umbrella.

16

Aging and Disease

Compare a sample of dogs from two different breeds. Even if all the dogs you are looking at were born at the same time, what you will almost always find is that animals from the two breeds are not responding to the aging process in the same way. At any given age, one breed will often be more active and will have suffered fewer of the problems associated with aging than the other. Dogs from these different breeds are all the same age, but aging affects the two breeds differently.

While play behavior is often a luxury of youth, disease and physical breakdown are the scourge of later years. In this chapter, we will first cover aging, and then disease. We will begin by examining aging, senescence, and their relation to animal behavior. **Senescence** is defined as an age-specific decline in survival, and it is said to occur when the probability of dying, or reproducing fewer or less-healthy offspring per year increases with increasing age (Promislow, 1991; Figure 16.1). It is possible for an organism to get older and older but never to senesce. For example, it might be that in a population of animals, the probability that an organism survives from year x to year $x + 1$ is always 80 percent. That is, whether we are calculating the chance of a three-year-old organism making it to age four or a twenty-year-old making it to age twenty-one, the odds are four in five. In that case, clearly individuals are *aging*, but they are not senescing.

To get a better idea of how ethologists study senescence, let us briefly examine this subject in red deer (Nussey et al., 2006). One theory of senescence, which we will delve into in more detail later in the chapter, suggests that when individuals invest a great deal of energy in reproduction early in life, rates of senescence should increase (Kirkwood, 1977; Kirkwood and Holliday, 1979; Kirkwood and Rose, 1991). Essentially, the effort expended early in life is paid for later in life by an increased rate of senescence.

Bill at age 20 → 0.95 → Bill at age 21

Bill at age 50 → 0.75 → Bill at age 51

FIGURE 16.1. Aging and senescence. Bill is shown here at four different ages: 20, 21, 50, and 51. If the probability of Bill's surviving from age 20 to 21 (which in this case is shown as 0.95) is greater than the corresponding probability of surviving from age 50 to 51 (shown here as 0.75), then senescence is occurring.

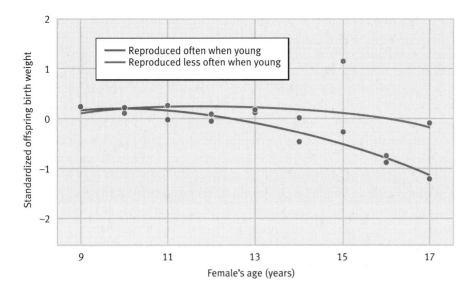

FIGURE 16.2. Senescence in red deer populations. After a female reaches about eight years old, senescence is seen in the lowered birthrate of the calves she produces. Senescence was greater in females that had reproduced often when they were young (green points and regression curve show lower birth weights in their offspring) compared to females that had produced fewer calves when young (orange points and regression curve show heavier birth weights in their offspring). *(From Nussey et al., 2006, p. 1348)*

In a long-term study of red deer on the Scottish island of Rum, Daniel Nussey, Tim Clutton-Brock, and their colleagues tested whether early reproduction led to increased rates of senescence. Nussey's team used two evolutionary measures of senescence, including whether the birth weight of calves—a good indicator of calf survival—decreased with increasing age of the mother, and if so, at what age this started.

Female red deer in the Rum population begin senescing at about eight years of age—that is, before age eight, the weight of the calves a female gives birth to tends to increase each year that the female has offspring. After age eight, the average weight of calves starts to decrease for all females. The key comparison to test the theory that early reproduction leads to increased senescence requires a comparison of the birth weights of the calves of eight-year-old (or older) females that differed in how many offspring they had produced when they were young. As predicted by senescence theory, females that reproduced often when they were young showed the greatest decrease in calf weight over time (Figure 16.2).

In this chapter, we will touch on the following age- and disease-related topics:

▸ Do animals in the wild live long enough to undergo senescence?
▸ What theories have been put forth to explain senescence and aging?
▸ What does the empirical literature reveal about the various theories of senescence and aging?
▸ How do animals respond to disease?

Senescence in the Wild?

As we have seen in earlier chapters, animal life in the wild is often fraught with danger and obstacles. As such, natural historians and ethologists long believed that senescence was rare in nature, since the prevailing wisdom was that animals rarely live long enough to begin senescing. Despite the fact that some observational work suggested that this view may in fact be wrong (Nesse, 1988),

FIGURE 16.3. Senescence and age of maturity. In a sample of twenty-six species of mammals, most do not show signs of senescence until after the age of maturity. Both the x-axis and the y-axis are measured on a log scale. The solid line represents the points at which age of maturity and senescence occur at the same time. Points above the line indicate species that senesce after maturity. *(Based on Promislow, 1991, p. 1874)*

it was not until Daniel Promislow undertook a rigid and systematic approach that ethologists realized that senescence occurred in animals in the wild, and more importantly, recognized some clues that explained patterns of senescence (Promislow, 1991, 2003).

Promislow analyzed detailed demographic data on forty-nine different species of mammals in fifty-six populations to examine whether individuals in natural populations senesce or not (Promislow, 1991). Using various mathematical models that corrected for errors made by prior investigators, he found evidence for senescence in forty-six of the fifty-six populations (in twenty-six of these cases, the mortality rate declined at a statistically significant rate; Figure 16.3). In addition, Promislow found that senescence often did not begin until sexual maturity and accelerated in species in which individuals either produced many litters (as we saw in the case of red deer) or began reproduction at an early age. In a follow-up analysis, Promislow also hypothesized that one reason that females often show slower rates of senescence in many species (including humans) is that male-male competition for access to breeding females is energetically costly, as are male traits that arise to attract females (for example, large antlers in male deer or colorful plumage in male birds). This increases rates of senescence in males as compared to females (Promislow, 2003; Figure 16.4).

Theoretical and Empirical Perspectives on Senescence

In this section, we will review two theories for the evolution of senescence—the antagonistic pleiotropy model and the disposable soma model—and we will examine a few case studies testing these models.

FIGURE 16.4. Mate choice and senescence. A schematic for the many ways that sexual selection in polyandrous species might affect senescence, including sexual conflict, female mate choice, and costs of reproduction. In the path indicated by the green arrows, female mate choice favors the evolution of costly traits in males, which, in turn, leads to higher rates of senescence in males. *(From Promislow, 2003, p. 196)*

FIGURE 16.5. Pleiotropy. Pleiotropy can act in two different ways. Here we have gene 1 acting on two different traits during the ontogeny of an organism, either **(A)** at the same time, or **(B)** at two different times.

THE ANTAGONISTIC PLEIOTROPY MODEL

Developed by George Williams in 1957, the **antagonistic pleiotropy theory** is the most well-known theory of senescence (Williams, 1957). Williams's model is based on a genetic phenomenon known as **pleiotropy**. A gene is pleiotropic when it has more than one effect on an organism; "antagonistic pleiotropy" refers to instances in which the multiple effects of a single gene have opposite (antagonistic) effects on fitness.

Pleiotropic effects can be manifested in at least two very different ways. First, a pleiotropic gene can affect more than one trait at any given time. For example, gene 1 might affect both hunting behavior and mating behavior in adult organisms. Second, the effects of pleiotropic genes can be manifest sequentially. In this case, gene 1 can affect trait 1 at time 1 and trait 2 at time 2 (Figure 16.5). The antagonistic pleiotropic model of senescence focuses on the latter (sequential) effects (Fisher, 1930; Haldane, 1941; Medawar, 1952).

Williams's model begins with the idea that natural selection should act more strongly on traits that manifest themselves early in life, rather than later. The reason is that younger individuals, by definition, have more of their reproductive life ahead of them, and since successful reproduction is the currency of evolution, selection will act more strongly on traits that appear in earlier stages of an individual's reproductive life.

To see how this might work, let's imagine that a gene has two separate effects on an individual, but that both these effects occur at time 1, and that time 1 represents youth. For example, suppose our gene makes individuals bigger and also reduces their visual acuity. Suppose further that being bigger provides individuals with a 10 percent increase in mating success, but reduced visual acuity reduces mating success by 10 percent. In this scenario, selection should be neutral with respect to the gene of interest. Now imagine that a mutation occurs such that our gene still makes younger individuals bigger, but now the negative effects of reduced visual acuity are not manifest until the organism is older. All of a sudden, selection favors our gene, as its positive effects occur early in life, when most reproduction is still to come, while its negative effects are not manifest until an age when much less lies ahead in terms of reproduction (Figure 16.6). Switch the scenario—make the negative effect occur early in life and the positive effect later in life—and selection should eliminate our hypothetical pleiotropic gene. In the context of the antagonistic pleiotropy model, senescence is conceptualized as the accumulation of negative effects of pleiotropic genes in aging animals. Work in the area of animal senescence suggests that genes with such antagonistic effects (with the negative effects occurring later in life) may be quite common (Leroi et al., 2005).

Effect of gene 1 early in life	Effect of gene 1 late in life
+	+
+	−
−	+
−	−

FIGURE 16.6. The effect of timing. If gene 1 has an effect (+ or −) both early and late in life, four possible scenarios exist. The boxed combinations should be favored by natural selection.

FIGURE 16.7. Fruit flies and the *abnormal abdomen* gene. The *abnormal abdomen* gene, expressed here in *Drosophila mercatorum*, increases early reproduction, but it also accelerates senescence and decreases longevity. *(Photo credit: Alan Templeton)*

Michael Rose has suggested that one obvious way to test the antagonistic pleiotropy model of senescence is to look for genes that have positive effects early in life and negative effects later in life (Rose, 1991; Rose et al., 2004). The *abnormal abdomen* gene in fruit flies (*Drosophila mercatorum*) may be just such a pleiotropic gene (Templeton et al., 1985; Figure 16.7). The effect of the *abnormal abdomen* gene is to cause the juvenile cuticle (the outer layer of the exoskeleton) of the fruit fly to remain in place into adulthood. For a number of reasons, including changes in egg-to-adult development time, early ovarian development, as well as early age at first oviposition, the *abnormal abdomen* gene has just the sort of antagonistic effects described in the Williams model—it greatly increases early reproduction in the fruit fly, but it also speeds up senescence and decreases longevity.

DISPOSABLE SOMA THEORY AND LONGEVITY

One aspect of senescence that has long fascinated ethologists, evolutionary biologists, and the general public alike is longevity. We are intensely interested in how long we live, and more generally, in how long all creatures live. Part of this interest stems from a never-ending desire to figure out how to increase our life span. But whatever the reason, this interest has translated into a fair share of work on longevity in both humans and nonhumans. It is important for us to keep in mind that longevity and senescence, though usually strongly related to one another, can interact in complex ways. Consider males and females in some population being studied in nature. Suppose that male age-specific mortality went from 0.01 to 0.02 to 0.04 over three years, while over the same time course, female age-specific mortality went from 0.2 to 0.21 to 0.22. In this example, males are senescing faster, as their age-specific mortality is doubling each year, while female age-specific mortality is increasing at a considerably slower rate. At the same time, however, males are also living lives that are, on average, longer than those of females, as their absolute age-specific mortality is lower than that of females. That is, while it is usually the case that high rates of senescence and decreased longevity will occur together, this example shows that this need not always be true.

One theory that addresses the evolution of longevity is called **disposable soma theory** (Drenos and Kirkwood, 2005; Kirkwood, 1977; Kirkwood and Holliday, 1979; Kirkwood and Rose, 1991). The disposable soma theory suggests that, under some circumstances, it may be beneficial for organisms to divert some energy and resources away from normal maintenance and repair associated with traits that have little connection to reproduction (that is, somatic traits) and instead invest that energy on traits related to reproduction. Decreased longevity is simply the consequence of such a diversion of resources—ignore maintenance and repair, and the body will start to fall apart sooner.

The disposable soma theory and the antagonistic pleiotropy theory are sometimes confused with one another because both focus on fitness effects at two different stages in the life of an organism. But they differ in that the disposable soma theory does not assume that a single gene has multiple effects, as does the antagonistic pleiotropy theory, just that allocation decisions are made with respect to somatic repair and maintenance. Yet, it is important to realize that just because the disposable soma theory does not assume pleiotropic effects, it does not mean that this theory can't accommodate pleiotropic effects. Rather, when the reallocation of resources that is at the heart of the disposable soma theory is due to pleiotropic effects, then the disposable soma theory becomes a subset of the antagonistic pleiotropy theory.

The disposable soma theory predicts that longevity should be generally lower in: (1) species where large investments are made in traits relating to reproduction, and (2) the sex that invests more in reproduction. Let us examine some of the evidence for each of these claims.

DISPOSABLE SOMA THEORY AND HUMAN LONGEVITY. From an evolutionary perspective, there are only two ways to spend one's resources: (1) on reproduction and reproduction-related activities—that is, on traits related to making new copies of genes for the next generation, or (2) on growth and normal body maintenance—that is, on traits related to sustaining what already exists. Given finite resources (food, energy, and so on) the disposable soma theory predicts that, on average, the more an individual reproduces, the shorter its life span. If you have only so much to spend, any resources you use on reproduction are not available for maintenance, and this should lead to a shorter life span (Le Bourg, 2007).

To test the disposable soma theory, John Lycett and his colleagues used demographic information from a historical population of 16,500 families that inhabited the Krummhorn region of Germany between 1720–1870 (Lycett et al., 2000; Figure 16.8). They focused on two fundamental predictions of the disposable soma theory: (1) that married women should have shorter life spans than their unmarried counterparts, and (2) that there should be a negative relationship between fecundity (number of offspring produced) and life span. The first of these tests—married versus unmarried—is a coarse test of the theory in that married women should have more children and hence live shorter lives, while the second is a specific test of the disposable soma theory. In order to gauge the impact of economic class on the predictions of the disposable soma theory, Lycett and his colleagues further divided up their population sample into three economic strata based on land holdings: wealthy farmers, intermediate small landowners, and the poor landless.

FIGURE 16.8. Evolution and human aging. The photograph shows the family of Wiardus Alberts Ohling (1804–1868), a wealthy farmer from the Krummhorn region of Germany. *(Photo credit: Eckart Voland)*

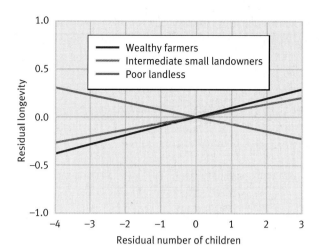

FIGURE 16.9. Longevity and number of children. The relationship between longevity and number of children in three classes of the Krummhorn population. *(Based on Lycett et al., 2000)*

When Lycett and his team analyzed the data, they found no difference in average age at death between married and unmarried women in any economic class, nor could they discern any pattern between fecundity and life span. What's more, it wasn't even the case that wealthy women with fewer children lived any longer than poor women with many children.

Lycett and his group next examined whether other factors may have confounded their analysis and masked evidence for the disposable soma theory. They realized that women who married late might live longer and have fewer children. Thus, duration of marriage per se might be important in the sense that it might have masked the effect predicted from the disposable soma theory.

When duration of marriage was removed from the analysis (using statistical techniques), a very interesting pattern emerged. For the wealthy farmer class, women who had lots of children lived *longer*, for small landowners there was no statistically significant relationship between reproduction and life span, and for those on the lowest rung of the economic ladder, more children did indeed translate into *earlier* death for the mother (Figure 16.9). Lycett and his colleagues interpreted this as partial support for the disposable soma theory in that one might expect the negative relationship between childbearing and longevity to be most pronounced when economic deprivation was greatest. To further support this interpretation, they found that there was a higher cost of reproduction in their study population in the early 1700s, when economic conditions were really severe, than later on, when living conditions improved overall.

Some, but not all, other studies of the disposable soma theory and longevity have also produced partial support for this theory, but further work is needed to get a more comprehensive understanding of the trade-off between reproduction and longevity in our own species (Le Bourg, 2007).

TSETSE FLIES AND LONGEVITY. Tim Clutton-Brock and Peter Langley tested the predictions of the disposable soma theory in a series of laboratory experiments using tsetse flies (*Glossina morsitans morsitans*) (Clutton-Brock and Langley, 1997; Figure 16.10). They began by examining whether just being mated had any impact on a female tsetse fly's life span. In this experiment, females were either mated with a male or remained unmated, and all females were raised in cages separately from males. That is to say, females who mated with males were separated from their mate, as well as from all other males, twenty-four hours

FIGURE 16.10. Tsetse longevity. The life span of this fly depends, in part, on the sex ratio of the group it finds itself in. *(Photo credit: Ann and Rob Simpson)*

FIGURE 16.11. Mated versus unmated females. Over several replications of the experiment (as represented by different lines on the graphs), no significant differences in longevity were found between **(A)** mated and **(B)** unmated tsetse flies when males were absent from the experimental cages. *(Based on Clutton-Brock and Langley, 1997)*

after mating. Somewhat surprisingly, unmated and mated females lived equally long (Figure 16.11). In their second, and more critical experiment, Clutton-Brock and Langley raised males and females together in circular cages. Some cages were very male biased (twenty-five males and five females), other cages were highly biased toward females (twenty-five females and five males), and others spanned the gamut between the extremes (Figure 16.12).

The results were striking. In cages in which females were in the vast minority, female longevity was significantly reduced. Females were constantly courted by so many males so much of the time that it actually shortened their

FIGURE 16.12. Longevity and sex ratios. The experimental protocol in Clutton-Brock and Langley's study was to manipulate sex ratios to examine the effect of courtship on longevity in tsetse flies.

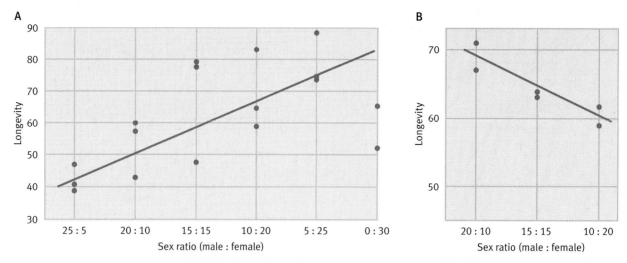

FIGURE 16.13. The effect of sex ratios on longevity in females and males. (A) Female longevity is strongly related to sex ratio. The more biased the sex ratio is toward females, the longer the females live. **(B)** Male longevity is also affected by sex ratio. When sex ratios are skewed toward males, their longevity increases. *(Based on Clutton-Brock and Langley, 1997)*

life spans significantly (Figure 16.13A). On the other hand, when males were in the minority, it was their life spans, and not those of females, that were reduced (Figure 16.13B). In female-biased cages, females were not harassed and could afford to be choosier about the males with whom they mated. The few males present, then, needed to court females vigorously to have any chance of obtaining a mate—so vigorously that it decreased their average life spans from about seventy to sixty days. Merely shifting the sex ratio of the fruit flies changed the costs of courtship and who paid those costs dramatically (Cordts and Partridge, 1996; Partridge and Farquhar, 1981; Partridge and Fowler, 1990; Partridge et al., 1986, 1987).

CROSS-SPECIES TESTS OF THE DISPOSABLE SOMA THEORY. In Chapter 6, we learned that sexual selection is often strongest in the male sex, and this can lead to male-male combat, as well as to the very exaggerated traits (horns, colors, and so on) seen in males. Daniel Promislow used this relationship between reproduction and male traits to test some of the basic predictions of the disposable soma theory (Promislow, 1992). More specifically, he examined the relationship between sexual size dimorphism and mortality in males and females across many species.

Using data on thirty-five natural populations of mammals, Promislow used the difference in size between males and females as a measure for the strength of sexual selection. The idea underlying this assumption is that, when competition between males is strongest, selection based on male size should be greatest, thus producing a big discrepancy between male and female size. Because more resources are needed to reach the large size, the disposable soma theory predicts that this should translate into a greater cost of reproduction in males, and hence a shorter average life span for males than for females (Carranza et al., 2004). Results were clear—when differences between male and female body size were plotted against differences in male and female life expectancy, the result was a strong positive relationship. The greater the difference in size between the sexes, the greater the difference in life expectancy between females and males.

Hormones, Heat-Shock Proteins, and Aging

In this section, we will look at some of the proximate underpinnings of aging. This is a very active field of research—particularly with respect to human aging—and we can only touch on the tip of the iceberg here. To do this, we will focus on the effects of stress hormones and heat-shock proteins on the aging process in animals.

GLUCOCORTICOIDS, STRESS, AND AGING

Glucocorticoids—"stress" hormones—are a family of hormones that are critically important in many of the adaptive responses animals use when placed in stressful situations (for example, being attacked by a predator, aggressive interactions, environmental shock, and so on) (Nelson, 2005). But excessive, prolonged exposure to glucocorticoids can have serious adverse effects on an animal's health, leading to such diseases as diabetes and hypertension (Sapolsky, 1999). In addition, high levels of glucocorticoids are often associated with suppression of the immune system (Munck et al., 1984; Sapolsky, 1996). Robert Sapolsky has argued that many of these symptoms are characteristic of the damage associated with aging, and that, as a consequence, a better understanding of the adverse effects of glucocorticoids will lead to a more thorough understanding of some of the proximate causes of aging (Sapolsky, 1999, 2004, 2005; Sapolsky et al., 1986, 2000; Sorrells and Sapolsky, 2007).

The neurological impact of glucocorticoids on the hippocampus often mimics normal hippocampal deterioration associated with senescence (Sapolsky, 1999; Sapolsky et al., 1986). Studies of the effect of glucocorticoids on hippocampal-dependent learning normally take one of three forms (Sapolsky, 1999). "Replication" studies address whether administering glucocorticoids to younger animals at levels normally found in older animals will cause degeneration of the hippocampus in the younger animals. In contrast, "prevention" studies examine whether creating the glucocorticoid milieu typically associated with that of young individuals can prevent the normal degeneration of hippocampal function in older individuals. Finally, "correlation" studies examine whether prior exposure to glucocorticoids predicts degeneration of the hippocampus in older animals.

In a review of glucocorticoids, stress, aging, and neurobiology, Sapolsky uncovered a number of general patterns emerging from studies on animals (particularly rats) and humans. In particular, Sapolsky reviewed work that demonstrates that exposure to high levels of glucocorticoids may disrupt hippocampal-dependent learning, inhibit nerve growth, increase the probability that neuron repair will fail, and facilitate neuron death. Many of these effects are similar to the way that neuron loss occurs with normal degeneration of the hippocampus with aging, and so studies on stress and glucocorticoids will likely continue to inform research in ethology and animal aging (Finch and Rose, 1995).

HEAT-SHOCK PROTEINS AND AGING

Heat-shock proteins (hsp) may play an important role in understanding the proximate underpinnings of aging and senescence in animals and humans (Feder, 1999; Feder and Hoffmann, 1999; Soti et al., 2003). When environmental factors such as heat stress cause certain proteins to assume a structure that differs from their normal structure, this can have devastating effects, such as the buildup of proteins that are now toxic to cells. The heat-shock proteins are inducible (that is, activated) by heat, and they act as "molecular chaperones" that minimize damage to other proteins facing a particular stress (for example, heat). Molecular chaperones such as the heat-shock proteins bind to such deformed and dangerous proteins and, via a number of different pathways, defuse the danger. Heat-shock proteins are universal, they play a diverse set of roles in response to stress, and they are very similar across many species.

In mammals, a number of studies have found a correlation between senescence and heat-shock proteins. Older rats, for example, are unable to transcribe heat-shock proteins (hsp70) at the same rate as younger rats (Blake et al., 1991; Gutsmann-Conrad et al., 1998; Udelsman et al., 1993). These correlational sorts of studies, however, make arrows of causality impossible to draw. That is, it is not possible to determine whether the process of senescence caused hsp70 to be less effective, whether less effective hsp70 promoted senescence, or whether both processes were acting simultaneously. To better understand the relationship between hsp and senescence, Marc Tatar and his colleagues inserted twelve extra copies of hsp70 genes into one strain of fruit flies. They also had a control line that retained its normal complement of hsp70 genes, but Tatar's team inserted dummy (not functioning) genetic sequences into this line's genome (Tatar et al., 1997). They found that, when heat shock was applied to both groups at four days of age, the group of flies with extra copies of the hsp70 gene had reduced mortality rates over time. Exposure to the heat appears to activate hsp70 genes in a manner that decreases mortality.

Disease and Animal Behavior

Animals tend to be more susceptible to disease as they age, and at least some of the age-specific increase in mortality we discussed earlier is a result of disease. Ethologists' and evolutionary biologists' interest in disease, however, is not limited to the impact of disease on senescence. What makes disease so interesting to researchers in these fields is that, compared to the animals they infect, the microbes that cause disease are both superabundant and reproduce extraordinarily quickly. This means that animals are in a constant struggle with newly evolving, and potentially very dangerous, diseases. In this section, we will examine the behavioral means available to animals in their constant struggle against disease. In particular, we will examine whether animals:

- avoid areas that contain disease-causing agents,
- avoid sick conspecifics,
- self-medicate.

AVOIDANCE OF DISEASE-FILLED HABITATS

Given that virulent diseases can wipe out entire populations of animals, we might expect that natural selection would act strongly on any behavioral trait that helps to minimize an animal's exposure to disease. The two most likely ways this might occur are through (1) the avoidance of areas that contain pathogens, and (2) the avoidance of individuals who are already ill. We will touch on the former here, and return to the latter mechanism in the next section.

One means by which individuals may reduce the risk of infection from parasitic diseases is by producing offspring in areas that have low parasite levels (Kiesecker and Skelly, 2000). Amphibians are particularly good for testing whether such disease behaviors are in play, as they host many parasitic pathogens (Blaustein and Bancroft, 2007; Kiesecker et al., 2001, 2004) and are able distinguish between oviposition sites based on a wide variety of characteristics (Duellman and Trueb, 1994).

Joseph Kiesecker and David Skelly examined whether gray treefrogs (*Hyla versicolor*) base their oviposition decisions on levels of parasite infection by trematode parasites that are known to affect both larval performance and mortality (Kiesecker and Blaustein, 1997, 1999; Kiesecker and Skelly, 2000). The ponds used by *H. versicolor* are also home to the snail *Pseudosuccinea columella*, which is an intermediate host for a trematode parasite. The presence of this snail may serve as a cue to the frogs that an oviposition area is risky in terms of trematode infections (Figure 16.14).

Kiesecker and Skelly addressed two related questions in their study of ethology and disease avoidance in frogs: (1) Do ovipositing frogs distinguish between sites with and without *P. columella* snails, and (2) do frogs respond

A

B

FIGURE 16.14. Oviposition and parasite infection level. (A) The gray treefrog (*Hyla versicolor*) bases choice of oviposition site on parasite infection level. **(B)** A trematode parasite uses the snail *Pseudosuccinea columella* as an intermediate host. Frogs attempt to oviposit in sites with low trematode levels. *(Photo credits: Joseph Kiesecker)*

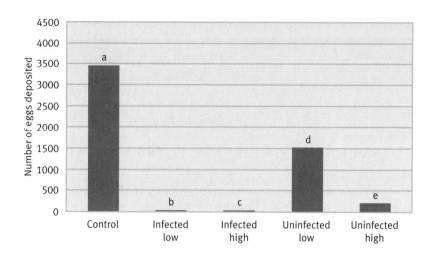

FIGURE 16.15. **Parasites and oviposition sites.** *Hyla versicolor* laid more eggs at control sites (with no snails) (a) than at sites with experimentally low (b) or high (c) levels of parasites. Frogs also preferred sites with low densities of snails (d) rather than high densities of snails (e), even if the snails were uninfected. *(Based on Kiesecker and Skelly, 2000, p. 2941)*

to the density of these snails (Kiesecker and Skelly, 2000)? To address these questions, they set up twenty-five artificial ponds and five treatments: no snails (control), five infected snails, five uninfected snails, ten infected snails, and ten uninfected snails (Figure 16.15). The researchers then assessed oviposition behavior of naturally occurring gray treefrogs. Despite the fact that controls (ponds with no snails) made up only 20 percent of the ponds, 66.1 percent of all eggs deposited by *H. versicolor* were laid in such ponds, demonstrating clearly that gray treefrogs were favoring ponds with no snails. In addition, the frogs also responded to the density treatments, with ponds containing uninfected snails receiving 33.5 percent of the eggs laid, and ponds containing infected snails receiving only 0.4 percent of the eggs laid.

AVOIDANCE OF DISEASED INDIVIDUALS

In Chapter 6, we learned that females in some species prefer to mate with males that have low parasite loads. Outside the context of mating, however, the broader question of whether individuals avoid diseased conspecifics, and how such avoidance is manifested, has been much less widely investigated, despite the fact that natural selection should clearly favor individuals who avoid diseased conspecifics (Brown and Brown, 1992; Dugatkin et al., 1994; Kiesecker et al., 1999).

Kiesecker and his colleagues studied avoidance of diseased conspecifics in the bullfrog, *Rana catesbeina* (Kiesecker et al., 1999; Figure 16.16). In *Rana*, as well as in a number of other amphibian genera, individuals are often infected with the intestinal pathogen *Candida humicola*, which can spread quickly, decrease growth rate, and increase mortality (Beebee, 1995; Beebee and Wong, 1992; Griffiths, 1995). Kiesecker and his team tested whether *R. catesbeina* individuals recognized and avoided infected groupmates, and if so, how they knew that others were infected.

Because tadpoles that are in close proximity to infected individuals are also likely to become infected, Kiesecker and his colleagues examined whether uninfected individuals avoided interactions with infected tadpoles. In order to determine whether tadpoles behaviorally "quarantine" infected individuals, the researchers undertook the sort of choice experiment that we discussed in Chapter 6. A "stimulus" tadpole was placed in each end of a long rectangular

FIGURE 16.16. **Bullfrog quarantine.** Healthy bullfrogs prefer to associate with other individuals that are not infected with intestinal pathogens. *(Photo credit: Ken Lucas/Visuals Unlimited)*

plastic arena behind a mesh partition. One of these stimulus tadpoles was infected with *C. humicola* and the other was not. The researchers placed a "focal" tadpole in the center of this arena, and then they recorded the amount of time that it spent near each of the other tadpoles. Kiesecker and his colleagues found that uninfected focal individuals showed a strong preference to spend time near the uninfected stimulus tadpole (Figure 16.17). In an interesting twist, *infected* individuals did not display a preference for either infected or uninfected individuals. Presumably, once frogs were infected, the choice presented by the researcher had no fitness consequences, and so no preference was uncovered.

Kiesecker's team followed up their initial experiment to better understand how focal individuals were determining whether or not conspecifics were ill. The experimental protocol was identical to their initial experiment, with a few important exceptions. First, based on the results from their initial experiment, they opted to test only uninfected focals. Second, in addition to the choice test they initially ran—a test that allowed for both visual and chemical cues—they now ran a treatment that allowed for only visual or only chemical cues. In addition to replicating the results of their first experiment (that is, avoidance of infected stimulus individuals when both types of cues were available), the researchers found that tadpoles were assessing illness by chemical, not visual cues.

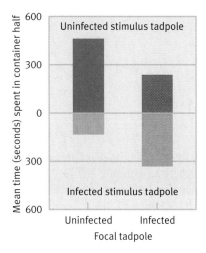

FIGURE 16.17. Infectious association. Infected and uninfected focal animals were given a choice to associate with another infected or uninfected tadpole. Uninfected focal tadpoles preferred to associate with uninfected conspecifics, while infected focals showed no preference. *(Based on Kiesecker et al., 1999)*

SELF-MEDICATION

Intriguing evidence is starting to mount that animals may modify their diet in a way that has the effect of self-medicating (Hart, 2005; Huffman, 1997, 2007; Janzen, 1978; Lozano, 1998; Rodriguez and Wrangham, 1993). Self-medicating behavior falls into one of two broad categories: (1) preventative—that is, behaviors taken to prevent sickness, and (2) therapeutic—that is, behaviors taken to alleviate sickness once an animal is ill (Johns, 1999; Lozano, 1998). Let's briefly examine some instances of animal behavior that *may* represent preventative self-medication.

In some species of birds and mammals, individuals add potentially antibacterial plant substances to their nests (Clark and Mason, 1985, 1988; Dawson, 2004; Hemmes et al., 2002; Lafuma et al., 2001; Thomas and Shutler, 2001; Wimberger, 1984). For example, starlings add fresh herbs, which are rich in potentially antimicrobial chemicals, to their nests. A comparison of nests that had such herbs experimentally added with those that did not found that chicks from the nests with herbs had fewer bacteria, and nestlings fledged at a higher body weight (Gwinner and Berger, 2005). Similar results were found with respect to protection against mites when green herbs were added to the nests of tree swallows. But it is important to note that tree swallows do not normally add herbs to their nests (Shutler and Campbell, 2007).

The consumption of clay, dirt, and rock may also be an example of preventative self-medication (Callahan, 2003; Krishnamani and Mahaney, 2000; Mahaney and Krishnamani, 2003). Although clay contains virtually no nutritional value, the ingestion of clay—technically called geophagy—is common not only in many human societies around the world, but also in many nonhuman species (Krishnamani and Mahaney, 2000). At least thirty-eight different species of primates are known to engage in geophagy. Clay may function to prevent indigestion, may serve as an antidiarrheal mechanism,

FIGURE 16.18. Preventative self-medication with soil. Here a chimpanzee grabs some soil from a termite mound to place in his nest. The soil contains an antibiotic fungus that will keep his nest free from mold. He may also eat the soil (geophagy) to self-medicate. *(Photo credit: Michael Huffman)*

and may absorb dangerous plant compounds (Huffman, 2007; Krishnamani and Mahaney, 2000; Figure 16.18). In fact, all of the clay samples that have been gathered from geophagous populations of both humans and animals have a chemical composition that is very similar to medicines that are sold for gastrointestinal relief (Huffman, 2007).

Two related types of possible self-medication in animals are "anting" and "fur rubbing." Anting has been studied most extensively in birds and involves crushing ants and rubbing them onto feathers (Clunie, 1976; Craig, 1999; Ehrlich et al., 1986; Eisner et al., 2005; Potter, 1970; Figure 16.19). Anting behavior has also been documented in mammals, including squirrels and primates, who apply the crushed ants to their fur (Bagg, 1952; Hauser, 1964; Longino, 1984). Tufted capuchin monkeys (*Cebus apella*), for example, crush carpenter ants (*Camponotus rufipes*) and apply the secretion from the ants—a secretion rich in formic acid—onto their fur. This behavior is used most often during seasons when tick infestations are highest, and it appears to reduce the number of ticks that infest the tufted capuchin monkeys (Verderane et al., 2007). "Fur

A   **B**

FIGURE 16.19. Anting by birds. Birds may actively rub crushed ants through their feathers or passively sit on anthills because the ants secrete formic acid, which may soothe irritated skin or protect the bird from parasites. **(A)** a jay sitting on ants, and **(B)** closeup of a jay's wing, with an ant crawling through the feathers. *(Photo credits: Andrew Cooper/naturepl.com)*

FIGURE 16.20. Fur rubbing in primates. These white-faced capuchins have oranges that they are rubbing against their fur. One possible function of fur rubbing is to reduce parasite infestation. *(Photo credit: Helene Meunier)*

rubbing" in primates is similar to anting, except that, instead of rubbing ants, the primates crush fruits, leaves, and vines, and rub them against their fur (Figure 16.20). The substances produced by fur rubbing have antimicrobial effects, but it is still unclear whether these effects are the primary driving force behind the evolution of fur rubbing or whether the crushed fruits, leaves, and vines serve some other function (Huffman, 2007).

With respect to therapeutic self-medication, it has long been thought that chimpanzees undertake certain forms of leaf swallowing as a means to suppress parasite infection. To test this idea, Richard Wrangham examined the relationship between leaf swallowing and the presence or absence of tapeworms in the guts of chimpanzees (Wrangham, 1995). He found that, during a seven-month period when tapeworm infestation was high (no tapeworms were found outside this time period), chimps showed extremely high levels of leaf swallowing compared to when tapeworms were absent (Figure 16.21). While it is not clear how effective a self-medicating procedure this is, chimps nonetheless appear to modify their diet in ways commensurate with self-medication. Similar sorts of work on self-

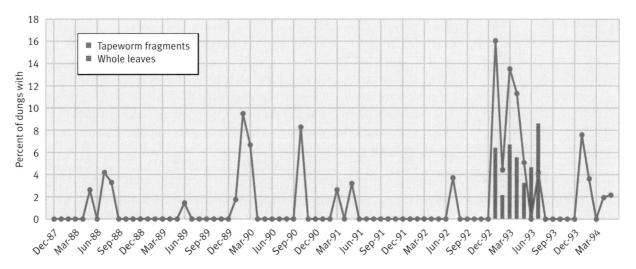

FIGURE 16.21. Tapeworms and chimp self-medication. Chimps increased consumption of whole leaves in concordance with an increase in tapeworm fragments found in their dung. *(Based on Wrangham, 1995)*

FIGURE 16.22. Therapeutic self-medication with leaves. By chewing the bitter pith of *Vernonia amygdalina* plants, this adult male chimpanzee from the Mahale Mountains in Tanzania can suppress parasitic infection. *(Photo credit: Michael Huffman)*

medication have been undertaken in chimpanzees of the Gombe and Mahale chimp populations of Africa, as well as in pygmy chimpanzees (bonobos) (Dupain et al., 2002; Huffman, 1993; Huffman and Wrangham 1994; Krief et al., 2006; Wrangham and Goodall, 1989; Figure 16.22).

Some evidence exists that neighboring groups of primates use the exact same plant species for the sorts of preventative self-medication mentioned above. There are a number of possible explanations for this finding. One possibility is that the preference for using plants as preventative medicine is a heritable trait. A second possibility is that each individual independently assesses which plants work best, and that they converge on a similar decision, both within and between populations. A third possibility is that individuals learn which plants to use in preventative medicine by copying the behavior of others in their group. Moreover, females move from group to group and may spread their plant preferences to members of their new group via cultural transmission. These three possibilities are not mutually exclusive, and one, two, or all three may be occurring simultaneously. Indeed, when Michael Huffman and Satoshi Hirata exposed chimps with no experience to leaves that help expel parasites, two individuals—let's call them A and B—folded up the leaves and ate them on the first encounter. They did so, even though the leaves of the test plant, *Helianthus tuberosus*, were covered with bristles and spines. Another four individuals were initially reluctant to eat the leaves, but did so after watching A and B eat these leaves many times—in all likelihood, this represents a case of social learning in the four animals. Six chimpanzees never ate the leaves at all (Huffman and Hirata, 2004).

Clearly, the study of self-medicating in nonhumans needs more investigation. Nonetheless, since the same plants are often used for medicinal reasons in humans and other primates, ethological work may shed light on the nature of self-medication in early hominids (Huffman, 2007; Lozano, 1998).

WHY SOME LIKE IT HOT

Humans are quite concerned about how their diet affects their health, including the effect of diet on disease and disease prevention. From an evolutionary perspective, studying the effect of diet on disease requires us to imagine how such an effect would have been manifest before modern-day conveniences, such as refrigeration, came into use. How might hunter/gatherers during the time before refrigerators have decided what to eat or not eat to prevent disease? One obvious decision would have been to avoid eating rotting meat—clearly repulsion to smells associated with decaying food would be strongly selected. But are there equally useful, if perhaps more subtle, ways that diet could be used to prevent disease in humans? For example, could spices, which are used in virtually every human culture, be a tool to fight disease?

To address this question, Jennifer Billing and Paul Sherman examined forty-three spices in meat-based cuisines from thirty countries (Billing and Sherman, 1998). Using data from 4,578 recipes, and scouring the literature for studies on the antimicrobial functions of the spices they studied, Billing and Sherman came up with some rather amazing findings. Let's start by taking a look at what does *not* explain the pattern of spice use across the world. The most obvious prediction regarding spice is that people simply eat the spices that are native to their region. Yet, people from areas of greater spice availability do not eat more spices, ruling out that hypothesis. Furthermore, Billing and Sherman

FIGURE 16.23. Spicy temperatures. A strong relationship exists between temperature and **(A)** the proportion of meat recipes calling for one or more spices, **(B)** the mean number of spices per recipe, and **(C)** the total number of spices used in the thirty-four countries that were examined. *(Based on Billing and Sherman, 1998, p. 15)*

ruled out several other alternative hypotheses. It turns out that the patterns of spice use cannot be explained by the nutritional value of spices, the odors they omit (potentially masking nasty smells), or the ability of spices to make people perspire and thus feel more comfortable in hot climates.

What Billing and Sherman did find was that all forty-three spices they examined had some antibacterial properties—that is, each of these spices inhibited the growth of various disease-causing microbes. Billing and Sherman found that, as mean annual temperature increases and food spoilage and bacterial diseases become more likely, the proportion of recipes containing spices increases, as does the number of spices per recipe (Figure 16.23). Similarly, with increasing temperature, the total number of spices used in recipes increases and reliance on the spices with the strongest antibacterial properties increases (Billing and Sherman, 1998; Sherman and Billing, 1999; Sherman and Flaxman, 2001; Sherman and Hash, 2001).

Billing and Sherman go on to show that the exception can sometimes prove the rule. In addition to antimicrobial properties, spices also have the negative effect of slightly increasing mutation rates in those who consume them. For the vast majority of people, the benefits of destroying potentially deadly diseases outweigh the slight increase in mutation rate, but for some groups this might not be the case. Following up some work done by Margie Profet, Billing and Sherman suggest that the costs of spice intake for two groups that are particularly susceptible to the dangers of increased mutation rate—pregnant women and young children—might explain why such individuals often have strong aversions to spices (Profet, 1992; Sherman and Flaxman, 2002).

In this chapter, we have discussed various theories of aging and senescence, including the antagonistic pleiotropy and disposable soma theories, both of which have been tested in animals and humans. We have also looked at the behavioral means by which animals combat disease—behaviors such as avoiding areas where infection is likely, avoiding infected conspecifics, and self-medicating. In the last chapter of the book, we will turn to work on animal personalities.

INTERVIEW WITH

Dr. Richard Wrangham

How did you ever think to test whether chimps ate leaves to fight tapeworm infections? What other sorts of things were you working on when this idea hit you?

The possibility of a relationship between leaf swallowing and tapeworm infestation emerged while my research team was working to habituate two "new" communities of wild chimpanzees in Kibale National Park in Uganda. Since the chimpanzees themselves were still too shy to allow observation, we studied their feeding habitats partly through fecal analysis. Infections by the tapeworm *Bertiella* are very obvious in chimpanzees, because they often lead to a thick white worm-like object being egested in the feces. This worm-like thing is a terminal segment of the tapeworm called a proglottid. *Bertiella* proglottids are remarkable because they are mobile, scattering fertilized eggs as they loop along on the forest floor. So when we found the feces quickly, the proglottid was still present and very obvious—it's up to 2–3 cm long. The evidence of leaf swallowing was equally clear. There's no mistaking it for leaf eating, because instead of finding barely recognizable fragments of chewed leaf, we found entire leaves that had passed through the chimpanzee gut without receiving a single tooth mark. They were always from the same few species of plant, none of which we saw being eaten until a few years later, when the chimpanzees were sufficiently well habituated to allow us to watch them closely at dawn. I soon noticed that

the presence of proglottids was associated with whole leaves in the dung. Having previously suspected that the function of leaf swallowing by chimpanzees in Gombe National Park in Tanzania was to expel worms, I was primed to look for this kind of correlation, of course.

How did it feel watching chimps apparently self-medicate? Were you shocked at what you were seeing?

It was exciting, naturally enough, because nothing like it had been reported before. Why would chimpanzees put all this care into selecting leaves of a particular and rather uncommon species, and then swallow them slowly one by one, despite their rough texture and considerable size? Admittedly, the behavior wasn't completely surprising. In the 1960s, Jane Goodall had found whole leaves of *Aspilia* in chimpanzee feces. But because no one at that time saw chimpanzees swallowing these leaves, none of the observers had paid

any attention to the problem of why the leaves hadn't been chewed, or what they meant to the chimpanzees. It took seeing the swallowing itself to focus my attention.

The puzzle was exacerbated by the peculiar time of day that chimpanzees swallowed their leaves. Normally when chimpanzees leave their night nests, the first thing that they do is to walk directly to a productive fruit tree, where they feed for an hour or more. But on leaf-swallowing days, they would postpone their morning meal. They would walk in the gray dawn to a patch of *Aspilia* and spend 20 minutes or more selecting and picking leaves that were very rough and obviously difficult to swallow. Sometimes they grimaced as they did it, so it seemed to take an effort to swallow the leaves. I found these leaves completely tasteless, unlike everything else they ate. There had to be a good reason for this postponement of feeding and ingestion of an apparently rather unpleasant object, but no ordinary explanations fit. So whatever the explanation was going to be—selection of a rare nutrient, psychoactive drug, or self-medication—it would obviously be fascinating.

How do the chimps know to eat more leaves when they are infected with tapeworms? Do they learn this from watching others?

There's no experimental evidence about how tapeworm infections make chimpanzees feel (and for ethical reasons, I trust there never will be). So we can only guess how chimpanzees learn to swallow leaves when infected. Different populations of chimpanzees swallow different species of leaves, in a pattern that suggests observational learning of the particular tradition of choice. Certainly infants see their mothers swallowing leaves from an early age, and they have a strong tendency to try unusual behaviors for themselves. They are also very interested in their mother's bodies. For instance, they pay strong attention to their mother's fresh wounds. Perhaps the most reasonable possibility is that infants copy their mother's behavior, and eventually learn for themselves that if they are not feeling well, a few swallowed leaves will make them feel better.

Aside from the case of leaf eating, what is the best case of self-medication you know of in nonhumans?

Once again, the most intriguing evidence comes from chimpanzees. In the Mahale Mountains in Tanzania, Michael Huffman has studied why chimpanzees occasionally chew the juicy tips of young stems of a particular shrub, *Vernonia amygdalina*. Like the leaf-swallowing case, this "bitter pith chewing" is odd because the rate of ingestion is slow compared to ordinary feeding. In addition, the *Vernonia* pith is intensely bitter, much more so than any other chimpanzee foods. I once saw a chimpanzee "gag" after chewing *Vernonia* pith. Finally, *Vernonia* pith is selected very rarely. On the basis of a few detailed observations, Huffman has hypothesized that chimpanzees chew *Vernonia* pith only when they have gut infections of pathogenic bacteria, responsible for diarrhea and lethargy. His cases are so striking that my guess is he's right.

If animals do indeed self-medicate, is it possible we can learn something valuable about fighting illness in humans by watching animals?

One of the most exciting possibilities when we first investigated leaf swallowing by chimpanzees was that they might have been selecting leaves that contained drugs that humans could also use. Unfortunately for that idea, there's now good evidence that leaf swallowing works through physical, not chemical, actions.

> One of the most exciting possibilities when we first investigated leaf swallowing by chimpanzees was that they might have been selecting leaves that contained drugs that humans could also use.

Chemical extracts of the leaves have no special toxins, and don't harm parasitic worms. But the leaves are all peculiarly rough-surfaced, and probably remove worms partly by scouring the wall of the small intestine. Other cases of self-medication, however, point clearly to the potential importance of specific chemicals. For example, *Vernonia amygdalina* contains a cocktail of powerful toxins that appear to follow the delicate medical principle of a drug being a poison that's a little worse for the pathogen than for the host. Huffman's team is investigating whether any of the components of *Vernonia amygdalina* pith might have medicinal value for people.

In a similar way, various birds line their nests with leaves. Toxins in the leaves appear to reduce pathogen loads for the chicks. Examples like this could provide ideas for human application.

Do chimps show any sign of using *preventative* medicine—i.e., do they appear to act in ways to reduce the chance of getting ill in the first place?

There's no indication yet of preventative medicine exactly. But like many other frugivores (including monkeys and parrots), chimpanzees regularly eat small amounts of termite-mound clays and other soils. People used to think of this as a way to get rare minerals, but it turns out that the only mineral consistently common in the soils eaten by chimpanzees is iron, which is not in short supply. On the other hand, all of the soil types eaten by chimpanzees have the kaolin-like property of being effective anti-toxins. In Kibale, chimpanzees tend to eat a walnut-sized chunk of soil late in the day, mostly after 3 p.m., around the time when they tend to start eating more leaves and piths. They take the soil off the root mass of a fallen tree, or from sinkholes where they can select below the humus layer. The cationic properties of these soils enable them to absorb toxins such as alkaloids and terpenes. It's still not clear what regulates this form of soil ingestion, but since it happens almost daily, one possibility is that the chimpanzees are systematically dosing themselves against the possibility of a high toxin load while eating vegetable matter in their evening meals.

Dr. Richard Wrangham is a professor at Harvard University. His long-term studies on primates in their natural habitat have reshaped the way ethologists view primate (including human) behavior. Some of this work is described in his immensely readable book Demonic Males *(Mariner Books, 1997), written with Dale Peterson.*

SUMMARY

1. With respect to aging, it is important to separate how long an animal lives from the process of senescence. Senescence is an age-specific decline in survival.

2. Natural historians and ethologists long believed that senescence was rare in nature, since they believed that animals rarely lived long enough to begin senescing. Despite the fact that some observational work suggests that this view may in fact be wrong, very few rigid and systematic tests on senescence in natural populations have been undertaken. Promislow's work involving forty-nine species of mammals suggests that senescence does in fact occur in wild animals.

3. One prominent model for senescence is the "antagonistic pleiotropy" model. Pleiotropic genes are those that have more than one effect on an organism, and antagonistic pleiotropy refers to the case when these effects work in opposite directions with respect to fitness. In the antagonistic pleiotropy model, senescence is conceptualized as the accumulation of negative effects of pleiotropic genes in aging animals.

4. Disposable soma theory suggests that, under some circumstances, it may pay for organisms to divert energy and resources from normal maintenance and repair to traits related to reproduction. Under this theory, decreased longevity is simply the consequence of such a diversion of resources.

5. Work has been done examining glucocorticoids and heat-shock proteins as proximate factors in the process of aging and senescence.

6. With respect to disease and animal behavior, two means by which individuals may reduce the risk of infection from parasitic diseases are: (a) preferentially producing offspring in areas that have low parasite levels, and (b) avoiding parasitized conspecifics.

7. Evidence is starting to mount that animals may modify their diet in a way that has the effect of self-medicating. This may be preventative or therapeutic self-medication.

8. Potential cases involving preventative self-medication in nonhumans include: (a) antibacterial plant substances in bird nests, (b) eating soil, dirt, and rocks as an antidiarrheal mechanism, (c) "anting" behavior in birds and primates, and (d) "fur rubbing" in primates.

DISCUSSION QUESTIONS

1. What is the difference between aging and senescence? Given the definition in the chapter, is it possible that animals may not only fail to senesce, but they may actually have survival probabilities that are the exact opposite of those associated with senescence? What would a chart of survival probabilities look like? Do you think this is likely in nature? Why or why not?

2. What might be an adaptationist's most basic argument against the antagonistic pleiotropy hypothesis? Hint: This hypothesis assumes that pleiotropic effects cannot be broken down.

3. If glucocorticoids are linked to disease, senescence, and aging, why has natural selection significantly reduced the levels of these hormones?

4. If animals, particularly primates, use self-medication, what impact might this have on the relationship between conservation biology and the medical sciences?

5. Imagine you are working with some species of fish in which individuals form associations with other group members when foraging, avoiding predators, and so on. How might you go about constructing laboratory experiments to examine how important avoiding disease conspecifics is when compared to other factors in choosing associates?

SUGGESTED READING

Austad, S. (1997). *Why we age: What science is discovering about the body's journey through life.* New York: Wiley. A popular book on aging in animals and humans.

Huffman, M. (2007). Primate self-medication. In C. Campbell, A. Fuentes, K. MacKinnon, M. Panger, & S. Bearder (Eds.), *Primates in perspective* (pp. 677–690). Oxford: Oxford University Press. A nice review on self-medication in our closest relatives.

Nussey, D. H., Kruuk, L. E. B., Donald, A., Fowlie, M., & Clutton-Brock, T. H. (2006). The rate of senescence in maternal performance increases with early-life fecundity in red deer. *Ecology Letters, 9,* 1342–1350. A recent case study of early lifetime reproduction and senescence.

Rose, M., Matos, M., & Passananti, H. (2004). *Methuselah flies: A case study in the evolution of aging.* Singapore: World Scientific Publishing Company. This book employs classic case studies on flies to understand the evolution of aging.

Sapolsky, R. M. (1998). *Why zebras don't get ulcers: A guide to stress, stress-related diseases and coping.* New York: Freeman. A trade book that ties aging to the idea of stress in wild populations of animals.

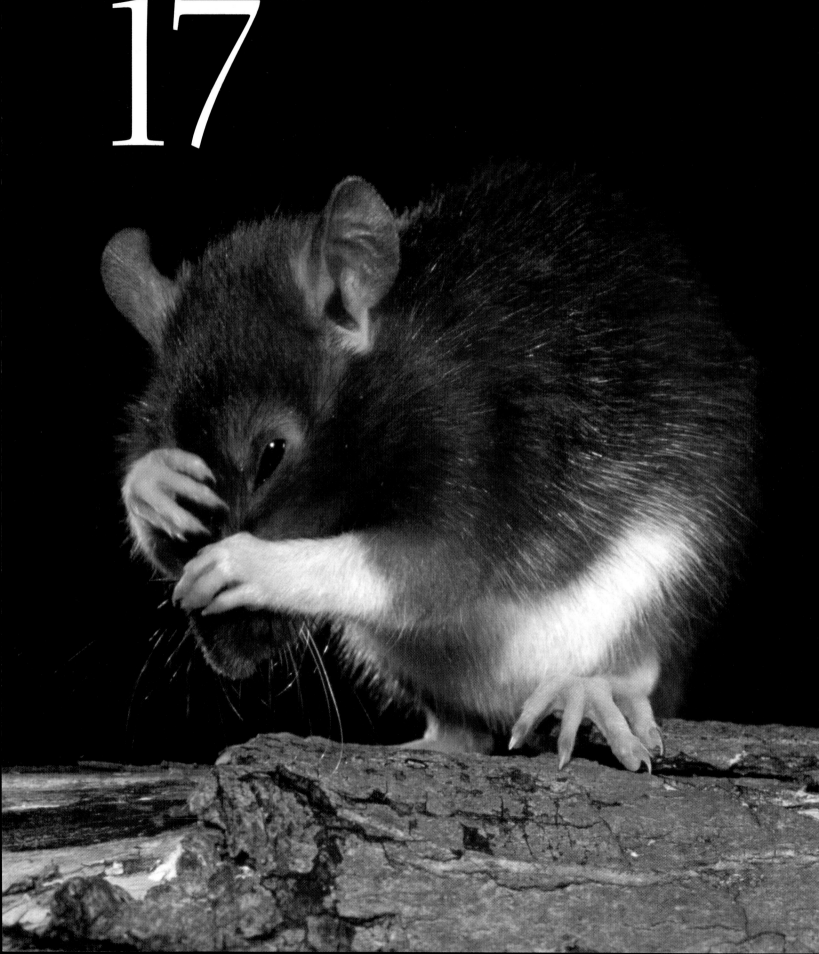

17

Animal Personalities

atch almost any group of animals long enough, and you will start noticing individual differences among group members. For example, some primatologists will tell you that chimpanzees have personalities in the same way that you and I do. Once you get to know a chimp's personality, you can even predict, in a general fashion, how it will act when placed in a new behavioral scenario. For example, take a chimp with an "anxious" personality and place it in a novel environment, and it will act differently than a chimp with a "bold" personality. The same general argument can be made with respect to many animals, most of whom are not nearly as closely related to humans as chimps are. For example, in the sticklebacks that are discussed numerous times throughout this book, we can find what might arguably be called "bold" and "inhibited" personalities. If we test a series of sticklebacks over and over again in the presence of danger, we end up with very distinct behavioral types. Some fish are willing to take risks and inspect the source of this danger, and others aren't.

Although there are certainly instances in which a single behavior is the optimal solution to a problem faced by an animal, oftentimes multiple behavioral solutions to problems co-exist. Animals can be cooperative or uncooperative, aggressive or passive, and so on—that is, a combination of different behaviors can often exist concurrently in a population. Here we will extend this concept even further and consider the possibility that consistent behavioral differences among individuals can amount to "personalities," which are sometimes also referred to as **coping styles**, or alternatively as "behavioral syndromes" or "temperaments" in the ethological literature (Bell, 2007; Dall et al., 2004; Dingemanse and Reale, 2005; Reale et al., 2007; Sih et al., 2004a, 2004b).

We will conceptualize **personality differences** as consistent long-term phenotypic behavioral differences among individuals (Bell, 2007; Caro and Bateson, 1986; Clark and Ehlinger, 1987; Dingemanse and Reale, 2005; Pervin and John, 1997; Schleidt, 1976; Slater, 1981; Stamps, 2007). This definition is close to what most psychologists mean when they speak of personality in humans. In fact, there is a growing psychological literature that relies on animal models to understand personality in the broadest sense, as well as to help cure human personality "disorders" (Gosling, 2001; Henry and Stephens, 1977; Koolhaas et al., 1999; McGuire and Troisi, 1998; Stevens and Price, 1996; Wenegrat, 1984; Zuckerman, 1996).

Our discussion of animal personalities can be cast in a theoretical mold by viewing individual differences in the language of evolutionary game theory (Dall et al., 2004). Recall that game theory models often produce a solution that contains more than one behavioral strategy—for example, hawks and doves, or cooperators and defectors. If individuals adopt strategies for long periods of time, such strategies can be thought of as personality variables. To see how this might work, let's return to the producers and scroungers we first encountered in Chapter 10. When it comes to foraging in groups, animals often adopt one of two very different strategies. Producers search for food, and so they accrue the costs associated with uncovering new food patches. Scroungers, on the other hand, watch producers, and learn where new food patches are by parasitizing the work of producers.

Chris Barnard and Richard Sibly constructed a game theory model of the producer-scrounger scenario that we can use as a model of personality types (producers and scroungers) (Barnard and Sibly, 1981; Figure 17.1). The

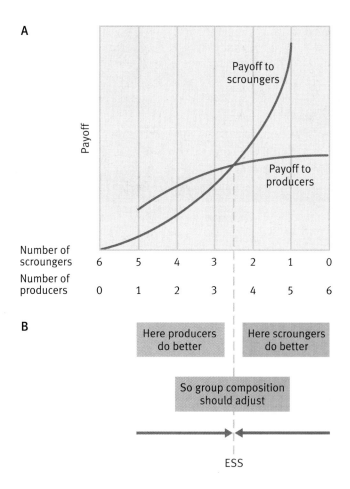

A

Payoff to
scroungers

Payoff

Payoff to
producers

| Number of scroungers | 6 | 5 | 4 | 3 | 2 | 1 | 0 |
| Number of producers | 0 | 1 | 2 | 3 | 4 | 5 | 6 |

B

Here producers
do better

Here scroungers
do better

So group composition
should adjust

ESS

FIGURE 17.1. Producers and scroungers. (A) Hypothetical payoff to producers and scroungers as a function of group composition, and **(B)** the ESS, given the payoffs in A. *(From Barnard and Sibly, 1981)*

solution to this game is some combination of both producers and scroungers, with the equilibrium frequency of each strategy depending on the exact costs and benefits associated with producing and scrounging. As with any game theory model, solutions that contain more than one behavioral strategy can be thought of in at least two ways. Imagine that the equilibrium frequency of producers is 75 percent, and the equilibrium frequency of scroungers is 25 percent. This might translate into each individual in a group using the producer strategy 75 percent of the time and the scrounger strategy the remaining 25 percent of the time. Alternatively, we might see 75 percent of the individuals in a group consistently adopting the producer strategy, and 25 percent of the individuals adopting the scrounger strategy (Figure 17.2). When this is the case—and it often is—the producer-scrounger game can be thought of in terms of predicting personality traits (Giraldeau and Caraco, 2000).

Food producers and scroungers are, of course, only one way in which personality traits manifest themselves in animals and humans. In this chapter, we will examine:

▸ bold and inhibited personality types,
▸ a series of case studies of personality across a wide array of species and ecological conditions,
▸ differences in coping styles,
▸ practical implications of animal personalities.

A

75% of individuals
are producers

25% of individuals
are scroungers

B

75%   25%

Individual produces
75% of the time...

...and scrounges
25% of the time

FIGURE 17.2. Behavioral strategies. Suppose a model predicts an equilibrium of 75 percent producers and 25 percent scroungers. This can occur by either **(A)** having 75 percent of the individuals play producer and 25 percent of the individuals play scrounger, or **(B)** having individuals act as producers 75 percent of the time and as scroungers 25 percent of the time.

Boldness and Shyness

Psychologists have long argued that where an individual falls on the continuum from very shy to very bold behavior is one of the most stable personality variables yet studied. If you are shy when you are young, chances are very good that you will be shy when you get older (Kagan, 1994; Kagan et al., 1987, 1988, 1989). While definitions of shyness and boldness vary considerably, **boldness** usually refers to the tendency to take risks in both familiar and unfamiliar situations, while **shyness** refers to the reluctance to take such risks, or even a reluctance to engage in unfamiliar activity at all. In the language of psychology, shyness is similar to behavioral inhibition, while boldness is similar to "sensation seeking" (Zuckerman, 1979, 1994).

Psychologists often speak of boldness and inhibition as overarching personality traits—individuals who are bold in one context are likely to be bold in other contexts, and likewise for shy individuals. Evolutionarily based ethologists argue, however, that there is no reason that natural selection should necessarily select for boldness or shyness as overarching personality traits. Rather, individuals may be bold in some contexts and shy in others, depending on the costs and benefits associated with the behavioral contexts being examined (Coleman and Wilson, 1998; Rodel et al., 2006; Wilson and McLaughlin, 2007; Wilson and Stevens, 2005; Wilson et al., 1993, 1994). This is the perspective that we will be taking here. Adopting such a view might lead us to think that shyness and boldness are not truly personality traits, as they are not generalizable across different contexts. There is, however, no reason that the context-specific term "bold forager," for example, should not be considered a personality trait, as long as individuals are *consistent* about being bold when foraging.

It is a promising sign that one emerging area of common interest between behavioral ecologists and those in the mental health community is the *evolution* of behaviorally inhibited versus bold personality types (Kagan, 1994; Kagan et al., 1988; Marks, 1987; Marks and Nesse, 1994; McGuire and Troisi, 1998; Nesse and Williams, 1995; Stevens and Price, 1996; Wilson et al., 1994; Zuckerman, 1994). While a great deal of work has been undertaken to examine both inhibition and boldness from psychological, psychiatric, and physiological perspectives, until recently little in the way of controlled experimental work examined the *costs and benefits* of inhibition and boldness (Gerra et al., 1999; Kogan and Wallach, 1964; Koopsman et al., 1995; Moller et al., 1998; Zuckerman, 1979, 1991, 1994, 1996). From an ethological perspective, this omission is striking, as a thorough understanding of the evolution of inhibition and boldness can only be attained through knowledge of the costs and benefits associated with these traits. As such, we will examine two species in which the costs and benefits of boldness and inhibition have been studied in depth.

FIGURE 17.3. Bold and shy fish. Pumpkinseed sunfish have been studied extensively in order to understand the evolution of boldness and shyness. *(Photo credit: Dwight R. Kuhn)*

BOLD AND SHY PUMPKINSEEDS

David Sloan Wilson, Christine Coleman, and their colleagues have studied shyness and boldness in pumpkinseed sunfish (*Lepomis gibbosus*) (Figure 17.3). Wilson and his team used an ingenious trapping method that allowed them to segregate shy and bold fish from natural populations (Wilson et al., 1993). They trapped sunfish from a pond using two techniques (Figure 17.4). The first technique was to place traps in the water. In effect, these underwater traps were meant to mimic the "novel object" test that psychologists use to classify humans along the shy-bold continuum. These traps were designed so that a pumpkinseed fish would have to actively swim into them to be collected, but once a fish was inside, the construction of the trap was such that it was very difficult for the fish to get out. Presumably, this technique would primarily capture bold sunfish, who would be the only ones willing to enter the trap in the first place.

The second technique involved dragging a large net called a seine through the pond. Seining occurred immediately after all underwater traps were collected,

FIGURE 17.4. Experimental set-up to study bold and shy fish. To examine boldness and shyness in pumpkinseed sunfish, David Sloan Wilson and his colleagues used two different experimental techniques. In one, a large seine was dragged through a pond; in the other, underwater traps were used to capture fish.

and it was undertaken in such a manner as to capture every sunfish in the vicinity of the traps. Seining, then, should capture a combination of both inhibited and bold fish, while the trapping method should have captured, on average, bolder fish than the seining method. In addition, the researchers ran an ingenious control in which trapped fish were placed in a seine and run through the pond for thirty seconds (approximately how long it takes to run the seine through a pond). This was done to test whether the seining process itself was more traumatic than the trapping process, and hence might account for any differences found between seined and trapped fish. The results indicate that it was not.

Wilson and his colleagues next examined the diets of trapped and seined fish, their parasite loads, and their growth rates. In addition, they tagged and released fish back into the pond, and then made detailed observations of these marked fish. In one experiment in which both trapped and seined fish were tagged and released back into their pond, behavioral observations indicated that trapped fish were less likely than the seined fish to flee from human observers, as might be expected from bolder fish. Behavioral observations of pumpkinseeds in their natural habitat suggest that the researchers indeed collected different proportions of bold and inhibited fish using the two techniques.

In ponds, trapped fish were more likely to forage away from other fish, and their diet contained three times as many copepods (small crustaceans that are the usual food of pumpkinseeds) as did the diet of seined fish (Ehlinger and Wilson, 1988; Wilson et al., 1996). In addition, trapped and seined fish differed in terms of the parasites they carried, suggesting different habitat use based on personality types. The diet and parasite data in conjunction with the behavioral observations suggest that trapped and seined fish, though caught from the same population, behave quite differently in nature. But trapped and seined fish were not segregating into groups—that is, forming groups of bold fish and groups of shy fish—when swimming in natural aggregations in ponds.

Once seined and trapped fish were brought into the laboratory, Wilson and his colleagues ran a barrage of behavioral and physiological tests on them over the course of approximately three months (Wilson et al., 1993). Wilson's team found no differences between trapped and seined fish with respect to age or sex (close to a 1:1 ratio was found in both groups). They did find that trapped fish acclimated to feeding in the lab more quickly than did seined fish, as might be expected if in fact trapped fish were bolder (Figure 17.5). Wilson and his colleagues ran a series of behavioral and physiological post-acclimation tests of the trapped and seined fish twenty-five days after they were captured. These tests included a "response to handling," a novel object test, aggressive contests between seined and trapped fish, and physiological tests of stress. In no case did the trapped and seined fish differ from each other in any of these experiments.

Exactly how all the variables measured by Wilson's team interact to produce the frequency of shy and bold individuals seen in nature is complex and difficult to pin down. Despite this, Wilson suggests that a true bold/inhibited continuum does exist in pumpkinseeds, both in nature and in the lab, and that where individuals fall along this continuum affects such as differences in diet, safety, and parasite load. That being said, when fish were housed in individual aquaria in the laboratory, the differences between trapped and seined fish disappeared after thirty days of social and ecological isolation. While there are numerous possible explanations for the disappearance of differences across samples over time in the laboratory, Wilson and his colleagues hypothesize that ecologically and socially relevant cues may solidify the differences between bold and inhibited

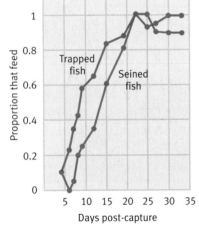

FIGURE 17.5. Feeding and boldness.
Two techniques were used by Wilson and his colleagues to capture pumpkinseed sunfish: trapping, which caught the boldest fish, and seining, which caught a mixture of bold and shy fish. Once brought into the lab, trapped fish acclimated to feeding more quickly than seined fish (this effect disappears with time). *(Based on D. S. Wilson et al., 1993)*

fish and that, in the laboratory, where such cues may be absent, differences in boldness and inhibition may either disappear or become too small to notice.

In a follow-up study, Coleman and Wilson collected and tagged trapped and seined fish in ponds and exposed them to three stimuli in their ponds— a red-tipped stick extended toward the fish, a novel food source, and a new predator (Coleman and Wilson, 1998). For each stimulus, consistent individual differences were found, with some fish bolder than others. The most important result, however, was that fish that were consistently bold when exposed to one stimulus were not necessarily bold when exposed to another stimulus. That is, boldness and inhibition were found to be context-specific, as evolutionary models predict they often will be.

GUPPIES, BOLDNESS, AND PREDATOR INSPECTION

Predator inspection behavior in fish (Chapters 2, 9, and 11) is a good behavioral scenario for measuring the costs and benefits of inhibition and boldness (Brown et al., 2005; Dugatkin and Alfieri, 2003; Fraser et al., 2001). Individual guppies differ in their tendency to inspect a predator, but variability of inspection behavior in a particular individual is relatively low—both inspectors and non-inspectors are consistent in their behavior when predators are present (Dugatkin and Alfieri, 1991b; Dugatkin and Wilson, 2000; Figure 17.6). Because of this consistency, we will speak of guppies that approach predators often and closely as bold, and those that do not as inhibited.

As we learned in our discussion of cooperation and predator inspection in Chapter 9, approaching a predator is dangerous, especially for those who inspect the predator most often and most closely (refer back to Figure 9.6). From an adaptationist perspective, one would hypothesize that there must be some compensating benefits(s) obtained by bold individuals, or natural selection would have culled this trait from the population. Jean-Guy Godin and I uncovered one such benefit in a study of inspection and mate choice (Godin and Dugatkin, 1996). In each trial of this experiment, a pair of males was placed in a large tank. On one side of this tank was another aquarium that served as housing for a pike cichlid predator. In some trials, the predator was present; in other trials,

FIGURE 17.6. Variation in risk taking. Guppies are ranked by their risk-taking scores during predator inspection. Significant differences in boldness exist between individuals, but fish were fairly consistent in their risk-taking tendencies over time. *(Based on Dugatkin and Alfieri, 1991b)*

FIGURE 17.7. Color, boldness, and attractiveness. (A) When observed by females, brightly colored males inspected a predator more often than did drab males. The difference disappears if the predator is removed from his tank. **(B)** The difference between colorful and drab males in terms of boldness exists only when female guppies are observing males. **(C)** When color and boldness are experimentally decoupled in male guppies, females prefer bolder individuals, regardless of color. *(Based on Godin and Dugatkin, 1996)* **(D)** To experimentally decouple boldness and color patterns in guppies, a motorized pulley system was built. Using this system, either colorful or drab males could be made bold by placing them in a small tube that was moved back and forth. The orange arrow indicates that the female preferred the bolder male as a mate. *(Based on Dugatkin and Godin, 1998)*

its tank was empty. In addition, in the large tank containing the male guppies, a clear partition was placed on the side of the aquarium farthest from the predator tank. In some trials, females were placed behind this see-through partition, and in some trials, this section remained empty. We found that more colorful male guppies were more likely to inspect predators (Figure 17.7A), but that differences in inspection behavior between colorful and drab males were manifest only when females were observing—no differences in inspection were found when males could not see females observing them (Figure 17.7B). Females also preferred colorful, bold males as potential mates. When we experimentally uncoupled color from boldness, it was a male's boldness, and not his color, that made him attractive to females (Figures 17.7C and 17.7D).

This study suggests that one benefit to being bold (versus inhibited) is that it makes males attractive as potential mates. Are there any other benefits associated with being a bold fish? To explore this question, my colleague Michael Alfieri and I tested male guppies both in terms of their boldness during inspection and their ability to associate a cue with a particular food source (Dugatkin and Alfieri, 2003). Two treatments were undertaken. In treatment I, males were evaluated as to their boldness first, and then they were given the learning task. In treatment II, the order of testing was reversed. Results suggest that bolder male guppies learn more quickly than do behaviorally inhibited individuals. But for this advantage to appear, bold behaviors must be expressed prior to the learning opportunities. It appears that predator inspection itself either "primes" bold fish to learn better, or it has a negative effect on learning in behaviorally inhibited inspectors. Whether behaviorally inhibited inspectors have higher levels of stress-related hormones after exposure to a predator than do bold individuals, and whether this difference in hormone levels translates into lowered rates of learning, remains an interesting area for future exploration.

Some Case Studies

Compared to most of the subjects we have examined in this book, animal personality is an understudied area of ethology, and there is no standard methodology used across studies. That said, the number of studies on this subject is growing each year, and in this section, we will examine a few case studies to better understand the dynamics of animal personality.

HYENA PERSONALITIES

Spotted hyenas (*Crocuta crocuta*) are native to African savannas and live in stable clans that often engage in cooperative hunting (Figure 17.8). Females hold the alpha (top-ranked) status in groups, dominance is inherited maternally, and the overall dynamics of social life in hyenas are complex (Engh et al., 2000; Frank, 1986a, 1986b; Gosling, 1998; Holekamp and Smale, 1998; Holekamp et al., 1996; Zabel et al., 1992). This complexity set the stage for Sam Gosling's study of personality in the spotted hyena (Gosling, 1998).

Gosling studied thirty-four hyenas to determine whether or not personality could be distilled down to a few variables in this group-living species—that is, he wanted to examine whether hyenas who displayed behavior x were more or less likely to display behaviors y, z, and so forth. As far as animal behavior studies go, Gosling's work on hyenas began in a somewhat unconventional manner. At the start of this work, three experts on hyena behavior were provided with a list of forty-two traits that had been employed in other studies on animal personality, and they were asked which traits they believed would apply to hyenas. Then these experts were provided with a list of forty traits used in human personality

FIGURE 17.8. Hyena personalities. Gosling studied forty-four personality traits in spotted hyenas. A detailed analysis revealed that hyena personalities are most easily understood in terms of assertiveness, excitability, human-directed agreeableness, sociability, and curiosity. *(Photo credit: E. R. Degginger/ Color-Pic, Inc.)*

work, and they were asked which applied to hyenas. Based on the replies of the three experts, Gosling amassed a master list of sixty personality traits. Finally, two other hyena experts were asked to go through this master list and to remove any redundancies (for example, "fearful" and "apprehensive" covered the same trait), and forty-four traits remained after this final culling process.

Four observers then used the traits to score the behavior of thirty-four hyenas. Next, Gosling ran a principle component statistical analysis to determine if certain traits grouped together, and whether such groupings made any sense in terms of hyena personality attributes. Results of this analysis suggest that hyena personalities are most easily understood in terms of five aggregate traits—assertiveness (which incorporated fifteen of the original forty-four traits), excitability (twelve of the original traits), human-directed agreeableness (seven of the original traits), sociability (four of the original traits), and curiosity (six of the original traits) (Table 17.1).

Gosling examined whether any of these aggregate personality traits correlated with an individual's sex, age, or rank in the hierarchy. Neither age nor dominance rank correlated with these aggregate traits. Females were more assertive than males, however, as might be expected in a social system with matriarchal dominance hierarchies.

In order to get a broader picture of what the hyena work meant for personality research in animals, Gosling compared the five aggregate traits that he uncovered in hyenas with major traits found in two studies of rhesus monkeys and in one study of gorillas (Bolig et al., 1992; Gold and Maple, 1994; Stevenson-Hinde et al., 1980; Stevenson-Hinde and Zunz, 1978). Except for "human-directed agreeableness," which was not measured in the primate studies, hyenas and nonhuman primates shared major personality traits, suggesting some cross-species commonalities.

OCTOPUS AND SQUID PERSONALITIES

The vast majority of work on animal personality work has been undertaken in vertebrates. This may reflect an inherent bias in the way we think about the complex nature of personality, but whatever the reason, such a focus leads us to ignore a large portion of the animal world—the invertebrates. Yet, a comparative approach to personality in vertebrates and invertebrates may lead us to new insights on the evolution of personality, and as such, research is now being conducted in this area. For example, Jennifer Mather and Roland Anderson have argued that, because learning plays a fundamental role in their development and because they display an array of complex behaviors, cephalopods, such as octopuses and squids, are ideal subjects for a sortie into personality in invertebrates (Mather, 1995; Mather and Anderson, 1993, 1999).

To obtain a sense of what, if anything, personality might encompass in octopuses, Mather and Anderson tested the response of forty one-year-old *Octopus rubescens* to three different treatments that were labeled alert, threat, and feed (Mather and Anderson, 1993). In the "alert" treatment, an experimenter opened the lid to an octopus tank, and brought her head down to where the octopus could see it. The threat treatment involved using a brush to touch, and presumably frighten, an octopus, and the "food" treatment recorded an octopus's response when a food item (a shore crab) was put into its tank. The nineteen octopus behaviors displayed across these three treatments were

TABLE 17.1. Hyena personality traits. A list of the forty-four variables Gosling used in his study of hyena personality. Trait labels with high absolute values clustered together to form five aggregate personality indices. The clusters can be identified by the groups of boldface numbers in each column. *(Based on Gosling, 1998, p. 110)*

TRAIT LABELS	ASSERTIVENESS	EXCITABILITY	HUMAN-DIRECTED AGREEABLENESS	SOCIABILITY	CURIOSITY
Assertive	**0.95**	−0.08	−0.14	−0.01	−0.01
Argumentative	**0.93**	0.13	−0.10	−0.02	−0.17
Aggressive	**0.90**	0.11	−0.22	0.03	−0.15
Bold	**0.88**	−0.32	0.08	0.11	0.05
Confident	**0.88**	−0.25	0.00	0.01	0.13
Persistent	**0.84**	0.07	−0.03	0.08	0.38
Fearful	**−0.80**	0.34	−0.31	−0.14	−0.08
Jealous	**0.79**	0.41	0.15	0.09	−0.09
Strong	**0.77**	−0.08	0.05	0.21	0.34
Irritable	**0.74**	0.19	−0.39	−0.27	−0.27
Greedy	**0.69**	0.27	0.20	0.00	0.19
Careful	**−0.66**	−0.25	−0.17	0.29	−0.30
Scapegoating	**0.65**	0.25	−0.27	−0.08	−0.23
Opportunistic	**0.62**	−0.06	0.31	0.18	0.52
Friendly	**−0.57**	−0.32	0.41	0.38	0.27
Vigilant	0.05	**0.88**	0.09	0.15	0.07
Excitable	0.34	**0.87**	−0.09	0.03	0.08
High strung	−0.23	**0.84**	−0.27	−0.23	0.08
Slow	0.06	**−0.82**	0.24	−0.01	−0.17
Calm	−0.01	**−0.82**	0.06	0.36	0.20
Active	0.03	**0.81**	−0.21	0.10	0.28
Lazy	0.00	**−0.75**	0.25	−0.18	−0.30
Vocal	0.16	**0.73**	0.46	0.09	0.13
Nervous	−0.44	**0.71**	−0.34	−0.15	−0.06
Moody	0.27	**0.67**	−0.41	−0.17	−0.25
Nurturant	0.01	**−0.52**	0.11	0.23	0.50
Eccentric	0.15	**0.50**	0.45	0.24	0.17
Testing	0.22	0.21	**−0.83**	−0.01	0.11
Social	0.04	0.01	**0.81**	0.47	0.04
Tame	−0.12	−0.37	**0.78**	0.22	−0.10
Warm	−0.08	−0.11	**0.75**	0.50	0.05
Obedient	0.26	0.08	**0.75**	−0.12	0.40
Deceitful	0.18	0.36	**−0.69**	−0.18	0.00
Flexible	0.28	−0.20	**0.68**	−0.02	0.44
Warm	−0.08	0.09	0.16	**0.86**	0.15
Affiliative	0.15	0.16	0.19	**0.86**	0.03
Sociable	0.18	−0.10	−0.04	**0.85**	0.20
Cold	0.14	0.10	−0.45	**−0.79**	−0.06
Exploratory	0.09	0.23	0.17	0.00	**0.79**
Impulsive	0.13	0.31	−0.29	0.06	**0.73**
Curious	0.07	0.22	0.44	0.02	**0.61**
Imaginative	0.00	−0.13	0.29	0.34	**0.52**
Playful	−0.13	0.12	−0.08	0.14	**0.51**
Intelligent	0.22	−0.19	0.35	0.32	**0.37**

TABLE 17.2. Octopus personality traits. Three "factors" (or dimensions) incorporate the personality variables used in Mather and Anderson's work on personality in *Octopus rubescens*. *(Based on Mather and Anderson, 1993)*

DIMENSION	PREDICTOR BEHAVIOR
Factor 1: Activity (active/inactive)	In den[a]
	At rest[a]
	Grasp[b]
Factor 2: Reactivity (anxious/calm)	Squirt[b]
	Shrink[b]
	Swim[b]
	Crawl[b]
Factor 3: Avoidance (bold/inhibited)	In den[b]
	In den[c]
	Color change[a]
	Ink[b]
	Alert[c]

[a]Alerting test. [b]Threat test. [c]Feeding test.

subject to a principle component statistical analysis, and three "components" of octopus personality emerged—active versus inactive, anxious versus calm, and bold versus inhibited (Table 17.2). Individual octopuses were very consistent with respect to these three personality traits, and these traits accounted for 45 percent of all the behavioral variance uncovered in the experimental treatments (Mather, 1991; Mather and Anderson, 1993; Figure 17.9).

It is interesting to note that the three components underlying octopus personality are quite similar to those documented in human infant development, as

FIGURE 17.9. Octopus personalities. Studies on personality in the red octopus *(Octopus rubescens)* represent some of the only work on invertebrates done in this field. *(Photo credit: Keith Clements/www. emeralddiving.com)*

well as in rhesus monkey personality, providing further support for some cross-species similarities in terms of personality variables (Buss and Plomin, 1986; Stevenson-Hinde et al., 1980).

Personality traits have also been explored in the dumpling squid (*Euprymna tasmanica*). David Sinn and Natalie Moltschaniwskyj examined the behavior of these squid in two different contexts—threat situations and feeding situations (Sinn et al., 2006; Sinn and Moltschaniwskyj, 2005). Each squid was tested four times in each context, and Sinn and Moltschaniwskyj then used principal component statistical analysis to determine whether any consistent personality traits could be detected. As in the red octopus, shy versus bold and active versus inactive emerged as two personality types in the dumpling squid. Personality traits in squid were again context-specific—that is, a squid that was consistently bold in the threat treatment was not any more likely to be bold in the feeding treatment than was a squid that was shy in the threat treatment.

RUFF SATELLITES

Let us return to the alternative male mating strategies of ruff birds (*Philomachus pugnax*), which we discussed in Chapter 2 (Figure 17.10). Here we will reexamine this phenomenon, but in light of personality. Recall that "independent" males form leks and actively guard an area within such a lek from other independent males. "Satellite" males, on the other hand, temporarily share an independent's lek spot (Lank et al., 1999) with that independent male. Independents and satellites differ not only in mating strategy, but in coloration and body mass, with satellites being generally smaller and in possession of lighter plumage (Bachman and Widemo, 1999; Hogan-Warburg, 1966). Alliances between independent and satellite males may be favored by natural selection, as females appear to prefer lek areas that contain both morphs (Hugie and Lank, 1997; Widemo, 1998).

Behavioral and morphological differences between independent and satellite ruffs are stable throughout an individual's life—indeed, in Chapter 2, we learned that such differences may be primarily due to genetic variance at a single locus—and so we will consider independent and satellite as two different types of ruff personality.

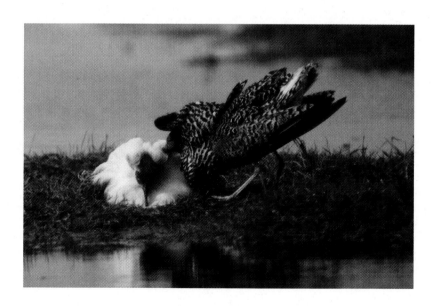

FIGURE 17.10. Two types of ruffs. Two male ruffs of different morphs co-occupying a single display court on a lek. The dark male is an independent territory holder, while the white male is a nonterritorial satellite male. The independent resident male defends the court against other independent males, but satellite males have access to all courts. The independent resident male benefits from having a satellite on his territory because females prefer to visit and mate on co-occupied courts. Nonetheless, independent residents also incur reproductive costs, because visiting females may mate with the satellite instead, or mate with both males. As seen here, the independent male often tries to dominate the satellite by standing with his bill, which is a weapon, over the satellite's head. *(Photo credit: Oene Moedt, courtesy of David Lank)*

The personality differences we discussed above are seen only in males, but prior work has shown that male mating strategy was *not* inherited via the sex chromosome. This might seem counterintuitive—since only males display this polymorphism (satellite versus independent), we might assume that the trait would be linked to the sex chromosome. Yet, this need not be the case if females carry the gene for the trait of interest but simply don't express the phenotype associated with that gene. Genetic analysis has suggested that this is true for ruffs (Lank et al., 1995).

David Lank and his colleagues examined whether there was any way to produce similar phenotypic differences in females, who normally express neither the independent nor satellite personality traits (Lank et al., 1999). If the satellite and independent strategies are not sex-linked, then in principle it should be possible for these personality traits to be expressed in females. Bird systems are particularly good models for these sorts of experiments, as prior work has demonstrated that testosterone implants in female birds can induce phenotypes that are usually only expressed in males (Emlen and Lorenz, 1942; Witschi, 1961). In addition, in ruffs, males that are castrated fail to molt into breeding plumage, further suggesting a critical role for testosterone in the expression of traits normally only expressed in males (van Oordt and Junge, 1936).

Lank and his colleagues examined females with known pedigrees (lines of descent indicating male and female relatives), who had received testosterone implants, to determine whether they could induce the independent and satellite personality types in females (Figure 17.11). The use of females with known pedigrees was particularly helpful, as without such knowledge, researchers could only have ascertained whether male phenotypes could be expressed in females, but not whether a particular female expressed the phenotype that one would expect based on the *genotypes* of males in her family. In other words, with a pedigree analysis, Lank and his colleagues could test not just whether females expressed independent or satellite morphology and behavior, but also whether females expressed the morphology and behavior that might be expected

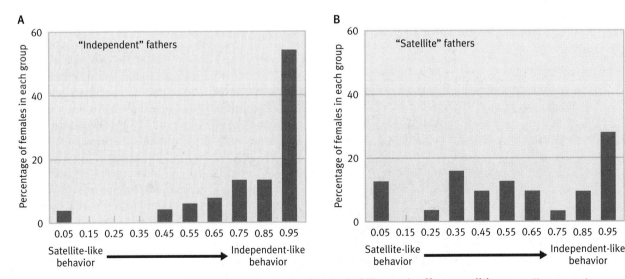

FIGURE 17.11. Hormones, heritability, and ruff personalities. In ruffs, two male phenotypes, independent and satellite, are well established. No such divergence in females is typically found. When females have testosterone experimentally implanted, **(A)** those from "independent" fathers display independent male-like behaviors to a much greater degree than do **(B)** those from "satellite" fathers. *(Based on Lank et al., 1999, p. 2327)*

based on the independent or satellite genotypes of males in their family. They hypothesized that females with male relatives that were independents would be more likely to express the independent strategy after being injected with testosterone than females who had male relatives that were satellites.

Two days after testosterone implants, female ruffs (known as reeves) were displaying typical male behavior, and a week later they were actually forming leks. After three to five weeks, these reeves had grown neck ruffs and male-like display feathers, leaving no doubt about the effects of testosterone on both female behavior and morphology.

Results from the pedigree analysis of the reeves were remarkably similar to those found in Lank's genetic study of male strategies, in which he uncovered two alleles, S and s, associated with the strategy that a male used. S is dominant to s, and so SS and Ss males were satellites, while only ss males were independents. This means that females with independent fathers should express the independent phenotype, while females with satellite fathers should be a mix of satellites and independents. This is, in fact, what Lank and his colleagues found. Females that had independent fathers nearly always displayed the independent personality type. The distribution of personality types from reeves that had satellite fathers was much flatter, with some females displaying satellite behavior, and some displaying much more independent traits. These results strongly suggest that, at least in some cases, the inheritance of differences in personality can be understood using a simple genetic model of dominant and recessive genes.

FIGURE 17.12. **Personality types in great tit birds.** In great tit birds, two personality types, fast and slow, appear to exist. Fast individuals approach novel objects quickly and spend little time with them. Slow individuals approach novel objects more reluctantly, but learn more about such items. *(Photo credit: Roy Glenn/www.Ardea.com)*

NATURAL SELECTION AND PERSONALITY IN GREAT TIT BIRDS

In a long-term study of exploratory behavior and reaction to novel objects in great tits (*Parus major*), Pieter Drent, M. E. Verbeek, and their colleagues have uncovered two very different personality types in juvenile birds (Verbeek et al., 1994; Figure 17.12). "Fast" birds quickly approach novel objects and explore new environments in a rapid manner, spending relatively short periods in any particular area. These birds are also aggressive, and once they develop a food-searching pattern, they are unlikely to change that pattern (Verbeek et al., 1996, 1999). On the other end of the behavioral spectrum, "slow" birds are reluctant to approach novel objects, vary their foraging routine often, display for long periods of time to potentially aggressive conspecifics but are not physically aggressive, and are slow to approach members of the opposite sex (Figure 17.13).

Besides documenting behavioral variation, Christian Both, Drent, and their colleagues have also gathered data on the two other prerequisites for natural selection to operate: fitness differences and heritability. In terms of measuring fitness, these researchers measured the reproductive success of slow and fast birds in a number of different types of environments (Both et al., 2005). Using detailed measurements of marked birds in a natural population of great tits in the Netherlands, they found that reproductive success was greatest when pairs of birds had similar personalities—that is, slow-slow and fast-fast pairings led to production of the healthiest chicks. Other work by Drent, Kees van Oers, Arie van Noordwijk, and Neils Dingemanse has shown that, in addition to having fitness consequences, personality in the great tit is also a heritable trait (Dingemanse et al., 2002; Drent et al., 2002; van Oers et al., 2004a, 2004b).

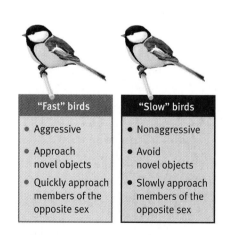

"Fast" birds	"Slow" birds
• Aggressive	• Nonaggressive
• Approach novel objects	• Avoid novel objects
• Quickly approach members of the opposite sex	• Slowly approach members of the opposite sex

FIGURE 17.13. **Fast and slow birds.** An overview of Verbeek's study on "fast" and "slow" great tit birds.

Indeed, a recent review of temperament and personality in nonhumans found evidence for heritability of these traits in twenty species (Reale et al., 2007).

In addition to measuring the three prerequisites for natural selection in the great tit system, Drent's team has also examined personality in the context of learning. For example, slow birds, while taking longer to explore an environment, also spend more time learning about each aspect of a new environment. In order to better understand whether other aspects of tit behavior correlate with fast-slow personality types, Chiara Marchetti and Drent examined whether birds could learn about changes in their foraging environment from watching a "tutor" bird (Marchetti and Drent, 2000). The theoretical backdrop for the protocol they devised was that slow birds might be similar to the producers of the producer-scrounger game (see Chapter 9), while fast birds might map onto the scrounger strategy.

After giving both slow and fast birds the opportunity to see a demonstrator bird forage, they found that although slow birds change feeders often when alone, they do not use the information provided by tutors to help them uncover new food sources (Marchetti and Drent, 2000). Conversely, fast birds, though reluctant to change feeders once they have established a routine of their own, are quick to change their foraging habits when paired with tutors who provide them with information about new food sources. Slow tits behave like producers, while fast birds act more like scroungers.

CHIMPANZEE PERSONALITIES AND CULTURAL TRANSMISSION

In the context of human personality studies, it would not strike anyone as surprising to hear that the society an individual lives in affects his or her personality. In certain limited conditions, this appears to be true for other primates as well. By far the best-documented case of cultural transmission of information affecting animal personality involves seven long-term studies of chimpanzees in Africa, studies that ranged from seven to thirty years in length (Whiten, 2005; Whiten and Boesch, 2001; Whiten et al., 1999, 2005). Senior researchers in these projects constructed a list of sixty-five behaviors that qualified as "cultural variants" that were almost certainly spread by imitation. These variants ranged from using leaves as sponges to picking out bone marrow to displaying at the start of a rainstorm (Figure 17.14). Somewhat remarkably, of these sixty-five behaviors, thirty-nine were present at some sites, but completely absent at others. In addition, this list includes only culturally transmitted behaviors that were, in principle, possible at all sites. For example, since "algae fishing" is not possible when algae are absent, as it is at some chimpanzee sites, algae fishing is not included among these thirty-nine variants.

If you were to visit these seven sites in Africa and watch the chimpanzees for years and years, you would see relatively stable innovative behavior patterns being spread within each group, but across groups you would observe very different suites of behaviors being used. Chimps in different populations use different behaviors to reconcile after fighting, they groom one another in different ways, and they search for food in unique, but different manners. Because we are talking about a long list of behaviors, and since individual behavior is fairly consistent within sites, it seems fair to conclude that the personalities of chimps across these seven African sites are very different, and that such differences are the result of the cultural transmission of behavior.

FIGURE 17.14. Chimpanzee culture. Cultural transmission of behaviors affecting animal personality has been examined in seven long-term studies of chimpanzees in Africa. Variants of similar behaviors are often shown in different populations of chimpanzees. These behaviors include chimpanzees that **(A)** groom while touching their hands above their heads, and **(B)** use leaves as sponges to get water out of tree trunks or out of shallow puddles. *(Photo credits: World Foto/Alamy; Danita Delimont/Alamy)*

It is admittedly frustrating that it is hard to say more about chimpanzee personality per se than what was said above. That is, given the large database available on chimps in the wild, why can't we say more about personality variables that appear to be under cultural control? While there are some anecdotes on specific personality traits in specific individuals, the controlled experimental studies of personality per se that we see in other parts of this chapter have simply not been undertaken on a large scale for chimps. There are many reasons for this, including the ethical considerations of personality work in chimps, the tendency to want to minimize experimental work in natural populations, the long generation time of chimpanzees, and perhaps the fear that personality work on chimpanzees would be viewed as an attempt to anthropomorphize animal behavior.

Coping Styles

One aspect of an animal's personality is how it handles stress in the environment, because how an animal copes with everyday, as well more extreme, stressors can have a profound impact on its health, and hence its reproductive success (Bartolomucci, 2007; Cavigelli, 2005; Koolhaas et al., 2007; Overli et al., 2007; Table 17.3). In their review of the literature on personality, stress, and coping, Jaap Koolhaas and his colleagues found two coping styles that they labeled **proactive** (sometimes called the active response) and **reactive** (also known as the conservation-withdrawal response) (Cannon, 1915; Engel and Schmale, 1972; Henry and Stephens, 1977; Koolhaas et al., 1999). The proactive personality

TABLE 17.3. Coping styles. A list of species in which individual differences in coping style have been studied. Some studies examined behavioral variables; others examined physiological variables. A single plus indicates a single-parameter study; two pluses indicate a multi-parameter study. *(Based on Koolhaas et al., 1999, p. 926)*

SPECIES	BEHAVIORAL PARAMETERS	PHYSIOLOGICAL PARAMETERS
Mouse (*Mus musculus domesticus*)	+ +	+ +
Rat (*Rattus novegicus*)	+ +	+ +
Pig (*Sus scrofa*)	+ +	+ +
Tree shrew (*Tupaja belangeri*)	+ +	+ +
Cattle (*Bos taurus*)	+	+ +
Great tit (*Parus major*)	+ +	
Chicken (*Gallus domesticus*)	+	+ +
Beech marten (*Martes foina*)	+	
Stickleback (*Gasterosteus aculeatus*)	+ +	
Rainbow trout (*Oncorhynchus mykiss*)	+	+
Rhesus monkey (*Macaca mulatta*)	+ +	+ +
Human (*Homo sapiens*)	+ +	+ +
Octopus (*Octopus rubescens*)	+ +	

type is characterized by territorial control and aggression, while the reactive style is characterized by immobility and low levels of aggression (Koolhaas et al., 1999; Table 17.4).

Proactive animals are also more likely to remove negative stimuli from their environment, while reactive animals are more likely to hide from any new negative stimulus. Frans Sluyter, for example, studied different strains of rats that had been selected for proactive or reactive coping styles (Sluyter et al., 1995). First, male rats were exposed to an intruder in an experiment in which another male was placed in an individual's home cage. Proactive rats were very aggressive toward intruders, while reactive rats most often attempted to hide from such intruders (Figure 17.15). The rats were then tested in a "defensive

TABLE 17.4. Proactive and reactive coping styles. A summary of the behavioral differences between proactive and reactive male rats and mice. *(Based on Koolhaas et al., 1999)*

BEHAVIORAL CHARACTERISTICS	PROACTIVE	REACTIVE
Attack latency	Low	High
Defensive burying	High	Low
Nest-building	High	Low
Routine formation	High	Low
Cue dependency	Low	High
Conditioned immobility	Low	High
Flexibility	Low	High

FIGURE 17.15. Proactive and reactive rats. **(A)** Proactive mice and rats tend to be territorial and aggressive, while **(B)** reactive mice and rats tend to be timid and become immobile or hide when threatened. *(Photo credits: Tom McHugh/Photo Researchers, Inc.; Joe McDonald/Corbis)*

burying" experiment. In the defensive burying experiment, a small electric prod was placed in a male's cage, and if the male investigated the prod and touched it, he received a mild shock. Once shocked, a rat had two ways to avoid future shock: he could either bury the prod under his bedding or significantly curtail his movements. The researchers found that individuals from the proactive strain of mice were much more likely to bury the prod than were mice from the reactive strain, suggesting that the two coping styles map nicely onto personality types.

The underlying proximate mechanisms associated with proactive and reactive strains have also been examined (Sluyter et al., 1995). Proactive and reactive mice were exposed to two different stressors—a five-minute forced swim or long-term stress associated with frequent handling. Alexa Veenema, Ronald de Kloet, Koolhaas, and their colleagues took a series of neuroendocrinological measurements of mice in the proactive and reactive strains, both before and after exposure to stress (Veenema et al., 2004, 2007).

Before exposure to stress conditions, corticosterone levels were fairly stable in reactive mice, but the levels fluctuated in proactive mice. Once they were stressed, reactive mice showed a dramatic increase in corticosterone levels, as compared to proactive mice. The "freeze response" and reduced aggression and territoriality in reactive mice might be linked to such increases in corticosterone. Compared to proactive mice, reactive mice also showed reduced cell growth in the hippocampal region of the brain, suggesting that the proximate differences between coping styles may also affect learning and memory (Veenema et al., 2004, 2007).

Proactive and reactive personalities have been found not only in laboratory and natural populations of animals, but also in domesticated animals such as pigs and cows (Hopster, 1998; Prelle et al., 2004; Spoolder et al., 1996; Weiss et al., 2004). While data on the costs and benefits of these two coping styles are scant, there is some evidence that proactive and reactive animals differ in their susceptibility to diseases such as hypertension, atherosclerosis, gastric ulcers, and immunosuppressive capabilities (Ely, 1981; Henry et al., 1993; Hessing et al., 1994; Sgoifo et al., 2005; Weiss, 1972).

Some Practical Applications of Animal Personality Research

The study of animal personality has potential practical implications for conservation biology, human-animal interactions, farming, and many other areas. Here we will examine the practical implications of animal personality work for preventing the death of livestock and aiding people with disabilities.

PREDATORS AND DOMESTICATED PREY

Farmers and breeders have long been interested in the processes of natural and artificial selection with respect to both the anatomy and behavior of domesticated livestock. An understanding of these processes can provide a road map for breeding programs designed to produce fruits, vegetables, flowers, meat, milk, and so forth. But an ethological understanding of personality traits may also prove beneficial for ranchers in that it can help minimize the number of their animals killed by large predators that have been deemed "problem individuals" (Linnell et al., 1999, 2000).

As a result of species recovery and conservation plans, a number of large carnivores have been successfully reintroduced into the wild, or have had their natural population numbers increase dramatically over the last few decades. The downside of this conservation success has been the rekindling of an old rivalry between herders and large carnivores that feed on their animals (Blanco et al., 1992; Cozza et al., 1996; Kaczensky, 1996; Oli et al., 1994; Quigley and Cragshaw, 1992). Reducing this conflict may be facilitated by an understanding of the ethology of the carnivores that are causing the problem.

Because there is widespread opposition to large-scale killing of carnivore populations, one way that this problem has been tackled is to focus on "problem individuals"—carnivore individuals that repeatedly attack and kill livestock. The data on particular aspects of the hunting behavior of large carnivores preying on domestic prey are difficult to obtain, but studies of hunting behavior in cougars, leopards, lions, and bears suggest that certain individuals are more likely to prey upon domesticated animals (Claar et al., 1986; Mitzutani, 1993; Ross et al., 1997; Stander, 1990). If such individuals do in fact exist, and if their behavior is both consistent and markedly different from that of their groupmates, then a case can be made for personality differences in carnivores, at least with respect to their hunting tactics.

Exactly how to use the information on personality differences and problem individuals, should it prove to be a general phenomenon, is still a matter of debate (Linnell et al., 1999, 2000). For example, one possibility would be to use the personality attributes of "problem" predators to design new traps specifically for these sorts of individuals.

GUIDE DOG PERSONALITIES

Humans have had a close mutualistic relationship with dogs since we began domesticating grey wolves in Asia about fifteen thousand years ago (Savolainen et al., 2002; Vila et al., 1997). On top of our immense practical experience with dog behavior, we have now completed sequencing the entire genome of the domestic dog, and many studies have been undertaken on the behavioral genetics of dogs (Lindblad-Toh et al., 2005; Saetre et al., 2006). And so, dogs seem like a good species for studying many aspects of animal personality. Here we will focus on dog personality as it applies to guide dogs for the blind (Ley and Bennett, 2007; Serpell and Hsu, 2001).

In order to become a guide dog for the blind, dogs must pass a very rigorous test. Data suggest that most dogs can, in fact, learn the difficult tasks needed to complete their training. Fear often interferes with a dog's performance, however, and is the single most common reason dogs fail to qualify to aid the blind (Baillie, 1972; Goddard and Beilharz, 1982, 1983; Scott and Bielfelt, 1976). This is not only an interesting finding in itself, but it suggests that a personality trait—fear or fearlessness—underlies which individuals become guide dogs and which do not (Boissy, 1995).

In order to understand the genetics of fear more completely and to suggest a good breeding program for guide dogs, M. E. Goddard and R. G. Beilharz crossbred four breeds of dogs—Labrador retrievers, Australian kelpies, boxers, and German shepherds (Goddard and Beilharz, 1985). Puppies from all crosses were allowed to remain with their mothers until they were six weeks old, at which point they were weaned and moved to the Guide Dog Association's kennel. At twelve weeks of age, the animals were given to "puppy walkers," who began training them to become guide dogs.

Fear and fearlessness were measured using thirty-eight different behaviors that were subsequently transformed into twelve components via principle component statistical analysis. The first three of these components map onto "general fearfulness," "fearfulness of objects," and "inhibited response to fear" (Goddard and Beilharz, 1984). Individual dog scores were consistent on these three components when the dogs were tested at six and twelve months of age.

Based on the observations of the puppy walkers and the individuals who tested the dogs on the guide dog exam, only general fearfulness was a good predictor of which animals would pass their final guide dog exam. This is particularly important because only "general fearfulness" has a strong underlying genetic component, whereas environmental factors explain much of the variance in the other two components of fear in these four species (Leotta et al., 2006; Wilsson and Sundgren, 1997). The genetic crosses also show that Labrador retrievers were most easily trained to be guide dogs (German shepherds were the most difficult to train). Goddard and Beilharz used the genetics of fear, along with the ethologically based information described above, to suggest a breeding program for guide dogs (Goddard and Beilharz, 1985).

Research on animal personality—consistent behavioral differences among individuals—is an active area in ethology, and it includes studies in everything from fish and octopuses to mice and primates. Much, but not all, of this work has focused on the bold-shy continuum, as well as on proactive and reactive personality types. These studies incorporate both proximate and ultimate perspectives, and they consider the role of both individual learning and social learning in shaping personality. Research in the area of animal personality has numerous practical implications, including preventing the death of livestock and aiding people with disabilities.

INTERVIEW WITH

Dr. Jerome Kagan

Why study personality?

The study of personality has theoretical and practical significance because the variation among humans in stable mood and behavior has consequences for the individual's adaptation, location of choice, and the risk for psychopathology. Unfortunately, current conclusions about basic personality types are based primarily on questionnaire evidence rather than behavioral observations combined with biological measurements. It is likely therefore that the currently popular categories are too general and will be replaced with a larger number of personality types, and these will take into account the contexts in which the person acts.

Your long-term study of shyness in children has uncovered many new, important findings. How did you first get started with this study at Harvard? What is the single most unexpected result you obtained?

Our study of inhibited and uninhibited children had its origins in three different sets of observations. In the book *Birth to Maturity*, which summarized in 1962 the longitudinal sample at the Fells Research Institute, the only profile stable from early childhood to adulthood resembled the children we call inhibited. The second observation came from our study of the effects of day care in a sample of Boston children that contained different ethnic groups. The temperamentally inhibited infants preserved their profile, which seemed

to be minimally affected by whether they were attending a day-care center or being raised at home. The third result came from Cynthia Garcia-Coll's thesis, over twenty years ago, which demonstrated that children selected to be inhibited or uninhibited in the second year preserved their respective behavioral styles. The most unexpected result of our work

over the last twenty-five years was the observation that four-month-old infants who showed vigorous motor activity and crying to varied classes of stimuli were biased to become inhibited children in the second year.

How has an evolutionary framework changed the way you study human personality?

The importance of an evolutionary framework derives from the fact that

closely related species or strains differ in their typical behavior to appropriate incentives. In addition, there is early evidence that these differences are derived from inherited differences in brain neurochemistry.

Darwin wrote *The Expression of Emotions in Man and Animals* more than 125 years ago. Why did it take so long for the serious study of animal personality to develop?

Investigators of animal behavior were not interested in variation because they saw each species as an essential prototype and were more interested in species differences than in differences within a species. Further, there had been no interest in predicting differential adaptation in animals reared in a laboratory because the context was identical for all animals.

What is the single most important thing psychologists studying human personality have gleaned from work on animal personality?

The most important fact gleaned from work on animals is the demonstration of different biological features correlated with different behavioral preferences.

What is the single most important thing psychologists studying animal personality have gleaned from work on human personality?

I believe that those investigators studying animals have been motivated to study the approach-avoidance categories because of the work on human personality types.

Could you talk a little about the role of color in the study of animal personality?

I have little to say about the role of color in animal behavior. The structures that produce differential coloration of skin or fur are ectodermal in origin and therefore might be expected to correlate with behavior. One of the most relevant studies comes from Belayev's study of silver fox on a Siberian farm. After twenty generations of breeding tame fox, the offspring were likely to be tame, and showed changes in the distribution of melanin in the fur.

How do you define "temperament"? How does this differ from other related concepts?

Temperament is defined as an inherited biological profile that is linked initially to preferences for emotions and behavior. The initial bias is acted on by others to produce personality types. Thus, by two years of age, it is difficult to see the original temperamental bias, for it has become integrated with experience to produce a personality profile.

> The most important fact gleaned from work on animals is the demonstration of different biological features correlated with different behavioral preferences.

How do you think the various genome-sequencing projects will affect our understanding of personality in humans and nonhumans?

The Genome Project will make an important contribution to our understanding of personality because it will eventually provide evidence regarding the inherited neurochemical profiles that create a large number of human temperaments.

What's the next frontier in the study of animal personality?

The next frontier in the study of animals will be the detection of a large number of specific functional relations among the neurobiology of the animal, associated behavioral profiles, and the contexts in which the animal acts.

Dr. Jerome Kagan is a professor at Harvard University. He is currently conducting the longest-running study ever on personality development in humans. Dr. Kagan's work, as represented in his book Galen's Prophecy: Temperament in Nature *(Basic Books, 1994), integrates evolutionary approaches into what has historically been an area reserved for cognitive and developmental psychologists.*

SUMMARY

1. Personality differences can be conceptualized as consistent long-term phenotypic behavioral differences among individuals.
2. Boldness/shyness is one of the most stable personality variables. But, evolutionarily based animal behaviorists argue that there is no reason that natural selection should necessarily select for boldness or shyness as a general personality trait. Rather, individuals may be bold in some contexts and shy in others, depending on the costs and benefits associated with the behavioral contexts being examined.
3. The best documented case of cultural transmission of information affecting animal personality involves seven long-term studies of chimpanzees in Africa. Stable innovative patterns of behavior are spread within groups of chimpanzees through imitation. But behaviors and personalities across populations are very different.
4. How an animal copes with everyday, as well more extreme, stressors can have a profound impact on its health. Two general coping styles emerge from studies across a wide variety of animals. These two styles are referred to as the proactive or "active response" and the reactive or "conservation-withdrawal response." The proactive coping style entails territorial control and aggression, while the reactive coping style is characterized by immobility and low levels of aggression.
5. The study of animal personality has potential practical implications for conservation biology, human-animal interactions, farming, and many other areas, including preventing the death of livestock and aiding people with disabilities.

DISCUSSION QUESTIONS

1. Go to the monkey exhibit at your local zoo and pick four individual monkeys to observe for at least four hours. Or go to a working farm and pick four individual cows or horses. Record all the information you can on each individual ("grooms," "eats," "attacks," "retreats," "sleeps," "plays," and so on), and if possible, note the proximity of the animals you are studying to others in the group. From your observations, can you suggest a list of behaviors that you might focus on during a longer, more controlled, study of personality in the population you are observing?
2. How would you construct an experiment to examine whether boldness and/or behavioral inhibition are heritable traits?
3. Besides the ones mentioned in this chapter, what general costs and benefits might you associate with being bold or inhibited? Pick a particular species you are familiar with and create a list of the potential costs and benefits of boldness and shyness in that species.
4. Pick up a few recent issues of the journal *Animal Behaviour* and scan the titles for anything on "alternative strategies." Once you have found one or two such articles, read them in detail. Is there any mention of personality in these papers? If not, how might you reanalyze the data to see whether the alternative strategies could be construed in light of the work on animal personalities? What other sorts of data could you collect to better understand whether the alternative strategies studied represent personality types?

5. Besides preventing the death of livestock and selecting guide dogs, can you think of any other practical applications of personality work in animals? How might you construct some experiments to better understand whether the applications you suggest are feasible?

SUGGESTED READING

Buss, D. (2007). *Evolutionary psychology* (3rd ed.). Boston: Allen and Bacon. A textbook on the evolution of traits traditionally studied by psychologists.

Jones, A. C., & Gosling, S. D. (2005). Temperament and personality in dogs (*Canis familiaris*): A review and evaluation of past research. *Applied Animal Behaviour Science, 95,* 1–53. An excellent review article on personality in dogs.

van Oers, K., de Jong, G., van Noordwijk, A. J., Kempenaers, B., & Drent, P. J. (2005). Contribution of genetics to the study of animal personalities: A review of case studies. *Behaviour, 42,* 1185–1206. A review of work on genetics and personality, with an emphasis on the great tit bird.

Whiten, A., & Boesch, C. (2001). The culture of chimpanzees. *Scientific American*, January 2001, 60–67. Interesting review suggesting how culture can potentially explain some personality traits seen within and across chimp populations.

Wilson, D. S., Clark, A. B., Coleman, K., & Dearstyne, T. (1994). Shyness and boldness in humans and other animals. *Trends in Ecology and Evolution, 9,* 442–446. A short, but thought-provoking article.

Glossary

adaptation A trait that results in the highest fitness among a specified set of behaviors in a particular environment. Adaptations are typically the result of the process of natural selection.

allele A gene variant; one of two or more alternative forms of a gene.

alliance A long-term coalition. *See also* coalition.

allogrooming The grooming of another individual, usually by scratching or licking an area of skin, often to remove parasites, but also to solidify social bonds. Also known as social grooming.

analogous traits Traits that are similar as a result of similar selection pressures rather than common descent.

antagonistic pleiotropy The case in which the multiple pleiotropic effects of a single gene work in opposite directions with respect to fitness. *See also* pleiotropy.

appetitive stimulus Any stimulus that is considered positive, pleasant, or rewarding.

arena mating *See* leks.

artificial selection Selection in which man is the selective agent and chooses certain varieties of an organism over others for breeding. *See also* natural selection.

audience effect An effect that occurs when individuals involved in aggressive interactions change their behavior as a function of being watched by others.

aversive stimulus Any stimulus (for example, a shock or noxious odor) that is associated with an unpleasant experience.

axons Nerve cell fibers that transmit electrical information from one nerve cell to another.

Bateman's principle The idea that, since eggs require greater energy to produce than sperm, females should be the choosier sex and this should result in greater variance in the reproductive success of males.

behavioral genetics The study of the genetic variance associated with behavior.

blocking When an association between an unconditioned stimulus (US1) and a response prevents an individual from responding to another stimulus (US2) or causes the individual to respond less strongly to the US2.

boldness The tendency to take risks in both familiar and unfamiliar situations.

brood parasitism A form of behavioral parasitism in which females place their eggs in the nests of others, often from another species, who raise the young as their own.

byproduct mutualism A type of cooperation in which an individual pays an immediate cost or penalty for not acting cooperatively, such that the immediate net benefit of cooperating outweighs that of cheating.

bystander effect An effect that occurs when observers of an aggressive interaction between two other individuals change their estimation of the fighting ability of those they are watching as a function of what they observe.

classical conditioning *See* Pavlovian conditioning.

coalition Cooperative action taken by at least two individuals or groups against another individual or group. *See also* cooperation.

communication The transfer of information from a signaler to a receiver.

conceptual approach An approach that usually entails integrating ideas generated in different disciplines and combining them in a new, cohesive way.

conditioned response (CR) The learned response to a conditioned stimulus.

conditioned stimulus (CS) A stimulus that initially fails to elicit a particular response, but comes to do so when it is associated with a second (unconditioned) stimulus.

convergent evolution The process whereby different populations or species converge on the same phenotypic characteristics as a result of similar selection pressures.

cooperation An outcome that, despite possible costs to the individual, provides some benefits to others. "To cooperate" means to behave in a way to make cooperation possible.

coping style A set of behavioral and related stress responses that are consistent over time.

copying Behavior that occurs when an observer repeats the actions of a demonstrator. The copier is often rewarded for whatever behavior it has copied.

cross-fostering experiment An experiment undertaken to measure the relative contributions of genetic and environmental variation on the expression of behavioral traits. This experiment often involves removing young individuals from their parent(s), and having them raised by adults that are not their genetic relatives.

cryptic Hidden through camouflage, and thus blending into the environment and avoiding predators. Also a form of hidden mate choice (cryptic mate choice), wherein females select which sperm transferred during copulation are used in actual fertilization.

cultural transmission The transfer of information from individual to individual through teaching or social learning—both within and between generations of animals. *See also* social learning; teaching.

dendrites Nerve cell fibers that receive electrical information from other cells.

developmental stability A measure of how well an organism handles changing environments as it matures.

disposable soma theory The theory that, under certain conditions, it may be beneficial for organisms to divert some energy and resources away from the normal maintenance and repair that is associated with traits that have little connection to reproduction (that is, somatic traits) and invest such energy in traits related to reproduction.

DNA fingerprint A molecular genetic technique often used to examine the genetic relatedness among individuals.

dominance hierarchy The relationship between individuals in a group as a result of aggressive behaviors and the response to aggressive behaviors.

dominant allele An allele that is expressed in heterozygote individuals. Allele A is dominant to allele a if the Aa genotype is identical to the AA genotype. *See also* allele.

dyadic interactions Interactions involving only two individuals.

ecology The study of the interaction of organisms with their environment.

empirical approach An approach that entails gathering data in one form or another and drawing inferences from that data. Empirical work in ethology can take many forms, but most often it is either observational or experimental.

endocrine system A communication network of ductless glands that secrete chemical messengers called hormones.

ethology The scientific study of animal behavior.

eusociality An extreme form of sociality in which there is cooperative brood care, division of labor, and overlapping generations.

evolutionarily stable strategy (ESS) A strategy that, if used by almost everyone in a population, will not decrease in frequency when new, mutant strategies arise. "Mutant" refers to a new strategy introduced into a population at a very low frequency.

excitatory conditioning When a conditioned stimulus leads to an action (for example, searching for food or hiding). Sometimes (incorrectly) used as a synonym for Pavlovian conditioning.

extinction curves Graphs that depict how long an animal will remember some paired association once the pairing itself has stopped.

extrapair copulations Copulations that occur outside the context of a pair bond.

female defense polygyny A mating system in which males aggressively guard females who are found in spatial clusters, obtaining sole reproductive access to such "harems" of females.

fitness Lifetime reproductive success that is usually measured in relative terms.

flight initiation distance The distance at which prey begin to flee from a predator.

foraging Feeding and all behaviors associated with feeding.

gene expression The expression of a gene as a result of environmental or behavioral triggers.

genetic recombination A recombination of genes during cell division in sexually reproducing organisms that involves sections of one chromosome "crossing over" and swapping positions with sections of the homologous chromosome. This swapping can create new genetic variation.

genetic variation Variation caused by genetic differences.

genotype The genetic makeup of an individual.

goal-directed learning *See* instrumental conditioning.

good genes model A model of sexual selection in which females choose to mate with males that possess traits that are indicators of good health and vigor—that is, traits that are best suited to their particular environment. Females who choose the males with such genes receive "indirect" benefits, in the sense that their offspring receive some of the good genes that led their mother to choose a male as a mate in the first place.

group selection A hierarchical model in which natural selection operates at two levels: within-group selection and between-group selection.

habitat choice models Models that examine how animals distribute themselves in space and time with respect to some resource (for example, food, mates, refuge from predators) in their environment.

habituation Becoming less sensitive to stimuli over time.

hawk-dove game In this game theory model of aggression, hawk is a strategy in which the individual escalates and continues to escalate until either it is injured or its opponent concedes, and dove is a strategy in which the individual bluffs, initially displaying as if it will escalate, but actually retreating and ceding the resource if its opponent escalates.

heritability The proportion of variance in a trait that is due to genetic variance.

home range A delineated, undefended area in which an animal spends most of its time.

homologous traits Traits that are shared by two or more species as a result of common descent.

homoplasy A trait that is present in two or more species but that is not due to common descent but rather results from natural selection acting independently on each species. *See also* analogous traits.

honest indicators principle The idea that traits that are costly to produce are more difficult to fake and hence truly indicate the "genetic quality" of an individual.

horizontal cultural transmission Cultural transmission in which information is passed across individuals of the same age or peer group. *See also* cultural transmission.

ideal free distribution (IFD) model A mathematical model developed to predict how animals will distribute themselves among habitats with varying levels of resource availability.

imitation The acquisition of a topographically novel response through observation of a demonstrator making that response.

inclusive fitness A measure of fitness that takes into account not only the effect a gene has on its bearer, but also the effect it has on its genetic relatives.

individual learning A relatively permanent change in behavior as a result of experience. Individual learning differs from social learning in that it does not involve learning from others.

inhibitory conditioning When a conditioned stimulus suppresses or inhibits behavior.

instrumental conditioning Learning that occurs when a response made by an animal is reinforced by reward or punishment. An animal must undertake some action or response in order for the conditioning process to produce learning.

intersexual selection A form of sexual selection in which individuals of one sex choose which individuals of the other sex to take as mates. *See also* sexual selection.

intrasexual selection A form of sexual selection whereby members of one sex compete with each other for access to the other sex. *See also* sexual selection.

kamikaze sperm hypothesis The hypothesis that natural selection might favor sperm that are designed to kill (or otherwise incapacitate) other males' sperm rather than to fertilize eggs.

kin recognition matching models Models in which an individual uses an internal template to gauge its genetic relatedness to others.

kin selection *See* inclusive fitness.

law of effect A principle that maintains that if a response in the presence of a stimulus is followed by a satisfying event, the association between the stimulus and the response will be strengthened.

leks Areas in which groups of males set up and defend small, temporary territorial patches and in which they display to females, specifically to attract females to mate with them. The result is called lekking or arena mating.

local enhancement A phenomenon in which an individual is drawn to a particular area because it observed another individual in that location.

locomotor play Play behaviors in which animals leap, jump, twist, shake, whirl, somersault, roll, or chase their tails. Also known as locomotor rotational play.

loser effect The increased probability of losing a fight at time T, based on losing at time T-1, T-2, and so on, respectively.

marginal value theorem A mathematical model developed to predict how long a forager will spend in a patch of food before moving on to new patches.

mate-choice copying The act of copying the mate choice of others.

migration The movement of organisms over long distances (often in a seasonal manner).

mobbing A type of antipredator behavior in which groups of prey join together, approach a predator, and aggressively attempt to chase it away.

monogamous mating system A mating system in which a male and female mate only with one another during a given breeding season.

mushroom bodies A cluster of small neurons located at the front of the brain of some invertebrates and associated with spatial navigation.

mutation Any change in genetic structure.

mutualism Any interaction that benefits all parties involved. Interspecies cooperation is often referred to as a mutualism.

natural selection The process at the heart of Darwin's theory of evolution. Natural selection occurs when variants of a trait that best suit an organism to its environment, and that are heritable, increase in frequency over evolutionary time. This process requires variation, fitness differences, and heritability.

neural plasticity The ability of neurons to undergo change as a function of experience.

neuroeconomics A collaborative research effort between economists, neurobiologists, and evolutionary biologists that uses brain-imaging technology to understand proximate (and eventually ultimate) questions regarding behavior.

neurohormones Though most hormones are produced by ductless glands, neurohormones are secreted directly into the bloodstream by nerve cells.

nomads Individuals who lack a home range or a territory and who rarely frequent the same area over time. Occasionally, reference will be made to a nomadic species.

nuptial gifts Prey presented by members of one sex to members of the other sex during courtship.

object play A kind of play that centers on the use of inanimate objects such as sticks, rocks, leaves, feathers, fruit, and human-provided objects, and the pushing, throwing, tearing, or manipulating of such objects.

oblique cultural transmission A form of cultural transmission in which information is passed across generations, but not from parent to offspring.

operant learning *See* instrumental conditioning.

operant response A learned action that an animal makes to change its environment.

optimal foraging theory (OFT) A family of mathematical models developed to predict animal foraging behavior. Models based on this theory examine questions concerning what to eat, where to eat, how long to eat, and so forth.

optimal skew theory A family of models that predicts the distribution of breeding within a group, as well as the degree of cooperation or conflict over reproductive activities.

overshadowing A situation in which the learned response to an unconditioned stimulus (US1) is stronger when it is presented alone versus when it is paired with a second unconditioned stimulus (US2).

parental investment The amount of energy parents invest in raising their offspring.

parent-offspring conflict A zone of conflict between how much a given offspring wants in terms of parental resources and how much a parent is willing to give.

parent-offspring regression A technique for measuring heritability that involves measuring a trait in parents and offspring.

parsimony analysis A technique for choosing among alternative phylogenetic trees by selecting the tree that requires the fewest character changes.

Pavlovian conditioning The experimental pairing of a conditioned and unconditioned stimulus. *See also* conditioned stimulus; unconditioned stimulus.

personality differences Consistent long-term phenotypic behavioral differences among individuals.

phenotype The observable characteristics of an organism.

phenotypic plasticity The ability of an organism to produce different phenotypes depending on environmental conditions.

phylogenetic tree The depiction of phylogeny by using branching, tree-like diagrams.

phylogeny Evolutionary history via common descent.

play Typically defined as motor activity performed during development that appears to be purposeless.

play markers Behavioral indicators that denote that some action that is about to be undertaken should be considered playful, not dangerous. Also known as play signals, they may serve to initiate play or to indicate the desire to keep playing.

pleiotropy The case wherein a gene has more than one effect (either at one time or sequentially).

polarity The historical direction of change in the appearance of different varieties of a trait so as to determine which were ancestral (appearing first) and which were derived from earlier varieties of the trait.

polyadic interactions Interactions involving more than two individuals.

polyandry A mating system wherein females mate with more than one male per breeding season.

polygamy A mating system in which either males or females have multiple mates during a given breeding season.

polygenic Caused by the action of more than one gene.

polygynandry A mating system wherein several males form pair bonds with several females simultaneously.

polygyny A mating system wherein males mate with more than one female per breeding season.

polygyny threshold model A model developed to predict the conditions under which a mating system will move from monogamy to polygyny (or vice versa).

predator inspection An antipredator behavior in which one to a few individuals break away from a group and slowly approach a potential predator to obtain various sorts of information.

preexisting bias *See* sensory exploitation.

prisoner's dilemma A game theory payoff matrix that is used to study the evolution of cooperation.

proactive coping style A personality type characterized by territorial behavior and various forms of aggression; animals with this personality are more likely to remove negative stimuli from their environment. This style is sometimes referred to as the active response.

producers Individuals that find and procure food.

promiscuity A type of mating system in which both polyandry and polygyny are occurring. In one form of promiscuity, both males and females mate with many partners and no pair bonds are formed. In the second type of promiscuous breeding system, labeled polygynandry, several males form pair bonds with several females simultaneously. *See also* polyandry; polygynandry; polygyny.

proximate analysis Analysis based on asking questions that focus on immediate causation.

reactive coping style A personality type characterized by immobility and low levels of aggression; animals with this personality are more likely to become immobile or to hide when exposed to a new negative stimulus. Also known as the conservation-withdrawal response.

recessive allele An allele in heterozygote individuals that is not expressed when combined with a dominant allele. Allele a is recessive to allele A if a is not expressed in the Aa genotype.

reciprocal altruism The exchange of altruistic acts.

resource holding power A measure of an animal's fighting ability.

risk-sensitive optimal foraging models A family of mathematical models that examines how variance in food supplies affects foraging behavior.

role reversal Behavior wherein older individuals allow subordinate, younger animals to take on the dominant role during play, or in which older individuals perform some act that is at a level clearly below that of which the older individual is capable. Also known as self-handicapping.

runaway sexual selection A model of sexual selection in which the genes for mate choice in the female and the genes for preferred traits in males become genetically linked.

scroungers Individuals that obtain a portion of their diet by parasitizing the food that others (producers) have uncovered. *See also* producers.

search image As predators encounter prey over and over, they form some sort of representation—a search image—of the prey. This representation becomes more detailed with experience.

self-handicapping *See* role reversal.

senescence An age-specific decline in the probability of survival.

sensitization Becoming more sensitive to stimuli over time.

sensory bias *See* sensory exploitation.

sensory exploitation A theory of sexual selection that posits that females may initially prefer male traits that elicit the greatest amount of stimulation from their sensory systems. Also known as sensory exploitation, sensory drive, or preexisting bias.

sequential assessment model A model of fighting in which an individual continually assesses its opponent's fighting ability during different stages of an aggressive interaction, and decides whether or not to continue in such an interaction based on the assessment it has made.

sexual selection A form of natural selection that, according to Darwin (1871), involves "a struggle between the individuals of one sex, generally the males, for the possession of the other sex."

sexy-son hypothesis A hypothesis that females select among males based on genetic traits in the males that will lead to the production of sons that are attractive to the opposite sex.

shyness The reluctance to take risks or to engage in unfamiliar activity.

sibling rivalry Aggressive interactions among siblings.

social facilitation When the mere presence of a model, regardless of what it does, facilitates learning on the part of an observer.

social grooming The grooming of another individual, usually by scratching or licking an area of skin, often to remove parasites, but also to solidify social bonds. Also known as allogrooming.

social learning Learning via the observation of others. Observation is used in a broad sense and can include obtaining information through olfaction and other senses besides sight.

social play Playing with others, which may lead to the forging of long-lasting social bonds, may provide social skills (including practice in fighting, hunting, and mating), and may help in the development of cognitive skills.

sperm competition A form of sexual selection that occurs directly between sperm after insemination.

symmetry A measure of the similarity of the left and right sides of the body. Sometimes referred to as bilateral symmetry.

teaching A behavior that occurs when one individual serves as an instructor and at least one other individual acts as a student who learns from the instructor. Teachers have a much more active and complicated role than just being a model that others mimic (as in social learning).

territory A delineated, defended area.

theoretical approach An approach that entails the generation of a model—usually a mathematical model—of some behavior.

tit for tat (TFT) A behavioral strategy that instructs a player to initially cooperate with a new partner, and subsequently to do whatever that partner does.

truncation selection experiment An experimental procedure that measures heritability by allowing only those with extreme forms of a trait to breed and then tracking changes in that trait across generations.

ultimate analysis Analysis based on asking questions that relate to the evolution of a trait.

unconditioned stimulus (US) A stimulus that elicits a vigorous response in the absence of training.

vertical cultural transmission Cultural transmission in which information is passed directly from parent(s) to offspring. *See also* cultural transmission.

waggle dance A dance performed by forager bees. The waggle dance provides information on the spatial location of food located at some distance from the hive.

war of attrition model A model of fighting in which animals display aggressively to one another without actually fighting, and the winner of the encounter is the individual that displays the longest.

winner effect The increased probability of winning a fight at time T, based on victories at times T-1, T-2, and so on.

worker policing Behavior that involves workers in a social insect species destroying the haploid eggs laid by other workers.

xenophobia The fear of strangers or those from outside one's group.

References

Able, K. P. (1999). *Gatherings of angels: Migrating birds and their ecology.* Ithaca, NY: Comstock Books.

Adams, E., & Mesterton-Gibbons, M. (1995). The cost of threat displays and the stability of deceptive communication. *Journal of Theoretical Biology, 175,* 405–421.

Agnarsson, I., Aviles, L., Coddington, J. A., & Maddison, W. P. (2006). Sociality in Theridiid spiders: Repeated origins of an evolutionary dead end. *Evolution, 60,* 2342–2351.

Ågren, G. (1984). Pair formation in the Mongolian gerbil. *Animal Behaviour, 32,* 528–535.

Alatalo, R. V., Hoglund, J., Lundberg, A., & Sutherland, W. J. (1992). Evolution of black grouse leks: Female preferences benefit males in larger leks. *Behavioral Ecology, 3,* 53–59.

Alcock, J. (1998). *Animal behavior* (6th ed.). Sunderland, MA: Sinauer.

Alcock, J. (2001). *The triumph of sociobiology.* New York: Oxford University Press.

Alcock, J. (2003). A textbook history of animal behaviour. *Animal Behaviour, 65,* 3–10.

Alcock, J., & Sherman, P. (1994). The utility of the proximate-ultimate dichotomy in ethology. *Ethology, 96,* 58–62.

Alderson, A. L., & Novack, T. A. (2002). Neurophysiological and clinical aspects of glucocorticoids and memory: A review. *Journal of Clinical and Experimental Neuropsychology, 24,* 335–355.

Alerstam, T. (1990). *Bird migration.* Cambridge: Cambridge University Press.

Alerstam, T., Hedenstrom, A., & Akesson, S. (2003). Long-distance migration: Evolution and determinants. *Oikos, 103,* 247–260.

Alexander, R. D. (1979). *Darwinism and human affairs.* Seattle: University of Washington Press.

Alexander, R. D. (1991). Social learning and kin recognition. *Ethology and Sociobiology, 12,* 387–399.

Alexander, R. D., & Tinkle, D. W. (Eds). (1981). *Natural selection and social behavior.* New York: Chiron Press.

Allan, S., & Suthers, R. (1994). Lateralization and motor stereotypy of song production in the brown-headed cowbird. *Journal of Neurobiology, 25,* 1154–1166.

Allee, W. (1951). *Cooperation among animals with human implications.* New York: Henry Schuman.

Allen, G. (1879). *The color sense: Its origin and development.* London: Trubner.

Allman, H. M. (1998). *Evolving brains.* New York: Scientific American Library.

Altmann, S. A. (1956). Avian mobbing behavior and predator recognition. *Condor, 58,* 241–253.

Altmann, S. (1962). Social behavior of anthropoid primates: Analysis of recent concepts. In E. Bliss (Ed.), *Roots of behavior* (pp. 277–285). New York: Harper and Brothers.

Altmann, S. A. (1979). Altruistic behaviour: The fallacy of kin deployment. *Animal Behaviour, 27,* 958–959.

Amat, J., Baratta, M. V., Paul, E., Bland, S. T., Watkins, L. R., & Maier, S. F. (2005). Medial prefrontal cortex determines how stressor controllability affects behavior and dorsal raphe nucleus. *Nature Neuroscience, 8,* 365–371.

Andersson, M. (1994). *Sexual selection.* Princeton: Princeton University Press.

Andersson, M., & Simmons, L. W. (2006). Sexual selection and mate choice. *Trends in Ecology & Evolution, 21,* 296–302.

Apfelbach, R., Blanchard, C. D., Blanchard, R. J., Hayes, R. A., & McGregor, I. S. (2005). The effects of predator odors in mammalian prey species: A review of field and laboratory studies. *Neuroscience and Biobehavioral Reviews, 29,* 1123–1144.

Aquilino, W. (1991). Family structure and home leaving: A further specification of the relationship. *Journal of Marriage and the Family, 53,* 999–1010.

Aragona, B. J., Liu, Y., Curtis, T., Stephan, F. K., & Wang, Z. X. (2003). A critical role for nucleus accumbens dopamine in partner-preference formation in male prairie voles. *Journal of Neuroscience, 23,* 3483–3490.

Aragona, B. J., Liu, Y., Yu, Y. J., Curtis, J. T., Detwiler, J. M., Insel, T. R., & Wang, Z. X. (2006). Nucleus accumbens dopamine differentially mediates the formation and maintenance of monogamous pair bonds. *Nature Neuroscience, 9,* 133–139.

Archer, J. (1988). *The behavioural biology of aggression.* Cambridge: Cambridge University Press.

Arnold, W., & Trillmich, F. (1985). Time budget in Galapagos fur seals: The influence of mother's presence and absence on pup activity and play. *Behaviour, 92,* 302–321.

Arnqvist, G., & Rowe, L. (2005). *Sexual conflict.* Princeton: Princeton University Press.

Atance, C. M., & Meltzoff, A. N. (2005). My future self: Young children's ability to anticipate and explain future states. *Cognitive Development, 20*, 341–361.

Atkinson, D., & Begon, M. (1987). Reproductive variation and adult size in two co-occurring grasshopper species. *Ecological Entomology, 12*, 119–127.

Attwell, D., & Laughlin, S. B. (2001). An energy budget for signaling in the grey matter of the brain. *Journal of Cerebral Blood Flow and Metabolism, 21*, 1133–1145.

Aubin, T., & Jouventin, P. (1998). Cocktail-party effect in king penguin colonies. *Proceedings of the Royal Society of London, Series B, 265*, 1665–1673.

Aubin, T., & Jouventin, P. (2002). How to vocally identify kin in a crowd: The penguin model. *Advances in the Study of Behavior, 31*, 243–277.

Aubin, T., Jouventin, P., & Hildebrand, C. (2000). Penguins use the two-voice system to recognize each other. *Proceedings of the Royal Society of London, Series B, 267*, 1081–1087.

Aviles, L., & Maddison, W. (1991). When is the sex ratio biased in social spiders? Chromosome studies of embryos and male meiosis in *Anelosimus* species (Aranae, Theridiidae). *Journal of Arachnology, 19*, 126–135.

Aviles, L., McCormack, J., Cutter, A., & Bukowski, T. (2000). Precise, highly female-biased sex ratios in a social spider. *Proceedings of the Royal Society of London, Series B, 267*, 1445–1449.

Aviles, L., Varas, C. & Dyreson, E. (1999). Does the African social spider *Stegodyphus dumicola* control the sex of individual offspring? *Behavioral Ecology and Sociobiology, 46*, 237–243.

Axelrod, R. (1984). *The evolution of cooperation.* New York: Basic Books.

Axelrod, R., & Hamilton, W. D. (1981). The evolution of cooperation. *Science, 211*, 1390–1396.

Bachman, G., & Widemo, F. (1999). Relationships between body composition, body size and alternative reproductive tactics in a lekking sandpiper, the ruff (*Philomachus pugnax*). *Functional Ecology, 13*, 411–416.

Badyaev, A. V., & Hill, G. E. (2002). Paternal care as a conditional strategy: Distinct reproductive tactics associated with elaboration of plumage ornamentation in the house finch. *Behavioral Ecology, 13*, 591–597.

Baerends, G. P., Wanders, J., & Vodegel, R. (1986). The relationship between marking patterns and motivational state in pre-spawning behavior of the cichlid fish *Chromidotilapia guentheri* (Sauvage). *Netherlands Journal of Zoology, 36*, 88–116.

Baerends-van Roon, J., & Baerends, G. (1979). *The morphogenesis of the behavior of the domestic cat, with special emphasis on the development of prey-catching.* Amsterdam: New Holland.

Bagg, A. (1952). Anting not exclusively an avian trait. *Journal of Mammalogy, 33*, 243.

Baillie, J. (1972). The behavioural requirements necessary for guide dogs for the blind in the United Kingdom. *British Veterinary Journal, 128*, 477.

Baker, R. R. (1978). *The evolutionary ecology of animal migration.* New York: Holmes & Meier Publishers.

Baker, R. R., & Bellis, M. A. (1988). Kamikaze sperm in mammals. *Animal Behaviour, 36*, 936–939.

Baker, R. R., & Bellis, M. A. (1993). Sperm competition: Ejaculate adjustment by males and the function of masturbation. *Animal Behaviour, 46*, 861–885.

Balaban, E., Alper, J. S., & Kasamon, Y. L. (1996). Mean genes and the biology of aggression: A critical review of recent animal and human research. *Journal of Neurogenetics, 11*, 1–43.

Balda, R., & Kamil, A. (1989). A comparative study of cache recovery by three corvid species. *Animal Behaviour, 38*, 486–495.

Balda, R., & Kamil, A. (1992). Long-term spatial memory in Clark's nutcracker, *Nucifraga columbiana. Animal Behaviour, 44*, 761–769.

Balda, R., Pepperberg, I., & Kamil, A. (Eds.). (1998). *Animal cognition in nature.* San Diego: Academic Press.

Baldwin, J. (1969). The ontogeny of social behavior of squirrel monkeys (*Saimiri sciureus*) in a seminatural environment. *Folia Primologica, 11*, 35–79.

Baldwin, J. (1971). The social organization of a semifree-ranging troop of squirrel monkeys (*Saimiri sciureus*). *Folia Primologica, 14*, 23–50.

Ball, G. F. (1993). The neural integration of environmental information by seasonally breeding birds. *American Zoologist, 33*, 185–199.

Ball, N., Amlaner, C., Shaffery, J., & Opp, M. (1988). Asynchronous eye-closure and unihemispheric quiet sleep of birds. In W. Koella, F. Obal, H. Schulz, & P. Visser (Eds.), *Sleep '86* (pp. 151–153). New York: Gustav Fischer Verlag.

Bandura, A. (1977). *Social learning theory.* Englewood Cliffs, NJ: Prentice Hall.

Bandura, A. (1986). *Social foundations of thought and action.* Englewood Cliffs, NJ: Prentice Hall.

Bandura, A., Ross, D., & Ross, S. (1961). Transmission of aggression through imitation of aggressive models. *Journal of Abnormal and Social Psychology, 63*, 572–582.

Barash, D. P. (1975). Marmot alarm calling and the question of altruistic behavior. *American Midland Naturalist, 94*, 468–470.

Barber, J. R., & Conner, W. E. (2007). Acoustic mimicry in a predator-prey system. *Proceedings of the National Academy of Sciences, 104*, 9331–9334.

Barkley, R., Neill, W., & Gooding, R. (1978). Skipjack tuna, *Katuwonus pelamis*, habitat based in temperature and oxygen requirements. *U.S. Fish and Wildlife Service Fishery Bulletin, 76*, 653–662.

Barlow, G. W. (1963). Ethology of the Asian teleost Badis badis. II. Motivation and signal value of colour patterns. *Physiological Zoology, 11*, 97–105.

Barnard, C. J. (Ed.). (1984). *Producers and scroungers.* London: Croom Helm/Chapman Hall.

Barnard, C. J., & Brown, C. A. (1984). A payoff asymmetry in resident-resident disputes between shrews. *Animal Behaviour, 32*, 302–304.

Barnard, C. J., & Sibly, R. M. (1981). Producers and scroungers: A general model and its application to captive flocks of house sparrows. *Animal Behaviour, 29*, 543–550.

Barron, A. B., & Robinson, G. E. (2005). Selective modulation of task performance by octopamine in honey bee (*Apis mellifera*) division of labour. *Journal of Comparative Physiology A, 191,* 659–668.

Barros, N. B. (1993). *Feeding ecology and foraging strategies of bottlenose dolphins of the Central East Coast of Florida.* Miami: University of Miami.

Bartolomucci, A. (2007). Social stress, immune functions and disease in rodents. *Frontiers in Neuroendocrinology, 28,* 28–49.

Bass, A. (1992). Dimorphic male brains and alternative reproductive tactics in a vocalizing fish. *Trends in Neurosciences, 15,* 139–145.

Bass, A. H. (1996). Shaping brain sexuality. *American Scientist, 84,* 352–363.

Bass, A. H. (1998). Behavioral and evolutionary neurobiology: A pluralistic approach. *American Zoologist, 38,* 97–107.

Bass, A., & Baker, R. (1990). Sexual dimorphisms in the vocal control system of a teleost fish: Morphological and physiological identified cells. *Journal of Neurobiology, 21,* 1155–1168.

Bass, A., & Baker, R. (1991). Adaptive modification of homologous vocal control traits in teleost fishes. *Brain, Behavior and Evolution, 38,* 240–254.

Bass, A., & Marchaterre, M. (1989). Sound-generating (sonic) motor system in a teleost fish (*Porichths notatus*): Sexual polymorphism in the ultrastructure of myofibrils. *Journal of Comparative Neurology, 286,* 141–153.

Bass, A. H., & McKibben, J. R. (2003). Neural mechanisms and behaviors for acoustic communication in teleost fish. *Progress in Neurobiology, 69,* 1–26.

Bass, A. H., & Zakon, H. H. (2005). Sonic and electric fish: At the crossroads of neuroethology and behavioral neuroendocrinology. *Hormones and Behavior, 48,* 360–372.

Bateman, A. J. (1948). Intra-sexual selection in *Drosophila. Heredity, 2,* 349–368.

Bateson, P. (1978). Early experience and sexual preferences. In J. B. Hutchinson (Ed.), *Biological determinants of sexual behavior* (pp. 29–53). New York: Wiley.

Bateson, P. (1990). Choice, preference and selection. In M. Bekoff & D. Jamieson (Eds.), *Interpretation and explanation in the study of animal behaviour* (Vol. 1, Interpretation, intentionality and communication, pp. 149–156). Boulder: Westview Press.

Bauer, G. B. (2005). Research training for releasable animals. *Conservation Biology, 19,* 1779–1789.

Baxter, D. A., & Byrne, J. H. (1990). Differential effects of cAMP and serotonin on membrane current, action potential duration, and excitability in somata of pleural sensory neurons of Aplysia. *Journal of Neurophysiology, 64,* 978–990.

Beacham, J. L. (2003). Models of dominance hierarchy formation: Effects of prior experience and intrinsic traits. *Behaviour, 140,* 1275–1303.

Beason, R. C., & Nichols, J. E. (1984). Magnetic orientation and magnetically sensitive material in a transequatorial migratory bird. *Nature, 309,* 151–153.

Beatty, W., Costello, K., & Berry, S. (1984). Suppression of play fighting by amphetamines: Effects of catecholamine antagonists, agonists and synthesis inhibitors. *Pharmacology Biochemistry and Behavior, 20,* 747–755.

Beatty, W. W., Dodge, A. M., Traylor, K. L., & Meaney, M. J. (1981). Temporal boundary of the sensitive period for hormonal organization of social play in juvenile rats. *Physiology & Behavior, 26,* 241–243.

Beauchamp, G. (1997). Determinants of interspecific brood amalgamation in waterfowl. *Auk, 114,* 11–21.

Beaugrand, J. P., & Zayan, R. (1985). An experimental model of aggressive dominance in *Xiphophorus helleri. Behavioural Processes, 10,* 1–52.

Beck, B. (1980). *Animal tool behavior: The use and manufacture of tools by animals.* New York: Garland STPM Press.

Beebee, T. (1995). Tadpole growth: Is there an interference effect in nature? *Herpetological Journal, 5,* 204–205.

Beebee, T., & Wong, A. (1992). Prototheca-mediated interference competition between anuran larvae operates by resource diversion. *Physiological Zoology, 65,* 815–831.

Beecher, M. D., Beecher, I., & Hahn, S. (1981a). Parent-offspring recognition in bank swallows: II. Development and acoustic basis. *Animal Behaviour, 29,* 95–101.

Beecher, M. D., Beecher, I., & Lumpkin, S. (1981b). Parent-offspring recognition in bank swallows: I. Natural history. *Animal Behaviour, 29,* 86–94.

Beecher, M. D., & Brenowitz, E. A. (2005). Functional aspects of song learning in songbirds. *Trends in Ecology and Evolution, 20,* 143–149.

Beecher, M. D., Campbell, S. E., & Nordby, J. C. (1998). The cognitive ecology of song communication and song learning in the song sparrow. In R. Dukas, R. (Ed.), *Cognitive ecology* (pp. 175–199). Chicago: University of Chicago Press.

Beecher, M. D., Medvin, B., Stoddard, P., & Loesch, P. (1986). Acoustic adaptations for parent-offspring recognition in swallows. *Experimental Biology, 45,* 179–193.

Beissinger, S. R. (1996). On the limited breeding opportunities hypothesis for avian clutch size. *American Naturalist, 147,* 655–658.

Bekoff, M. (1977). Social communication in canids: Evidence for the evolution of a stereotyped mammalian display. *Science, 1971,* 1097–1099.

Bekoff, M. (1995). Play signals as punctuation: The structure of play in social canids. *Behaviour, 132,* 419–429.

Bekoff, M. (2000). Social play behavior: Cooperation, fairness, trust, and the evolution of morality. *Journal of Consciousness Studies, 8,* 81–90.

Bekoff, M. (2004). Wild justice and fair play: Cooperation, forgiveness, and morality in animals. *Biology & Philosophy, 19,* 489–520.

Bekoff, M. (2007). *The emotional lives of animals: A leading scientist explores animal joy, sorrow, and empathy.* Novato, CA: New World Library.

Bekoff, M., & Allen, C. (1998). Intentional communication and social play: How and why animals negotiate and agree to play. In M. Bekoff & J. Byers, J. (Eds.), *Animal play: Evolutionary, comparative and ecological perspectives* (pp. 97–114). Cambridge: Cambridge University Press.

Bekoff, M., & Byers, J. (1981). A critical reanalysis of the ontogeny and phylogeny of mammalian social and locomotor play: An ethological hornet's nest. In K. Immelman, G. Barlow, L. Petrinivich, & M. Main (Eds.), *Behavioral development* (pp. 296–337). Cambridge: Cambridge University Press.

Bekoff, M., & Byers, J. (Eds.). (1998). *Animal play: Evolutionary, comparative and ecological perspectives.* Cambridge: Cambridge University Press.

Bell, A. M. (2007). Future directions in behavioural syndromes research. *Proceedings of the Royal Society of London, Series B, 274,* 755–761.

Bell, G. (1997). *Selection: The mechanism of evolution.* New York: Chapman and Hall.

Bellis, M. A., Baker, R. R., & Gage, M. J. G. (1990). Variation in rat ejaculates consistent with the kamikaze sperm hypothesis. *Journal of Mammalogy, 71,* 479–480.

Bellrose, F., & Holm, D. (1994). *Ecology and management of the wood duck.* Mechanicsburg, PA: Stackpole Books.

Belovsky, G. E. (1978). Diet optimization in a generalist herbivore: The moose. *Theoretical Population Biology, 14,* 105–134.

Ben-Shahar, Y., Dudek, N. L., & Robinson, G. E. (2004). Phenotypic deconstruction reveals involvement of manganese transporter malvolio in honey bee division of labor. *Journal of Experimental Biology, 207,* 3281–3288.

Benavides, T., & Drummond, H. (2007). The role of trained winning in a broodmate dominance hierarchy. *Behaviour, 144,* 1133–1146.

Bennett, A., Cuthill, I. C., Partridge, J. C., & Maier, E. (1996). Ultraviolet vision and mate choice in zebra finches. *Nature, 380,* 433–435.

Bercovitch, F. (1988). Coalitions, cooperation and reproductive tactics among adult male baboons. *Animal Behaviour, 36,* 1198–1209.

Bereczkei, T., Gyuris, P., & Weisfeld, G. E. (2004). Sexual imprinting in human mate choice. *Proceedings of the Royal Society of London, Series B, 271,* 1129–1134.

Berger, J. (1979). Weaning conflict in desert and mountain bighorn sheep: An ecological interpretation. *Zeitschrift fur Tierpsychologie, 50,* 187–200.

Berger, J. (1980). The ecology, structure and function of social play in bighorn sheep (*Ovis canedensis*). *Journal of Zoology (London), 192,* 531–542.

Berger, R. J., & Phillips, N. H. (1995). Energy conservation and sleep. *Behavioural Brain Research, 69,* 65–73.

Berglund, A., & Rosenqvist, G. (2003). Sex role reversal in pipefish. *Advances in the Study of Behavior, 32,* 131–167.

Bergman, A., & Feldman, M. (1995). On the evolution of learning: Representation of a stochastic environment. *Theoretical Population Biology, 48,* 251–276.

Bernasconi, G., & Strassmann, J. E. (1999). Cooperation among unrelated individuals: The ant foundress case. *Trends in Ecology and Evolution, 14,* 477–482.

Berthold, P. (1990). Wegzugbeginn und Einsetzen der zugunruhe bei 19 Vogelpopulationen: Eine vergleichende untersuchung. In R. van den Elzen, K. Schuchmann, K. Schmidt-Koenig, K. (Eds.), *Proceedings of the International Centennial Meeting of the DO-G, Current topics in avian biology* (pp. 217–22). Bonn: DO-G.

Bertram, B. (1978). Living in groups: Predators and prey. In J. R. Krebs & N. B. Davies (Eds.), *Behavioural ecology: An evolutionary approach* (pp. 64–96). Oxford: Blackwell Science.

Biardi, J. E., Chien, D. C., & Coss, R. G. (2005). California ground squirrel (*Spermophilus beecheyi*) defenses against rattlesnake venom digestive and hemostatic toxins. *Journal of Chemical Ecology, 31,* 2501–2518.

Biardi, J. E., Chien, D. C., & Coss, R. G. (2006). California ground squirrel (*Spermophilus beecheyi*) defenses against rattlesnake venom digestive and hemostatic toxins. *Journal of Chemical Ecology, 32,* 137–154.

Biardi, J. E., Coss, R. G., & Smith, D. G. (2000). California ground squirrel (*Spermophilus beecheyi*) blood sera inhibits crotalid venom proteolytic activity. *Toxicon, 38,* 713–721.

Biben, M. (1986). Individual- and sex-related strategies of wrestling play in captive squirrel monkeys. *Ethology, 71,* 229–241.

Biben, M. (1998). Squirrel monkey playfighting: Making the case for a cognitive function for play. In M. Bekoff & J. Byers (Eds.), *Animal play: Evolutionary, comparative and ecological perspectives* (pp. 161–182). Cambridge: Cambridge University Press.

Bildstein, K. L. (1983). Why white-tailed deer flag their tails. *American Naturalist, 121,* 709–715.

Billen, J., & Morgan, E. D. (1997). Pheromonal communication in social insects: Sources and secretions. In R. Vander Meer, M. Breed, K. Espelie, & M. Winston (Eds.), *Pheromonal communication in social insects* (pp. 3–33). Boulder, CO: Westview Press.

Billing, J., & Sherman, P. W. (1998). Antimicrobial functions of spices: Why some like it hot. *Quarterly Review of Biology, 73,* 3–49.

Birkhead, T., & Møller, A. (1992). *Sperm competition in birds.* London: Academic Press.

Birkhead, T., & Møller, A. (1998). *Sperm competition and sexual selection.* London: Academic Press.

Birkhead, T. R., & Pizzari, T. (2002). Postcopulatory sexual selection. *Nature Reviews Genetics, 3,* 262–273.

Bischof, H. J., & Clayton, N. (1991). Stabilization of sexual preferences by sexual experience in male zebra finches, *Taeniopygia guttata castanotis. Behaviour, 118,* 144–154.

Bischof, H. J., & Rollenhagen, A. (1999). Behavioural and neurophysiological aspects of sexual imprinting in zebra finches. *Behavioural Brain Research, 98,* 267–276.

Bishop, D. T., Cannings, C., & Maynard Smith, J. (1978). The war of attrition with random rewards. *Journal of Theoretical Biology, 74,* 377–388.

Bishop, J. M., Jarvis, J. U. M., Spinks, A. C., Bennett, N. C., & O'Ryan, C. (2004). Molecular insight into patterns of colony composition and paternity in the common mole-rat *Cryptomys hottentotus hottentotus. Molecular Ecology, 13,* 1217–1229.

Bitterman, M. (1975). The comparative analysis of learning. *Science, 188,* 699–709.

Blackburn, J., Pfaus, J., & Phillips, A. (1992). Dopamine functions in appetitive and defensive behaviors. *Progress in Neurobiology, 39,* 247–249.

Blaffer-Hrdy, S. B. (1977). Infanticide as a primate reproductive strategy. *American Scientist, 65,* 40–49.

Blaffer-Hrdy, S. (1979). Infanticide among animals. *Ethology and Sociobiology, 1,* 13–40.

Blake, M., Udelsman, R., Feulner, G., Norton, D., & Holbrook, N. (1991). Stress induced shock protein 70 expression in adrenal cortex: An adrenocorticotropic hormone-sensitive, age-dependent response. *Proceedings of the National Academy of Sciences, U.S.A.*, 88, 9873–9877.

Blanco, J., Reig, S., & Cuesta, L. (1992). Distribution, status and conservation problems of the wolf (*Canis lupis*) in Spain. *Biological Conservation*, 60, 73–80.

Blaustein, A. (1983). Kin recognition mechanisms: Phenotype matching or recognition alleles. *American Naturalist, 121*, 749–754.

Blaustein, A. R., & Bancroft, B. A. (2007). Amphibian population declines: Evolutionary considerations. *Bioscience*, 57, 437–444.

Bloch, G., Toma, D. P., & Robinson, G. E. (2001). Behavioral rhythmicity, age, division of labor and period expression in the honey bee brain. *Journal of Biological Rhythms*, 16, 444–456.

Boehm, C. (1992). Segmentary warfare and management of conflict: A comparison of East African chimpanzees and patrilineal-patrilocal humans. In A. H. Harcourt & F. B. M. de Waal (Eds.), *Coalitions and alliances in humans and other animals* (pp. 137–173). Oxford: Oxford University Press.

Boesch, C. (1994a). Cooperative hunting in wild chimpanzees. *Animal Behaviour*, 48, 653–667.

Boesch, C. (1994b). Hunting strategies of Gombe and Tai chimpanzees. In R. W. Wrangham, W. C. McGrew, F. B. M. de Waal, & P. G. Heltne (Eds.), *Chimpanzee cultures* (pp. 77–91). Cambridge, MA: Harvard University Press.

Boesch, C. (2002). Cooperative hunting roles among Tai chimpanzees. *Human Nature, 13*, 27–46.

Boesch, C., & Boesch, H. (1989). Hunting behavior of wild chimpanzees in the Tai National Park. *American Journal of Physical Anthropology*, 78, 547–573.

Boissy, A. (1995). Fear and fearfulness in animals. *Quarterly Review of Biology*, 70, 165–191.

Bolig, R., Price, C., O'Neill, P., & Suomi, S. (1992). Subjective assessment of reactivity level and personality traits of rhesus monkeys. *International Journal of Primatology*, 13, 287–306.

Bonabeau, E., Theraulaz, G., & Deneubourg, J. L. (1996). Mathematical model of self-organizing hierarchies in animal societies. *Bulletin of Mathematical Biology*, 58, 661–717.

Bonabeau, E., Theraulaz, G., & Deneubourg, J. L. (1999). Dominance orders in animal societies: The self-organization hypothesis revisited. *Bulletin of Mathematical Biology*, 61, 727–757.

Bonner, J. T. (1980). *The evolution of culture in animals*. Princeton: Princeton University Press.

Borgerhoff-Mulder, M. (1988). Kipsigis bridewealth payments. In L. Betzig, M. Borgerhoff-Mulder, & P. Turke (Eds.), *Human reproductive behaviour: A Darwinian perspective* (pp. 65–82). Cambridge: Cambridge University Press.

Borgerhoff-Mulder, M. (1990). Kipsigis women's preferences for wealthy men: Evidence for female choice in mammals. *Behavioral Ecology and Sociobiology*, 27, 255–264.

Both, C., Dingemanse, N. J., Drent, P. J., & Tinbergen, J. M. (2005). Pairs of extreme avian personalities have highest reproductive success. *Journal of Animal Ecology*, 74, 667–674.

Bottger, K. (1974). Zur biologie von *Sphaerodema grassei ghesquieri*. Studien an zentralafrikanischen belostomatiden (Heteroptera: Insecta) I. *Archive fur Hydrobiologie*, 74, 100–122.

Boucher, D. (Ed). (1985). *The biology of mutualism: Ecology and evolution*. Oxford: Oxford University Press.

Boulton, M. J. (1991). Partner preferences in middle school children's playful fighting and chasing. *Ethology and Sociobiology*, 12, 177–193.

Boyd, R., & Richerson, P. J. (1985). *Culture and the evolutionary process*. Chicago: University of Chicago Press.

Boyd, R., & Richerson, P. J. (2004). *Not by genes alone*. Chicago: University of Chicago Press.

Boyd, R., & Richerson, P. J. (2005). *The origin and evolution of cultures*. New York: Oxford University Press.

Boyse, E., Beauchamp, G., Yamazaki, K., & Bard, J. (1991). Genetic components of kin recognition in mammals. In P. G. Hepper (Ed.), *Kin recognition* (pp. 162–219). Cambridge: Cambridge University Press.

Bradbury, J. W., & Vehrencamp, S. (1977). Social organization and foraging in emballonurid bats. III. Mating systems. *Behavioural Ecology and Sociobiology*, 2, 1–17.

Braithwaite, V. A., & de Perera, T. B. (2006). Short-range orientation in fish: How fish map space. *Marine and Freshwater Behaviour and Physiology*, 39, 37–47.

Brantley, R., & Bass, A. (1994). Alternative male spawning tactics and acoustic signalling in the plainfin midshipman fish, *Porichtys notatus*. *Ethology*, 96, 213–232.

Brass, M., & Heyes, C. (2005). Imitation: Is cognitive neuroscience solving the correspondence problem? *Trends in Cognitive Sciences*, 9, 489–495.

Braude, S. (2000). Dispersal and new colony formation in wild naked mole-rats: Evidence against inbreeding as the system of mating. *Behavioral Ecology*, 11, 7–12.

Bray, J. (1988). Children's development during early remarriage. In E. M. Hetherington & J. D. Arasteh (Eds.), *Impact of divorce, single parenting and stepparenting on children* (pp. 279–298). Hillsdale, NJ: Lawrence Erlbaum Associates.

Brenowitz, E. A. (1997). Comparative approaches to the avian song system. *Journal of Neurobiology*, 33, 517–531.

Brick, O. (1999). A test of the sequential assessment game: The effect of increased cost of sampling. *Behavioral Ecology*, 10, 726–732.

Brightsmith, D. J. (2005). Competition, predation and nest niche shifts among tropical cavity nesters: Phylogeny and natural history evolution of parrots (Psittaciformes) and trogons (Trogoniformes). *Journal of Avian Biology*, 36, 64–73.

Bronstein, J. L. (1994). Our current understanding of mutualism. *Quarterly Review of Biology*, 69, 31–51.

Broom, M., & Ruxton, G. D. (2003). Evolutionarily stable kleptoparasitism: Consequences of different prey types. *Behavioral Ecology*, 14, 23–33.

Brown, C. R. (1986). Cliff swallow colonies as information centers. *Science*, 234, 83–85.

Brown, C. (1988). Social foraging in cliff swallows: Local enhancement, risk sensitivity and the avoidance of predators. *Animal Behaviour*, 36, 780–792.

Brown, C. R., & Brown, M. B. (1992). Ectoparasitism as a cause of natal dispersal in cliff swallows. *Ecology*, 73, 1718–1723.

Brown, C., & Brown, M. B. (2000). Heritable basis for choice of group size in a colonial bird. *Proceedings of the National Academy of Sciences, U.S.A., 97*, 14825–14830.

Brown, C. R., & Brown, M. B. (2004a). Empirical measurement of parasite transmission between groups in a colonial bird. *Ecology, 85*, 1619–1626.

Brown, C. R., & Brown, M. B. (2004b). Group size and ectoparasitism affect daily survival probability in a colonial bird. *Behavioral Ecology and Sociobiology, 56*, 498–511.

Brown, C., Brown, M. B., & Shaffer, M. L. (1991). Food-sharing signals among socially foraging cliff swallows. *Animal Behaviour, 42*, 551–564.

Brown, C., Jones, F., & Braithwaite, V. (2005). In situ examination of boldness-shyness traits in the tropical poeciliid, *Brachyraphis episcopi. Animal Behaviour, 70*, 1003–1009.

Brown, C., & Laland, K. N. (2002). Social learning of a novel avoidance task in the guppy: Conformity and social release. *Animal Behaviour, 64*, 41–47.

Brown, J. L. (1969). The buffer effect and productivity in tit populations. *American Naturalist, 103*, 347–354.

Brown, J. L. (1974). Alternate routes to sociality in jays with a theory for the evolution of altruism and communal breeding. *Amerian Zoologist, 14*, 63–80.

Brown, J. L. (1975). *The evolution of behavior.* New York: Norton.

Brown, J. L. (1982). Optimal group size in territorial animals. *Journal of Theoretical Biology, 95*, 793–810.

Brown, J. L. (1983). Cooperation: A biologist's dilemma. In J. S. Rosenblatt (Ed.), *Advances in the study of behavior* (Vol. 13, pp. 1–37). New York: Academic Press.

Brown, J. L. (1987). *Helping and communal breeding in birds.* Princeton: Princeton University Press.

Brown, J. L., Brown, E., Brown, S. D., & Dow, D. D. (1982). Helpers: Effects of experimental removal on reproductive success. *Science, 215*, 421–422.

Brown, J. S., & Rosenzweig, M. L. (1985). Habitat selection in slowly regenerating environments. *Journal of Theoretical Biology, 123*, 151–171.

Brown, M., Hopkins, W., & Keynes, R. (1991). *Essentials of neural development.* Cambridge: Cambridge University Press.

Brumm, H., & Slabbekoorn, H. (2005). Acoustic communication in noise. *Advances in the Study of Behavior, 35*, 151–209.

Bruner, J., Jolly, A., & Sylva, K. (Eds.). (1976). *Play: Its role in development and evolution.* New York: Basic Books.

Brush, A. (1990). Metabolism of carotenoid pigments in birds. *Federation of American Societies for Experimental Biology Journal, 4*, 2969–2977.

Brush, A., & Power, D. (1976). House finch pigmentation, carotenoid pigmentation and the effect of diet. *Auk, 93*, 725–739.

Brush, F. R. (2003). Selection for differences in avoidance learning: The Syracuse strains differ in anxiety, not learning ability. *Behavior Genetics, 33*, 677–696.

Brush, F. R., Gendron, C. M., & Isaacson, M. D. (1999). A selective genetic analysis of the Syracuse high- and low-avoidance (SHA/Bru and SLA/Bru) strains of rats (*Rattus norvegicus*). *Behavioural Brain Research, 106*, 1–11.

B'shary, R., & Bronstein, J. L. (2004). Game structures in mutualistic interactions: What can the evidence tell us about the kind of models we need? *Advances in the Study of Behavior, 34*, 59–101.

B'shary, R., Wickler, W., & Fricke, H. (2002). Fish cognition: A primate's eye view. *Animal Cognition, 5*, 1–13.

Burgdorf, J., Panksepp, J., Brudzynski, S. M., Kroes, R., Moskal, J. R. (2005). Breeding for 50–kHz positive affective vocalization in rats. *Behavior Genetics, 35*, 67–72.

Burgess, J. W. (1976). Social spiders. *Scientific American,* March 1976, 100–106.

Burghardt, G. (1988). Precocity, play and the ectotherm-endotherm transition. *Behaviour, 36*, 246–257.

Burghardt, G. (1998). The evolutionary origins of play revisited: Lessons from turtles. In M. Bekoff & J. Byers (Eds.), *Animal play: Evolutionary, comparative and ecological perspectives* (pp. 1–26). Cambridge: Cambridge University Press.

Burghardt, G. (2005). *The genesis of animal play: Testing the limits.* Cambridge, MA: MIT Press.

Buss, A., & Plomin, R. (1986). The EAS approach to temperament. In R. Plomin & J. Dunn (Eds.), *The study of temperament: Changes, continuities and challenges* (pp. 67–79). Hillsdale, NJ: Lawrence Erlbaum Associates.

Busse, C. (1978). Do chimps hunt cooperatively? *American Naturalist, 112*, 767–770.

Butcher, G., & Rohwer, S. (1989). The evolution of conspicuous and distinctive coloration for communication in birds. *Current Ornithology, 6*, 51–107.

Byers, J. (1984). Play in ungulates. In P. K. Smith (Ed.), *Play in animals and humans* (pp. 43–65). Oxford: Blackwell Science

Byers, J. (1998). Biological effects of locomotor play: Getting into shape or something more specific. In M. Bekoff & J. Byers (Eds.), *Animal play: Evolutionary, comparative and ecological perspectives* (pp. 205–220). Cambridge: Cambridge University Press.

Byers, J. A., Moodie, J. D., & Hall, N. (1994). Pronghorn females choose vigorous mates. *Animal Behaviour, 47*, 33–43.

Byers, J., & Waits, L. (2006). Good genes sexual selection in nature. *Proceedings of the National Academy of Sciences, U.S.A., 103*, 16343–16345.

Byers, J., & Walker, C. (1995). Refining the motor training hypothesis for the evolution of play. *American Naturalist, 146*, 25–40.

Bygott, J. D. (1979). Agonistic behavior, dominance and social structure in wild chimpanzees of the Gombe National Park. In D. A. Hamburg & E. R. McCown (Eds.), *The great apes.* Menlo Park, CA: Benjamin/Cummings.

Bygott, J. D., Bertram, B., & Hanby, J. P. (1979). Male lions in large coalitions gain reproductive advantages. *Nature, 282*, 839–841.

Byrne, P. G., Simmons, L. W., & Roberts, J. D. (2003). Sperm competition and the evolution of gamete morphology in frogs. *Proceedings of the Royal Society of London, Series B, 270*, 2079–2086.

Byrne, R. W. (1993). Do larger brains mean greater intelligence? *Behavioral and Brain Sciences, 16*, 696–697.

Byrne, R. W. (2002). Imitation of novel complex actions: What does the evidence from animals mean? *Advances in the Study of Behavior, 31*, 77–105.

Cafaro, M. J., & Currie, C. R. (2005). Phylogenetic analysis of mutualistic filamentous bacteria associated with fungus-growing ants. *Canadian Journal of Microbiology, 51*, 441–446.

Cahan, S., & Julian, G. E. (1999). Fitness consequences of cooperative colony founding in the desert leaf-cutter ant *Acromyrmex versicolor*. *Behavioral Ecology, 10*, 585–591.

Caldwell, R. (1986). Withholding information on sexual condition as a competitive mechanism. In L. Drickamer, *Behavioral ecology and population biology* (pp. 83–88). Toulouse: Privat.

Caldwell, R. (1992). Recognition, signalling and reduced aggression between former mates in a stomatopod. *Animal Behaviour, 44*, 11–19.

Callahan, G. N. (2003). Eating dirt. *Emerging Infectious Diseases, 9*, 1016–1021.

Cameron, E., Day, T., & Rowe, L. (2003). Sexual conflict and indirect benefits. *Journal of Evolutionary Biology, 16*, 1055–1060.

Campbell, C., Steffen-Campbell, J., & Werren, J. H. (1993). Phylogeny of the *Nasonia* species complex (Hymenoptera: Pteromalidae) inferred from internal transcribed spacer (T2) and 28s rDNA sequences. *Insect Molecular Biology, 2*, 225–237.

Campbell, T., Lin, S., DeVries, C., & Lambert, K. (2003). Coping strategies in male and female rats exposed to multiple stressors. *Physiology and Behavior, 78*, 495–504.

Cannon, W. (1915). *Bodily changes in pain, hunger, fear and rage.* New York: Appleton.

Capaldi, E. A., Robinson, G. E., & Fahrbach, S. E. (1999). Neuroethology of spatial learning: The birds and the bees. *Annual Review of Psychology, 50*, 651–682.

Caraco, T. (1979). Time budgeting and group size: A test of theory. *Ecology, 60*, 618–627.

Caraco, T. (1980). On foraging time allocation in a stochastic environment. *Ecology, 61*, 119–128.

Caraco, T., Martindale, S., & Whitham, M. (1980). An empirical demonstration of risk sensitive foraging preferences. *Animal Behaviour, 28*, 820–830.

Carlier, P., & Lefebvre, L. (1996). Differences in individual learning between group-foraging and territorial *Zenaida* doves. *Behaviour, 133*, 1197–1207.

Caro, T. (1980). Effects of the mother, object play and adult experience on predation in cats. *Behavioural and Neural Biology, 29*, 29–51.

Caro, T. (1994a). *Cheetahs of the Serengeti Plains.* Chicago: University of Chicago Press.

Caro, T. M. (1994b). Ungulate antipredator behavior: Preliminary and comparative data from African bovids. *Behaviour, 128*, 189–228.

Caro, T. M. (1995a). Pursuit-deterrence revisited. *Trends in Ecology & Evolution, 10*, 500–503.

Caro, T. M. (1995b). Short-term costs and correlates of play in cheetahs. *Animal Behaviour, 49*, 333–345.

Caro, T. M., & Bateson, P. (1986). Organization and ontogeny of alternative tactics. *Animal Behaviour, 34*, 1483–1499.

Caro, T. M., Graham, C. M., Stoner, C. J., & Vargas, J. K. (2004). Adaptive significance of antipredator behaviour in artiodactyls. *Animal Behaviour, 67*, 205–228.

Caro, T. M., & Hauser, M. D. (1992). Is there teaching in nonhuman animals? *Quarterly Review of Biology, 67*, 151–174.

Caro, T. M., Lombardo, L., Goldizen, A. W., & Kelly, M. (1995). Tail-flagging and other antipredator signals in white deer: New data and synthesis. *Behavioral Ecology, 6*, 442–450.

Carpenter, C. R. (1934). A field study of the behavior and social relations of howling monkeys. *Comparative Psychology Monographs, 10*, 1–168.

Carpenter, C. R. (1942). Sexual behavior of free-ranging rhesus monkeys, *M. mulatta*. *Journal of Comparative Psychology, 33*, 113–162.

Carranza, J., Alarcos, S., Sanchez-Prieto, C. B., Valencia, J., & Mateos, C. (2004). Disposable-soma senescence mediated by sexual selection in an ungulate. *Nature, 432*, 215–218.

Carroll, S. (2007). *The making of the fittest.* New York: Norton.

Carter, C. S., Devries, A. C., & Getz, L. L. (1995). Physiological substrates of mammalian monogamy: The prairie vole model. *Neuroscience and Biobehavioral Reviews, 19*, 303–314.

Cassey, P., Blackburn, T. M., Sol, S., Duncan, R. P., & Lockwood, J. L. (2004). Global patterns of introduction effort and establishment success in birds. *Proceedings of the Royal Society of London, Series B, 271*, S405–S408.

Catchpole, C., & Slater, P. (Ed). (1995). *Bird song: Biological themes and variation.* New York: Cambridge University Press.

Cavalli-Sforza, L. L., & Feldman, M. W. (1981). *Cultural transmission and evolution: A quantitative approach.* Princeton: Princeton University Press.

Cavigelli, S. A. (2005). Animal personality and health. *Behaviour, 142*, 1223–1244.

Chamberlin, T. (1897). The method of multiple working hypotheses. *Journal of Geology, 5*, 837–848.

Chapais, B. (1992). The role of alliances in social inheritance of rank among female primates. In A. H. Harcourt & F. B. M. de Waal (Eds.), *Coalitions and alliances in humans and other animals* (pp. 29–59). Oxford: Oxford University Press.

Charnov, E. L. (1976). Optimal foraging, the marginal value theorem. *Theoretical Population Biology, 9*, 129–136.

Charnov, E. L., & Krebs, J. R. (1975). The evolution of alarm calls: Altruism or manipulation? *American Naturalist, 109*, 107–112.

Chase, I. (1974). Models of hierarchy formation in animal societies. *Behavioral Science, 19*, 374–382.

Chase, I. D. (1982). Dynamics of hierarchy formation: The sequential development of dominance relationships. *Behaviour, 80*, 218–240.

Chase, I. D. (1985). The sequential analysis of aggressive acts during hierarchy formation: An application of the "jigsaw puzzle" approach. *Animal Behaviour, 33*, 86–100.

Chase, I., Bartolomeo, C., & Dugatkin, L. A. (1994). Aggressive interactions and inter-contest interval: How long do winners keep winning? *Animal Behaviour, 48*, 393–400.

Cheney, D. L., & Seyfarth, R. M. (1990). *How monkeys see the world.* Chicago: University of Chicago Press.

Chesser, R. T., & Levey, D. J. (1998). Austral migrants and the evolution of migration in new world birds: Diet, habitat, and migration revisited. *American Naturalist, 152*, 311–319.

Chinen, A., Matsumoto, Y., & Kawamura, S. (2005). Reconstitution of ancestral green visual pigments of zebrafish and molecular mechanism of their spectral differentiation. *Molecular Biology and Evolution, 22*, 1001–1010.

Chivers, D. P., Wisenden, B. D., & Smith, R. J. F. (1996). Damselfly larvae learn to recognize predators from chemical cues in the predator's diet. *Animal Behaviour, 52*, 315–320.

Choleris, E., Gustafsson, J. A., Korach, K. S., Muglia, L. J., Pfaff, D. W., & Ogawa, S. (2003). An estrogen-dependent four-gene micronet regulating social recognition: A study with oxytocin and estrogen receptor-alpha and -beta knockout mice. *Proceedings of the National Academy of Sciences, U.S.A., 100*, 6192–6197.

Choleris, E., Kavaliers, M., & Pfaff, D. W. (2004). Functional genomics of social recognition. *Journal of Neuroendocrinology, 16*, 383–389.

Christensen, J. W., Rundgren, M., & Olsson, K. (2006). Training methods for horses: Habituation to a frightening stimulus. *Equine Veterinary Journal, 38*, 439–443.

Church, S., Bennett, A., Cuthill, I., & Partridge, J. (1998). Ultraviolet cues affect the foraging behaviour of blue tits. *Proceedings of the Royal Society of London, Series B, 265*, 1509–1514.

Claar, j., Klaver, R., & Servheen, C. (1986). Grizzly bear management on the Flathead Indian Reservation, Montana. *International Conference of Bear Research and Management, 6*, 203–208.

Clark, A. B., & Ehlinger, T. J. (1987). Pattern and adaptation in individual behavioral differences. In P. P. G. Bateson & P. H. Klopfer (Eds.), *Perspectives in ethology* (Vol. 7, pp. 1–45). New York: Plenum Press.

Clark, L., & Mason, J. (1985). Use of nest material as insecticidal and antipathogenic agents by the European starling. *Oecologia, 67*, 169–176.

Clark, L., & Mason, J. (1988). Effect of biologically active plants used as nest material and the derived benefit to starling nestlings. *Oecologia, 77*, 174–180.

Clark, M., Crews, D., & Galef, B. (1991). Concentrations of sex steroid hormones in pregnant and fetal Mongolian gerbils. *Physiology and Behavior, 49*, 239–243.

Clark, M., & Galef, B. (1999). A testosterone mediated trade-off between parental care and sexual effort in male Mongolian gerbils, *Meriones unguiculatus. Journal of Comparative Psychology, 113*, 388–395.

Clark, M., & Galef, B. (2000). Why some male Mongolian gerbils may help at the nest: Testosterone, asexuality and alloparenting. *Animal Behaviour, 59*, 801–806.

Clark, M. M., Johnson, J., & Galef, B. G. (2004). Sexual motivation suppresses paternal behaviour of male gerbils during their mates' postpartum oestrus. *Animal Behaviour, 67*, 49–57.

Clark, M., vom Saal, F., & Galef, B. (1992a). Fetal intrauterine position correlates with endogenous testosterone levels of adult Mongolian gerbils. *Physiology and Behavior, 51*, 957–960.

Clark, M. M., Tucker, L., & Galef, B. G. (1992b). Stud males and dud males: Intrauterine position effects on the reproductive success of male gerbils. *Animal Behaviour, 43*, 215–221.

Clark, M., Vonk, J., & Galef, B. (1998). Intrauterine position, parenting and nest-sites attachment in male Mongolian gerbils. *Developmental Psychobiology, 32*, 177–181.

Clarke, J. A. (1983). Moonlight's influence on predator/prey interactions between short-eared owls (*Asio flammeus*) and deer mice (*Peromyscus maniculatus*). *Behavioral Ecology and Sociobiology, 13*, 205–209.

Clayton, D. F. (2004). Songbird genomics: Methods, mechanisms, opportunities, and pitfalls. In H. P. Zeigler & P. Marler (Eds.), *Behavioral neurobiology of birdsong* (Vol. 1016, pp. 45–60). New York: New York Academy of Sciences.

Clayton, N. S., & Dickinson, A. (1998). Episodic-like memory during cache recovery by scrub jays. *Nature, 395*, 272–274.

Clemens, L. G., Gladue, B. A., & Coniglio, L. P. (1978). Prenatal endogenous androgenic influences on masculine sexual behavior and genital morphology in male and female rats. *Hormones and Behavior, 10*, 40–53.

Clements, K. C., & Stephens, D. W. (1995). Testing models of non-cooperation: Mutualism and the prisoner's dilemma. *Animal Behavior, 50*, 527–535.

Close, R. (1972). Dynamic properties of fast and slow skeletal muscles of the rat during development. *Journal of Physiology, 173*, 74–95.

Clotfelter, E. D., O'Hare, E. P., McNitt, M. M., Carpenter, R. E., & Summers, C. H. (2007). Serotonin decreases aggression via 5–HT1A receptors in the fighting fish *Betta splendens. Pharmacology Biochemistry and Behavior, 87*, 222–231.

Clunie, F. (1976). Jungle mynah "anting" with a millipede. *Notornis, 23*, 77.

Clutton-Brock, T., & Albon, S. (1979). The roaring of red deer and the evolution of honest advertising. *Behaviour, 49*, 145–169.

Clutton-Brock, T., Albon, S., Gibson, S., & Guinness, F. (1979). The logical stag: Adaptive aspects of fighting in the red deer. *Animal Behaviour, 27*, 211–225.

Clutton-Brock, T., & Harvey, P. (1980). Primates, brain and ecology. *Journal of Zoology, London, 190*, 309–323.

Clutton-Brock, T. H., & Langley, P. (1997). Persistent courtship reduces male and female longevity in captive tsetse flies *Glossina morsitans morsitans* Westwood (Diptera: Glossinidae). *Behavioral Ecology, 8*, 392–395.

Coccaro, E. (1992). Impulsive aggression and central serotonergic system function in humans: An example of a dimensional brain-behavior relationship. *International Clinical Psychopharmacology, 7*, 3–12.

Coleman, K., & Wilson, D. S. (1998). Shyness and boldness in pumpkinseed sunfish: Individual differences are context-specific. *Animal Behaviour, 56*, 927–936.

Coleman, R., Gross, M., & Sargent, R. C. (1985). Parental investment decision rules: A test in bluegill sunfish. *Behavioral Ecology and Sociobiology, 18*, 59–66.

Connor, R. (1992). Dolphin alliances and coalitions. In A. H. Harcourt, & F. B. M. de Waal (Eds.), *Coalitions and alliances in humans and other animals* (pp. 415–443). Oxford: Oxford University Press.

Connor, R. C. (1995). The benefits of mutualism: A conceptual framework. *Biological Review, 70*, 427–457.

Connor, R. C., Heithaus, M. R., & Barre, L. M. (2001). Complex social structure, alliance stability and mating access in a bottlenose dolphin "super-alliance." *Proceedings of the Royal Society of London, Series B, 268*, 263–267.

Connor, R. C., Smolker, R. A., & Richards, A. F. (1992). Two levels of alliance formation among male bottleneck dolphins. *Proceedings of the National Academy of Sciences, U.S.A., 89*, 987–990.

Cook, M., & Mineka, S. (1989). Observational conditioning of fear to fear relevant versus fear-irrelevant stimuli in rhesus monkeys. *Journal of Abnormal Psychology, 98*, 448–459.

Cook, M., Mineka, S., Wolkenstein, B., & Laitsch, K. (1985). Observational conditioning of snake fear in unrelated rhesus monkeys. *Journal of Abnormal Psychology, 94*, 591–610.

Cooke, F., Finney, G. H., & Rockwell, R. (1976). Assortative mating in lesser snow geese (*Anser carulescens*). *Behavioral Genetics, 6*, 127–139.

Cooke, F., & McNally, C. (1975). Mate selection and color preferences in lesser snow geese. *Behaviour, 53*, 151–170.

Cooke, F., Mirsky, P., & Seiger, M. (1972). Color preferences in lesser snow geese and their possible role in mate selection. *Canadian Journal of Zoology, 50*, 529–536.

Cordero, C. (1996). On the evolutionary origin of nuptial seminal gifts in insects. *Journal of Insect Behavior, 9*, 969–974.

Cords, M. (1995). Predator vigilance costs of allogrooming in wild blue monkeys. *Behaviour, 132*, 559–569.

Cordts, R., & Partridge, L. (1996). Courtship reduces longevity of male *Drosophila melanogaster*. *Animal Behaviour, 52*, 269–278.

Coss, R. G. (1991). Context and animal behavior III. The relationship between early development and evolutionary persistence of ground squirrel antisnake behavior. *Ecological Psychology, 3*, 277–315.

Coss, R. G., & Owings, D. H. (1985). Restraints on ground squirrel antipredator behavior: Adjustments over multiple time scales. In T. D. Johnston & A. T. Pietrewicz (Eds.), *Issues in the ecological study of learning* (pp. 167–200). Hillsdale, NJ: Lawrence Erlbaum Associates.

Coultier, S., Beaugrand, J. P., & Lague, P. C. (1996). The role of individual differences and patterns of resolution in the formation of dominance orders in domestic hen triads. *Behavioural Processes, 38*, 227–239.

Cowie, R. (1977). Optimal foraging in great tits. *Nature, 268*, 137–139.

Cox, C., & Le Boeuf, B. J. (1977). Female incitation of male competition: A mechanism in sexual selection. *American Naturalist, 111*, 317–335.

Cozza, K., Fico, R., Batistini, L. & Rogers, E. (1996). The damage-conservation interface illustrated by predation on domestic livestock in Italy. *Biological Conservation, 78*, 329–336.

Craig, A. (1999). Anting in Afrotropical birds: A review. *Ostrich, 70*, 203–207.

Crawley, M. (1983). *Herbivory*. Oxford: Blackwell Science.

Creel, S. (2001). Cooperative hunting and sociality in African wild dogs, *Lycaon pictus*. In L. Dugatkin (Ed.), *Model systems in behavioral ecology*. Princeton: Princeton University Press.

Crockford, C., & Boesch, C. (2003). Context-specific calls in wild chimpanzees, Pan troglodytes versus analysis of barks. *Animal Behaviour, 66*, 115–125.

Croft, D. P., James, R., Thomas, P. O. R., Hathaway, C., Mawdsley, D., Laland, K. N., & Krause, J. (2006). Social structure and co-operative interactions in a wild population of guppies (*Poecilia reticulata*). *Behavioral Ecology and Sociobiology, 59*, 644–650.

Crowl, T., & Covich, A. (1990). Predator-induced life-history traits in a freshwater snail. *Science, 247*, 949–951.

Crowley, P. H., Gillett, S., & Lawton, J. H. (1988). Contests between larval damselflies: Empirical steps toward a better ESS model. *Animal Behaviour, 36*, 1496–1510.

Crozier, R. (1987). Genetic aspects of kin recognition: Concepts, models and synthesis. In D. C. Fletcher & C. D. Michener (Eds.), *Kin recognition in animals* (pp. 55–74). Chichester, UK: Wiley.

Curio, E., Ernest, U., & Vieth, W. (1978). Cultural transmission of enemy recognition: One function of mobbing. *Science, 202*, 899–901.

Curio, E., Klump, G., & Regelmann, K. (1983). An anti-predator response in the great tit (Parus major): Is it tuned to predator risk? *Oecologia, 60*, 83–88.

Curio, E., & Regelmann, K. (1985). The behavioral dynamics of great tits (*Parus major*) approaching a predator. *Zeitschrift fur Tierpsychologie, 69*, 3–18.

Currie, C. R., Mueller, U. G., & Malloch, D. (1999a). The agricultural pathology of ant fungus gardens. *Proceedings of the National Academy of Sciences, U.S.A., 96*, 7998–8002.

Currie, C. R., Scott, J. A., Summerbell, R. C., & Malloch, D. (1999b). Fungus-growing ants use antibiotic-producing bacteria to control garden parasites. *Nature, 398*, 701–704.

Curtsinger, J. W. (1986). Stay times in *Scatophaga* and the theory of evolutionarily stable strategies. *American Naturalist, 128*, 130–136.

Dall, S. R. X., Houston, A. I., & McNamara, J. M. (2004). The behavioural ecology of personality: Consistent individual differences from an adaptive perspective. *Ecology Letters, 7*, 734–739.

Dally, J. M., Emery, N. J. & Clayton, N. S. (2006). Food-caching western scrub-jays keep track of who was watching when. *Science, 312*, 1662–1665.

Daly, M., & Wilson, M. (1988). *Homicide*. New York: Aldine de Gruyter.

Daly, M., & Wilson, M. (1994). Some differential attributes of lethal assaults on small children by stepfathers versus genetic fathers. *Ethology and Sociobiology, 15*, 207–217.

Daly, M., & Wilson, M. (1996). Violence against stepchildren. *Current Directions in Psychological Science, 5*, 77–81.

Daly, M., & Wilson, M. (1999). *The truth about Cinderella : A Darwinian view of parental love*. New Haven: Yale University Press.

Danchin, E., Giraldeau, L. A., Valone, T. J., & Wagner, R. H. (2004). Public information: From nosy neighbors to cultural evolution. *Science, 305*, 487–491.

Darwin, C. (1845). *The voyage of the Beagle*. London: J. Murray.

Darwin, C. (1859). *On the origin of species*. London: J. Murray.

Darwin, C. (1871). *The descent of man and selection in relation to sex*. London: J. Murray.

Davies, N. B. (1976). Food, flocking and territorial behavior in the pied wagtail Motacilla alba in winter. *Journal of Animal Ecology, 45*, 235–254.

Davies, N. B. (1978). Territorial defence in the speckled wood butterfly (*Parage aegeria*): The resident always wins. *Animal Behaviour, 26*, 138–147.

Davies, N. B. (1986). Reproductive success of dunnocks in a variable mating system. II. Factors influencing provisioning rate, nestling weight and fledgling success. *Journal of Animal Ecology, 55,* 123–138.

Davies, N. B. (1991). Mating systems. In J. R. Krebs & N. B. Davies (Eds.), *Behavioural ecology: An evolutionary approach* (3rd ed., pp. 263–299). Oxford: Blackwell Science.

Davies, N. B. (1992). *Dunnock behaviour and social evolution.* Oxford: Oxford University Press.

Davies, N., & Halliday, T. (1978). Deep croaks and fighting assessment in toads, *Bufo bufo. Nature, 391,* 56–58.

Davies, N. B., & Houston, A. I. (1981). Owners and satellites: The economics of territory defence in the pied wagtail *Motacilla alba. Journal of Animal Ecology, 50,* 157–180.

Davies, N. B., & Lundberg, A. (1984). Food distribution and a variable mating system in the dunnock. *Journal of Animal Ecology, 53,* 895–912.

Davis, D. (1942). The phylogeny of social nesting in the Crotophaginae. *Quarterly Review of Biology, 17,* 115–134.

Davis, J., & Daly, M. (1997). Evolutionary theory and the human family. *Quarterly Review of Biology, 72,* 407–435.

Davis, R. (1993). Mushroom bodies and Drosophila learning. *Neuron, 11,* 1–14.

Dawkins, R. (1976). *The selfish gene.* Oxford: Oxford University Press.

Dawkins, R. (1979). Twelve misunderstandings of kin selection. *Zeitschrift fur Tierpsychologie, 51,* 184–200.

Dawkins, R. (1982). *The extended phenotype.* Oxford: Oxford University Press.

Dawkins, R. (1987). *The blind watchmaker.* New York: Norton.

Dawkins, R. (2006). *The selfish gene* (30th anniversary edition). Oxford: Oxford University Press.

Dawkins, R., & Krebs, J. R. (1978). Animal signals: Information for manipulation? In J. R. Krebs & N. B. Davies (Eds.), *Behavioural ecology: An evolutionary approach* (pp. 282–309). Oxford: Blackwell Science.

Dawkins, R., & Krebs, J. (1979). Arms races between and within species. *Proceedings of the Royal Society of London, Series B, 205,* 489–511.

Dawson, A. (2002). Photoperiodic control of the annual cycle in birds and comparison with mammals. *Ardea, 90,* 355–367.

Dawson, R. D. (2004). Does fresh vegetation protect avian nests from ectoparasites? An experiment with tree swallows. *Canadian Journal of Zoology-Revue Canadienne De Zoologie, 82,* 1005–1010.

Dayrat, B. (2005). Ancestor-descendant relationships and the Reconstruction of the Tree of Life. *Paleobiology, 31,* 347–353.

Dean, J. (1980a). Effects of thermal and chemical components of bombardier beetle chemical defense: Glossopharyngeal response in two species of toad (*Bufo americanus, Bufo marinus*). *Journal of Comparative Physiology, 135,* 51–59.

Dean, J. (1980b). Encounters between bombardier beetles and 2 species of toads (*Bufo americanus, Bufo marinus*): Speed of prey capture does not determine success. *Journal of Comparative Physiology, 135,* 41–50.

De Backer, C. J. S., & Gurven, M. (2006). Whispering down the lane: The economics of vicarious information transfer. *Adaptive Behavior, 14,* 249–264.

Decety, J., Chaminade, T., Grezes, J., & Meltzoff, A. N. (2002). A PET exploration of the neural mechanisms involved in reciprocal imitation. *Neuroimage, 15,* 265–272.

Dejong, G. (1994). The fitness of fitness concepts and the description of natural selection. *Quarterly Review of Biology, 69,* 3–29.

de Kloet, E. R., Grootendorst, J., Karssen, A. A., & Oitzl, M. S. (2002). Gene x environment interaction and cognitive performance: Animal studies on the role of corticosterone. *Neurobiology of Learning and Memory, 78,* 570–577.

de Kloet, E. R., Oitzl, M. S., & Joels, M. (1999). Stress and cognition: Are corticosteroids good or bad guys? *Trends in Neuroscience, 22,* 422–426.

de Kloet, E. R., Vreugdenhil, E., Oitzl, M. S., & Joels, M. (1998). Brain corticosteroid receptor balance in health and disease. *Endocrine Reviews, 19,* 269–301.

de Kort, S. R., & Clayton, N. S. (2006). An evolutionary perspective on caching by corvids. *Proceedings of the Royal Society of London, Series B, 273,* 417–423.

De Laet, J. (1985). Dominance and anti-predator behavior of great tits *Parus major*: A field study. *Ibis, 127.*

Delph, L., & Havens, K. (1998). Pollen competition in flowering plants. In T. Birkhead & A. Møller(Eds.), *Sperm competition and sexual selection* (pp. 149–173). London: Academic Press.

Delsuc, F., Brinkmann, H., & Philippe, H. (2005). Phylogenomics and the reconstruction of the tree of life. *Nature Reviews Genetics, 6,* 361–375.

Denison, R. F., Kiers, E. T., & West, S. A. (2003). Darwinian agriculture: When can humans find solutions beyond the reach of natural selection? *Quarterly Review of Biology, 78,* 145–168.

de Quervain, D. J. F. (2006). Glucocorticoid-induced inhibition of memory retrieval: Implications for posttraumatic stress disorder. In R. Yehuda, *Psychobiology of posttraumatic stress disorder: A decade of progress* (Vol. 1071, pp. 216–220). New York: Annals of the New York Academy of Sciences.

de Quervain, D. J. F., Fischbacher, U., Treyer, V., Schelthammer, M., Schnyder, U., Buck, A., & Fehr, E. (2004). The neural basis of altruistic punishment. *Science, 305,* 1254–1258.

de Quervain, D. J. F., Roozendaal, B., & McGaugh, J. L. (1998). Stress and glucocorticoids impair retrieval of long-term spatial memory. *Nature, 394,* 787–790.

de Quervain, D. J. F., Roozendaal, B., Nitsch, R. M., McGaugh, J. L., & Hock, C. (2000). Acute cortisone administration impairs retrieval of long-term declarative memory in humans. *Nature Neuroscience, 3,* 313–314.

DeSalle, R., & Schierwater, B. (Eds.). (1998). *Molecular approaches to ecology and evolution.* Basel: Birkhauser Verlag.

de Waal, F. (1989). *Peacemaking among primates.* Cambridge, MA: Harvard University Press.

de Waal, F. B. M. (1992). Coalitions as part of reciprocal relations in the Arnhem chimpanzee colony. In A. Harcourt & F. B. M. de Waal (Eds.), *Coalitions and alliances in humans and other animals* (pp. 233–257). Oxford: Oxford University Press.

de Waal, F. (1997). The chimpanzee's service economy: Food for grooming. *Evolution and Human Behavior, 18,* 375–386.

Dewey, M. J., & Dawson, W. D. (2001). Deer mice: "The drosophila of North American mammalogy." *Genesis, 29,* 105–109.

Dewsbury, D. (1992). On problems studied in ethology, comparative psychology and animal behavior. *Ethology, 92,* 89–107.

Dewsbury, D. (1994). On the utility of the proximate-ultimate distinction in the study of animal behavior. *Ethology, 96,* 63–68.

Dill, L. (1974). The escape response of the zebra Danio (*Brachydanio rerio*) II. The effect of experience. *Animal Behaviour, 22,* 723–730.

Dill, L. (1983). Adaptive flexibility in the foraging behavior of fishes. *Canadian Journal of Fisheries and Aquatic Sciences, 40,* 398–408.

Dill, L., & Fraser, A. (1984). Risk of predation and the feeding behaviour of juvenile Coho salmon (*Oncorynchus kisutch*). *Behavioral Ecology and Sociobiology, 16,* 65–72.

DiMarco, F. P., & Hanlon, R. T. (1997). Agonistic behavior in the squid *Loligo plei* (Loliginidae, Teuthoidea): Fighting tactics and the effects of size and resource value. *Ethology, 103,* 89–108.

Dingemanse, N. J., Both, C., Drent, P. J., Van Oers, K., & Van Noordwijk, A. J. (2002). Repeatability and heritability of exploratory behaviour in great tits from the wild. *Animal Behaviour, 64,* 929–938.

Dingemanse, N. J., & Reale, D. (2005). Natural selection and animal personality. *Behaviour, 142,* 1159–1184.

Dingle, H. (1996). *Migration: The biology of life on the move.* New York: Oxford University Press.

Dingle, H., & Caldwell, R. (1972). Reproductive and maternal behavior of the mantis shrimp *Gonodactylus bredini Manning* (Crustacea: Stomatopoda). *Biological Bulletin, 142,* 417–426.

Dittman, A., & Quinn, T. P. (1996). Homing in Pacific salmon: Mechanisms and ecological basis. *Journal of Experimental Biology, 199,* 83–91.

Dittman, A. H., Quinn, T. P., Nevitt, G. A., Hacker, B., & Storm, D. R. (1997). Sensitization of olfactory guanylyl cyclase to a specific imprinted odorant in coho salmon. *Neuron, 19,* 381–389.

Dodson, J. J. (1988). The nature and role of learning in the orientation and migratory behavior of fishes. *Environmental Biology of Fishes, 23,* 161–182.

Domjan, M. (1992). Adult learning and mate choice: Possibilities and experimental evidence. *American Zoologist, 32,* 48–61.

Domjan, M. (1998). *The principles of learning and behavior* (4th ed.). Pacific Grove, CA: Brooks/Cole.

Domjan, M. (2005). Pavlovian conditioning: A functional perspective. *Annual Review of Psychology, 56,* 179–206.

Domjan, M. (2006). *The principles of learning and behavior: Active learning edition* (5th ed.). Belmont, CA: Thomson/Wadsworth.

Domjan, M., Blesbois, E., & Williams, J. (1998). The adaptive significance of sexual conditioning: Pavlovian control of sperm release. *Psychological Science, 9,* 411–415.

Domjan, M., Cusato, B., & Villarreal, R. (2000). Extensions, elaborations, and explanations of the role of evolution and learning in the control of social behavior. *Behavioral and Brain Sciences, 23,* 269–282.

Domjan, M., & Hollis, K. L. (1988). Reproductive behavior: A potential model system for adaptive specializations in learning. In R. C.

Bolles & M. D. Beecher (Eds.), *Evolution and learning* (pp. 213–237): Hillsdales, NJ: Lawrence Erlbaum Associates.

Domjan, M., Lyons, R., North, N., & Bruell, J. (1986). Sexual Pavlovian conditioned approach behavior in male Japanese quail (*Coturnix coturnix japonica*). *Journal of Comparative Psychology, 100,* 413–421.

Dopazo, H., Gordon, M. B., Perazzo, R., & Risau-Gusman, S. (2003). A model for the emergence of adaptive subsystems. *Bulletin of Mathematical Biology, 65,* 27–56.

Dornhaus, A., Collins, E. J., Dechaume-Moncharmont, F. X., Houston, A. I., Franks, N. R., & McNamara, J. M. (2006). Paying for information: Partial loads in central place foragers. *Behavioral Ecology and Sociobiology, 61,* 151–161.

Douglas-Hamilton, I., & Douglas-Hamilton, O. (1975). *Among the elephants.* Glasgow: Collins.

Doutrelant, C., McGregor, P., & Oliveira, R. (2001). The effect of an audience on intra-sexual communication in male Siamese fighting fish, *Betta splendens. Behavioral Ecology, 12,* 283–286.

Drenos, F., & Kirkwood, T. B. L. (2005). Modellng the disposable soma theory of ageing. *Mechanisms of Ageing and Development, 126,* 99–103.

Drent, P., van Oers, K., & van Noordwijk, A. J. (2002). Realized heritability of personalities in the great tit (*Parus major*). *Proceedings of the Royal Society of London, Series B, 270,* 45–51.

Drent, P. J., van Oers, K., & van Noordwijk, A. J. (2003). Realized heritability of personalities in the great tit (*Parus major*). *Proceedings of the Royal Society of London, Series B, 270,* 45–51.

Drevets, W. C. (2000). Functional anatomical abnormalities in limbic and prefrontal cortical structures in major depression. In H. B. M. Uylings, C. G. van Eden, J. P. C. de Bruin, M. G. P. Feenstra, & C. M. A. Pennartz (Eds.), *Cognition, emotion and autonomic responses: The integrative role of the prefrontal cortex and limbic structures* (pp. 413–431): Elsevier.

Drickamer, L. C. (1996). Intra-uterine position and anogenital distance in house mice: Consequences under field conditions. *Animal Behaviour, 51,* 925–934.

Drummond, H. (2006). Dominance in vertebrate broods and litters. *Quarterly Review of Biology, 81,* 3–32.

Drummond, H., & Canales, C. (1998). Dominance between booby nestlings involves winner and loser effects. *Animal Behaviour, 55,* 1669–1676.

Drummond, H., & Osorno, J. L. (1992). Training siblings to be submissive losers: Dominance between booby nestlings. *Animal Behaviour, 44,* 881–893.

Duckworth, R. A., Mendonca, M. T., & Hill, G. E. (2001). A condition dependent link between testosterone and disease resistance in the house finch. *Proceedings of the Royal Society of London, Series B, 268,* 2467–2472.

Duckworth, R. A., Mendonca, M. T., & Hill, G. E. (2004). Condition-dependent sexual traits and social dominance in the house finch. *Behavioral Ecology, 15,* 779–784.

Duellman, W. E., & Trueb, L. (1994). *Biology of amphibians.* New York: Johns Hopkins University Press.

Dugatkin, L. A. (1991). Dynamics of the TIT FOR TAT strategy during predator inspection in guppies. *Behavioral Ecology and Sociobiology, 29,* 127–132.

Dugatkin, L. A. (1992a). Sexual selection and imitation: Females copy the mate choice of others. *American Naturalist, 139*, 1384–1389.

Dugatkin, L. A. (1992b). Tendency to inspect predators predicts mortality risk in the guppy, *Poecilia reticulata. Behavioral Ecology, 3*, 124–128.

Dugatkin, L. A. (1995). Formalizing Allee's idea on dominance hierarchies: An intra-demic selection model. *American Naturalist, 146*, 154–160.

Dugatkin, L. A. (1996a). Copying and mate choice. In C. Heyes & G. Galef (Eds.), *Social learning in animals: The roots of culture* (pp. 85–105). New York: Academic Press.

Dugatkin, L. A. (1996b). The interface between culturally-based preferences and genetic preferences: Female mate choice in *Poecilia reticulata. Proceedings of the National Academy of Sciences, U.S.A., 93*, 2770–2773.

Dugatkin, L. A. (1997a). *Cooperation among animals: An evolutionary perspective.* New York: Oxford University Press.

Dugatkin, L. A. (1997b). Winner effects, loser effects and the structure of dominance hierarchies. *Behavioral Ecology, 8*, 583–587.

Dugatkin, L. A. (1998a). A model of coalition formation in animals. *Proceedings of the Royal Society of London, Series B, 265*, 2121–2125.

Dugatkin, L. A. (1998b). Breaking up fights between others: A model of intervention behaviour. *Proceedings of the Royal Society of London, Series B, 265*, 443–437.

Dugatkin, L. A. (2000). *The imitation factor: Evolution beyond the gene.* New York: Free Press.

Dugatkin, L. A. (2001a). Bystander effects and the structure of dominance hierarchies. *Behavioral Ecology, 12*, 348–352.

Dugatkin, L. A. (Ed). (2001b). *Model systems in behavioral ecology: Integrating conceptual, theoretical and empirical perspectives.* Princeton: Princeton University Press.

Dugatkin, L. A. (2001c). Preface. In L. A. Dugatkin (Ed.), *Model systems in behavioral ecology: Integrating conceptual, theoretical and empirical perspectives.* Princeton: Princeton University Press.

Dugatkin, L. A. (2006). *The altruism equation: Seven scientists search for the origins of goodness.* Princeton: Princeton University Press.

Dugatkin, L. A., & Alfieri, M. (1991a). Guppies and the TIT FOR TAT strategy: Preference based on past interaction. *Behavioral Ecology and Sociobiology, 28*, 243–246.

Dugatkin, L. A., & Alfieri, M. (1991b). TIT FOR TAT in guppies: The relative nature of cooperation and defection during predator inspection. *Evolutionary Ecology, 5*, 300–309.

Dugatkin, L. A., & Alfieri, M. (1992). Interpopulational differences in the use of the Tit for Tat strategy during predator inspection in the guppy. *Evolutionary Ecology, 6*, 519–526.

Dugatkin, L. A., & Alfieri, M. (2003). Boldness, behavioral inhibition and learning: An evolutionary approach. *Ethology, Ecology & Evolution, 15*, 43–49.

Dugatkin, L. A., FitzGerald, G. J., & Lavoie, J. (1994). Juvenile three-spined sticklebacks avoid parasitized conspecifics. *Environmental Biology of Fishes, 39*, 215–218.

Dugatkin, L. A., & Godin, J.-G. J. (1992). Prey approaching predators: A cost-benefit perspective. *Annales Zoologici Fennici, 29*, 233–252.

Dugatkin, L. A., & Godin, J.-G. J. (1998). How females choose their mates. *Scientific American*, April 1998, 46–51.

Dugatkin, L. A., Mesterton-Gibbons, M., & Houston, A. I. (1992). Beyond the prisoner's dilemma: Towards models to discriminate among mechanisms of cooperation in nature. *Trends in Ecology & Evolution, 7*, 202–205.

Dugatkin, L. A., & Reeve, H. K. (1994). Behavioral ecology and levels of selection: Dissolving the group selection controversy. *Advances in the Study of Behaviour, 23*, 101–133.

Dugatkin, L. A., & Reeve, H. K. (Eds.). (1998). *Game theory and animal behavior.* Oxford: Oxford University Press.

Dugatkin, L. A., & Wilson, D. S. (2000). Assortative interactions and the evolution of cooperation in guppies. *Evolutionary Ecology, 2*, 761–767.

Dukas, R. (Ed). (1998a). *Cognitive ecology.* Chicago: University of Chicago Press.

Dukas, R. (1998b). Constraints on information processing and their effects on behavior. In R. Dukas (Ed.), *Cognitive ecology* (pp. 89–127). Chicago: University of Chicago Press.

Dukas, R. (2006). Learning in the context of sexual behaviour in insects. *Animal Biology, 56*, 125–141.

Dukas, R., & Bernays, E. A. (2000). Learning improves growth rate in grasshoppers. *Proceedings of the National Academy of Sciences, 97*, 2637–2640.

Dukes, J. P., Deaville, R., Bruford, M. W., Youngson, A. F., & Jordan, W. C. (2004). Odorant receptor gene expression changes during the parr-smolt transformation in Atlantic salmon. *Molecular Ecology, 13*, 2851–2857.

Dumond, F. (1968). The squirrel monkey in a seminatural environment. In L. Rosenblum & R. Cooper (Eds.), *The squirrel monkey* (pp. 87–145). New York: Academic Press.

Dunbar, R. (1992). Neocortex size as a constraint on group size in primates. *Journal of Human Evolution, 20*, 469–493.

Dupain, J., Van Elsacker, L., Nell, C., Garcia, P., Ponce, F., & Huffman, M. A. (2002). New evidence for leaf swallowing and Oesophagostomum infection in bonobos (*Pan paniscus*). *International Journal of Primatology, 23*, 1053–1062.

Dyer, F. (1998). Cognitive ecology of navigation. In R. Dukas (Ed.), *Cognitive ecology* (pp. 201–260). Chicago: University of Chicago Press.

Eadie, J., Sherman, P., & Semel, B. (1998). Conspecific brood parasitism, population dynamics and the conservation of cavity-nesting birds. In T. Caro (Ed.), *Behavioral ecology and conservation biology* (pp. 306–340). New York: Oxford University Press.

Earley, R., & Dugatkin, L. A. (2002). Eavesdropping on visual cues in green swordtails (*Xiphophorus helleri*): A case for networking. *Proceedings of the Royal Society of London, Series B, 269*, 943–952.

Earley, R., & Dugatkin, L. A. (2005). Fighting, mating and networking: Pillars of poeciliid sociality. In P. McGregor (Ed.), *Animal communication networks* (pp. 84–113). Cambridge: Cambridge University Press.

Eason, P. K., Cobbs, G. A., & Trinca, K. G. (1999). The use of landmarks to define territorial boundaries. *Animal Behaviour, 58,* 85–91.

East, M. (1981). Alarm calling and parental investment in the robin *Erithacus rubecula. Ibis, 123,* 223–230.

Eberhard, W. (1996). *Female control: Sexual selection by cryptic female choice.* Princeton: Princeton University Press.

Edgerton, V. (1978). Mammalian muscle fibers and their adaptability. *American Zoologist, 18,* 113–125.

Edwards, D. H., & Spitzer, N. (2006). Social dominance and serotonin receptor genes in crayfish. *Current Topics in Developmental Biology, 74,* 177–199.

Edwards, S. V., & Hedrick, P. W. (1998). Evolution and ecology of MHC molecules: From genomics to sexual selection. *Trends in Ecology and Evolution, 13,* 305–311.

Edwards, S. V., & Naeem, S. (1993). The phylogenetic component of cooperative breeding in perching birds. *American Naturalist, 141,* 754–789.

Eggebeen, D., & Hogan, D. (1990). Giving between generations in American families. *Human Nature, 1,* 211–232.

Ehlinger, T. J., & Wilson, D. S. (1988). Complex foraging polymorphism in bluegill sunfish. *Proceedings of the National Academy of Sciences, U.S.A., 85,* 1878–1882.

Ehrlich, P., Dobkin, D., & Wheye, D. (1986). The adaptive significance of anting. *Auk, 103,* 835.

Eibesfeldt, I., & Eible-Eibesfeldt, E. (1967). Das parasitenabwehren der minima-arbeiterinnen der blattschneider-ameise (*Atta cephalotes*). *Zeitschrift fur Tierpsychologie, 24,* 278–281.

Eichenbaum, H., Stewart, C., & Morris, R. G. M. (1990). Hippocampal representation in place learning *Journal of Neuroscience, 10,* 3531–3542.

Eisenberg, J. F. (1966). The social organization of mammals. *Handbook of Zoology, 10,* 1–92.

Eisner, T., & Aneshansley, D. (1999). Spray aiming in the bombardier beetle: Photographic evidence. *Proceedings of the National Academy of Sciences, U.S.A., 96,* 9705–9709.

Eisner, T., & Aneshansley, D. J. (1982). Spray aiming in bombardier beetles: Jet deflection by the coanda effect. *Science, 215,* 83–85.

Eisner, T., Aneshansley, D. J., Eisner, M., Attygalle, A. B., Alsop, D. W., & Meinwald, J. (2000). Spray mechanism of the most primitive bombardier beetle (*Metrius contractus*). *Journal of Experimental Biology, 203,* 1265–1275.

Eisner, T., & Dean, J. (1976). Ploy and counterploy in predator-prey interactions: Orb-weaving spiders versus bombardier beetles *Proceedings of the National Academy of Sciences, U.S.A., 73,* 1365–1367.

Eisner, T., Eisner, M., & Aneshansley, D. (2005). Pre-ingestive treatment of bombardier beetles by jays: Food preparation by "anting" and "sand-wiping." *Chemoecology, 15,* 227–233.

Ekman, J., & Askenmo, C. (1984). Social rank and habitat use in willow tit groups. *Animal Behaviour, 32,* 508–14.

Elekonich, M. M., Schulz, D. J., Bloch, G., & Robinson, G. E. (2001). Juvenile hormone levels in honey bee (*Apis mellifera L.*) foragers: Foraging experience and diurnal variation. *Journal of Insect Physiology, 47,* 1119–1125.

Elgar, M. (1986). House sparrows establish foraging flocks by giving chirrup calls if the resource is divisible. *Animal Behaviour, 34,* 169–174.

Elgar, M., & Crespi, B. (Eds.). (1992). *Cannibalism: Ecology and evolution among diverse taxa.* Oxford: Oxford University Press.

Elgar, M., & Pierce, N. (1988). Mating success and fecundity in an ant-tended lycaenid butterfly. In T. Clutton-Brock (Ed.), *Reproductive success* (pp. 59–75). Chicago: University of Chicago Press.

Ely, D. (1981). Hypertension, social rank and aortic arteriosclerosis in CBA/J mice. *Physiology and Behavior, 26,* 655–661.

Emery, N. J. (2006). Cognitive ornithology: The evolution of avian intelligence. *Philosophical Transactions of the Royal Society of London, Series B, 361,* 23–43.

Emlen, J. M. (1966). The role of time and energy in food preference. *American Naturalist, 100,* 611–617.

Emlen, J. T. ,& Lorenz, F. W. (1942). Pairing responses of free-living valley quail to sex hormone pellet tablets. *Auk, 59.*

Emlen, S. T. (1967). Migratory orientation in the Indigo bunting, *Passerina cyanea. II.* Mechanisms of celestial orientation. *Auk, 84,* 463–469.

Emlen, S. T. (1970). Celestial rotation: Its importance in the development of migratory orientation. *Science, 170,* 1198–1201.

Emlen, S. T. (1975). The stellar-orientation system of a migratory bird. *Scientific American, 233,* 102–111.

Emlen, S. T. (1982a). The evolution of helping: An ecological constraints model. *American Naturalist, 119,* 29–39.

Emlen, S. T. (1982b). The evolution of helping: II. The role of behavioral conflict. *American Naturalist, 119,* 40–53.

Emlen, S. T. (1995a). An evolutionary theory of the family. *Proceedings of the National Academy of Sciences, U.S.A., 92,* 8092–8099.

Emlen, S. T. (1995b). Can avian biology be useful to the social sciences? *Journal of Avian Biology, 26,* 273–276.

Emlen, S. T., & Oring, L. W. (1977). Ecology, sexual selection and evolution of mating systems. *Science, 197,* 215–223.

Emlen, S. T., & Wrege, P. H. (1992). Parent-offspring conflict and the recruitment of helpers among bee-eaters. *Nature, 356,* 331–333.

Emlen, S. T., Wrege, P. H., & Webster, M. (1998). Cuckoldry as a cost of polyandry in the sex-reversed wattled jacana, *Jacana jacana. Proceedings of the Royal Society of London, Series B, 265,* 2359–2364.

Enard, W., Przeworski, M., Fisher, S. E., Lai, C. S. L., Wiebe, V., Kitano, T., Monaco, A. P., & Paabo, S. (2002). Molecular evolution of FOXP2, a gene involved in speech and language. *Nature, 418,* 869–872.

Endler, J. (1986). *Natural selection in the wild.* Princeton: Princeton University Press.

Endler, J. (1995). Multiple trait co-evolution and environmental gradients in guppies. *Trends in Ecology and Evolution, 10,* 22–29.

Endler, J. (1999). Adaptive genetic variation in the wild: Concluding remarks. In T. Mousseau, B. Sinervo, & J. Endler (Eds.), *Adaptive genetic variation in the wild* (pp. 251–260). New York: Oxford University Press.

Endler, J., & McLellan, T. (1988). The process of evolution: Toward a newer synthesis. *Annual Review of Ecology and Systematics, 19*, 395–421.

Engel, G., & Schmale, A. (1972). Conservation-withdrawal: A primary regulatory process for organic homeostasis. In R. Porter, & J. Knight, (Eds.), *Physiology, emotions and psychosomatic illness* (pp. 57–75). Amsterdam: Elsevier.

Engh, A. L., Esch, K., Smale, L., & Holekamp, K. E. (2000). Mechanisms of maternal rank "inheritance" in the spotted hyaena, *Crocuta crocuta. Animal Behaviour, 60*, 323–332.

Enquist, M., & Leimar, O. (1983). Evolution of fighting behavior: Decision rules and assessment of relative strength. *Journal of Theoretical Biology, 102*, 387–410.

Enquist, M., & Leimar, O. (1987). Evolution of fighting behavior: The effect of variation in resource value. *Journal of Theoretical Biology, 127*, 185–207.

Enquist, M., & Leimar, O. (1990). The evolution of fatal fighting. *Animal Behaviour, 39*, 1–9.

Enquist, M., Leimar, O., Ljungberg, T., Mallner, Y., & Segardahl, N. (1990). A test of the sequential assessment game: Fighting in the cichlid fish, *Nannacara anomala. Animal Behaviour, 40*, 1–15.

Enquist, M., Ljungberg, T., & Zandor, A. (1987). Visual assessment of fighting ability in the cichlid fish *Nanacara anomala. Animal Behaviour, 35*, 1262–1263.

Ens, B. J., & Goss-Custard, J. (1984). Interference among oyster catchers (*Haematopus ostraleugus*) feeding on mussels (*Mytilus edulis*) on the Exe Estuary. *Journal of Animal Ecology, 53*, 217–231.

Erber, J., Kloppenburg, P., & Scheidler, A. (1993). Neuromodulation by serotonin and octopamine in the honeybee: Behavior, neuroanatomy and electrophysiology. *Experientia, 49*, 1073–1083.

Essapian, F. S. (1963). Observations on abnormalities of partuition in captive bottle-nosed dolphins. *Journal of Mammalogy, 44*, 405–414.

Estes, R. D., & Goddard, J. (1967). Prey selection and hunting behavior of the African dog. *Journal of Wildlife Management, 31*, 52–70.

Evans, C. S., & Marler, P. (1994). Food calling and audience effects in male chickens, *Gallus gallus*: Their relationships to food availability, courtship and social facilitation. *Animal Behaviour, 47*, 1159–1170.

Even, M., Dahr, M., & vom Saal, F. (1992). Transport of steroids between fetuses via amniotic fluid in relation to the intrauterine position in rats. *Journal of Reproduction and Fertility, 96*, 709–712.

Ewald, P. (1985). Influences of asymmetries in resource quality and age on aggression and dominance in black-chinned hummingbirds. *Animal Behaviour, 33*, 705–719.

Ewald, P. W. (1994). *Evolution of infectious diseases*. New York: Oxford University Pres.

Ewald, P. W. (2000). *Plague time*. New York: Free Press.

Ewer, R. (1969). The "instinct to teach." *Nature, 222*, 698.

Ewing, A. W., & Bennet-Clark, H. C. (1968). The courtship songs of Drosophila. *Behaviour, 31*, 288–301.

Fagen, R. M. (1981). *Animal play behavior*. Oxford: Oxford University Press.

Fagen, R., & Fagen, J. (2004). Juvenile survival and benefits of play behaviour in brown bears, *Ursus arctos. Evolutionary Ecology Research, 6*, 89–102.

Fahrbach, S. E. (2006). Structure of the mushroom bodies of the insect brain. *Annual Review of Entomology, 51*, 209–232.

Feder, M. (1999). Organismal, ecological and evolutionary aspects of heat-shock proteins and the stress response: Established conclusion and unresolved issues. *American Zoologist, 39*, 857–864.

Feder, M. E., Bennett, A. F., & Huey, R. B. (2000). Evolutionary physiology. *Annual Review of Ecology and Systematics, 31*, 315–341.

Feder, M., & Hoffmann, G. (1999). Heat-shock proteins, molecular chaperones and the stress response: Evolutionary and ecological physiology and the stress response: Established conclusion and unresolved issues. *Annual Review of Physiology, 61*, 243–282.

Feener, D. H., & Moss, K. A. (1990). Defense against parasites by hitchhikers in leaf-cuttting ants: A quantitative assessment. *Behavioral Ecology and Sociobiology, 26*, 17–29.

Felsenstein, J. (1985). Phylogenies and the comparative method. *American Naturalist, 125*, 1–15.

Felsenstein, J. (2004). *Inferring phylogenies*. Sunderland, MA: Sinauer.

Ferguson, J. N., Aldag, J. M., Insel, T. R., & Young, L. J. (2001). Oxytocin in the medial amygdala is essential for social recognition in the mouse. *Journal of Neuroscience, 21*, 8278–8285.

Ferguson, J. N., Young, L. J., Hearn, E. F., Matzuk, M. M., Insel, T. R., & Winslow, J. T. (2000). Social amnesia in mice lacking the oxytocin gene. *Nature Genetics, 25*, 284–288.

Fernandez, A., & Morris, M. (2007). Sexual selection and trichromatic color vision in primates: Statistical support for the preexisting bias hypothesis. *American Naturalist, 170*, 10–20.

Fernandez-Teruel, A., Escorihuela, R. M., Gray, J. A., Aguilar, R., Gil, L., Gimenez-Llort, L., Tobena, A., Bhomra, A., Nicod, A., Mott, R., Driscoll, P., Dawson, G. R., & Flint, J. (2002). A quantitative trait locus influencing anxiety in the laboratory rat. *Genome Research, 12*, 618–626.

Ferrari, M. C. O., Capitania-Kwok, T., & Chivers, D. P. (2006a). The role of learning in the acquisition of threat-sensitive responses to predator odours. *Behavioral Ecology and Sociobiology, 60*, 522–527.

Ferrari, M. C. O., & Chivers, D. P. (2006). Learning threat-sensitive predator avoidance: How do fathead minnows incorporate conflicting information? *Animal Behaviour, 71*, 19–26.

Ferrari, M. C. O., Messier, F., & Chivers, D. P. (2006b). The nose knows: Minnows determine predator proximity and density through detection of predator odours. *Animal Behaviour, 72*, 927–932.

Ferrari, M. C. O., Trowell, J. J., Brown, G. E., & Chivers, D. P. (2005). The role of learning in the development of threat-sensitive predator avoidance by fathead minnows. *Animal Behaviour, 70*, 777–784.

Ficken, M. S., Witkin, S. R., & Weise, C. M. (1980). Associations among members of a black-capped chickadee flock. *Behavioral Ecology and Sociobiology, 8*, 245–249.

Fiedler, K., & Maschwitz, U. (1988). Functional analysis of the myrmecophilous relationships between ants (Hymenoptea: formicidae) and lycaenids (Lepidotera: Lycaenidae). *Oecologia, 75*, 204–206.

Field, E. F., Whishaw, I. Q., Pellis, S. M., & Watson, N. V. (2006). Play fighting in androgen-insensitive tfm rats: Evidence that androgen receptors are necessary for the development of adult playful attack and defense. *Developmental Psychobiology, 48,* 111–120.

Field, S. A., Calbert, G., & Keller, M. A. (1998). Patch defence in the parasitoid wasp *Trissolcus basalis* (Insecta: Scelionidae): The time structure of pairwise contests, and the "waiting game." *Ethology, 104,* 821–840.

Finch, C., & Rose, M. (1995). Hormones and the physiological architecture of life history evolution. *Quarterly Review of Biology, 70,* 1–52.

Fisher, J. (1954). Evolution and bird sociality. In J. Huxley, A.C. Hardy, & E. B. Ford (Eds.), *Evolution as a process* (pp. 71–83). London: Allen and Unwin.

Fisher, J., & Hinde, R. (1949). The opening of milk bottles by birds. *British Birds, 42,* 347–357.

Fisher, R. A. (1915). The evolution of sexual preference. *Eugenics Review, 7,* 184–192.

Fisher, R. A. (1930). *The genetical theory of natural selection.* New York: Dover.

Fisher, R. A. (1958). *The genetical theory of natural selection* (2nd ed.). New York: Dover.

Fitzgibbon, C. D. (1994). The costs and benefits of predator inspection behaviour in Thomson's gazelles. *Behavioral Ecology and Sociobiology, 34,* 139–148.

Fitzpatrick, J. W., & Woolfenden, G. E. (1984). The helpful shall inherit the scrub. *Natural History, 93,* 55–63.

Fitzpatrick, J. W., & Woolfenden, G. E. (1988). Components of lifetime reproductive success in the Florida scrub jay. In T. H. Clutton-Brock (Ed.), *Reproductive success* (pp. 305–320). Chicago: University of Chicago Press.

Fitzpatrick, M. J., Ben-Shahar, Y., Smid, H. M., Vet, L. E. M., Robinson, G. E., & Sokolowski, M. B. (2005). Candidate genes for behavioural ecology. *Trends in Ecology & Evolution, 20,* 96–104.

Fleishman, L., Lowe, E., & Leal, M. (1993). Ultraviolet vision in lizards. *Nature, 365,* 397.

Fletcher, D., & Michener, C. (Ed). (1987). *Kin recognition in animals.* New York: Wiley.

Flint, J., Corley, R., DeFries, J., Fulker, D., Gray, J., Miller, S., & Collins, A. C. (1995). A simple genetic basis for a complex psychological trait in mice. *Science, 269,* 1432–1435.

Foltz, D. (1981). Genetic evidence for long-term monogamy in a small rodent, *Peromyscus polionotus. American Naturalist, 117,* 665–675.

Ford, R., & McLauglin, F. (1983). Variation of male fidelity in monogamous birds. In R. Johnstone (Ed.), *Current ornithology* (pp. 329–356). New York: Plenum.

Forslund, P. (2000). Male-male competition and large size mating advantage in European earwigs, *Forficula auricularia. Animal Behaviour, 59,* 753–762.

Foster, K. R., &Wenseleers, T. (2006). A general model for the evolution of mutualisms. *Journal of Evolutionary Biology, 19,* 1283–1293.

Fox, A. D., & Madsen, J. (1997). Behavioural and distributional effects of hunting disturbance on waterbirds in Europe: Implications for refuge design. *Journal of Applied Ecology, 34,* 1–13.

Fragasy, D. M., & Perry, S. (2003). *The biology of traditions: Models and evidence.* Cambridge: Cambridge University Press.

Franck, D., Klamroth, B., Taebel-Hellwig, A., & Schartl, M. (1998). Home ranges and satellite tactics of male green swordtails (*Xiphophorus helleri*) in nature. *Behavioural Processes, 43,* 115–123.

Frank, L. G. (1986a). Social organization of the spotted hyena (*Crocuta crocuta*). 1. Demography. *Animal Behaviour, 34,* 1500–1509.

Frank, L. G. (1986b). Social organization of the spotted hyena (Crocuta crocuta). 2. Dominance and reproduction. *Animal Behaviour, 34,* 1510–1527.

Franks, N. R., & Richardson, T. (2006). Teaching in tandem-running ants. *Nature, 439,* 153–153.

Fraser, D. F., Gilliam, J. F., Daley, M., Le, A., & Skalski, G. (2001). Explaining leptokurtic movement distributions: Intrapopulation variance in boldness and exploration. *American Naturalist, 158,* 124–135.

Freake, M. J., Muheim, R., & Phillips, J. B. (2006). Magnetic maps in animals: A theory comes of age? *Quarterly Review of Biology, 81,* 327–347.

Freeberg, T. M. (1998). The cultural transmission of courtship patterns in cowbirds, *Molothrus ater. Animal Behaviour, 56,* 1063–1073.

Freeberg, T. M. (2004). Social transmission of courtship behavior and mating preferences in brown-headed cowbirds, *Molothrus ater. Learning & Behavior, 32,* 122–130.

Freeberg, T. M., King, A. P., & West, M. J. (2001). Cultural transmission of vocal traditions in cowbirds (*Molothrus ater*) influences courtship patterns and mate preferences. *Journal of Comparative Psychology, 115,* 201–211.

Fretwell, S. (1972). *Populations in a seasonal environment.* Princeton: Princeton University Press.

Fretwell, S., & Lucas, H. (1970). On territorial behavior and other factors influencing habitat distribution in birds. I. Theoretical development. *Acta Biotheoretica, 19,* 16–36.

Frommen, J. G., Luz, C., & Bakker, T. C. M. (2007). Kin discrimination in sticklebacks is mediated by social learning rather than innate recognition. *Ethology, 113,* 276–282.

Fry, C. (1977). The evolutionary significance of cooperative breeding in birds. In B. Stonehouse & C. Perrins (Eds.), *Evolutionary ecology.* London: MacMillan.

Gadagkar, R. (1997). *Survival strategies: Cooperation and conflict in animal societies.* Cambridge, MA: Harvard University Press.

Gaffrey, G. (1957). Zur fortpflanzungsbiologie bei hunden. *Zoological Garten, Jena, 23,* 251.

Galef, B. G. (1996). Social enhancement of food preferences in Norway rats: A brief review. In C. M. Heyes & B. G. Galef (Eds.), *Social learning in animals: The roots of culture* (pp. 49–64). London: Academic Press.

Galef, B. G. (2004). Approaches to the study of traditional behaviors of free-living animals. *Learning & Behavior, 32,* 53–61.

Galef, B. G., & Giraldeau, L. A. (2001). Social influences on foraging in vertebrates: Causal mechanisms and adaptive functions. *Animal Behaviour, 61,* 3–15.

Galef, B. G., & Laland, K. N. (2005). Social learning in animals: Empirical studies and theoretical models. *Bioscience, 55,* 489–499.

Galef, B. G., Manzig, L., & Field, R. (1986). Imitation learning in budgerigars: Dawson and Foster Revisted. *Behavioral Processes, 13,* 191–202.

Galef, B. G., Whiskin, E. E., & Dewar, G. (2005). A new way to study teaching in animals: Despite demonstrable benefits, rat dams do not teach their young what to eat. *Animal Behaviour, 70,* 91–96.

Galef, B. G., & Wigmore, S. (1983). Transfer of information concerning distant foods: A laboratory investigation of the "information-centre" hypothesis. *Animal Behaviour, 31,* 748–758.

Gallagher, J. (1976). Sexual imprinting: Effects of various regimens of social experience on the mate preference in Japanese quail (*Coturnix coturnix japonica*). *Behaviour, 57,* 91–115.

Gallese, V., Fadiga, L., Fogassi, L., & Rizzolatti, G. (1996). Action recognition in the premotor cortex. *Brain, 119,* 593–609.

Gamboa, G. J., Reeve, H. K., & Pfennig, D. W. (1986). The evolution and ontogeny of nestmate recognition in social wasps. *Annual Review of Entomology, 31,* 431–454.

Gangestad, S. W., & Simpson, J. A. (2000). Trade-offs, the allocation of reproductive effort, and the evolutionary psychology of human mating. *Behavioral and Brain Sciences, 23,* 624–644.

Gangestad, S. W., & Thornhill, R. (1998). Menstrual cycle variation in women's preferences for the scent of symmetrical men. *Proceedings of the Royal Society of London, Series B, 265,* 927–933.

Gangestad, S. W., Thornhill, R., & Garver-Apgar, C. E. (2005). Women's sexual interests across the ovulatory cycle depend on primary partner developmental instability. *Proceedings of the Royal Society of London, Series B, 272,* 2023–2027.

Gannon, D. P., Barros, N. B., Nowacek, D. P., Read, A. J., Waples, D. M., & Wells, R. S. (2005). Prey detection by bottlenose dolphins, *Tursiops truncatus*: An experimental test of the passive listening hypothesis. *Animal Behaviour, 69,* 709–720.

Garcia, J., Ervin, F., & Koelling, R. (1966). Learning with prolonged delay of reinforcement. *Psychonomic Science, 5,* 121–122.

Garcia, J., & Koelling, R. (1966). Relation of cue to consequence in avoidance learning. *Psychonomic Science, 4,* 123–124.

Garcia, J., McGowan, B., & Green, K. (1972). Biological constraints on conditioning. In A. Black & W. Prokasy (Eds.), *Classical conditioning II: Current theory and research* (pp. 3–27). New York: Appleton.

Gaston, A. J. (1973). Ecology and behavior of long-tailed tit. *Ibis, 115,* 330–351.

Gaulin, S. J. C., & Fitzgerald, R. W. (1986). Sex-differences in spatial ability: An evolutionary hypothesis and test. *American Naturalist, 127,* 74–88.

Gaulin, S. J. C., & Fitzgerald, R. W. (1989). Sexual selection for spatial-learning ability. *Animal Behaviour, 37,* 322–331.

Gauthreaux, S. (Ed). (1980). *Animal migration, orientation, and navigation.* New York: Academic Press.

Gauthreaux, S. (Ed). (1997). *Animal migration, orientation, and navigation* (2nd ed.). New York: Academic Press.

Geist, V. (1966). The evolution of horn-like organs. *Behaviour, 27,* 175–224.

Geist, V. (1974a). On fighting strategies in animal combat. *Nature, 250,* 354.

Geist, V. (1974b). The development of social behavior through play in the Stellar sea lion. *American Zoologist, 14,* 205–220.

Gelowitz, C., Mathis, A., & Smith, R. J. F. (1993). Chemosensory recognition of northern pike (*Esox lucius*) by brook stickleback (*Culaea inconstans*): Population differences and the influence of predator diet. *Behaviour, 127,* 106–118.

George, C. (1960). *Behavioral interactions in the pickerel and the mosquitofish.* Unpublished Ph.D., Harvard University.

Gerra, G., Avanzini, P., Zaimovic, A., Sartor, I. R., Bocchi, C., Timpano, M., Zambelli, U., Delsignore, R., Gardini, F., Talarico, E., & Brambilla, F. (1999). Neurotransmitters, neuroendocrine correlates of sensation seeking temperament in normal humans. *Neuropsycholobiology, 39,* 207–213.

Getty, T. (1987). Dear enemy and the prisoner's dilemma: Why should territorial neighbors form defensive coalitions. *American Zoology, 27,* 327–336.

Giancola, P. R., & Chermack, S. T. (1998). Construct validity of laboratory aggression paradigms: A response to Tedeschi and Quigley (1996). *Aggression and Violent Behavior, 3,* 237–253.

Gibson, R. M., Bradbury, J. W., & Vehrencamp, S. L. (1991). Mate choice in lekking sage grouse: The roles of vocal display, female site fidelity and copying. *Behavioral Ecology, 2,* 165–180.

Giraldeau, L. A., & Caraco, T. (2000). *Social foraging theory.* Princeton: Princeton University Press.

Giraldeau, L. A., & Lefebvre, L. (1986). Exchangeable producer and scrounger roles in a captive flock of feral pigeons: A case for the skill pool effect. *Animal Behaviour, 34,* 797–803.

Giraldeau, L. A., & Lefebvre, L. (1987). Scrounging prevents cultural transmission of food-finding in pigeons. *Animal Behaviour, 35,* 387–394.

Giske, J., Huse, G., & Fiksen, O. (1998). Modelling spatial dynamics of fish. *Reviews in Fish Biology and Fisheries, 8,* 57–91.

Gleason, J. M., Nuzhdin, S. V., & Ritchie, M. G. (2002). Quantitative trait loci affecting a courtship signal in *Drosophila melanogaster*. *Heredity, 89,* 1–6.

Glimcher, P. (2004). *Decisions, uncertainty, and the brain: The science of neuroeconomics.* Cambridge, MA: MIT Press.

Glimcher, P. W., & Rustichini, A. (2004). Neuroeconomics: The consilience of brain and decision. *Science, 306,* 447–452.

Godard, R. (1991). Long-term memory of neighbors in a migratory songbird. *Nature, 350,* 228–229.

Goddard, M. E., & Beilharz, R. (1982). Genetic and environmental factors affecting the suitability of dogs as guide dogs for the blind. *Theoretical and Applied Genetics, 62,* 97–102.

Goddard, M. E., & Beilharz, R. (1983). Genetics of traits which determine the suitability of dogs as guide dogs for the blind. *Applied Animal Ethology, 9,* 299–315.

Goddard, M. E., & Beilharz, R. (1984). A factor analysis of fearfulness in potential guide dogs. *Applied Animal Behaviour Science, 12,* 253–265.

Goddard, M. E., & Beilharz, R. (1985). A multivariate analysis of the genetics of fearfulness in potential guide dogs. *Behavior Genetics, 15,* 69–89.

Godin, J. G. (Ed). (1997). *Behavioural ecology of fishes.* Oxford: Oxford University Press.

Godin, J. G. J., & Dugatkin, L. A. (1996). Female mating preference for bold males in the guppy, *Poecilia reticulata. Proceedings of the National Academy of Sciences, U.S.A., 93,* 10262–10267.

Gold, K. C., & Maple, T. (1994). Personality assessment in the gorilla and its utility as a management tool. *Zoo Biology, 13,* 509–522.

Goldstein, L., Rasmussen, A., Bunney, B., & Roth, R. (1996). Role of the amygdala in the coordination of behavioral, neuroendocrine and prefrontal cortical monoamine responses to psychological stress in the rat. *Journal of Neuroscience, 16,* 4787–4798.

Gomendio, M., Harcourt, A., & Roldan, E. (1998). Sperm competition in mammals. In T. Birkhead & A. Moller (Eds.), *Sperm competition and sexual selection* (pp. 667–756). London: Academic Press.

Gonzalez-Voyer, A., Szekely, T., & Drummond, H. (2007). Why do some siblings attack each other? Comparative analysis of aggression in avian broods. *Evolution, 61,* 1946–1955.

Goodall, J. (1986). *The chimpanzees of Gombe: Patterns of behavior.* Cambridge, MA: Belknap Press.

Goodson, J. L., & Bass, A. H. (2001). Social behavior functions and related anatomical characteristics of vasotocin/vasopressin systems in vertebrates. *Brain Research Reviews, 35,* 246–265.

Goodwin, D. (1986). *Crows of the world* (2nd ed). London: British Museum.

Goodwin, N. B., Balshine-Earn, S., & Reynolds, J. D. (1998). Evolutionary transitions in parental care in cichlid fish. *Proceedings of the Royal Society of London, Series B, 265,* 2265–2272.

Goodwin, T. (1950). Carotenoids and reproduction. *Biological Reviews of the Cambridge Philosophical Society, 25,* 391–413.

Gosling, S. D. (1998). Personality dimensions in spotted hyenas (*Crocuta crocuta*). *Journal of Comparative Psychology, 112,* 107–118.

Gosling, S. D. (2001). From mice to men: What can we learn about personality from animal research? *Psychological Bulletin, 127,* 45–86.

Gould, S. J., & Lewontin, R. (1979). The spandrels of San Marcos and the Paglossian paradigm: A critique of the adaptationist programme. *Proceedings of the Royal Society of London, Series B, 205,* 581–598.

Grafe, T. U., Dobler, S., & Linsenmair, K. E. (2002). Frogs flee from the sound of fire. *Proceedings of the Royal Society of London, Series B, 269,* 999–1003.

Grafen, A. (1984). Natural selection, kin selection and group selection. In J. R. Krebs & N. B. Davies (Eds.), *Behavioural ecology: An evolutionary approach* (2nd ed., pp. 62–84). Oxford: Blackwell Science.

Grafen, A. (1988). On the uses of data on lifetime reproductive success. In T. Clutton-Brock (Ed.), *Reproductive success* (pp. 454–471). Chicago: University of Chicago Press.

Grafen, A. (1990a). Biological signals as handicaps. *Journal of Theoretical Biology, 144,* 517–546.

Grafen, A. (1990b). Sexual selection unhandicapped by the Fisher Process. *Journal of Theoretical Biology, 144,* 473–476.

Grafen, A., & Ridley, M. (Eds). (2006). Richard Dawkins: How a scientist changed the way we think. New York: Oxford University Press.

Graham, J., & Desjardins, C. (1980). Classical conditioning: Induction of luteinizing and testosterone secretion in anticipation of sexual activity. *Science, 210,* 1039–1041.

Grant, B. R., & Grant, P. R. (1996). Cultural inheritance of song and its role in the evolution of Darwin's finches. *Evolution, 50,* 2471–2487.

Grant, P. R., & Grant, B. R. (1997). Hybridization, sexual imprinting, and mate choice. *American Naturalist, 149,* 1–28.

Grant, P. R., & Grant, R. (1994). Phenotypic and genetic effects of hybridization in Darwin's finches. *Evolution, 48,* 297–316.

Greenewalt, C. (1968). *Bird song: Acoustics and physiology.* Washington, DC: Smithsonian Press.

Greenough, W., & Juraska, J. (1979). Experience-induced changes in brain fine structure: Their behavioral implications. In M. Hahn, C. Jensen, & B. Dudek (Eds.), *Development and evolution of brain size: Behavioral implications* (pp. 295–320). New York: Academic Press.

Grezes, J., Armony, J. L., Rowe, J., & Passingham, R. E. (2003). Activations related to "mirror" and "canonical" neurons in the human brain: An fMRI study. *Neuroimage, 18,* 928–937.

Grezes, J., & Decety, J. (2001). Functional anatomy of execution, mental simulation, observation, and verb generation of actions: A meta-analysis. *Human Brain Mapping, 12,* 1–19.

Griffin, D. (1959). *Listening in the dark.* New Haven: Yale University Press.

Griffith, S. C., Owens, I. P. F., & Thuman, K. A. (2002). Extra pair paternity in birds: A review of interspecific variation and adaptive function. *Molecular Ecology, 11,* 2195–2212.

Griffiths, R. (1995). Determining competition mechanisms in tadpole assemblages. *Herpetological Journal, 5,* 208–210.

Grobecker, D., & Pietsch, T. (1978). Crows use automobiles as nutcrackers. *Auk, 95,* 760.

Gross, C., Zhuang, X. X., Stark, K., Ramboz, S., Oosting, R., Kirby, L., Santarelli, L., Beck, S., & Hen, R. (2002). Serotonin(1A) receptor acts during development to establish normal anxiety-like behaviour in the adult. *Nature, 416,* 396–400.

Gross, M. R. (1982). Sneakers, satellites, and parentals: Polymorphic mating strategies in North American sunfishes. *Zeitschrift fur Tierpsychologie, 60,* 1–26.

Gross, M. (1985). Disruptive selection for alternative life histories in salmon. *Nature, 313,* 47–48.

Gross, M., & Charnov, R. (1980). Alternative male life histories in bluegill sunfish. *Proceedings of the National Academy of Sciences, U.S.A., 77,* 6937–6940.

Gross, M. R., & Sargent, R. C. (1985). The evolution of male and female parental care in fishes. *American Zoologist, 25,* 807–822.

Guthrie, D. M., & Muntz, W. (1993). Role of vision in fish behavior. In T. Pitcher (Ed.), *Behaviour of teleost fishes.* New York: Chapman and Hall.

Guthrie, R. D. (1971). A new theory of mammalian rump patch evolution. *Behaviour, 38,* 132–145.

Gutierrez, G., & Domjan, M. (1996). Learning and male-male sexual competition in Japanese quail (*Coturnix japonica*). *Journal of Comparative Psychology, 110,* 170–175.

Gutsmann-Conrad, A., Heydari, A., You, S., & Richardson, A. (1998). The expression of heat shock protein 70 decreases with cellular senescence in vitro and in cells derived from young and old human subjects. *Experimental Cell Research, 241,* 404–413.

Gwinner, H., & Berger, S. (2005). European starlings: Nestling condition, parasites and green nest material during the breeding season. *Journal of Ornithology, 146,* 365–371.

Hack, M. A. (1997). Assessment strategies in the contests of male crickets, *Acheta domesticus* (L). *Animal Behaviour, 53,* 733–747.

Haesler, S., Wada, K., Nshdejan, A., Morrisey, E. E., Lints, T., Jarvis, E. D., & Scharff, C. (2004). FoxP2 expression in avian vocal learners and non-learners. *Journal of Neuroscience, 24,* 3164–3175.

Hagenguth, H., & Rembold, H. (1978). Identification of juvenile hormone 3 as the only JH homolog in all developmental stages of the honey bee. *Zeitschrift fur Naturforschun C, 33,* 847–850.

Haig, D. (1993). Genetic conflicts in human pregnancy. *Quarterly Review of Biology, 68,* 495–532.

Hailman, J. (1982). Ontogeny: Toward a general theoretical framework for ethology. *Perspectives in Ethology, 5,* 133–189.

Hain, T., & Neff, B. (2006). Promiscuity drives self-referent recognition. *Current Biology, 16,* 1807–1811.

Haldane, J. B. S. (1941). *New paths in genetics.* London: Allen and Unwin.

Hall, K. R., & Devore, I. (1965). Baboon social behavior. In I. Devore (Ed.), *Primate behavior: Field studies of monkeys and apes* (pp. 53–110). New York: Holt, Rinehart and Winston.

Hall, S. (1998). Object play by adult animals. In M. Bekoff & J. Byers (Eds.), *Animal play: Evolutionary, comparative and ecological perspectives* (pp. 45–60). Cambridge: Cambridge University Press.

Hamilton, W. D. (1963). The evolution of altruistic behavior. *American Naturalist, 97,* 354–356.

Hamilton, W. D. (1964). The genetical evolution of social behaviour. I and II. *Journal of Theoretical Biology, 7,* 1–52.

Hamilton, W. D. (1967). Extraordinary sex ratios. *Science, 156,* 477–487.

Hamilton, W. D., & Zuk, M. (1982). Heritable true fitness and bright birds: A role for parasites. *Science, 218,* 384–387.

Hammer, M., & Menzel, R. (1998). Multiple sites of associative odor learning as revealed by local brain microinjections of octopamine in honeybees. *Learning & Memory, 5,* 146–156.

Hammerstein, P., & Parker, G. A. (1982). The asymmetric war of attrition. *Journal of Theoretical Biology, 96,* 647–682.

Hanlon, R. T., & Messenger, J. B. (1988). Adaptive coloration in young cuttlefish (*Sepia officinalis*): The morphology and development of body patterns and their relation to behavior. *Philosophical Transactions of the Royal Society of London, Series B, 320,* 437–487.

Hanlon, R. T., Naud, M. J., Forsythe, J. W., Hall, K., Watson, A. C., & McKechnie, J. (2007). Adaptable night camouflage by cuttlefish. *American Naturalist, 169,* 543–551.

Harcourt, A. H., & de Waal, F. B. M. (Eds). (1992). *Coalitions and alliances in humans and other animals.* Oxford: Oxford University Press.

Harcourt, R. (1991). Survivorship costs of play in the South American fur seal. *Animal Behaviour, 42,* 509–511.

Hardy, J. (1961). Studies of behavior and phylogeny of certain New World jays (*Garrulinae*). *University of Kansas Science Bulletin, 42,* 13–149.

Hare, J. F., & Atkins, B. A. (2001). The squirrel that cried wolf: Reliability detection by juvenile Richardson's ground squirrels (*Spermophilus richardsonii*). *Behavioral Ecology and Sociobiology, 51,* 108–112.

Hariri, A. R., Mattay, V. S., Tessitore, A., Kolachana, B., Fera, F., Goldman, D., Egan, M. F., & Weinberger, D. R. (2002). Serotonin transporter genetic variation and the response of the human amygdala. *Science, 297,* 400–403.

Harlow, H. (1959). Learning set and error factor theory. In S. Koch (Ed.), *Psychology: A study of science* (pp. 429–537). New York: McGraw-Hill.

Harper, D. C. (1982). Competitive foraging in mallards: "Ideal free" ducks. *Animal Behaviour, 30,* 575–584.

Hart, B. L. (2005). The evolution of herbal medicine: Behavioural perspectives. *Animal Behaviour, 70,* 975–989.

Hart, B. L., & Hart, L. A. (1992). Reciprocal allogrooming in impala, *Aepyceros melampus. Animal Behaviour, 44,* 1073–1083.

Hartl, D., & Clark, A. (2006). *Principles of population genetics* (4th ed.). Sunderland, MA: Sinauer.

Harvell, C. (1998). Genetic variation and polymorphism in the inducible spines of a marine bryozoan. *Evolution, 52,* 80–86.

Harvell, C. D. (1991). Coloniality and inducible polymorphism. *American Naturalist, 138,* 1–14.

Harvell, C. D. (1994). The evolution of polymorphism in colonial invertebrates and social insects. *Quarterly Review of Biology, 69,* 155–185.

Hatchwell, B. J., Ross, D. J., Fowlie, M. K., & McGowan, A. (2001). Kin discrimination in cooperatively breeding long-tailed tits. *Proceedings of the Royal Society of London, Series B, 268,* 885–890.

Hatchwell, B. J., Russell, A. F., MacColl, A. D. C., Ross, D. J., Fowlie, M. K., & McGowan, A. (2004). Helpers increase long-term but not short-term productivity in cooperatively breeding long-tailed tits. *Behavioral Ecology, 15,* 1–10.

Hauber, M. E., Russo, S. A., & Sherman, P. W. (2001). A password for species recognition in a brood-parasitic bird. *Proceedings of the Royal Society of London, Series B, 268,* 1041–1048.

Hauser, D. (1964). Anting by gray squirrels. *Journal of Mammalogy, 45,* 136–138.

Hauser, M. (1997). *The evolution of communication.* Cambridge, MA: MIT Press.

Hauser, M. (2000). *Wild minds.* New York: Henry Holt.

Hauser, M., & Konishi, M. (Eds). (1999). *The design of animal communication.* Cambridge, MA: MIT Press.

Hausfater, G., & Blaffer-Hrdy, S. (Eds.). (1984). *Infanticide*. New York: Aldine.

Hawkins, R. D., Kandel, E. R., & Bailey, C. H. (2006). Molecular mechanisms of memory storage in *Aplysia*. *Biological Bulletin*, *210*, 174–191.

Hay, M., & Fuller, P. (1981). Seed escape from hetromyids rodents: The importance of microhabitat and seed preference. *Ecology*, *62*, 1395–1399.

Healey, S. (1992). Optimal memory: Toward an evolutionary ecology of animal cognition. *Trends in Ecology and Evolution*, *8*, 399–400.

Healey, S., & Krebs, J. R. (1992). Food storing and the hippocampus in corvids: Amount and volume are correlated. *Proceedings of the Royal Society of London, Series B*, *248*, 241–245.

Heape, W. (1931). *Emigration, migration and nomadism*. Cambridge: Cambridge University Press.

Hegner, R. (1985). Dominance and anti-predator behaviour in blue tits (*Parus caeruleus*). *Animal Behaviour*, *33*, 762–768.

Heinrich, B. (1988a). Why do ravens fear their food? *Condor*, *90*, 950–952.

Heinrich, B. (1988b). Winter foraging at carcasses by three sympatric corvids, with emphasis on recruitment by the raven, *Corvus corax*. *Behavioral Ecology and Sociobiology*, *23*, 141–156.

Heinrich, B. (1995). Neophilia and exploration in juvenile common ravens, *Corvus corax*. *Animal Behaviour*, *50*, 695–704.

Heinrich, B. (1999). *Mind of the raven*. New York: Harper Collins.

Heinrich, B., & Bugnyar, T. (2007). Just how smart are ravens? *Scientific American*, *296*, 64–71.

Heinrich, B., & Marzluff, J. M. (1991). Do common ravens yell because they want to attract others? *Behavioral Ecology and Sociobiology*, *28*, 13–21.

Heinrich, B., Marzluff, J., & Adams, W. (1996). Fear and food recognition in naive common ravens. *Auk*, *112*, 499–503.

Heinrich, B., & Smokler, R. (1998). Play in common ravens (*Corvus corax*). In M. Bekoff & J. Byers (Eds.), *Animal play: Evolutionary, comparative and ecological perspectives* (pp. 27–44). Cambridge: Cambridge University Press.

Hemelrijk, C. K., & Ek, A. (1991). Reciprocity and interchange of grooming and "support" in captive chimpanzees. *Animal Behaviour*, *41*, 923–935.

Hemmes, R. B., Alvarado, A., & Hart, B. L. (2002). Use of California bay foliage by wood rats for possible fumigation of nest-borne ectoparasites. *Behavioral Ecology*, *13*, 381–385.

Henrich, J., Boyd, R., Bowles, S., Camerer, C., Fehr, E., Gintis, H., McElreath, R., Alvard, M., Barr, A., Ensminger, J., Henrich, N. S., Hill, K., Gil-White, F., Gurven, M., Marlowe, F. W., Patton, J. Q., & Tracer, D. (2005). "Economic man" in cross-cultural perspective: Behavioral experiments in 15 small-scale societies. *Behavioral and Brain Sciences*, *28*, 795–855.

Henry, J., Liu, Y., Nadra, W., Qian, G., Mormede, P., Lemaire, V., Ely, D., & Hendley, E. (1993). Psychosocial stress can induce chronic hypertension in normotensive strains of rats. *Hypertension*, *21*, 714–723.

Henry, J., & Stephens, P. (1977). *Stress, health and the social environment: A sociobiological approach to medicine*. Berlin: Springer-Verlag.

Hepper, P. G. (Ed). (1991). *Kin recognition*. Cambridge: Cambridge University Press.

Hepper, P., & Cleland, J. (1998). Developmental aspects of kin recognition. *Genetica*, *104*, 199–205.

Herard, F., Keller, M. A., Lewis, W. J., & Tumlinson, J. H. (1988). Beneficial arthropod behavior mediated by airborne semiochemicals. 3. Influence of age and experience on flight chamber responses of *Microplitis demolitor Wilkinson* (Hymenoptera, Braconidae). *Journal of Chemical Ecology*, *14*, 1583–1596.

Herrero, A. I., Sandi, C., & Venero, C. (2006). Individual differences in anxiety trait are related to spatial learning abilities and hippocampal expression of mineralocorticoid receptors. *Neurobiology of Learning and Memory*, *86*, 150–159.

Hessing, M., Hagelso, A., Schouten, W., Wiepkema, P., & Van Beek, J. (1994). Individual, behavioral and physiological strategies in pigs. *Physiology and Behavior*, *55*, 39–46.

Heyes, C. M. (1994). Social learning in animals: Categories and mechanisms. *Biological Reviews of the Cambridge Philosophical Society*, *69*, 207–231.

Heyes, C. M., & Galef, B. G. (Eds.). (1996). *Social learning in animals: The roots of culture*. London: Academic Press.

Hill, G. (1990). Female house finches prefer colourful males: Sexual selection for a condition-dependent trait. *Animal Behaviour*, *40*, 563–572.

Hill, G. (1991). Plumage coloration is a sexually selected indicator of male quality. *Nature*, *350*, 337–339.

Hill, G. (1992). The proximate basis of variation in carotenoid pigmentation in male house finches. *Auk*, *109*, 1–12.

Hill, G. (1993a). Geographic variation in the carotenoid plumage pigmentation of male house finches (*Carpodacus mexicanus*). *Biological Journal of the Linnean Society*, *49*, 63–86.

Hill, G. (1993b). Male mate choice and the evolution of female plumage coloration in the house finch. *Evolution*, *47*, 1515–1525.

Hill, G. (1993c). The proximate basis of inter- and intra-population variation in female plumage coloration in the house finch. *Canadian Journal of Zoology*, *71*, 619–627.

Hill, G. E., & Farmer, K. L. (2005). Carotenoid-based plumage coloration predicts resistance to a novel parasite in the house finch. *Naturwissenschaften*, *92*, 30–34.

Hill, G. E., Inouye, C. Y., & Montgomerie, R. (2002). Dietary carotenoids predict plumage coloration in wild house finches. *Proceedings of the Royal Society of London, Series B*, *269*, 1119–1124.

Hill, G., & Pierce, N. (1989). The effect of adult diet on the biology of butterflies, 1: The common imperial blue, *Jalmenus evagoras*. *Oecologia*, *81*, 249–257.

Hill, H., & Bekoff, M. (1977). The variability of some motor components of social play and agonistic behavior in infant Eastern coyotes, *Canis latrans*. *Animal Behaviour*, *25*, 907–909.

Hillis, D. M., Bull, J. J., White, M. E., Badgett, M. R., & Molineux, I. J. (1992). Experimental phylogenetics: Generation of a known phylogeny. *Science*, *255*, 589–592.

Hinde, R. A. (1973). Nobel recognition for ethology. *Nature, 245,* 346.

Hinton, G., & Nowlan, S. (1987). How learning can guide evolution. *Complex Systems, 1,* 495–502.

Hiraiwa, M. (1975). Pebble collecting behavior in Japanese macaques. *Monkey, 19,* 24–25 (in Japanese).

Hirth, D. H., & McCullough, D. R. (1977). Evolution of alarm signals in ungulates with special reference to white-tailed deer. *American Naturalist, 111,* 31–42.

Hodge, M. A., & Uetz, G. (1995). A comparison of agonistic behaviour of colonial web-building spiders from desert and tropical habitats. *Animal Behaviour, 50,* 963–972.

Hoekstra, H. E. (2006). Genetics, development and evolution of adaptive pigmentation in vertebrates. *Heredity, 97,* 222–234.

Hoese, H. D. (1971). Dolphin feeding out of water in a salt marsh. *Journal of Mammalogy, 52,* 222–223.

Hofferth, S. L. (2006). Residential father family type and child well-being: Investment versus selection. *Demography, 43,* 53–77.

Hofferth, S. L., & Anderson, K. G. (2003). Are all dads equal? Biology versus marriage as a basis for paternal investment. *Journal of Marriage and the Family, 65,* 213–232.

Hoffman-Goetz, L., & Pedersen, B. (1994). Exercise and the immune system: A model of the stress response? *Immunology Today, 15,* 382–387.

Hoffmann, A. (1999). Laboratory and field heritabilities: Some lessons from Drosophila. In T. Mousseau, B. Sinervo, & J. Endler (Eds.), *Adaptive genetic variation in the wild* (pp. 200–218). New York: Oxford University Press.

Hogan, J. (1994). The concept of cause in the study of behavior. In J. Hogan & J. Bolhuis (Eds.), *Causal mechanisms of behavioural development* (pp. 3–15). Cambridge: Cambridge University Press.

Hogan-Warburg, A. J. (1966). Social behavior of the ruff, *Philomachus pugnax* (L). *Ardea, 54,* 109–229.

Hoglund, J. (2003). Lek-kin in birds: Provoking theory and surprising new results. *Annales Zoologici Fennici, 40,* 249–253.

Hoglund, J., & Alatalo, R. (1995). *Leks.* Princeton: Princeton University Press.

Hoglund, J., Alatalo, R., Gibson, R., & Lundberg, A. (1995). Mate-choice copying in black grouse. *Animal Behaviour, 49,* 1627–1633.

Hoglund, J., Alatalo, R. V., & Lundberg, A. (1990). Copying the mate choice of others? Observations on female black grouse. *Behaviour, 114,* 221–236.

Hoglund, J., Alatalo, R. V., Lundberg, A., Rintamaki, P. T., & Lindell, J. (1999). Microsatellite markers reveal the potential for kin selection on black grouse leks. *Proceedings of the Royal Society of London, Series B, 266,* 813–816.

Hoglund, J., Widemo, F., Sutherland, W. J., & Nordenfors, H. (1998). Ruffs, *Philomachus pugnax,* and distribution models: Can leks be regarded as patches? *Oikos, 82,* 370–376.

Hogstad, O. (1995). Alarm calling by willow tits, *Paras montanus,* as mate investment. *Animal Behaviour, 49,* 221–225.

Holden, P., & Sharrock, J. (1988). *The Royal Society for the Protection of Birds book. Book of the British Isles.* London: MacMillan.

Holekamp, K. E., & Smale, L. (1998). Behavioral development in the spotted hyena. *Bioscience, 48,* 997–1005.

Holekamp, K. E., Smale, L., & Szykman, M. (1996). Rank and reproduction in the female spotted hyaena. *Journal of Reproduction and Fertility, 108,* 229–237.

Holldobler, B., & Roces, F. (2001). The behavioral ecology of stridulatory communication in leaf cutting ants. In L. A. Dugatkin (Ed.), *Model systems in behavioral ecology.* Princeton: Princeton University Press.

Holldobler, B., & Wilson, E. O. (1990). *The ants.* Cambridge, MA: Harvard University Press.

Hollen, L. I., & Manser, M. B. (2006). Ontogeny of alarm call responses in meerkats, *Suricata suricatta:* The roles of age, sex and nearby conspecifics. *Animal Behaviour, 72,* 1345–1353.

Hollis, K. L. (1984). The biological function of Pavlovian conditioning: The best defense is a good offense. *Journal of Experimental Psychology–Animal Behavior Processes, 10, 413–425.*

Hollis, K. L., Cadieux, E. L., & Colbert, M. M. (1989). The biological function of Pavlovian conditioning: A mechanism for mating success in blue gourami (*Trichogaster trichopterus*). *Journal of Comparative Psychology, 103,* 115–121.

Hollis, K. L., Dumas, M., Singh, P., & Fackelman, P. (1995). Pavlovian conditioning of aggressive behavior in blue gourami fish (*Trichogaster trichopterus*): Winners become winners and losers stay losers. *Journal of Comparative Psychology, 109,* 123–133.

Holloway, W., & Thor, D. (1985). Interactive effects of caffeine, 2–cholroadenosine and haloperidol on activity, social investigation and play fighting of juvenile rats. *Pharmacology Biochemistry and Behavior, 22,* 421–426.

Holman, L., & Snook, R. R. (2006). Spermicide, cryptic female choice and the evolution of sperm form and function. *Journal of Evolutionary Biology, 19,* 1660–1670.

Holmes, W. G. (2004). The early history of Hamiltonian-based research on kin recognition. *Annales Zoologici Fennici, 41,* 691–711.

Holmes, W., & Sherman, P. W. (1983). Kin recognition in animals. *American Scientist, 71,* 46–55.

Hoogland, J. L. (1983). Nepotism and alarm calls in the black-tailed prarie dog (*Cynomys ludovicianus*). *Animal Behaviour, 31,* 472–479.

Hoogland, J. L. (1995). *The black-tailed prairie dog.* Chicago: University of Chicago Press.

Hoogland, J., & Sherman, P. W. (1976). Advantages and disadvantages of bank swallow coloniality. *Ecological Monographs, 46,* 33–58.

Hopster, H. (1998). *Coping strategies in dairy cows.* Wageningen: Agricultural University.

Hosoi, S. A., Rothstein, S. I., & O'Loghlen, A. L. (2005). Sexual preferences of female brown-headed cowbirds (*Molothrus ater*) for perched song repertoires. *Auk, 122,* 82–93.

Houde, A. E. (1988). Genetic difference in female choice in two guppy populations. *Animal Behaviour, 36,* 510–516.

Houde, A. E. (1992). Sex-linked heritability of a sexually selected character in a natural population of *Poecilia reticulata. Heredity, 69,* 229–235.

Houde, A. E. (1994). Effect of artificial selection on male colour patterns on mating preference of female guppies. *Proceedings of the Royal Society of London, Series B, 256,* 125–130.

Houde, A. E. (1997). *Sex, color and mate choice in guppies.* Princeton: Princeton University Press.

Houde, A. E., & Endler, J. A. (1990). Correlated evolution of female mating preference and male color pattern in the guppy, *Poecilia reticulata. Science, 248,* 1405–1408.

Howe, N., & Harris, L. (1978). Transfer of the sea anemone pheromone, anthropleurine, by the nudibranch *Acolidia papillosa. Journal of Chemical Ecology, 4,* 551–561.

Hrdy, S. (1999). *Mother nature: A history of mothers, infants, and natural selection.* New York: Pantheon Books.

Hsu, Y., Earley, R. L., & Wolf, L. (2005). Modulation of aggressive behavior by fighting experience: Mechanisms and contest outcomes. *Biological Reviews of the Cambridge Philosophical Society, 80,* 1–42.

Hsu, Y. Y., & Wolf, L. L. (1999). The winner and loser effect: Integrating multiple experiences. *Animal Behaviour, 57,* 903–910.

Hsu, Y. Y., & Wolf, L. L. (2001). The winner and loser effect: What fighting behaviours are influenced? *Animal Behaviour, 61,* 777–786.

Huber, R., & Kravitz, E. (1995). A quantitative analysis of agonistic behavior in juvenile American lobsters (*Homarus americanus*). *Brain, Behavior and Evolution, 46,* 72–83.

Huber, R., Smith, K., Delago, A., Isakson, K., & Kravitz, E. (1997). Serotonin and aggressive motivation in crustaceans: Altering the decision to retreat. *Proceedings of the National Academy of Sciences, U.S.A., 94,* 5939–5942.

Huffman, M. (1993). An investigation of the use of medicinals by chimpanzees: Current status and future prospects. *Primate Research, 9,* 179–187.

Huffman, M. (1996). Acquisition of innovative cultural behaviors in nonhuman primates: A case study of stone handling , a socially transmitted behavior in Japanese macaques. In C. M. Heyes, & B. G. Galef (Eds.), *Social learning in animals: The roots of culture* (pp. 267–289). London: Academic Press.

Huffman, M. (1997). Current evidence for self-medication in primates: A multidisciplinary perspective. *Yearbook of Physical Anthropology, 40,* 171–200.

Huffman, M. (2007). Primate self-medication. In C. Campbell, A. Fuentes, K. MacKinnon, M. Panger, & S. Bearder (Eds.), *Primates in perspective* (pp. 677–690). Oxford: Oxford University Press.

Huffman, M., & Wrangham , R. (1994). Diversity of medicinal plant use by chimpanzees in the wild. In R. Wrangham, W. C. McGrew, F. de Waal, & P. Heltne (Eds.), *Chimpanzee culture* (pp. 129–148). Cambridge: Harvard University Press.

Huffman, M. A., & Hirata, S. (2004). An experimental study of leaf swallowing in captive chimpanzees: Insights into the origin of a self-medicative behavior and the role of social learning. *Primates, 45,* 113–118.

Hughes, L., Chang, B., Wagner, D., & Pierce, N. (2000). Effects of mating history on ejaculate size, fecundity and copulation duration in the ant-tended lycaenid butterfly, *Jalmenus evagoras. Behavioral Ecology and Sociobiology, 47,* 119–128.

Hugie, D. M., & Lank, D. B. (1997). The resident's dilemma: A female choice model for the evolution of alternative mating strategies in lekking male ruffs (*Philomachus pugnax*). *Behavioral Ecology, 8,* 218–225.

Hulscher-Emeis, T. (1992). The variable patterns of *Tilapia zillii* (Cichlidae): Integrating ethology, chromatophore regulation and the physiology of stress. *Netherlands Journal of Zoology, 42,* 525–560.

Humphreys, A., & Einon, D. (1981). Play as a reinforcer for maze learning in juvenile rats. *Animal Behaviour, 29,* 259–270.

Humphreys, A., & Smith, P. (1987). Rough and tumble play, friendship and dominance in school children: Evidence for continuity and change with age. *Child Development, 58,* 201–212.

Huntingford, F. A. (1984). Some ethical issues raised by studies of predation and aggression. *Animal Behaviour, 32,* 210–215.

Huntingford, F., & Turner, A. (1987). *Animal conflict.* London: Chapman and Hall.

Huntingford, F. A., & Wright, P. J. (1992). Inherited population differences in avoidance conditioning in three-spined sticklebacks, *Gasterosteus aculeatu*s. *Behaviour, 122,* 264–273.

Hurd, P. (1997). Cooperative signalling between opponents in fish fights. *Animal Behaviour, 54,* 1309–1315.

Hurd, P. L. (2006). Resource holding potential, subjective resource value, and game theoretical models of aggressiveness signalling. *Journal of Theoretical Biology, 241,* 639–648.

Hutt, C. (1966). Exploration and play in children. *Zoological Society of London (Symposium), 18,* 61–81.

Hutt, C. (1970). Specific and diverse exploration. *Advances in Child Development and Behavior, 5,* 119–180.

Huttenlocher, P. (2002). *Neural plasticity: The effects of environment on the development of the cerebral cortex.* Cambridge. MA: Harvard University Press.

Huxley, J. (1938). Darwin's theory of sexual selection and the data subsumed by it, in light of recent research. *American Naturalist, 72,* 416–433.

Huxley, J. (1942). *Evolution: The modern synthesis.* New York: Harper.

Huxley, T. H. (1888). The struggle for existence: A programme. *Nineteenth Century, 23,* 161–180.

Iacoboni, M., Koski, L. M., Brass, M., Bekkering, H., Woods, R. P., Dubeau, M. C., Mazziotta, J. C., & Rizzolatti, G. (2001). Reafferent copies of imitated actions in the right superior temporal cortex. *Proceedings of the National Academy of Sciences, U.S.A., 98,* 13995–13999.

Immelmann, K. (1972). Sexual and other long-term aspects of imprinting in birds and other species. In D. S. Lehrman, R. A. Hinde, & E. Shaw (Eds.), *Advances in the study of behavior* (pp. 147–174). New York: Academic Press.

Immelmann, K., Prove, R., Lassek, R., & Bischof, H. J. (1991). Influence of adult courtship experience on the development of sexual preferences in zebra finches. *Animal Behaviour, 42,* 83–89.

Ims, R. A. (1987). Responses in social organization and behaviour manipulation of the food resource in the vole *Clethrionomys rufocanus. Journal of Animal Ecology, 56,* 585–596.

Inouye, C. Y., Hill, G. E., Stradi, R. D., & Montgomerie, R. (2001). Carotenoid pigments in male house finch plumage in relation to age, subspecies, and ornamental coloration. *Auk, 118,* 900–915.

Irwin, D. E., & Price, T. (1999). Sexual imprinting, learning and speciation. *Heredity, 82,* 347–354.

Jablonski, P. G., Lee, S. D., & Jerzak, L. (2006). Innate plasticity of a predatory behavior: Nonlearned context dependence of avian flush-displays. *Behavioral Ecology, 17,* 925–932.

Jacobs, G. H. (1992). Ultraviolet vision in vertebrates. *American Zoologist, 32,* 544–554.

Jacobs, L. F., Gaulin, S. J. C., Sherry, D. F., & Hoffman, G. E. (1990). Evolution of spatial cognition: Sex-specific patterns of spatial behavior predict hippocampal size. *Proceedings of the National Academy of Sciences, U.S.A., 87,* 6349–6352.

Jacobson, M. (1991). *Developmental neurobiology.* New York: Plenum Press.

Janik, V. M., Sayigh, L. S., & Wells, R. S. (2006). Signature whistle shape conveys identity information to bottlenose dolphins. *Proceedings of the National Academy of Sciences, U.S.A., 103,* 8293–8297.

Jansa, S. A., & Weksler, M. (2004). Phylogeny of muroid rodents: Relationships within and among major lineages as determined by IRBP gene sequences. *Molecular Phylogenetics and Evolution, 31,* 256–276.

Janzen, D. (1978). Complications in interpreting the chemical defenses of trees against tropical arboreal plant-eating vertebrates. In G. Montgomerie (Ed.), *The ecology of arboreal boliovores* (pp. 73–84). Washington, DC: Smithsonian Press.

Jarrard, H. E. (1997). Postembryonic changes in the structure of the olfactory bulb of the Chinook salmon (*Oncorhynchus tshawytscha*) across its life history. *Brain Behavior and Evolution, 49,* 249–260.

Jarvis, J. (1981). Eusociality in a mammal: Cooperative breeding in the naked mole-rat. *Science, 212,* 571–573.

Jeffreys, A., Wilson, V., & Thein, S. (1985). Hypervariable "minisatellite" regions in human DNA. *Nature, 314,* 67–73.

Jenkins, W. M., Merzenich, M. M., Ochs, M. T., Allard, T., & Guicrobles, E. (1990). Functional reorganization of primary somatosensory cortex in adult owl monkeys after behaviorally controlled tactile stimulation. *Journal of Neurophysiology, 63,* 82–104.

Jenni, D., & Collier, G. (1972). Polyandry in the American jacana (*Jacana spinosa*). *Auk, 89,* 743–765.

Jennions, M., & Backwell, P. (1996). Residency and size affect fight duration and outcome in the fiddler crab *Uca annulipes*. *Biological Journal of the Linnean Society, 57,* 293–306.

Jensen, P., & Yngvesson, J. (1998). Aggression between unacquainted pigs: Sequential assessment and effects of familiarity and weight. *Applied Animal Behavior Science, 58,* 49–61.

Johannesen, J., Hennig, A., Dommermuth, B., & Schneider, J. M. (2002). Mitochondrial DNA distributions indicate colony propagation by single matri-lineages in the social spider *Stegodyphus dumicola* (Eresidae). *Biological Journal of the Linnean Society, 76,* 591–600.

John, J. (1994). The avian spleen: A neglected organ. *Quarterly Review of Biology, 69,* 327–351.

Johns, T. (1999). The chemical ecology of human ingestive behaviors. *Annual Review of Anthropology, 28,* 27–50.

Johnson, R. N., Oldroyd, B. P., Barron, A. B., & Crozier, R. H. (2002). Genetic control of the honey bee (*Apis mellifera*) dance language: Segregating dance forms in a backcrossed colony. *Journal of Heredity, 93,* 170–173.

Johnsson, J., & Akerman, A. (1998). Watch and learn: Preview of the fighting ability of opponents alters contest behaviour in rainbow trout. *Animal Behaviour, 56,* 771–776.

Johnston, T. (Ed). (1985). *Issues in the ecological study of learning.* Hillsdale, NJ: Lawrence Erlbaum Associates.

Johnstone, R. A. (1995). Sexual selection, honest advertisement and the handicap principle: Reviewing the evidence. *Biological Reviews of the Cambridge Philosophical Society, 70,* 1–65.

Johnstone, R. A. (1998). Game theory and communication. In L. A. Dugatkin & H. K. Reeve (Eds.), *Game theory and animal behavior* (pp. 94–117). New York: Oxford University Press.

Johnstone, R., & Dugatkin, L. A. (2000). Coalition formation in animals and the nature of winner and loser effects. *Proceedings of the Royal Society of London, Series B, 267,* 17–21.

Johnstone, T. D. (1982). The selective costs and benefits of learning. *Advances in the Study of Behavior, 12,* 65–106.

Jolicoeur, P., Pirlot, P., Baron, G., & Stephan, H. (1984). Brain structure and correlation patterns in Insectivora, Chiroptera and Primates. *Systematic Zoology, 33,* 14–29.

Jones, G., Barabas, A., Elliott, W., & Parsons, S. (2002). Female greater wax moths reduce sexual display behavior in relation to the potential risk of predation by echolocating bats. *Behavioral Ecology, 13,* 375–380.

Jones, G., & Holderied, M. W. (2007). Bat echolocation calls: Adaptation and convergent evolution. *Proceedings of the Royal Society of London, Series B, 274,* 905–912.

Jones, G., & Teeling, E. C. (2006). The evolution of echolocation in bats. *Trends in Ecology & Evolution, 21,* 149–156.

Jones, T. M., Quinnell, R. J., & Balmford, A. (1998). Fisherian flies: Benefits of female choice in a lekking sandfly. *Proceedings of the Royal Society of London, Series B, 265,* 1651–1657.

Jouventin, P., & Aubin, T. (2002). Acoustic systems are adapted to breeding ecologies: Individual recognition in nesting penguins. *Animal Behaviour, 64,* 747–757.

Jouventin, P., Aubin, T., & Lengagne, T. (1999). Finding a parent in a king penguin colony: The acoustic system of individual recognition. *Animal Behaviour, 57,* 1175–1183.

Kacelnik, A., Krebs, J., & Bernstein, C. (1992). The ideal free distributions and predator-prey populations. *Trends in Ecology & Evolution, 7,* 50–55.

Kaczensky, P. (1996). *Livestock-carnivore conflicts in Europe.* Munich: Munich Wildlife Society.

Kaczmarek, L. (1993). Molecular biology of vertebrate learning: Is c-fos a new beginning? *Journal of Neuroscience Research, 34,* 377–381.

Kagan, J. (1994). *Galen's prophecy: Temperament in human nature.* New York: Basic Books.

Kagan, J., Reznick, J. S., & Gibbons, J. (1989). Inhibited and uninhibited types of children. *Child Development, 60,* 838–845.

Kagan, J., Reznick, J. S., & Snidman, N. (1987). Temperamental variation in response to the unfamiliar. In N. A. Krasnegor, E. M. Blass, M. A. Hofer, & W. P. Smotherman (Eds.), *Perinatal development: A psychobiological perspective* (pp. 397–419). New York: Academic Press.

Kagan, J., Reznick, J. S., & Snidman, N. (1988). Biological bases of childhood shyness. *Science, 240,* 167–171.

Kamil, A., & Balda, R. (1990). Spatial memory in food caching birds. *Psychology of Learning and Motivation, 26,* 1–25.

Kamil, A., Krebs, J., & Pulliam, H. R. (Eds.). (1987). *Foraging behavior.* New York: Plenum.

Kamil, A., & Yoerg, S. (1982). Learning and foraging behavior. *Perspectives in Ethology, 5,* 325–364.

Kamin, L. J. (1968). "Attention-like" processes in classic conditioning. In M. R. Jones (Ed.), *Miami symposium on the prediction of behavior: Aversive stimulation* (pp. 9–31). Miami: Miami University Press.

Kamin, L. J. (1969). Predictability, surprise, attention and conditioning. In B. Campbell & R. Church (Eds.), *Punishment and aversive behavior* (pp. 279–296). New York: Appleton-Century-Crofts.

Kandel, E. R. (2001). The molecular biology of memory storage: A dialogue between genes and synapses. *Science, 294,* 1030–1038.

Kandel, E., & Abel, T. (1995). Neuropeptides, adenylyl cyclase and memory storage. *Science, 268,* 825–826.

Kaplun, D., & Reich, R. (1976). The murdered child and his killers. *American Journal of Psychiatry, 133,* 809–813.

Kavaliers, M., Colwell, D. D., & Choleris, E. (2001). NMDA-mediated social learning of fear-induced conditioned analgesia to biting flies. *Neuroreport, 12,* 663–667.

Kavaliers, M., Colwell, D. D., Choleris, E., & Ossenkopp, K. P. (1999). Learning to cope with biting flies: Rapid NMDA-mediated acquisition of conditioned analgesia. *Behavioral Neuroscience, 113,* 126–135.

Kavaliers, M., Ossenkopp, K. P., Galea, L. A. M., & Kolb, B. (1998). Sex differences in spatial learning and prefrontal and parietal cortical dendritic morphology in the meadow vole, Microtus pennsylvanicus. *Brain Research, 810,* 41–47.

Kawai, M. (1965). Newly acquired precultural behavior of the natural troop of Japanese monkeys on Koshima Islet. *Primates, 6,* 1–30.

Kawamura, S. (1959). The process of sub-culture propagation among Japanese macaques. *Primates,* 43–60.

Kawamura, S., Blow, N., & Yokoyama, S. (1999). Genetic analyses of visual pigments of the pigeon (*Columba livia*). *Genetics, 153,* 1839–1850.

Kawanabe, H., Cohen, J., & Iwasaki, K. (Eds.). (1993). *Mutualism and community organization: Behavioural, theoretical, and food-web approaches.* New York: Oxford University Press.

Keefe, M. (1992). Chemically mediated avoidance behaviour in wild brook trout, *Salvelinus fontinalis*: The response to familiar and unfamiliar predaceous fishes and the influences of diet. *Canadian Journal of Zoology, 70,* 288–292.

Keenleyside, M. (1955). Some aspects of the schooling behavior of fish. *Behaviour, 8,* 83–248.

Keenleyside, M., & Yamamoto, F. (1962). Territorial behaviour of juvenile Atlantic salmon (*Salmo salar L.*). *Behaviour, 19,* 139–169.

Keeton, W. T. (1971). Magnets interfere with pigeon homing. *Proceedings of the American Philosophical Society, 68,* 102–106.

Kemp, D. J., & Wiklund, C. (2004). Residency effects in animal contests. *Proceedings of the Royal Society of London, Series, B, 271,* 1707–1711.

Kendal, R. L., Coolen, I., van Bergen, Y., & Laland, K. N. (2005). Trade-offs in the adaptive use of social and asocial learning. *Advances in the Study of Behavior, 35,* 333–379.

Kendziorski, C., & Wang, P. (2006). A review of statistical methods for expression quantitative trait loci mapping. *Mammalian Genome, 17,* 509–517.

Kennedy, M., & Gray, R. (1993). Can ecological theory predict the distribution of foraging animals? A critical analysis of experiments on the ideal free distribution. *Oikos, 68,* 158–166.

Ketterson, E. D., & Nolan, V. (1999). Adaptation, exaptation, and constraint: A hormonal perspective. *American Naturalist, 154,* S4–S25.

Keverne, E. B., Martel, F. L., & Nevison, C. M. (1996). Primate brain evolution: Genetic and functional considerations. *Proceedings of the Royal Society of London, Series B, 263,* 689–696.

Keverne, E. B., Martenz, N. D., & Tuite, B. (1989). Beta-endorphin concentration in cerebrospinal fluid of monkeys are influenced by grooming relationships. *Psychoneuroendocrinology, 14,* 155–161.

Kiesecker, J. M., Belden, L. K., Shea, K., & Rubbo, M. J. (2004). Amphibian decline and emerging disease. *American Scientist, 92,* 138–147.

Kiesecker, J., & Blaustein, A. (1997). Influences of egg-laying behavior on pathogenic infection of amphibian eggs. *Conservation Biology, 11,* 214–220.

Kiesecker, J. M., & Blaustein, A. R. (1999). Pathogen reverses competition between larval amphibians. *Ecology, 80,* 2442–2448.

Kiesecker, J. M., Blaustein, A. R., & Belden, L. K. (2001). Complex causes of amphibian population declines. *Nature, 410,* 681–684.

Kiesecker, J., & Skelly, D. K. (2000). Choice of oviposition site by gray treefrogs: The role of potential parasitic infection. *Ecology, 81,* 2939–2943.

Kiesecker, J. M., Skelly, D. K., Beard, K. H., & Preisser, E. (1999). Behavioral reduction of infection risk. *Proceedings of the National Academy of Sciences, U.S.A., 96,* 9165–9168.

Kilner, J. M., Paulignan, Y., & Blakemore, S. J. (2003). An interference effect of observed biological movement on action. *Current Biology, 13,* 522–525.

Kim, J. J., & Jung, M. W. (2006). Neural circuits and mechanisms involved in Pavlovian fear conditioning: A critical review. *Neuroscience and Biobehavioral Reviews, 30,* 188–202.

Kingsolver, J. G., Hoekstra, H. E., Hoekstra, J. M., Berrigan, D., Vignieri, S. N., Hill, C. E., Hoang, A., Gibert, P., & Beerli, P. (2001). The strength of phenotypic selection in natural populations. *American Naturalist, 157,* 245–261.

Kirchhof, J., & Hammerschmidt, K. (2006). Functionally referential alarm calls in tamarins (*Saguinus fuscicollis* and *Saguinus mystax*): Evidence from playback experiments. *Ethology, 112,* 346–354.

Kirkpatrick, M. (1982). Sexual selection and the evolution of female choice. *Evolution, 36,* 1–12.

Kirkpatrick, M., & Ryan, M. (1991). The evolution of mating preferences and the paradox of the lek. *Nature, 350,* 33–38.

Kirkwood, T. (1977). Evolution and ageing. *Nature, 270,* 301–304.

Kirkwood, T., & Holliday, R. (1979). The evolution of ageing and longevity. *Proceedings of the Royal Society of London, Series B, 205,* 531–546.

Kirkwood, T., & Rose, M. (1991). Evolution of senescence: Late survival sacrificed for reproduction. *Philosophical Transactions of the Royal Society of London, Series B, 332,* 15–24.

Kitchen, W. D. (1972). *The social behavior and ecology of the pronghorn.* University of Michigan.

Kleiman, D. (1977). Monogamy in mammals. *Quarterly Review of Biology, 52,* 39–69.

Kodric-Brown, A., & Brown, J. H. (1984). Truth in advertising: The kinds of traits favored by sexual selection. *American Naturalist, 124,* 309–323.

Koenig, W. D., & Pitelka, F. (1981). Ecological factors and kin selection in the evolution of cooperative breeding in birds. In R. Alexander & D. Tinkle (Eds.), *Natural selection and social behavior* (pp. 261–280). New York: Chiron Press.

Koenig, W., Pitelka, F. A., Carmen, W. J., Mumme, R. L., & Stanback, M. T. (1992). The evolution of delayed dispersal in cooperative breeders. *Quarterly Review of Biology, 67,* 111–150.

Kogan, N., & Wallach, M. (1964). *Risk taking.* New York: Holt, Rinehart and Winston.

Kokko, H., Brooks, R., Jennions, M. D., & Morley, J. (2003). The evolution of mate choice and mating biases. *Proceedings of the Royal Society of London, Series B, 270,* 653–664.

Kokko, H., & Lindstrom, J. (1996). Kin selection and the evolution of leks: Whose success do young males maximize? *Proceedings of the Royal Society of London, Series B, 263,* 919–923.

Kokko, H., Lopez-Sepulcre, A., & Morrell, L. J. (2006). From hawks and doves to self-consistent games of territorial behavior. *American Naturalist, 167,* 901–912.

Kokko, H., Sutherland, W. J., Lindstrom, J., Reynolds, J. D., & Mackenzie, A. (1998). Individual mating success, lek stability, and the neglected limitations of statistical power. *Animal Behaviour, 56,* 755–762.

Kolb, B., & Stewart, J. (1996). Sex-related differences in dendritic branching of cells in the prefrontal cortex of rats. *Behavioral Neuroscience, 110,* 1271–1281.

Komdeur, J. (1992). Importance of habitat saturation and territory quality for the evolution of cooperative breeding in the Seychelles warbler. *Nature, 358,* 493–495.

Komers, P. E. (1989). Dominance relationships between juvenile and adult black-billed magpies. *Animal Behaviour, 37,* 256–265.

Konopka, R., & Benzer, S. (1971). Clock mutants of *Drosophila melanogaster. Proceedings of the National Academy of Sciences, 68,* 2112–2116.

Koolhaas, J. M., de Boer, S. F., Buwalda, B., & van Reenen, K. (2007). Individual variation in coping with stress: A multidimensional approach of ultimate and proximate mechanisms. *Brain, Behavior and Evolution, 70,* 218–226.

Koolhaas, J. M., Korte, S. M., De Boer, S. F., Van Der Vegt, B. J., Van Reenen, C. G., Hopster, H., De Jong, I. C., Ruis, M. A. W., & Blokhuis, H. J. (1999). Coping styles in animals: Current status in behavior and stress-physiology. *Neuroscience and Biobehavioral Reviews, 23,* 925–935.

Koops, M. A., & Grant, J. W. A. (1993). Weight symmetry and sequential assessment in convict cichlid contests. *Canadian Journal of Zoology, 71,* 475–479.

Koopsman, J., Boomsma, D., Heath, A., & Vandoornen, L. (1995). A multivariate genetic analysis of sensation seeking. *Behavior Genetics, 25,* 349–356.

Kosfeld, M., Heinrichs, M., Zak, P. J., Fischbacher, U., & Fehr, E. (2005). Oxytocin increases trust in humans. *Nature, 435,* 673–676.

Koski, L., Wohlschlager, A., Bekkering, H., Woods, R. P., Dubeau, M. C., Mazziotta, J. C., & Iacoboni, M. (2002). Modulation of motor and premotor activity during imitation of target-directed actions. *Cerebral Cortex, 12,* 847–855.

Kovalzan, V., & Mukhametov, L. (1982). Temperature variations in the brain corresponding to unihemispheric slow wave sleep in dolphins. *Journal of Evolution and Biochemical Physiology (in Russian), 18,* 307–309.

Krams, I., Krama, T., & Igaune, K. (2006). Alarm calls of wintering great tits Parus major: Warning of mate, reciprocal altruism or a message to the predator? *Journal of Avian Biology, 37,* 131–136.

Kraus, W. F. (1989). Surface wave communication during courtship in the giant water bug, *Abedus-Indentatus* (Heteroptera, Belostomatidae). *Journal of the Kansas Entomological Society, 62,* 316–328.

Krause, J., & Ruxton, G. (2002). *Living in groups.* Oxford: Oxford University Press.

Kravitz, E. (1988). Hormonal control of behavior: Amines and the biasing of behavioral output in lobsters. *Science, 241,* 1775–1781.

Krebs, J. (1978). Optimal foraging: Decision rules for predators. In J. R. Krebs & N. B. Davies (Eds.), *Behavioural ecology: An evolutionary approach* (pp. 23–63). Oxford: Blackwell Science.

Krebs, J. R. (1980). Optimal foraging, predation risk and territory defence. *Ardea, 68,* 83–90.

Krebs, J. R., & Davies, N. B. (1987). *An introduction to behavioural ecology* (2nd ed.). Oxford: Blackwell Science.

Krebs, J. R., & Davies, N. B. (1993). *An introduction to behavioural ecology* (3rd ed.). Oxford: Blackwell Science.

Krebs, J. R., & Dawkins, R. (1984). Animal signals: Mind-reading and manipulation? In J. R. Krebs & N. B. Davies (Eds.), *Behavioural ecology: An evolutionary approach* (2nd ed., pp. 380–402). Oxford: Blackwell Science.

Krebs, J. R., Kacelnik, A., & Taylor, P. (1978). Test of optimal sampling in foraging great tits. *Nature, 275,* 27–31.

Krebs, J. R., & McCleery. (1984). Optimization in behavioural ecology. In J. R. Krebs & N. B. Davies (Eds.), *Behavioural ecology: An evolutionary approach* (2nd ed., pp. 91–121). Oxford: Blackwell Science.

Krebs, J. R., Sherry, D. F., Healey, S. D., Perry, V. H., & Vaccarino, A. L. (1989). Hippocampal specialization of food-storing birds. *Proceedings of the National Academy of Sciences, 86,* 1388–1392.

Krief, S., Huffman, M. A., Sevenet, T., Hladik, C. M., Grellier, P., Loiseau, P. M., & Wrangham, R. W. (2006). Bioactive properties of plant species ingested by chimpanzees (*Pan troglodytes schweinfurthii*) in the Kibale National Park, Uganda. *American Journal of Primatology, 68*, 51–71.

Krishnamani, R., & Mahaney, W. C. (2000). Geophagy among primates: Adaptive significance and ecological consequences. *Animal Behaviour, 59*, 899–915.

Kroeber, A. L., & Kluckhohn, C. (1952). Culture, a critical review of the concepts and definitions. *Papers of the Peabody Museum, 47*, 1–223. Cambridge, MA: Peabody Museum of American Archeology and Ethnology.

Kroodsma, D., & Byers, B. (1991). The function(s) of birdsong. *American Zoologist, 31*, 318–328.

Kropotkin, P. (1902). *Mutual aid* (3rd ed.). London: William Heinemann.

Krutzen, M., Mann, J., Heithaus, M. R., Connor, R. C., Bejder, L., & Sherwin, W. B. (2005). Cultural transmission of tool use in bottlenose dolphins. *Proceedings of the National Academy of Sciences, U.S.A. 102*, 8939–8943.

Krutzen, M., Sherwin, W. B., Connor, R. C., Barre, L. M., Van de Casteele, T., Mann, J., & Brooks, R. (2003). Contrasting relatedness patterns in bottlenose dolphins (*Tursiops sp.*) with different alliance strategies. *Proceedings of the Royal Society of London, Series B, 270*, 497–502.

Kuczaj, S. A., Gory, J. D. & Xitco, M. J. (1998). Using programs to solve problems: Imitation versus insight. *Behavioral and Brain Sciences, 21*, 695.

Kudo, H., Tsuneyoshi, Y., Nagae, M., Adachi, S., Yamauchi, K., Ueda, U., & Kawamura, H. (1994). Detection of thyroid hormone receptors in the olfactory system and brain of wild masu salmon, *Oncorhynchus maou* (Brevoort), during smolting by in vitro autoradiography. *Aquaculture and Fish Management, 25* 171–182.

Kuhn, T. (1962). *The structure of scientific revolutions*. Chicago: University of Chicago Press.

Kunz, T. H., Allgaier, A. L., Seyjagat, J., & Caligiuri, R. (1994). Allomaternal care: Helper-assisted birth in the Rodrigues fruit bat, *Pteropus rodricensis* (Chiroptera: Pteropodidae). *Journal of Zoology, London, 232*, 691–700.

Kurtz, J., Kalbe, M., Aeschlimann, P. B., Haberli, M. A., Wegner, K. M., Reusch, T. B. H., & Milinski, M. (2004). Major histocompatibility complex diversity influences parasite resistance and innate immunity in sticklebacks. *Proceedings of the Royal Society of London, Series B, 271*, 197–204.

Kutsukake, N., & Clutton-Brock, T. H. (2006). Social functions of allogrooming in cooperatively breeding meerkats. *Animal Behaviour, 72*, 1059–1068.

Kyriacou, C., Oldroyd, M., Wood, J., Sharp, M., & Hill, M. (1990). Clock mutations alter developmental timing in Drosophila. *Heredity, 64*, 395–401.

Lacey, E. A., & Sherman, P. W. (1991). Social organization of naked mole-rats: Evidence for divisions of labor. In P. W. Sherman, J. Jarvis, & R. D. Alexander (Eds.), *The biology of the naked mole-rat* (pp. 275–336). Princeton: Princeton University Press.

Lachlan, R. F., & Servedio, M. R. (2004). Song learning accelerates allopatric speciation. *Evolution, 58*, 2049–2063.

Lack, D. (1968). *Ecological adaptations for breeding in birds*. London: Methuen.

Lafuma, L., Lambrechts, M. M., & Raymond, M. (2001). Aromatic plants in bird nests as a protection against blood-sucking flying insects? *Behavioural Processes, 56*, 113–120.

Laiolo, P., & Rolando, A. (2003). The evolution of vocalisations in the genus Corvus: Effects of phylogeny, morphology and habitat. *Evolutionary Ecology, 17*, 111–123.

Laland, K. N., & Janik, V. M. (2006). The animal cultures debate. *Trends in Ecology & Evolution, 21*, 542–547.

Laland, K. N., & Williams, K. (1998). Social transmission of maladaptive information in the guppy. *Behavioral Ecology, 9*, 493–499.

Landau, H. G. (1951a). On dominance relations and the structure of animal societies: I. Effects of inherent characteristics. *Bulletin of Mathematical Biophysics, 13*, 1–19.

Landau, H. G. (1951b). On dominance relations and the structure of animal societies: II. Some effects of possible social causes. *Bulletin of Mathematical Biophysics, 13*, 245–262.

Langley, C. M. (1996). Search images: Selective attention to specific visual features of prey. *Journal of Experimental Psychology-Animal Behavior Processes, 22*, 152–163.

Lank, D. B., Coupe, M., & Wynne-Edwards, K. E. (1999). Testosterone-induced male traits in female puffs (*Philomachus pugnax*): Autosomal inheritance and gender differentiation. *Proceedings of the Royal Society of London, Series B, 266*, 2323–2330.

Lank, D. B., Smith, C. M., Hanotte, O., Burke, T., & Cooke, F. (1995). Genetic polymorphism for alternative mating behavior in lekking male ruff *Philomachus pugnax*. *Nature, 378*, 59–62.

Laughlin, S. B., van Steveninck, R. R. D., & Anderson, J. C. (1998). The metabolic cost of neural information. *Nature Neuroscience, 1*, 36–41.

Law, R., & Koptur, S. (1986). On the evolution of non-specific mutualism. *Biological Journal of the Linnean Society, 27*, 251–267.

Lawick-Goodall, J. (1968). The behaviour of free-living chimpanzees in the Gombe Stream Reserve. *Animal Behavior Monographs, 1*, 161–311.

Leadbeater, E., Raine, N. E., & Chittka, L. (2006). Social learning: Ants and the meaning of teaching. *Current Biology, 16*, R323–R325.

Le Boeuf, B. J. (1978). Social behaviour in some marine and terrestrial carnivores. In E. Reese & F. Lighter (Eds.), *Contrasts in behavior* (pp. 251–279). New York: Wiley.

Le Boeuf, B. J., & Reiter, J. (1988). Lifetime reproductive success on Northern elephant seals. In T. Clutton-Brock (Ed.), *Reproductive success*. Chicago: University of Chicago.

Le Bourg, E. (2007). Does reproduction decrease longevity in human beings? *Ageing Research Reviews, 6*, 141–149.

Lefebvre, L., Gaxiola, A., Dawson, S., Timmermans, S., Rosza, L., & Kabai , P. (1997a). Feeding innovations and forebrain size in Australasian birds. *Behaviour, 135*, 1077–1097.

Lefebvre, L., Whittle, P., Lascaris, E., & Finkelstein, A. (1997b). Feeding innovations and forebrain size in birds. *Animal Behaviour, 53*, 549–560.

Lefebvre, L., Gaxiola, A., Dawson, S., Timmermans, S., Rosza, L., & Kabai, P. (1998). Feeding innovations and forebrain size in Australasian birds. *Behaviour, 135,* 1077–1097.

Lefebvre, L., Reader, S. M., & Sol, D. (2004). Brains, innovations and evolution in birds and primates. *Brain Behavior and Evolution, 63,* 233–246.

Leffler, J. (1993). *An introduction to free radicals.* New York: Wiley.

Lehmann, L., & Keller, L. (2006). The evolution of cooperation and altruism: A general framework and a classification of models. *Journal of Evolutionary Biology, 19,* 1365–1376.

Leimar, O., Austad, S., & Enquist, M. (1991). A test of the sequential assessment game: Fighting in the bowl and doily spider *Frontinella pyramitela. Evolution, 45,* 862–874.

Leimar, O., & Enquist, M. (1984). Effects of asymmetries in owner-intruder conflicts. *Journal of Theoretical Biology, 111,* 475–491.

Leisler, B., Winkler, H., & Wink, M. (2002). Evolution of breeding systems in acrocephaline warblers. *Auk, 119,* 379–390.

Lema, S. C., & Nevitt, G. A. (2004). Evidence that thyroid hormone induces olfactory cellular proliferation in salmon during a sensitive period for imprinting. *Journal of Experimental Biology, 207,* 3317–3327.

Lemaire, V., Koehl, M., Le Moal, M., & Abrous, D. N. (2000). Prenatal stress produces learning deficits associated with an inhibition of neurogenesis in the hippocampus. *Proceedings of the National Academy of Sciences, U.S.A., 97,* 11032–11037.

Lengagne, T., Aubin, T., Jouventin, P., & Lauga, J. (2000). Perceptual salience of individually distinctive features in the calls of adult king penguins. *Journal of the Acoustical Society of America, 107,* 508–516.

Leonard, J. E. & Boake, C. R. B. (2006). Site-dependent aggression and mating behaviour in three species of *Nasonia* (Hymenoptera: Pteromalidae). *Animal Behaviour, 71,* 641–647.

Leopold, A. S. (1977). *The California quail.* Los Angeles: University of California Press.

Leotta, R., Voltini, B., Mele, M., Curadi, M. C., Orlandi, M., & Secchiari, P. (2006). Latent variable models on performance tests in guide dogs. 1. Factor analysis. *Italian Journal of Animal Science, 5,* 377–385.

Leroi, A. M., Bartke, A., De Benedictis, G., Franceschi, C., Gartner, A., Gonos, E., Feder, M. E., Kivisild, T., Lee, S., Kartal-Ozer, N., Schumacher, M., Sikora, E., Slagboom, E., Tatar, M., Yashin, A. I., Vijg, J., & Zwaan, B. (2005). What evidence is there for the existence of individual genes with antagonistic pleiotropic effects? *Mechanisms of Ageing and Development, 126,* 421–429.

Levey, D. J., & Stiles, F. G. (1992). Evolutionary precursors of long-distance migration: Resource availability and movement patterns in neotropical birds. *American Naturalist, 140,* 447–476.

Levins, R. (1968). *Evolution in changing environments.* Princeton: Princeton University Press.

Levitan, D. (2000). Sperm velocity and longevity trade off each other and influence fertilization in the sea urchin *Lytechinus variegatus. Proceedings of the Royal Society of London, Series B, 267,* 531–534.

Lewontin, R. C. (1961). Evolution and the theory of games. *Journal of Theoretical Biology, 1,* 382–403.

Ley, J. M., & Bennett, P. C. (2007). Understanding personality by understanding companion dogs. *Anthrozoos, 20,* 113–124.

Liers, E. (1951). Notes on the river otter (*Luta canadensis*). *Journal of Mammalogy, 32,* 1–9.

Lima, S. L. (1985). Foraging-efficiency-predation-risk trade-off in the grey squirrel. *Animal Behaviour, 33,* 155–165.

Lima, S. (1988a). Initiation and termination of daily feeding in dark-eyed juncos: Influences of predation risk and energy reserves. *Oikos, 53,* 3–11.

Lima, S. (1988b). Vigilance during the initiation of daily feeding in dark-eyed juncos. *Oikos, 53,* 12–16.

Lima, S. L. (1998). Stress and decision making under the risk of predation: Recent developments from behavioral, reproductive, and ecological perspectives. *Advances in the Study of Behavior, 27,* 215–290.

Lima, S., & Dill, L. (1990). Behavioral decisions made under the risk of predation: A review and prospectus. *Canadian Journal of Zoology, 68,* 619–640.

Lima, S. L., & Valone, T. J. (1986). Influence of predation risk on diet selection: A simple example in the grey squirrel. *Animal Behaviour, 34,* 536–544.

Lind, J., & Cresswell, W. (2005). Determining the fitness consequences of antipredation behavior. *Behavioral Ecology, 16,* 945–956.

Lindblad-Toh, K., Wade, C. M., Mikkelsen, T. S., Karlsson, E. K., Jaffe, D. B., Kamal, M., Clamp, M., Chang, J. L., Kulbokas, E. J., Zody, M. C., Mauceli, E., Xie, X. H., Breen, M., Wayne, R. K., Ostrander, E. A., Ponting, C. P., Galibert, F., Smith, D. R., deJong, P. J., Kirkness, E., Alvarez, P., Biagi, T., Brockman, W., Butler, J., Chin, C. W., Cook, A., Cuff, J., Daly, M. J., DeCaprio, D., Gnerre, S., Grabherr, M., Kellis, M., Kleber, M., Bardeleben, C., Goodstadt, L., Heger, A., Hitte, C., Kim, L., Koepfli, K. P., Parker, H. G., Pollinger, J. P., Searle, S. M. J., Sutter, N. B., Thomas, R., Webber, C., & Lander, E. S. (2005). Genome sequence, comparative analysis and haplotype structure of the domestic dog. *Nature, 438,* 803–819.

Lindenfors, P., Tullberg, B. S., & Biuw, M. (2002). Phylogenetic analyses of sexual selection and sexual size dimorphism in pinnipeds. *Behavioral Ecology and Sociobiology, 52,* 188–193.

Linnell, J. D. C., Odden, J., Smith, M. E., Aanes, R., & Swenson, J. E. (1999). Large carnivores that kill livestock: Do "problem individuals" really exist? *Wildlife Society Bulletin, 27,* 698–705.

Linnell, J. D. C., Swenson, J. E., & Andersen, R. (2000). Conservation of biodiversity in Scandinavian boreal forests: Large carnivores as flagships, umbrellas, indicators, or keystones? *Biodiversity and Conservation, 9,* 857–868.

Linsdale, J. (1946). *The California ground squirrel.* Berkeley: University of California Press.

Little, A. E. F., Murakami, T., Mueller, U. G., & Currie, C. R. (2003). The infrabuccal pellet piles of fungus-growing ants. *Naturwissenschaften, 90,* 558–562.

Little, A. E. F., Murakami, T., Mueller, U. G., & Currie, C. R. (2006). Defending against parasites: Fungus-growing ants combine specialized behaviours and microbial symbionts to protect their fungus gardens. *Biology Letters, 2,* 12–16.

Littledyke, M., & Cherrett, J. (1976). Direct ingestion of plant sap from leaves cut by the leaf-cutting ants *Atta cepholotes* and *Acromymex octospinus. Bulletin of Entomological Research, 66,* 205–217.

Liu, Y., & Wang, Z. X. (2003). Nucleus accumbens oxytocin and dopamine interact to regulate pair bond formation in female prairie voles. *Neuroscience, 121,* 537–544.

Lohmann, K. J., & Johnsen, S. (2000). The neurobiology of magnetoreception in vertebrate animals. *Trends in Neurosciences, 23,* 153–159.

Long, T. A. F. (2005). The influence of mating system on the intensity of parent-offspring conflict in primates. *Journal of Evolutionary Biology, 18,* 509–515.

Longino, J. (1984). True anting by a capuchin (*Cebus capucinus*). *Primates, 25,* 243–245.

Lorenz, K. (1935). Der Kumpan in der Umwelt des Vogels. *Journal of Ornithology, 83,* 137–213, 289–413.

Loup, F., Tribollet, E., Dubois-Dauphin, M., & Dreifuss, J. J. (1991). Localization of high-affinity binding sites for oxytocin and vasopressin in the human brain: An autoradiography study. *Brain Research, 555,* 220–232.

Low, B. (2000). *Why sex matters: A Darwinian look at human behaviour.* Princeton: Princeton University Press.

Lozano, G. (1998). Parasitic stress and self-medication in wild animals. *Advances in the Study of Behavior, 27,* 291–317.

Lubin, Y. D., & Crozier, R. H. (1985). Electrophoretic evidence for population differentiation in a social spider, *Achaearanea wau* (Theridiidae). *Insectes Sociaux, 32,* 297–304.

Lucas, N. S., Hume, E. M. & Henderson, H. (1937). On the breeding of the common marmoset (*Hapale jacchus*) in captivity when irradiated with ultra-violet rays. II. A ten-year family history. *Proceedings of the Zoological Society of London, Series A, 107,* 205–211.

Lucas, P. W., Darvell, B. W., Lee, P. K. D., Yuen, T. D. B., & Choong, M. F. (1998). Colour cues for leaf food selection by long-tailed macaques (*Macaca fascicularis*) with a new suggestion for the evolution of trichromatic colour vision. *Folia Primatologica, 69,* 139–152.

Lucas, P. W., Dominy, N. J., Riba-Hernandez, P., Stoner, K. E., Yamashita, N., Loria-Calderon, E., Petersen-Pereira, W., Rojas-Duran, Y., Salas-Pena, R., Solis-Madrigal, S., Osorio, D., & Darvell, B. W. (2003). Evolution and function of routine trichromatic vision in primates. *Evolution, 57,* 2636–2643.

Lyamin, O. I. & Chetyrbok, I. S. (1992). Unilateral Eeg activation during sleep in the cape fur seal, *Arctocephalus pusillus. Neuroscience Letters, 143,* 263–266.

Lycett, J., Dunbar, R., & Voland, E. (2000). Longevity and the costs of reproduction in a historical human population. *Proceedings of the Royal Society of London, Series B, 267,* 31–35.

MacArthur, R., & Pianka, E. (1966). On optimal use of a patchy environment. *American Naturalist, 100,* 603–609.

MacDougal-Shackleton, S. (1997). Sexual selection and the evolution of song repertoires. In V. Nolam, E. Ketterson, & C. Thompson (Eds.), *Current ornithology* (pp. 81–124). New York: Plenum.

Mace, G., Harvey, P., & Clutton-Brock, T. (1981). Brain size and ecology in small mammals. *Journal of Zoology, 193,* 333–354.

Mackenzie, A., Reynolds, J. D., Brown, V. J., & Sutherland, W. J. (1995). Variation in male mating success on leks. *American Naturalist, 145,* 633–652.

Macnair, M. R., & Parker, G. A. (1978). Models of parent-offspring conflict. 2. Promiscuity. *Animal Behaviour, 26,* 111–122.

Macphail, E. (1987). The comparative psychology of intelligence. *Behavioral and Brain Sciences, 10,* 645–695.

Maddison, P., & Maddison, W. (1992). *MacClade.* Sunderland, MA: Sinauer.

Maestripieri, D. (1993). Vigilance costs of allogrooming in macaque mothers. *American Naturalist, 141,* 744–753.

Maestripieri, D. (1995). Maternal encouragement in nonhuman primates and the question of animal teaching. *Human Nature, 6,* 361–378.

Magurran, A. E. (1990). The inheritance and development of minnow anti-predator behaviour. *Animal Behaviour, 39,* 834–842.

Magurran, A. E. (2005). *Evolutionary ecology: The Trinidadian guppy.* Oxford: Oxford University Press.

Magurran, A. E., & Higham, A. (1988). Information transfer across fish shoals under predator threat. *Ethology, 78,* 153–158.

Magurran, A. E., & Pitcher, T. J. (1987). Provenance, shoal size and the sociobiology of predator-evasion in minnow shoals. *Proceedings of the Royal Society of London, Series B, 229,* 439–465.

Magurran, A. E., & Seghers, B. H. (1990). Population differences in predator recognition and attack cone avoidance in the guppy *Poecilia reticulata. Animal Behaviour, 40,* 443–452.

Magurran, A. E., & Seghers, B. H. (1991). Variation in schooling and aggression amongst guppy populations (*Poecilia reticulata*) in Trinidad. *Behaviour, 118,* 214–234.

Magurran, A. E., Seghers, B. H., Carvalho, G. R., & Shaw, P. W. (1992). Behavioral consequences of an artificial introduction of guppies (*Poecilia reticulata*) in N. Trinidad: Evidence for the evolution of anti-predator behaviour in the wild. *Proceedings of the Royal Society of London, Series B, 248,* 117–122.

Magurran, A. E., Seghers, B. H., Carvalho, G. R., & Shaw, P. W. (1993). Evolution of adaptive variation in antipredator behaviour. *Marine Behaviour and Physiology, 23,* 29–44.

Magurran, A. E., Seghers, B. H., Shaw, P. W., & Carvalho, G. R. (1995). The behavioral diversity and evolution of guppy, *Poecilia reticulata,* populations in Trinidad. *Advances in the Study of Behavior, 24,* 155–202.

Mahaney, W. C., & Krishnamani, R. (2003). Understanding geophagy in animals: Standard procedures for sampling soils. *Journal of Chemical Ecology, 29,* 1503–1523.

Mahometa, M. J., & Domjan, M. (2005). Classical conditioning increases reproductive success in Japanese quail, *Coturnix japonica. Animal Behaviour, 69,* 983–989.

Mank, J. E., Promislow, D. E. L., & Avise, J. C. (2005). Phylogenetic perspectives in the evolution of parental care in ray-finned fishes. *Evolution, 59,* 1570–1578.

Mann, J., & Sargeant, B. L. (2003). Like mother, like calf: The ontogeny of foraging strategies in the wild Indian Ocean bottlenose dolphins (*Tursiops sp.*). In D. M. Fragasy & S. Perry (Eds.), *The biology of traditions: Models and evidence* (pp. 236–266). Cambridge: Cambridge University Press.

Manning, C. J., Dewsbury, D. A., Wakeland, E. K., & Potts, W. K. (1995). Communal nesting and communal nursing in house mice, *Mus musculus domesticus. Animal Behaviour, 50,* 741–751.

Manning, C. J., Wakeland, E. K., & Potts, W. K. (1992). Communal nesting patterns in mice implicate MHC genes in kin recognition. *Nature, 360,* 581–583.

Marchetti, C., & Drent, P. J. (2000). Individual differences in the use of social information in foraging by captive great tits. *Animal Behaviour, 60,* 131–140.

Margulis, S. W., Nabong, M., Alaks, G., Walsh, A., & Lacy, R. C. (2005). Effects of early experience on subsequent parental behaviour and reproductive success in oldfield mice, *Peromyscus polionotus. Animal Behaviour, 69,* 627–634.

Marinesco, S., Duran, K. L., & Wright, W. G. (2003). Evolution of learning in three aplysiid species: Differences in heterosynaptic plasticity contrast with conservation in serotonergic pathways. *Journal of Physiology-London, 550,* 241–253.

Markl, H. (1968). Die verstandigung durch stridulationssignale bei blattschneiderameisesn. II Erzeugung und eigenschaften der signale. *Zeitschrift fur Vergleichende Physiologie, 60,* 103–150.

Marks, I. (1987). *Fear, phobias and rituals.* New York: Oxford University Press.

Marks, I., & Nesse, R. (1994). Fear and fitness: An evolutionary analysis of anxiety disorders. *Ethology and Sociobiology, 15,* 247–261.

Marler, P. (1968). Visual systems. In T. Sebeok (Ed.), *Animal communications* (pp. 103–126). Bloomington: Indiana University Press.

Marler, P., & Griffin, D. R. (1973). The 1973 Nobel prize for physiology or medicine. *Science, 182,* 464–466.

Marler, P., & Terrace, H. (Eds.). (1984). *The biology of learning.* New York: Springer-Verlag.

Martel, F. L., Nevison, C. M., Rayment, F. D., Simpson, M. J. A., & Keverne, E. B. (1993). Opioid receptor blockade reduces maternal effect and social grooming in rhesus monkeys. *Psychoneuroendocrinology, 18,* 307–321.

Martin, P., & Caro, T. (1985). On the functions of play and its role in behavioral development. *Advances in the Study of Behavior, 15,* 59–103.

Martin, T. E. (1993). Evolutionary determinants of clutch size in cavity nesting birds: Nest predation or limited breeding opportunities? *American Naturalist, 142,* 937–946.

Martin, T. E. (1995). Avian life history in relation to nest sites, nest predation and food. *Ecological Monographs, 65,* 101–127.

Marzluff, J. M., Heinrich, B., & Marzluff, C. (1996). Raven roosts are mobile information centres. *Animal Behaviour, 51,* 89–103.

Masseti, M. (2000). Did the study of ethology begin in Crete 4000 years ago? *Ethology Ecology & Evolution, 12,* 89–96.

Mather, J. A. (1991). Foraging, feeding and prey remains in middens of juvenile *Octopus vulgaris* (Mollusca: Cephalopoda). *Journal of Zoology, London, 224,* 27–39.

Mather, J. A. (1995). Cognition in cephalopods. In P. Slater, J. Rosenblatt, C. Snowdon, & M. Milinski, *Advances in the study of behavior* (Vol. 24, pp. 317–353). New York: Academic Press.

Mather, J., & Anderson, R. (1993). Personalities of octopuses (*Octopus rubescens*). *Journal of Comparative Psychology, 107,* 336–340.

Mather, J. A., & Anderson, R. C. (1999). Exploration, play, and habituation in octopuses (*Octopus dofleini*). *Journal of Comparative Psychology, 113,* 333–338.

Mathis, A., & Smith, R. J. F. (1993a). Chemical labeling of northern pike (*Esox lucius*) by the alarm pheromone of fathead minnows (*Pimephales promelas*). *Journal of Chemical Ecology, 19,* 1967–1979.

Mathis, A., & Smith, R. J. F. (1993b). Fathead minnows, *Pimephales promelas*, learn to recognize northern pike, *Esox lucius*, as predators on the basis of chemical stimuli from minnows in the pike's diet. *Animal Behaviour, 46,* 645–656.

Maynard Smith, J. (1974). The theory of games and the evolution of animal conflicts. *Journal of Theoretical Biology, 47,* 209–221.

Maynard Smith, J. (1982). *Evolution and the theory of games.* Cambridge: Cambridge University Press.

Maynard Smith, J., & Parker, G. A. (1976). The logic of asymmetric contests. *Animal Behaviour, 24,* 159–175.

Maynard Smith, J., & Price, G. (1973). The logic of animal conflict. *Nature, 246,* 15–18.

Mayr, E. (1961). Cause and effect in biology. *Science, 134,* 1501–1506.

Mayr, E. (1982). *The growth of biological thought.* Cambridge, MA: Harvard University Press.

Mayr, E. (1983). How to carry out the adaptationist program. *American Naturalist, 121,* 324–334.

Mays, H. L., & Hill, G. E. (2004). Choosing mates: Good genes versus genes that are a good fit. *Trends in Ecology & Evolution, 19,* 554–559.

McCarthy, M. M. (1994). Molecular aspects of sexual differentiation of the rodent brain. *Psychoneuroendocrinology, 19,* 415–427.

McCullough, D. R. (1969). The tule elk: Its history, behavior and ecology. *University of California Publications in Zoology, 88,* 1–209.

McEwen, B., & Sapolsky, R. M. (1995). Stress and cognitive function. *Current Opinions in Neurobiology, 5,* 205–210.

McGill, B. (2005). A mechanistic model of a mutualism and its ecological and evolutionary dynamics. *Ecological Modelling, 187,* 413–425.

McGraw, K. J., Stoehr, A. M., Nolan, P. M., & Hill, G. E. (2001). Plumage redness predicts breeding onset and reproductive success in the house finch: A validation of Darwin's theory. *Journal of Avian Biology, 32,* 90–94.

McGregor, P. (2005). *Animal communication networks.* Cambridge: Cambridge University Press.

McGregor, P. K., & Peake, T. (2000). Communication networks: Social environments for receiving and signalling behaviour. *Acta Ethologica, 2,* 71–81.

McGuire, M., & Troisi, A. (1998). *Darwinian psychiatry.* New York: Oxford University Press.

McKinney, F., Cheng, K., & Bruggers, D. (1984). Sperm competition in apparently monogamous birds. In R. Smith (Ed.), *Sperm competition and the evolution of animal mating systems* (pp. 523–545). New York: Academic Press.

McLean, I. G., Holzer, C., & Studholme, B. J. S. (1999). Teaching predator-recognition to a naive bird: Implications for management. *Biological Conservation, 87,* 123–130.

McLean, I. G., Lundie-Jenkins, G., & Jarman, P. J. (1996). Teaching an endangered mammal to recognise predators. *Biological Conservation, 75,* 51–62.

McLean, I. G., Schmitt, N. T., Jarman, P. J., Duncan, C., & Wynne, C. D. L. (2000). Learning for life: Training marsupials to recognise introduced predators. *Behaviour, 137*, 1361–1376.

McMann, S. (1993). Contextual signaling and the structure of dyadic encounters in *Anolis carolinensis*. *Animal Behaviour, 46*, 657–668.

McNab, B. K. (1973). Energetics and distribution of vampires. *Journal of Mammalogy, 54*, 131–144.

McNamara, J. M., & Houston, A. I. (1992). Risk sensitive foraging: A review of the theory. *Bulletin of Mathematical Biophysics, 54*, 355–378.

Mead, L. S., & Arnold, S. J. (2004). Quantitative genetic models of sexual selection. *Trends in Ecology & Evolution, 19*, 264–271.

Medawar, P. (1952). *An unsolved problem in biology*. London: H. K. Lewis.

Mello, C., Nottebohm, F., & Clayton, D. (1995). Repeated exposure to one song leads to a rapid and persistent decline in an immediate early gene's response to that song in zebra finch telencephalon. *Journal of Neuroscience, 15*, 6919–6925.

Mello, C. V., Velho, T. A. F., & Pinaud, R. (2004). A window on song auditory processing and perception. In H. P. Zeigler & P. Marler (Eds.), *Behavioral neurobiology of birdsong* (Vol. 1016, pp. 263–281). New York: Annals of the New York Academy of Sciences.

Mello, C. V., Vicario, D. S., & Clayton, D. F. (1992). Song presentation induces gene expression in the songbird forebrain. *Proceedings of the National Academy of Sciences, U.S.A., 89*, 6818–6822.

Mendozagranados, D., & Sommer, V. (1995). Play in chimpanzees of the Arnhem Zoo: Self-serving compromises. *Primates, 36*, 57–68.

Mercer, A. R., Emptage, N. J., & Carew, T. J. (1991). Pharmacological dissociation of modulatory effects of serotonin in aplysia sensory neurons. *Science, 254*, 1811–1813.

Mery, F., & Kawecki, T. J. (2002). Experimental evolution of learning ability in fruit flies. *Proceedings of the National Academy of Sciences, U.S.A., 99*, 14274–14279.

Mery, F., & Kawecki, T. J. (2003). A fitness cost of learning ability in *Drosophila melanogaster*. *Proceedings of the Royal Society of London, Series B, 270*, 2465–2469.

Mesoudi, A., Whiten, A., & Laland, K. N. (2006). Towards a unified science of cultural evolution. *Behavioral and Brain Sciences, 29*, 329–381.

Mesterton-Gibbons, M. (1992). Ecotypic variation in an asymmetric hawk-dove game: When is bourgeois an ESS? *Evololutionary Ecology, 6*, 198–222.

Mesterton-Gibbons, M. (1999). On the evolution of pure winner and loser effects: A game-theoretic model. *Bulletin of Mathematical Biology, 61*, 1151–1186.

Mesterton-Gibbons, M., & Adams, E. (1998). Animal contests as evolutionary games. *American Scientist, 86*, 334–341.

Mesterton-Gibbons, M., & Dugatkin, L. A. (1992). Cooperation among unrelated individuals: Evolutionary factors. *Quarterly Review of Biology, 67*, 267–281.

Mesterton-Gibbons, M., & Sherratt, T. N. (2007). Coalition formation: A game-theoretic analysis. *Behavioral Ecology, 18*, 277–286.

Mettke-Hofmann, C., & Gwinner, E. (2003). Long-term memory for a life on the move. *Proceedings of the National Academy of Sciences, U.S.A., 100*, 5863–5866.

Miklosi, A. (1999). The ethological analysis of imitation. *Biological Reviews of the Cambridge Philosophical Society, 74*, 347–374.

Milinski, M. (1977). Do all members of a swarm suffer the same predation? *Zeitschrift fur Tierpsychologie, 45*, 373–378.

Milinski, M. (1979). An evolutionarily stable feeding strategy in sticklebacks. *Zeitschrift fur Tierpsychologie, 51*, 36–40.

Milinski, M. (1987). TIT FOR TAT and the evolution of cooperation in sticklebacks. *Nature, 325*, 433–435.

Milinski, M. (2006). The major histocompatibility complex, sexual selection, and mate choice. *Annual Review of Ecology, Evolution, and Systematics, 37*, 159–186.

Milinski, M., & Bakker, T. (1990). Female sticklebacks use male coloration in mate choice and hence avoid parasitized sticklebacks. *Nature, 344*, 330–333.

Milinski, M., Griffiths, S., Wegner, K. M., Reusch, T. B. H., Haas-Assenbaum, A., & Boehm, T. (2005). Mate choice decisions of stickleback females predictably modified by MHC peptide ligands. *Proceedings of the National Academy of Sciences, U.S.A.,102*, 4414–4418.

Milinski, M., Kulling, D., & Kettler, R. (1990). Tit for tat: Sticklebacks "trusting" a cooperating partner. *Behavioral Ecology, 1*, 7–12.

Milinski, M., Luthi, J., Eggler, R., & Parker, G. (1997). Cooperation under predation risk: Experiments on costs and benefits. *Proceedings of the Royal Society of London, Series B, 264*, 831–837.

Milinski, M., & Wedekind, C. (2001). Evidence for MHC-correlated perfume preferences in humans. *Behavioral Ecology, 12*, 140–149.

Miller, J., Crowder, L., & Moser, M. (1985). Migration and utilization of estuarine nurseries by juvenile fishes: An evolutionary perspective. In M. Rankin (Ed.), *Migration: Mechanisms and adaptive significance*. Austin, TX: Marine Science Center.

Mills, A. D., Crawford, L. L., Domjan, M., & Faure, J. (1997). The behavior of the Japanese or domestic quail, *Coturnix japonica*. *Neuroscience and Biobehavioral Reviews, 21*, 261–281.

Mineka, S., & Cook, M. (1986). Immunization against the observational conditioning of snake fear in rhesus monkeys. *Journal of Abnormal Psychology, 95*, 307–318.

Mineka, S., & Cook, M. (1988). Social learning and the acquisition of snake fear in monkeys. In T. Zentall & B. G. Galef (Eds.), *Social learning: Psychological and biological perspectives* (pp. 51–73). Hillsdale, NJ: Lawrence Erlbaum Associates.

Mineka, S., Davidson, M., Cook, M., & Keir, R. (1984). Observational conditioning of snake fear in rhesus monkeys. *Journal of Abnormal Psychology, 93*, 355–372.

Mitchell, W. A., & Valone, T. J. (1990). Commentary: The optimization approach - studying adaptations by their function. *Quarterly Review of Biology, 65*, 43–52.

Mitman, G. (1992). *The state of nature: Ecology, community and American social thought, 1900–1950*. Chicago: University of Chicago Press.

Mittlebach, G. (1984). Group size and feeding rate in bluegills. *Copeia, 4*, 998–1000.

Mitzutani, F. (1993). Home range of leopards and their impact on livestocks on Kenyan ranches. *Zoological Society of London (Symposium), 65*, 425–439.

Miyaki, C. Y., Matioli, S. R., Burke, T., & Wajntal, A. (1998). Parrot evolution and paleogeographical events: Mitochondrial DNA evidence. *Molecular Biology and Evolution, 15*, 544–551.

Miyatake, T., Katayama, K., Takeda, Y., Nakashima, A., Sugita, A., & Mizumoto, M. (2004). Is death-feigning adaptive? Heritable variation in fitness difference of death-feigning behaviour. *Proceedings of the Royal Society of London, Series B, 271*, 2293–2296.

Mock, D. (1980). White-dark polymorphism in herons. In D. L. Drawe (Ed.), *Proceedings of the first Welder Wildlife Symposium* (pp. 145–161). Sinton, TX: Welder Wildlife Foundation.

Mock, D. (2004). *More than kin and less than kind: The evolution of family conflict.* Cambridge, MA: Belknap Press.

Mock, D., & Parker, G. (1997). *The evolution of sibling rivalry.* New York: Oxford University Press.

Molina-Borja, M., Padron-Fumero, M., & Alfonso-Martin, T. (1998). Morphological and behavioural traits affecting the intensity and outcome of male contests in *Gallotia galloti galloti* (family Lacertidae). *Ethology, 104*, 314–322.

Møller, A. P. (1988). False alarm calls as a means of resource usurpation in the great tit *Parus major. Ethology, 79*, 25–30.

Møller, A. P. (1990). Deceptive use of alarm calls by male swallows, *Hirundo rustica*: A new paternity guard. *Behavioral Ecology, 1*, 1–6.

Møller, A. P., & Erritzøe, J. (1996). Parasite virulence and host immune defense: Host immune response is related to nest re-use in birds. *Evolution, 50*, 2066–2072.

Møller, A. P., & Erritzøe, J. (1998). Host immune defence and migration in birds. *Evolutionary Ecology, 12*, 945–953.

Møller, A., Hell, D., & Krober, H. L. (1998). Sensation seeking: A review of the theory and its applications. *Fortschritte der Neurologie Psychiatrie, 66*, 487–495.

Møller, A., & Jennions, M. (2001). How important are direct benefits of sexual selection. *Naturwissenschaften, 88*, 401–415.

Møller, A., & Swaddle, J. (1998). *Asymmetry, developmental stability, and evolution.* Oxford: Oxford University Press.

Møller, A. P., & Thornhill, R. (1998). Bilateral symmetry and sexual selection: A meta-analysis. *American Naturalist, 151*, 174–192.

Mollon, J. D. (1989). "Tho' she knnel'd in that place where they grew..." *Journal of Experimental Biology, 146*, 21–38.

Monkkonen, M., & Orell, M. (1997). Clutch size and cavity excavation in parids (Paridae): The limited breeding opportunities hypothesis tested. *American Naturalist, 149*, 1164–1174.

Montague, R. (2006). *Why choose this book? How we make decisions.* New York: Dutton.

Montgomerie, R., Lyon, B., & Holder, K. (2001). Dirty ptarmigan: Behavioral modification of conspicuous male plumage. *Behavioral Ecology, 12*, 429–438.

Moore, H. D. M., Martin, M., & Birkhead, T. R. (1999). No evidence for killer sperm or other selective interactions between human spermatozoa in ejaculates of different males in vitro. *Proceedings of the Royal Society of London, Series B, 266*, 2343–2350.

Mooring, M. S., & Hart, B. L. (1992). Reciprocal allogrooming in dam-reared and hand-reared impala fawns. *Ethology, 90*, 37–51.

Morgan, E. (1984). Chemical words and phrases in the language of pheromones for foraging and recruitment. In T. D. Lewis (Ed.), *Communication* (pp. 169–194). London: Academic Press.

Morgan, J., & Curran, T. (1991). Stimulus transmission using coupling in the nervous system: Involvement of the inducible proto-oncogenes fos and jun. *Annual Review of Neuroscience, 14*, 421–451.

Morris, D. W. (1994). Habitat matching: Alternatives and implications to populations and communities. *Evolutionary Ecology, 8*, 387–406.

Morris, R. G. M., Garrud, P., Rawlins, J. N. P., & Okeefe, J. (1982). Place navigation impaired in rats with hippocampal lesions. *Nature, 297*, 681–683.

Morse, D. H. (1970). Ecological aspects of some mixed species foraging flocks of birds. *Ecological Monographs, 4*, 119–168.

Morton, D., & Chiel, H. (1994). Neural architecture for adaptive behavior. *Trends in Neurosciences, 10*, 413–420.

Morton, E. S. (1977). On the occurrence and significance of motivation-structural rules in some bird and animal sounds. *American Naturalist, 111*, 855–869.

Moser, M. B., Trommald, M., & Andersen, P. (1994). An increase in dendritic spine density on hippocampal CA1 pyramidal cells following spatial learning in adult rats suggests the formation of new synapses. *Proceedings of the National Academy of Sciences, U.S.A., 91*, 12673–12675.

Mouritsen, H., & Frost, B., J. (2002). Virtual migration in tethered flying monarch butterflies reveals their orientation mechanisms. *Proceedings of the National Academy of Sciences, U.S.A., 99*, 10162–10166.

Mousseau, T. A., & Roff, D. A. (1987). Natural selection and the heritability of fitness components. *Heredity, 59*, 181–197.

Mousseau, T., Sinervo, B., & Endler, J. (Eds.). (1999). *Adaptive genetic variation in the wild.* New York: Oxford University Press.

Muhlau, M., Hermsdorfer, J., Goldenberg, G., Wohlschlager, A. M., Castrop, F., Stahl, R., Rottinger, M., Erhard, P., Haslinger, B., Ceballos-Baumann, A. O., Conrad, B., & Boecker, H. (2005). Left inferior parietal dominance in gesture imitation: An fMRI study. *Neuropsychologia, 43*, 1086–1098.

Mukhametov, L., Supin, A., & Lyamin, O. (1988). Interhemispheric asymmetrie of the EEG during sleep in marine mamals. In T. Oniani (Ed.), *Neurobiology of sleep-wakefulness cycle* (pp. 147–159). Tbilisi: Metsniereba.

Mulder, R., Dunn, P., Cockburn, A., Lazenby-Cohen, K., & Howell, M. (1994). Helpers liberate female fairy-wrens from constraints on extra-pair mate choice. *Proceedings of the Royal Society of London, Series B, 255*, 223–229.

Munafo, M. R., Clark, T. G., Moore, L. R., Payne, E., Walton, R., & Flint, J. (2003). Genetic polymorphisms and personality in healthy adults: A systematic review and meta-analysis. *Molecular Psychiatry, 8*, 471–484.

Munck, A., Guyre, P., & Holbrook, N. (1984). Physiological functions of glucocorticoids in stress and the relation to pharmacological actions. *Endocrine Reviews, 5*, 25–41.

Munn, C. A. (1986). Birds that "cry wolf." *Nature, 319*, 143–145.

Munz, T. (2005). The bee battles: Karl von Frisch, Adrian Wenner and the honey bee dance language controversy. *Journal of the History of Biology, 38*, 535–570.

Nahallage, C., & Huffman, M. (2007). Age-specific functions of stone handling, a solitary-object play behavior, in Japanese macaques (*Macaca fiscata*). *American Journal of Primatology, 69*, 267–81.

Nash, S., & Domjan, M. (1991). Learning to discriminate the sex of conspecifics in male Japanese quail (*Coturnix coturnix japonica*): Tests of "biological constraints." *Journal of Experimental Psychology: Animal Behavior Processes, 17*, 342–353.

Neff, B. D., Fu, P., & Gross, M. R. (2003). Sperm investment and alternative mating tactics in bluegill sunfish (*Lepomis macrochirus*). *Behavioral Ecology, 14*, 634–641.

Neff, B. D., & Sherman, P. W. (2004). Behavioral syndromes versus Darwinian algorithms. *Trends in Ecology & Evolution, 19*, 621–622.

Nelissen, M. (1985). Structure of the dominance hierarchy and dominance determining "group factors" in *Melanochromatis auratus*. *Behaviour, 94*, 85–107.

Nelson, D. A., Khanna, H., & Marler, P. (2001). Learning by instruction or selection: Implications for patterns of geographic variation in bird song. *Behaviour, 138*, 1137–1160.

Nelson, R. (2005). *An introduction to behavioral endocrinology* (3rd ed.). Sunderland, MA: Sinauer.

Nesse, R. M. (1988). Life table tests of evolutionary theories of senescence. *Experimental Gerontology, 23*, 445–453.

Nesse, R., & Williams, G. C. (1995). *Why we get sick: The new science of Darwinian medicine*. New York: Vintage Books.

Neudorf, D. L. H. (2004). Extrapair paternity in birds: Understanding variation among species. *Auk, 121*, 302–307.

Nevitt, G. A., Dittman, A. H., Quinn, T. P., & Moody, W. J. (1994). Evidence for a peripheral olfactory memory in imprinted salmon. *Proceedings of the National Academy of Science, U.S.A., 91*, 4288–4292.

Nielsen, C. R., Semel, B., Sherman, P. W., Westneat, D. F., & Parker, P. G. (2006). Host-parasite relatedness in wood ducks: Patterns of kinship and parasite success. *Behavioral Ecology, 17*, 491–496.

Niesink, R., & Van Ree, J. (1989). Involvement of opioid and dopaminergic systems in isolation-induced pinning and social grooming of young rats. *Neuropharmacology, 28*, 411–418.

Nishida, T. (1979). The social structure of chimpanzees of the Mahale Mountains. In D. A. Hamburg & E. R. McCown (Eds.), *The great apes*. Menlo Park, CA: Benjamin Cummings.

Nishida, T., Hiraiwa-Hasegawa, M., Hasegawa, T., & Takahata, Y. (1985). Group extinction and female transfer in wild chimpanzees in the Mahale National Park, Tanzania. *Zeitschrift fur Tierpsychologie, 67*, 284–301.

Nishida, T., Uehara, S., & Nyondo, R. (1983). Predatory behaviour among wild chimpanzees of the Mahale Mountains. *Primates, 20*, 1–20.

Nishida, T., & Wallauer, W. (2003). Leaf-pile pulling: An unusual play pattern in wild chimpanzees. *American Journal of Primatology, 60*, 167–173.

Noble, J. (1999). Cooperation, conflict and the evolution of communication. *Adaptive Behavior, 7*, 349–369.

Noe, R. (1986). Lasting alliances among adult male Savannah baboons. In J. Else & P. Lee, P. (Eds.), *Primate ontogeny, cognition and social behaviour* (pp. 381–392). Cambridge: Cambridge University Press.

Noe, R., & Hammerstein, P. (1995). Biological markets. *Trends in Ecology & Evolution, 10*, 336–339.

Noe, R., Van Hooff, J., & Hammerstein, P. (2002). *Economics in nature: Social dilemma, mate choice and biological markets*. Cambridge: Cambridge University Press.

Normansell, L., & Panksepp, J. (1990). Effects of morphine and naloxone on play-rewarded social discrimination in juvenile rats. *Developmental Psychobiology, 23*, 75–83.

Nottebohm, F., & Nottebohm, M. E. (1976). Left hypoglossal dominance in control of canary and white-crowned sparrow song. *Journal of Comparative Physiology, 108*, 1368–1370.

Nowacek, D. P. (2005). Acoustic ecology of foraging bottlenose dolphins (*Tursiops truncatus*), habitat-specific use of three sound types. *Marine Mammal Science, 21*, 587–602.

Nowak, M. (2006a). *Evolutionary dynamics: Exploring the equations of life*. Cambridge, MA: Harvard University Press.

Nowak, M. A. (2006b). Five rules for the evolution of cooperation. *Science, 314*, 1560–1563.

Nunes, S., Muecke, E. M., Anthony, J., & Batterbee, A. S. (1999). Endocrine and energetic mediation of play behavior in free-living Belding's ground squirrels. *Hormones and Behavior, 36*, 153–165.

Nussey, D. H., Kruuk, L. E. B., Donald, A., Fowlie, M., & Clutton-Brock, T. H. (2006). The rate of senescence in maternal performance increases with early-life fecundity in red deer. *Ecology Letters, 9*, 1342–1350.

Odling-Smee, L., & Braithwaite, V. A. (2003). The role of learning in fish orientation. *Fish and Fisheries, 4*, 235–246.

Odling-Smee, F. J., Laland, K. N., & Feldman, M. W. (2003). *Niche construction: The neglected process in evolution*. Princeton: Princeton University Press.

Ohno, T., & Miyatake, T. (2007). Drop or fly? Negative genetic correlation between death-feigning intensity and flying ability as alternative anti-predator strategies. *Proceedings of the Royal Society of London, Series B, 274*, 555–560.

O'Keefe, J., & Nadel, L. (1978). *The hippocampus as a cognitive map*. Oxford: Claredon.

Okuda, J., Fujii, T., Ohtake, H., Tsukiura, T., Tanji, K., Suzuki, K., Kawashima, R., Fukuda, H., Itoh, M., & Yamadori, A. (2003). Thinking of the future and past: The roles of the frontal pole and the medial temporal lobes. *NeuroImage, 19*, 1369–1380.

Olesen, K. M., Jessen, H. M., Auger, C. J., & Auger, A. P. (2005). Dopaminergic activation of estrogen receptors in neonatal brain alters progestin receptor expression and juvenile social play behavior. *Endocrinology, 146*, 3705–3712.

Oli, M., Taylor, K., & Rogers, M. (1994). Snow leopard (*Panthera uncia*) predation of livestock: An assessment of local perceptions in the Annapurna conservation area, Nepal. *Biological Conservation, 68*, 63–68.

Olioff, M., & Stewart, J. (1978). Sex differences in play behavior of prepubescent rats. *Physiology and Behavior, 20,* 113–115.

Oliveira, R. F., Carneiro, L. A., & Canario, A. V. M. (2005). No hormonal response in tied fights. *Nature, 437,* 207–208.

Oliveira, R. F., Hirschenhauser, K., Carneiro, L. A.. & Canario, A. V. M. (2002). Social modulation of androgen levels in male teleost fish. *Comparative Biochemistry and Physiology B-Biochemistry & Molecular Biology, 132,* 203–215.

Oliveira, R. F., Lopes, M., Carneiro, L. A., & Canario, A. V. M. (2001). Watching fights raises fish hormone levels: Cichlid fish wrestling for dominance induce an androgen surge in male spectators. *Nature, 409,* 475–475.

Oliveira, R. F., McGregor, P. K., & Latruffe, C. (1998). Know thine enemy: Fighting fish gather information from observing conspecific interactions. *Proceedings of the Royal Society of London, Series B, 265,* 1045–1049.

O'Loghlen, A. L. (1995). Delayed access to local songs prolongs vocal development in dialect populations of brown-headed cowbirds. *Condor, 97,* 402–414.

O'Loghlen, A. L., & Rothstein, S. I. (1993). An extreme example of delayed vocal development: Song learning in a population of wild brown-headed cowbirds. *Animal Behaviour, 46,* 293–304.

O'Loghlen, A. L., & Rothstein, S. I. (1995). Culturally correct song dialects are correlated with male age and female song preferences in wild populations of brown-headed cowbirds. *Behavioral Ecology and Sociobiology, 36,* 251–259.

O'Loghlen, A. L., & Rothstein, S. I. (2002). Ecological effects on song learning: Delayed development is widespread in wild populations of brown-headed cowbirds. *Animal Behaviour, 63,* 475–486.

Olsen, K. L., & Whalen, R. E. (1982). Estrogen binds to hypothalamic nuclei of androgen-insensitive (Tfm) rats. *Experientia, 38,* 139–140.

Oppliger, A., Naciri-Graven, Y., Ribi, G., & Hosken, D. J. (2003). Sperm length influences fertilization success during sperm competition in the snail *Viviparus ater. Molecular Ecology, 12,* 485–492.

Ord, T. J., Martins, E. P., Thakur, S., Mane, K. K., & Borner, K. (2005). Trends in animal behaviour research (1968–2002): Ethoinformatics and the mining of library databases. *Animal Behaviour, 69,* 1399–1413.

Orians, G. (1962). Natural selection and ecological theory. *American Naturalist, 96,* 257–263.

Orians, G. (1969). On the evolution of mating systems in birds and mammals. *American Naturalist, 103,* 589–603.

Ortega, C. (1998). *Cowbirds and other brood parasites.* University of Arizona Press.

Osuch, E. A., Ketter, T. A., Kimbrell, T. A., George, M. S., Benson, B. E., Willis, M. W., Herscovitch, P., & Post, R. M. (2000). Regional cerebral metabolism associated with anxiety symptoms in affective disorder patients. *Biological Psychiatry, 48,* 1020–1023.

Outlaw, D. C., & Voelker, G. (2006). Phylogenetic tests of hypotheses for the evolution of avian migration: A case study using the Motacillidae. *Auk, 123,* 455–466.

Outlaw, D. C., Voelker, G., Mila, B., & Girman, D. J. (2003). Evolution of long-distance migration in and historical biogeography of *Catharus* thrushes: A molecular phylogenetic approach. *Auk, 120,* 299–310.

Overli, O., Sorensen, C., Pulman, K. G. T., Pottinger, T. G., Korzan, W., Summers, C. H., & Nilsson, G. E. (2007). Evolutionary background for stress-coping styles: Relationships between physiological, behavioral, and cognitive traits in non-mammalian vertebrates. *Neuroscience and Biobehavioral Reviews, 31,* 396–412.

Owings, D. H., & Coss, R. G. (1977). Snake mobbing by California ground squirrels: Adaptive variation and ontogeny. *Behaviour, 62,* 50–69.

Owings, D. H., & Leger, D. W. (1980). Chatter vocalization of California ground squirrels: Predator- and social-role specificity. *Zeitschrift fur Tierpsychologie, 54,* 163–184.

Packard, A. (1972). Cephalopods and fish: Limits of convergence. *Biological Reviews of the Cambridge Philosophical Society, 47,* 241–307.

Packer, C. (1977). Reciprocal altruism in *Papio anubis. Nature, 265,* 441–443.

Packer, C., Gilbert, D., Pusey, A., & O'Brien, S. (1991). A molecular genetic analysis of kinship and cooperation in African lions. *Nature, 351,* 562–565.

Packer, C., Herbst, L., Pusey, A. E., Bygott, J. D., Hanby, J. P., Cairns, S. J., & Borgerhoff-Mulder, M. (1988). Reproductive success of lions. In T. H. Clutton-Brock (Ed.), *Reproductive success* (pp. 363–383). Chicago: University of Chicago Press.

Packer, C., Lewis, S., & Pusey, A. (1992). A comparative analysis of non-offspring nursing. *Animal Behaviour, 43,* 265–281.

Packer, C., & Pusey, A. E. (1982). Cooperation and competition within coalitions of male lions: Kin selection or game theory? *Nature, 296,* 740–742.

Palagi, E., Antonacci, D., & Cordoni, G. (2007). Fine-tuning of social play in juvenile lowland gorillas (*Gorilla gorilla gorilla*). *Developmental Psychobiology, 49,* 433–445.

Palameta, B., & Lefebvre, L. (1985). The social transmission of a food-finding technique in pigeons: What is learned? *Animal Behaviour, 33,* 892–896.

Panksepp, J. (2005). Beyond a joke: From animal laughter to human joy? *Science, 308,* 62–63.

Panksepp, J., & Burgdorf, J. (2003). "Laughing" rats and the evolutionary antecedents of human joy? *Physiology & Behavior, 79,* 533–547.

Panksepp, J., Siviy, S., & Normansell, L. (1984). The psychobiology of play: Theoretical and methodological considerations. *Neuroscience and Biobehavioral Reviews, 8,* 465–492.

Panksepp, J. B., Yue, Z. X., Drerup, C., & Huber, R. (2003). Amine neurochemistry and aggression in crayfish. *Microscopy Research and Technique, 60,* 360–368.

Papaj, D., & Lewis, A. (Ed). (1993). *Insect learning: Ecological and evolutionary perspectives.* New York: Chapman and Hall.

Papaj, D., Lewis, A., & Prokopy, R. (1989). Ecological and evolutionary aspects of learning in phytophagus insects. *Annual Review of Entomology, 34,* 315–340.

Parker, G. (1970a). Sperm competition and its evolutionary effect on copula duration in the fly *Scatophagua stercoraria. Journal of Insect Physiology, 16,* 1301–1328.

Parker, G. (1970b). Sperm competition and its evolutionary consequences in insects. *Biological Reviews of the Cambridge Philosophical Society, 45,* 525–567.

Parker, G. A. (1974a). Assessment strategy and the evolution of fighting behaviour. *Journal of Theoretical Biology, 47,* 223–243.

Parker, G. A. (1974b). Courtship persistence and female-guarding as male investment strategies. *Behaviour, 48,* 157–184.

Parker, G. A. (1974c). The reproductive behavior and nature of sexual selection in *Scatophaga stercoraria.* IX. Spatial distribution of fertilization rates and evolution of male search strategy within the reproductive area. *Evolution, 28,* 93–108.

Parker, G. A. (2001). Golden flies, sunlit meadows: A tribute to the yellow dungfly. In L. A. Dugatkin (Ed.), *Model systems in behavioral ecology: Integrating conceptual, theoretical and empirical perspectives* (pp. 3–26). Princeton: Princeton University Press.

Parker, G. A., & Macnair, M. R. (1979). Models of parent-offspring conflict. 4. Suppression: Evolutionary retaliation by the parent. *Animal Behaviour, 27,* 1210–1235.

Parker, G. A., & Maynard Smith, J. (1987). The distribution of stay times in *Scatophaga:* A reply to Curtsinger. *American Naturalist, 129,* 621–628.

Parker, G. A., & Stuart, R. A. (1976). Animal behavior as a strategy optimizer: Evolution of resource assessment strategies and optimal emigration thresholds. *American Naturalist, 110,* 1055–1076.

Parker, G. A., & Sutherland, W. J. (1986). Ideal free distribution when individuals differ in competitive ability: Phenotype-limited ideal free models. *Animal Behaviour, 34,* 1222–1242.

Parker, G. A., & Thompson, E. (1980). Dung fly struggles: A test of the war of attrition. *Behavioral Ecology and Sociobiology, 7,* 37–44.

Parker, P. G., Waite, T. A., Heinrich, B., & Marzluff, J. M. (1994). Do common ravens share ephemeral food resources with kin? DNA fingerprinting evidence. *Animal Behaviour, 48,* 1085–1093.

Parmigian, S., & vom Saal, F. (Eds.). (1995). *Infanticide and parental care.* New York: Gordon and Breach Science Publishers.

Partridge, L., & Farquhar, M. (1981). Sexual activity reduces lifespan of male fruit flies. *Nature, 294,* 580–582.

Partridge, L., & Fowler, K. (1990). Non-mating costs of exposure to males in female *Drosophila melanogaster. Journal of Insect Physiology, 36,* 419–425.

Partridge, L., Fowler, K., Trevitt, S., & Sharp, W. (1986). An examination of the effects of males on the survival and egg-production rates of female *Drosophila melanogaster. Journal of Insect Physiology, 32,* 925–929.

Partridge, L., Green, A., & Fowler, K. (1987). Effects of egg production and of exposure to males on female survival in *Drosophila melanogaster. Journal of Insect Physiology, 33,* 745–749.

Paul, E. S., Harding, E. J., & Mendl, M. (2005). Measuring emotional processes in animals: The utility of a cognitive approach. *Neuroscience and Biobehavioral Reviews, 29,* 469–491.

Pavlov, I. P. (1927). *Conditioned reflexes.* New York: Oxford University Press.

Payne, R. (1977). The ecology of brood parasitism in birds. *Annual Review of Ecology and Systematics, 8,* 1–28.

Pedersen, C. A., & Boccia, M. L. (2002). Oxytocin maintains as well as initiates female sexual behavior: Effects of a highly selective oxytocin antagonist. *Hormones and Behavior, 41,* 170–177.

Pellegrini, A. D. (1995). Boys' rough-and-tumble play and social competence: Contemporaneous and longitudinal relations. In A. D. Pellegrini (Ed.), *The future of play theory: A multidisciplinary inquiry into the contributions of Brian Sutton-Smith* (pp. 107–126). Albany, NY: State University of New York Press.

Pellegrini, A. D., Dupuis, D., & Smith, P. K. (2007). Play in evolution and development. *Developmental Review, 27,* 261–276.

Pellis, S. M. (2002). Sex differences in play fighting revisited: Traditional and nontraditional mechanisms of sexual differentiation in rats. *Archives of Sexual Behavior, 31,* 17–26.

Pellis, S., Castenada, E., McKenna, M., Tran-Nguten, L., & Whishaw, I. B. (1993). The role of the striatum in organizing sequences of play fighting in neonatally dopamine depleted rats. *Neuroscience Letters, 158,* 13–15.

Pellis, S., & Iwaniuk, A. (1999). The roles of phylogeny and sociality in the evolution of social play in muroid rodents. *Animal Behaviour, 58,* 361–373.

Pellis, S., Pellis, V., & Kolb, B. (1992a). Neonatal testosterone augmentation increases juvenile play fighting but does not influence the adult dominance relationships of male rats. *Aggressive Behavior, 18,* 437–442.

Pellis, S., Pellis, V., & Whishaw, I. B. (1992b). The role of the cortex in play fighting by rats: Developmental and evolutionary implications. *Brain, Behavior and Evolution, 39,* 270–284.

Penn, D., & Potts, W. (1998). How do major histocompatibility complex genes influence odor and mating preferences? *Advances in Immunology, 69,* 411–436.

Penn, D., & Potts, W. (1999). The evolution of mating preferences and the major histocompatibility complex genes. *American Naturalist, 153,* 145–164.

Pepper, J. W., Braude, S. H., Lacey, E. A., & Sherman, P. W. (1991). Vocalizations of the naked mole-rat. In P. W. Sherman, J. Jarvis, & R. D. Alexander (Eds.), *The biology of the naked mole-rat* (pp. 243–274). Princeton: Princeton University Press.

Pereira, M. E., Rosat, R., Huang, C. H., Godoy, M. G. C., & Izquierdo, I. (1989). Inhibition by diazepam of the effect of additional training and of extinction on the retention of shuttle avoidance behavior in rats. *Behavioral Neuroscience, 103,* 202–205.

Perez, S. M., Taylor, O. R., & Jander, R. (1997). A sun compass in monarch butterflies. *Nature, 387,* 29.

Pervin, L., & John, O. P. (1997). *Personality: Theory and research.* New York: Wiley.

Petrie, M., Krupa, A., & Burke, T. (1999). Peacocks lek with relatives even in the absence of social and environmental cues. *Nature, 401,* 155–157.

Pfaus, J. G., Kippin, T. E., & Centeno, S. (2001). Conditioning and sexual behavior: A review. *Hormones and Behavior, 40,* 291–321.

Pfennig, D. W. (1995). Absence of joint nesting advantage in desert seed harvester ants: Evidence from a field experiment. *Animal Behaviour, 49,* 567–575.

Pfennig, D. W., Reeve, H. K., & Sherman, P. W. (1993). Kin recognition and cannibalism in spadefoot toads. *Animal Behaviour, 46,* 87–94.

Pfennig, D. W., & Sherman, P. W. (1995). Kin recognition. *Scientific American,* June 1995, 98–103.

Pfungst, O. (1911). *Clever Hans: The horse of Mr. Von Osten.* New York: Holt, Rinehart and Winston.

Philipp, D., & Gross, M. (1994). Genetic evidence for cuckoldry in bluegill *Lepomis macrochirus. Molecular Ecology, 3,* 563–569.

Piaget, J. (1951). *Play, dreams and imitation in childhood.* New York: Norton.

Pierce, N. E., Braby, M. F., Heath, A., Lohman, D. J., Mathew, J., Rand, D. B., & Travassos, M. A. (2002). The ecology and evolution of ant association in the *Lycaenidae* (Lepidoptera). *Annual Review of Entomology, 47,* 733–771.

Pierce, N., Kitchling, R., Buckley, R., Talor, M., & Benbow, K. (1987). The costs and benefits of cooperation between the Australian lycaenid butterfly, *Jalmenus evagoras,* and its attendant ants. *Behavioral Ecology and Sociobiology, 21,* 237–248.

Pietrewicz, A. T., & Kamil, A. C. (1979). Search image formation in the blue jay (*Cyanocitta cristata*). *Science, 204,* 1332–1333.

Pietrewicz, A., & Richards, J. (1985). Learning to forage: An ecological perspective. In T. Johnston & A. Pietrewicz (Eds.), *Issues in the ecological study of learning* (pp. 99–119). Hillsdale, NJ: Lawrence Erlbaum Associates.

Pitcher, T. (1986). Functions of shoaling behaviour. In T. Pitcher (Ed.), *The behavior of teleost fishes* (pp. 294–338). Baltimore: John Hopkins University Press.

Pitcher, T. (1992). Who dares wins: The function and evolution of predator inspection behaviour in shoaling fish. *Netherlands Journal of Zoology, 42,* 371–391.

Pitcher, T. J., Green, D. A., & Magurran, A. E. (1986). Dicing with death: Predator inspection behavior in minnow shoals. *Journal of Fish Biology, 28,* 439–448.

Platzen, D., & Magrath, R. D. (2005). Adaptive differences in response to two types of parental alarm call in altricial nestlings. *Proceedings of the Royal Society of London, Series B, 272,* 1101–1106.

Pleszczynska, W. K., & Hansell, R. (1980). Polygeny and decision theory: Testing of a model in lark buntings, *Calamospiza melanocorys. American Naturalist, 116,* 821–830.

Plomin, R., DeFries, J. C., Craig, I., & McGuffin, P. (2002). *Behavioral genetics in the post genomic era.* New York: American Psychological Association.

Plomin, R., DeFries, J. C., McClearn, G. E., & McGuffin, P. (2000). *Behavioral genetics.* New York: Worth.

Podos, J., Huber, S. K., & Taft, B. (2004). Bird song: The interface of evolution and mechanism. *Annual Review of Ecology, Evolution, and Systematics, 35,* 55–87.

Poirier, F. E., Stini, W. A., & Wreden, K. B. (1994). *In search of ourselves: An introduction to physical anthropology.* New York: Prentice Hall.

Polhemus, J. (1990). Surface wave communication in water striders. Field observations of unreported taxa (Heteroptera: Gerridae, Veliidae). *Journal of the New York Entomological Society, 98,* 383–384.

Polhemus, J., & Karunaratne, P. (1993). A review of the genus *Rhagadotarsus,* with descriptions of three new species (Heteroptera: Gerridae). *Raffles Bulletin of Zoology, 41,* 95–112.

Pollock, G. B., Cabrales, A., & Rissing, S. W. (2004). On suicidal punishment among *Acromyrmex versicolor* co-foundresses: The disadvantage in personal advantage. *Evolutionary Ecology Research, 6,* 891–917.

Poppleton, F. (1957). The birth of an elephant. *Oryx, 4,* 180–181.

Poran, N. S., & Coss, R. G. (1990). Development of antisnake defenses in California ground squirrels (*Spermophilus beecheyi*): I. Behavioral and immunological relationships. *Behaviour, 112,* 222–245.

Portmann, A. (1947). Etudes sur la cerebralisation des oiseaux: Les indices intra-cerebraux. *Alauda, 15,* 1–15.

Potegal, M., & Einon, D. (1989). Aggressive behaviors in adult rats deprived of playfighting experience as juveniles. *Developmental Psychobiology, 22,* 159–172.

Potter, E. (1970). Anting in wild birds, its frequency and probable purpose. *Auk, 87,* 692–713.

Poundstone, W. (1992). *Prisoner's dilemma: Jon Von Neuman, game theory and the puzzle of the bomb.* New York: Doubleday.

Power, T. G. (2000). *Play and exploration in children and animals.* Hillsdale, NJ: Lawrence Erlbaum Associates.

Pravosudov, V. V., & Clayton, N. S. (2002). A test of the adaptive specialization hypothesis: Population differences in caching, memory, and the hippocampus in black-capped chickadees (*Poecile atricapilla*). *Behavioral Neuroscience, 116,* 515–522.

Pravosudov, V. V., & Grubb, T. C. (1997). Energy management of passerine birds during the non-breeding season. *Current Ornithology, 14,* 189–234.

Pravosudov, V. V., Kitaysky, A. S., Wingfield, J. C., & Clayton, N. S. (2001). Long-term unpredictable foraging conditions and physiological stress response in mountain chickadees (*Poecile gambeli*). *General and Comparative Endocrinology, 123,* 324–331.

Prelle, I., Phillips, C. J. C., da Costa, M. J. P., Vandenberghe, N. C., & Broom, D. M. (2004). Are cows that consistently enter the same side of a two-sided milking parlour more fearful of novel situations or more competitive? *Applied Animal Behaviour Science, 87,* 193–203.

Prete, F. R. (1990). The conundrum of the honey-bees: One impediment to the publication of Darwin's theory. *Journal of the History of Biology, 23,* 271–290.

Prete, F. R. (1991). Can females rule the hive: The controversy over honey-bee gender roles in British beekeeping texts of the 16th-18th centuries. *Journal of the History of Biology, 24,* 113–144.

Price, J. J., & Lanyon, S. M. (2002a). A robust phylogeny of the oropendolas: Polyphyly revealed by mitochondrial sequence data. *Auk, 119,* 335–348.

Price, J. J., & Lanyon, S. M. (2002b). Reconstructing the evolution of complex bird song in the oropendolas. *Evolution, 56,* 1514–1529.

Price, J. J., & Lanyon, S. M. (2004a). Patterns of song evolution and sexual selection in the oropendolas and caciques. *Behavioral Ecology, 15,* 485–497.

Price, J. J., & Lanyon, S. M. (2004b). Song and molecular data identify congruent but novel affinities of the green oropendola (*Psarocolius viridis*). *Auk, 121,* 224–229.

Price, T., & Schulter, D. (1991). On the low heritability of life-history traits. *Evolution, 45,* 853–861.

Price, T., Schulter, D., & Heckman, N. E. (1993). Sexual selection when the female benefits directly. *Biological Journal of the Linnean Society, 48,* 187–211.

Profet, M. (1992). Pregnancy sickness as adaptation: A deterrent to maternal ingestion of teratogens. In J. Barkow, L. Cosmides, & J. Tooby (Eds.), *The adapted mind* (pp. 324–365). New York: Oxford University Press.

Profet, M. (1993). Menstruation as a defense against pathogens transported by sperm. *Quarterly Review of Biology, 68,* 335–386.

Promislow, D. E. (1991). Senescence in natural populations of mammals: A comparative study. *Evolution, 45,* 1869–1887.

Promislow, D. E. (1992). Costs of sexual selection in natural populations of mammals. *Proceedings of the Royal Society of London, Series B, 247,* 203–207.

Promislow, D. (2003). Mate choice, sexual conflict, and evolution of senescence. *Behavior Genetics, 33,* 191–201.

Pruett-Jones, S. G. (1992). Independent versus non-independent mate choice: Do females copy each other? *American Naturalist, 140,* 1000–1009.

Pruett-Jones, S., & Lewis, M. (1990). Sex ratio and habitat limitation promote delayed dispersal in superb fairy-wrens. *Nature, 348,* 541–542.

Pulido, F., Berthold, P., Mohr, G., & Querner, U. (2001). Heritability of the timing of autumn migration in a natural bird population. *Proceedings of the Royal Society of London, Series B, 268,* 953–959.

Pulliam, R. (1973). On the advantages of flocking. *Journal of Theoretical Biology, 38,* 419–422.

Purves, D., & Lichtman, J. (1980). Elimination of synapses in the developing nervous system. *Science, 210,* 153–157.

Purvis, K., Haug, E., Clausen, O. P. F., Naess, O., & Hansson, V. (1977). Endocrine status of testicular feminized male (Tfm) rats. *Molecular and Cellular Endocrinology, 8,* 317–334.

Pysh, J., & Weiss, G. (1979). Exercise during development induces an increase in Purkinje cell dendritic tree size. *Science, 206,* 230–231.

Queller, D. C. (1992). Quantitative genetics, inclusive fitness and group selection. *American Naturalist, 139,* 540–558.

Quigley, H., & Cragshaw, P. (1992). A conservation plan for the jaguar (*Panthera onca*) in the Pantanal region of Brazil. *Biological Conservation, 61,* 149–157.

Quinn, J. S., Woolfenden, G. E., Fitzpatrick, J. W., & White, B. N. (1999). Multi-locus DNA fingerprinting supports genetic monogamy in Florida scrub-jays. *Behavioral Ecology and Sociobiology, 45,* 1–10.

Quinn, T. (1984). Homing and straying in Pacific salmon. In J. McCleave, G. Arnold, J. Dodson, & W. Neill, W. (Eds.), *Mechanisms of migration in fishes* (pp. 357–362). New York: Plenum Press.

Quinn, T. P., & Dittman, A. H. (1990). Pacific salmon migrations and homing: Mechanisms and adaptive significance. *Trends in Ecology & Evolution, 5,* 174–177.

Raby, C. R., Alexis, D. M., Dickinson, A., & Clayton, N. S. (2007). Planning for the future by western scrub-jays. *Nature, 445,* 919–921.

Raleigh, M., & McGuire, M. (1991). Bidirectional relationships between tryptophan and social behavior in vervet monkeys. In R. Schwarcz, S. N. Young, & R. R. Brown (Eds.), *Kynurenine and serotonin pathway: Progress in tryptophan research, advances in experimental medicine and biology* (pp. 289–298). New York: Plenum Press.

Raleigh, M., McGuire, M., Brammer, G., Pollack, D., & Yuwiler, A. (1991). Serotonergic mechanisms promote dominance in adult vervet monkeys. *Brain Research, 559,* 181–190.

Ramenofsky, M., & Wingfield, J. C. (2007). Regulation of migration. *Bioscience, 57,* 135–143.

Rammensee, H., Bachmann, J., & Stefanovic, S. (1997). *MHC ligands and peptide motifs.* Georgetown, TX: Landes Biosciences.

Ratnieks, F. L. (1995). Evidence for queen-produced egg-marking pheromone and its use in worker policing in the honey bee. *Journal of Apicultural Research, 34,* 31–37.

Ratnieks, F. L., & Visscher, P. K. (1988). Reproductive harmony via mutual policing by workers in eusocial hymenoptera. *American Naturalist, 132,* 217–236.

Ratnieks, F. L., & Visscher, P. K. (1989). Worker policing in the honeybee. *Nature, 342,* 796–797.

Rattenborg, N., Lima, S., & Amlaner, C. (1999a). Facultative control of avian unihemispheric sleep under the risk of predation. *Behavioral Brain Research, 105,* 163–172.

Rattenborg, N., Lima, S., & Amlaner, C. (1999b). Half-awake to the risk of predation. *Nature, 397,* 397–398.

Rattenborg, N. C., Amlaner, C. J., & Lima, S. L. (2000). Behavioral, neurophysiological and evolutionary perspectives on unihemispheric sleep. *Neuroscience and Biobehavioral Reviews, 24,* 817–842.

Reader, S. M. (2004). Don't call me clever. *New Scientist, 183,* 34–37.

Reader, S. M., Kendal, J. R., & Laland, K. N. (2003). Social learning of foraging sites and escape routes in wild Trinidadian guppies. *Animal Behaviour, 66,* 729–739.

Reader, S. M., & Laland, K. (Ed). (2003). *Animal innovation.* Oxford: Oxford University Press.

Reader, S. M., & Laland, K. N. (2002). Social intelligence, innovation and enhanced brain size in primates. *Proceedings of the National Academy of Sciences, U.S.A., 99,* 4436–4441.

Real, L., & Caraco, T. (1986). Risk and foraging in stochastic environments. *Annual Review of Ecology and Systematics, 17,* 371–390.

Reale, D., Reader, S. M., Sol, D., McDougall, P. T., & Dingemanse, N. J. (2007). Integrating animal temperament within ecology and evolution. *Biological Reviews, 82,* 291–318.

Reby, D., McComb, K., Cargnelutti, B., Darwin, C., Fitch, W. T., & Clutton-Brock, T. (2005). Red deer stags use formants as assessment cues during intrasexual agonistic interactions. *Proceedings of the Royal Society of London, Series B, 272,* 941–947.

Reeve, H. K. (1989). The evolution of conspecific acceptance thresholds. *American Naturalist, 133,* 407–435.

Reeve, H. K. (1992). Queen activation of lazy workers in colonies of the eusocial naked mole-rat. *Nature, 358,* 147–149.

Reeve, H. K., & Ratnieks, F. L. (1993). Queen-queen conflicts in polygynous societies: Mutual tolerance and reproductive skew. In L. Keller (Ed.), *Queen number and sociality in insects* (pp. 45–86). Oxford: Oxford University Press.

Reeve, H. K., & Sherman, P. W. (1991). Intracolonial aggression and nepotism by the breeding female naked mole rat. In P. W. Sherman, J. Jarvis, & R. D. Alexander (Eds.), *The biology of the naked mole-rat* (pp. 337–357). Princeton: Princeton University Press.

Reeve, H. K., & Sherman, P. W. (1993). Adaptation and the goals of evolutionary research. *Quarterly Review of Biology, 68*, 1–32.

Reeve, H. K., Westneat, D. F., Noon, W. A., Sherman, P. W., & Aquadro, C. F. (1990). DNA "fingerprinting" reveals high levels of inbreeding in colonies of the eusocial naked mole rat. *Proceedings of the National Academy of Sciences, U.S.A., 87*, 2496–2500.

Reeve, H. K., Westneat, D. F., & Queller, D. C. (1992). Estimating average within-group relatedness from DNA fingerprints. *Molecular Ecology, 2*, 223–232.

Reid, P. J., & Shettleworth, S. J. (1992). Detection of cryptic prey: Search image or search rate. *Journal of Experimental Psychology: Animal Behavior Processes, 18*, 273–286.

Remage-Healey, L., & Bass, A. H. (2007). Plasticity in brain sexuality is revealed by the rapid actions of steroid hormones. *Journal of Neuroscience, 27*, 1114–1122.

Remage-Healey, L., Nowacek, D. P., & Bass, A. H. (2006). Dolphin foraging sounds suppress calling and elevate stress hormone levels in a prey species, the Gulf toadfish. *Journal of Experimental Biology, 209*, 4444–4451.

Reusch, T. B. H., Haberli, M. A., Aeschlimann, P. B., & Milinski, M. (2001). Female sticklebacks count alleles in a strategy of sexual selection explaining MHC polymorphism. *Nature, 414*, 300–302.

Reznick, D. (1996). Life history evolution in guppies: A model system for the empirical study of adaptation. *Netherlands Journal of Zoology, 46*, 172–190.

Reznick, D., Brygaa, H., & Endler, J. (1990). Experimentally induced life-history evolution in a natural population. *Nature, 346*, 357–359.

Ribas, C. C., & Miyaki, C. Y. (2004). Molecular systematics in Aratinga parakeets: Species limits and historical biogeography in the "solstitialis" group, and the systematic position of Nandayus nenday. *Molecular Phylogenetics and Evolution, 30*, 663–675.

Richards, R. J. (1987). *Darwin and the emergence of evolutionary theories of mind and behavior.* Chicago: University of Chicago.

Ridley, M. (1996). *Evolution* (2nd ed.). Oxford: Blackwell Science.

Riechert, S. (1998). Game theory and animal contests. In L. A. Dugatkin & H. K. Reeve (Eds.), *Game theory and animal behavior* (pp. 64–93). New York: Oxford University Press.

Rilling, J., Gutman, D., Zeh, T., Pagnoni, G., Berns, G., & Kilts, C. (2002). A neural basis for social cooperation. *Neuron, 35*, 395–405.

Rissing, S., & Pollock, G. (1986). Social interaction among pleometric queens of *Veromessor pergandei* during colony foundation. *Animal Behaviour, 34*, 226–234.

Rissing, S., & Pollock, G. (1987). Queen aggression, pleometric advantage and brood raiding in the ant *Veromessor pergandei*. *Animal Behaviour, 35*, 975–982.

Rissing, S., & Pollock, G. (1991). An experimental analysis of pleometric advantage in *Messor pergandei*. *Insectes Sociaux, 63*, 205–211.

Rissing, S., Pollock, G., Higgins, M., Hagen, R., & Smith, D. (1989). Foraging specialization without relatedness or dominance among co-founding ant queens. *Nature, 338*, 420–422.

Rissing, S. W., Pollock, G. B., & Higgins, M. R. (1996). Fate of ant foundress associations containing "cheaters." *Naturwissenschaften, 83*, 182–185.

Ritchie, M. G., Halsey, E. J., & Gleason, J. M. (1999). Drosophila song as a species-specific mating signal and the behavioural importance of Kyriacou & Hall cycles in *D. melanogaster* song. *Animal Behaviour, 58*, 649–657.

Rizzolatti, G., & Craighero, L. (2004). The mirror-neuron system. *Annual Review of Neuroscience, 27*, 169–192.

Rizzolatti, G., Fadiga, L., Gallese, V., & Fogassi, L. (1996). Premotor cortex and the recognition of motor actions. *Cognitive Brain Research, 3*, 131–141.

Rizzolatti, G., Fogassi, L., & Gallese, V. (2001). Neurophysiological mechanisms underlying the understanding and imitation of action. *Nature Reviews Neuroscience, 2*, 661–670.

Rizzolatti, G., Fogassi, L., & Gallese, V. (2006). Mirrors in the mind. *Scientific American, 295*, 54–61.

Roberts, M., & Shapiro, M. (2002). NMDA receptor antagonists impair memory for nonspatial, socially transmitted food preference. *Behavioral Neuroscience, 116*, 1059–1069.

Robinson, G. (1985). Effects of a juvenile hormone analog on honey bee foraging behavior and alarm pheromone. *Journal of Insect Physiology, 31*, 277–282.

Robinson, G. (1987). Modulation of alarm pheromone perception in the honey bee: Evidence for division of labor based on hormonally regulated response thresholds. *Journal of Comparative Physiology. A., 160*, 613–619.

Robinson, G. E. (1992). Regulation of division of labor in insect societies. *Annual Review of Ecology and Systematics, 37*, 637–665.

Robinson, G. E., Grozinger, C. M., & Whitfield, C. W. (2005). Sociogenomics: Social life in molecular terms. *Nature Reviews Genetics, 6*, 257–271.

Robinson, G. E., Page, R. E., Strambi, C., & Strambi, A. (1989). Hormonal and genetic control of behavioral integration in honeybee colonies. *Science, 246*, 109–112.

Robinson, S., & Smotherman, W. (1991). Fetal learning: Implications for the development of kin. In P. G. Hepper (Ed.), *Kin recognition* (pp. 308–334). Cambridge: Cambridge University Press.

Roces, F., & Holldobler, B. (1995). Vibrational communication between hitchhikers and foragers in leaf-cutting ants (*Atta cephalotes*). *Behavioral Ecology and Sociobiology, 37*, 297–302.

Roces, F., & Holldobler, B. (1996). Use of stridulation in foraging leaf-cutting ants: Mechanical support during cutting or short-range recruitment signal? *Behavioral Ecology and Sociobiology, 39*, 293–299.

Roces, F., Tautz, J. & Holldobler, B. (1993). Stridulation in leaf-cutting ants: Short-range recruitment through plant-borne substances. *Naturwissenschaften, 80*, 521–524.

Rodd, F. H., Hughes, K. A., Grether, G. F., & Baril, C. T. (2002). A possible non-sexual origin of mate preference: Are male guppies mimicking fruit? *Proceedings of the Royal Society of London, Series B, 269*, 475–481.

Rodel, H. G., Monclus, R., & von Holst, D. (2006). Behavioral styles in European rabbits: Social interactions and responses to experimental stressors. *Physiology and Behavior, 89,* 180–188.

Rodriguez, E., & Wrangham, R. (1993). Zoopharmacognosy: The use of medicinal plants by animals. *Recent Advances in Phytochemistry, 27,* 89–105.

Roeloffs, R., & Riechert, S. E. (1988). Dispersal and population genetic structure of the cooperative spider, *Agelena consociata* in West African rainforests. *Evolution, 42,* 173–183.

Roguet, C., Dumont, B., & Prache, S. (1998). Selection and use of feeding sites and feeding stations by herbivores: A review. *Annales De Zootechnie, 47,* 225–244.

Rohwer, F. C., & Freeman, S. (1989). The distribution of conspecific nest parasitism in birds. *Canadian Journal of Zoology, 67,* 239–253.

Rohwer, S. (1982). The evolution of reliable and unreliable badges of fighting ability. *American Zoologist, 22,* 531–546.

Rollenhagen, A., & Bischof, H. J. (1991). Rearing conditions affect neuron morphology in a telecephalic area of the zebra finch. *Neuroreport, 2,* 711–714.

Rollenhagen, A., & Bischof, H. J. (1994). Phase specific morphological changes induced by social experience in two forebrain areas of the zebra finch. *Behavioural Brain Research, 65,* 83–88.

Romanes, G. J. (1884). *Mental evolution in animals.* New York: AMS Press.

Romanes, G. J. (1889). *Mental evolution in man.* New York: Appleton.

Romanes, G. J. (1898). *Animal intelligence* (7th ed). London: Kegan Paul, Trench, Trubner and Co.

Roper, K., Kaiser, D., & Zentall, T. (1995). True directed forgetting in pigeons may occur only when alternative working memory is required on forget-cue trials. *Animal Learning and Behavior, 23,* 280–285.

Roper, T. J. (1986). Badges of status in avian societies. *New Scientist, 109,* 38–40.

Rose, M. (1991). *The evolutionary biology of aging.* New York: Oxford University Press.

Rose, M., Matos, M., & Passananti, H. (2004). *Methuselah flies: A case study in the evolution of aging.* Singapore: World Scientific Publishing Company.

Rosenbaum, R. S., Kohler, S., Schacter, D. L., Moscovitch, M., Westmacott, R., Black, S. E., Gao, F. Q., & Tulving, E. (2005). The case of KC: Contributions of a memory-impaired person to memory theory. *Neuropsychologia, 43,* 989–1021.

Rosenthal, T., & Zimmerman, B. (1978). *Social learning and cognition.* New York: Academy Press.

Rosenzweig, M. (1981). A theory of habitat selection. *Ecology, 62,* 327–335.

Rosenzweig, M. (1985). Some theoretical aspects of habitat selection. In M. Cody (Ed.), *Habitat selection in birds* (pp. 517–540). New York: Academic Press.

Rosenzweig, M. (1990). Do animals choose habitats? In M. Bekoff & D. Jamieson (Eds.), *Interpretation and explanation in the study of animal behaviour* (pp. 157–179). Boulder: Westview Press.

Rosenzweig, M. (1991). Habitat selection and population interactions. *American Naturalist, 137,* S5–S28.

Ross, P., Jalkotzy, G., & Festa-Bianchet, M. (1997). Cougar predation on bighorn sheep in Southwestern Alberta during winter. *Canadian Journal of Zoology, 74,* 771–775.

Rothstein, S., & Pirotti, R. (1987). Distinctions among reciprocal altruism, kin selection and cooperation and a model for the initial evolution of beneficent behavior. *Ethology and Sociobiology, 9,* 189–209.

Rowden, J. (1996). The evolution of display behavior in the parrot genus *Neophema* (Aves: Psittaciformes). Durham, NC: Duke University.

Rowe, L., Repasky, R. R., & Palmer, A. R. (1997). Size-dependent asymmetry: Fluctuating asymmetry versus antisymmetry and its relevance to condition-dependent signaling. *Evolution, 51,* 1401–1408.

Rowland, W. J., & Sevenster, P. (1985). Sign stimuli in three-spined sticklebacks, (*Gasterosteus aculeatus*): A reexamination of some classic experiments. *Behaviour, 93,* 241–257.

Roy, R., Graham, S., & Peterson, J. (1988). Fiber type composition of the plantaflexors of giraffes (*Giriffa camelopardalis*) at different postnatal stages of development. *Comparative Biochemistry and Physiology A-Physiology, 91,* 347–352.

Rozin, P. (1988). The adaptive-evolutionary point of view in experimental psychology. In R. Atkinson, R Herrnstein, G. Lindzey, & R. Luce (Eds.), *Steven's handbook of experimental psychology* (pp. 503–546). New York: Wiley.

Russell, A. F., Clutton-Brock, T. H., Brotherton, P. N. M., Sharpe, L. L., McIlrath, G. M., Dalerum, F. D., Cameron, E. Z., & Barnard, J. A. (2002). Factors affecting pup growth and survival in co-operatively breeding meerkats *Suricata suricatta. Journal of Animal Ecology, 71,* 700–709.

Russello, M., & Amato, G. (2003). A molecular phylogeny of *Amazona*: Implications for Neotropical biogeography, taxonomy and conservation. *Molecular Phylogenetics and Evolution, 30,* 421–437.

Rutte, C., Taborsky, M., & Brinkhof, M. W. G. (2006). What sets the odds of winning and losing? *Trends in Ecology and Evolution, 21,* 16–21.

Ruxton, G., Sherrat, T., & Speed, M. (2004). *Avoiding attack: The evolutionary ecology of crypsis, warning signals and mimicry.* Oxford: Oxford University Press.

Ryan, B. C., & Vandenbergh, J. G. (2002). Intrauterine position effects. *Neuroscience and Biobehavioral Reviews, 26,* 665–678.

Ryan, K. K., & Altmann, J. (2001). Selection for male choice based primarily on mate compatibility in the oldfield mouse, *Peromyscus polionotus rhoadsi. Behavioral Ecology and Sociobiology, 50,* 436–440.

Ryan, M. (1985). *The tungara frog: A study in sexual selection and communication.* Chicago: University of Chicago Press.

Ryan, M. J. (1990). Sexual selection, sensory systems and sensory exploitation. *Oxford Surveys in Evolutionary Biology, 7,* 157–195.

Ryan, M. J., Fox, J., Wilczynski, W., & Rand, S. (1990). Sexual selection for sensory exploitation in the frog, *Physaleamus pustulosus. Nature, 343,* 66–67.

Ryan, M. J., & Keddy-Hector, A. (1992). Directional patterns of female mate choice and the role of sensory biases. *American Naturalist, 139,* S4–S35.

Ryan, M. J., & Rand, A. S. (1993). Sexual selection and signal evolution: Ghost of biases past. *Philosophical Transactions of the Royal Society of London, Series B, 340,* 187–195.

Ryti, R. T., & Case, T. J. (1984). Spatial arrangement and diet overlap between colonies of desert ants. *Oecologia, 62,* 401–404.

Sachs, J., Mueller, U. G., Wilcox, T., & Bull, J. J. (2004). The evolution of cooperation. *Quarterly Review of Biology, 79,* 135–160.

Saetre, P., Strandberg, E., Sundgren, P. E., Pettersson, U., Jazin, E., & Bergstrom, T. F. (2006). The genetic contribution to canine personality. *Genes, Brain and Behavior, 5,* 240–248.

Salamone, J. (1994). The involvement of nucleus accumbens dopamine in appetitive and aversive motivation. *Behavioural Brain Research, 61,* 117–133.

Salcedo, E., Zheng, L. J., Phistry, M., Bagg, E. E., & Britt, S. G. (2003). Molecular basis for ultraviolet vision in invertebrates. *Journal of Neuroscience, 23,* 10873–10878.

Salewsk, V., & Bruderer, B. (2007). The evolution of bird migration: A synthesis. *Naturwissenschaften, 4,* 268–279.

Sanfey, A. G., Loewenstein, G., McClure, S. M., & Cohen, J. D. (2006). Neuroeconomics: Cross-currents in research on decision-making. *Trends in Cognitive Sciences, 10,* 108–116.

Sansone, M. (1975). Benzodiazepines and amphetamines: Avoidance behavior in mice. *Archives Internationales de Pharmacodynamie et de Therapie, 218,* 125–132.

Sapolsky, R. M. (1996). Stress, glucocorticoids and damage to the nervous system: The current state of confusion. *Stress, 1,* 1–16.

Sapolsky, R. M. (1999). Glucocorticoids, stress, and their adverse neurological effects: Relevance to aging. *Experimental Gerontology, 34,* 721–732.

Sapolsky, R. M. (2003). Stress and plasticity in the limbic system. *Neurochemical Research, 28,* 1735–1742.

Sapolsky, R. M. (2004). Social status and health in humans and other animals. *Annual Review of Anthropology, 33,* 393–418.

Sapolsky, R. M. (2005). The influence of social hierarchy on primate health. *Science, 308,* 648–652.

Sapolsky, R. M., Krey, L., & McEwen, B. (1986). The endocrinology of stress and aging: The glucocorticoid cascade hypothesis. *Endocrine Reviews, 7,* 284–306.

Sapolsky, R. M., Romero, L. M., & Munck, A. U. (2000). How do glucocorticoids influence stress responses? Integrating permissive, suppressive, stimulatory, and preparative actions. *Endocrine Reviews, 21,* 55–89.

Sargeant, B. L., Mann, J., Berggren, P., & Krutzen, M. (2005). Specialization and development of beach hunting, a rare foraging behavior, by wild bottlenose dolphins (*Tursiops sp.*). *Canadian Journal of Zoology, 83,* 1400–1410.

Sasvari, L. (1985). Keypeck conditioning with reinforcement in two different locations in thrush, tit and sparrow species. *Behavioural Processes, 11,* 245–252.

Saunders, I., Sayer, M., & Goodale, A. (1999). The relationship between playfulness and coping in preschool children: A pilot study. *American Journal of Occupational Therapy, 53,* 221–226.

Sauro, M. D., Jorgensen, R. S., & Pedlow, C. T. (2003). Stress, glucocorticoids, and memory: A meta-analytic review. *Stress: The International Journal on the Biology of Stress, 6,* 235–245.

Savolainen, P., Zhang, Y. P., Luo, J., Lundeberg, J., & Leitner, T. (2002). Genetic evidence for an East Asian origin of domestic dogs. *Science, 298,* 1610–1613.

Sawaguchi, T., & Kudo, H. (1990). Neocortical development and social structure in primates. *Primates,* 283–290.

Schaller, G. (1967). *The deer and the tiger.* Chicago: University of Chicago Press.

Scheiner, R., Pluckhahn, S., Oney, B., Blenau, W., & Erber, J. (2002). Behavioural pharmacology of octopamine, tyramine and dopamine in honey bees. *Behavioural Brain Research, 136,* 545–553.

Schenkel, R. (1966). Play, exploration and territoriality in the wild lion. *Symposia of the Zoological Society of London, 18,* 11–22.

Schilcher, F. (1976a). The function of pulse song and sine song in the courtship of *Drosophila melanogaster. Animal Behaviour, 24,* 622–625.

Schilcher, F. (1976b). The role of auditory stimuli in the courtship song of *Drosophila melanogaster. Animal Behaviour, 24,* 18–26.

Schino, G. (2007). Grooming and agonistic support: A meta-analysis of primate reciprocal altruism. *Behavioral Ecology, 18,* 115–120.

Schino, G., Scuccio, S., Maestrippi, D., & Turillazzi, P. G. (1988). Allogrooming as a tension reduction mechanism: A behavioral approach. *American Journal of Primatology, 16,* 43–50.

Schleidt, W. (1976). On individuality: The constituents of distinctiveness. In P. Bateson & P. Klopfer (Eds.), *Perspectives in ethology* (pp. 299–310). New York: Plenum Press.

Schneider, K. (1984). Dominance, predation and optimal foraging in white-throated sparrow flocks. *Ecology, 65,* 1820–1827.

Schuett, G. (1997). Body size and agonistic experience affect dominance and mating success in male copperheads. *Animal Behaviour, 54,* 213–224.

Schuett, G. W., & Gillingham, J. C. (1989). Male-male agonistic behavior of the copperhead, *Agkistrodon contortrix. Amphibia-Reptilia, 10,* 243–266.

Schuett, G. W., & Grober, M. S. (2000). Post-fight levels of plasma lactate and corticosterone in male copperheads, *Agkistrodon contortrix* (Serpentes, Viperidae): Differences between winners and losers. *Physiology & Behavior, 71,* 335–341.

Schuett, G. W., Harlow, H. J., Rose, J. D., van Kirk, E. A., & Murdoch, W. J. (1996). Levels of plasma corticosterone and testosterone in male copperheads (*Agkistrodon contortrix*) following staged fights. *Hormones and Behavior, 30,* 60–68.

Schulz, D. J., Elekonich, M. M., & Robinson, G. E. (2003). Biogenic amines in the antennal lobes and the initiation and maintenance of foraging behavior in honey bees. *Journal of Neurobiology, 54,* 406–416.

Scott, J. P., & Bielfelt, S. W. (1976). Analysis of the puppy training program. In C. J. Pfaffenberger, J. P. Scott, J. L. Fuller, B. E. Ginsburg, & S. W. Bielfelt, (Eds.), *Guide dogs for the blind: Their selection, development and training* (pp. 39–75). Amsterdam: Elsevier.

Scott, S. (1987). *Field guide to the birds of North America.* Washington, DC: National Geographic Society.

Searby, A., Jouventin, P., & Aubin, T. (2004). Acoustic recognition in macaroni penguins: An original signature system. *Animal Behaviour, 67,* 615–625.

Searcy, W., Yasukawa, K., & Lanyon, S. (1999). Evolution of polygyny in the ancestors of red-winged blackbirds. *Auk, 116*, 5–19.

Sebeok, T., & Rosenthal, R. (Eds.). (1981). *The Clever Hans phenomenon: Communication with horses, whales, apes, and people.* New York: New York Academy of Sciences.

Seeley, T. (1985). *Honeybee ecology: A study of adaptation in social life.* Princeton: Princeton University Press.

Seeley, T. (1995). *The wisdom of the hive.* Cambridge, MA: Harvard University Press.

Seeley, T. (1997). Honey bee colonies are group-level adaptive units. *American Naturalist, 150 (supplement)*, S22–S41.

Seeley, T. D., & Tarpy, D. R. (2007). Queen promiscuity lowers disease within honeybee colonies. *Proceedings of the Royal Society of London, Series B, 274*, 67–72.

Seger, J. (1989). All for one, one for all, that is our device. *Nature, 338*, 374–375.

Seghers, B. H. (1973). An analysis of geographic variation in the antipredator adaptations of the guppy, *Poecilia reticulata.* University of British Columbia.

Selander, R., Smith, M., Yang, S., Johnson, W., & Gentry, J. (1971). Biochemical polymorphism and systematics in the genus *Peromyscus*: I. Variation of the oldfield mouse (*Peromyscus polionotus*). *Studies in Genetics, 6*, 49–90.

Seligman, M., & Hager, J. (1972). *Biological boundaries of learning.* New York: Appleton.

Selye, H. (1936). A syndrome produced by diverse nocuous agents. *Nature, 138*, 32–35.

Semel, B., & Sherman, P. (1986). Dynamics of nest parasitism in wood ducks. *Auk, 103*, 136–139.

Semel, B., Sherman, P., & Byers, S. (1988). Effects of brood parasitism and nest-box placement on wood duck breeding ecology. *Condor, 90*, 920–930.

Semel, B., Sherman, P., & Byers, S. (1990). Nest boxes and brood parasitism in wood ducks: A management dilemma. In L. H. Fredrickson, G. V. Burger, S. P. Havera, D. A. Graber, R. E. Kirkby, & T. S. Taylor (Eds.), *Proceedings of the 1988 North American Wood Duck Symposium* (pp. 163–170). St. Louis, MO.

Serpell, J. A., & Hsu, Y. Y. (2001). Development and validation of a novel method for evaluating behavior and temperament in guide dogs. *Applied Animal Behaviour Science, 72*, 347–364.

Seyfarth, R. M., & Cheney, D. L. (1986). Vocal development in vervet monkeys. *Animal Behaviour, 34*, 1640–1658.

Seyfarth, R. M., Cheney, D. L., & Marler, P. (1980). Vervet monkey alarm calls: Semantic communication in a free-ranging primate. *Animal Behaviour, 28*, 1070–1094.

Sgoifo, A., Costoli, T., Meerlo, P., Buwalda, B., Pico'Alfonso, M. A., De Boer, S., Musso, E., & Koolhaas, J. (2005). Individual differences in cardiovascular response to social challenge. *Neuroscience and Biobehavioral Reviews, 29*, 59–66.

Sharp, S. P., & Hatchwell, B. J. (2005). Individuality in the contact calls of cooperatively breeding long-tailed tits (*Aegithalos caudatus*). *Behaviour, 142*, 1559–1575.

Shaw, P. W., Carvalho, G. R., Seghers, B. H., & Magurran, A. E. (1992). Genetic consequences of an artificial introduction of guppies (*Poecilia reticulata*) in N. Trinidad. *Proceedings of the Royal Society of London, Series B, 248*, 111–116.

Sheard, M. (1983). Aggressive behavior: Effects of neural modulation by serotonin. In E. Simmell, M. Hahn, & J Walters (Eds.), *Aggressive behavior* (pp. 167–181). Hillsdale, NJ: Lawrence Erlbaum Associates.

Sherman, P. W. (1977). Nepotism and the evolution of alarm calls. *Science, 197*, 1246–1253.

Sherman, P. W. (1980). The meaning of nepotism. *American Naturalist, 116*, 604–606.

Sherman, P. W. (1981). Kinship, demography, and Belding's ground squirrel nepotism. *Behavioral Ecology and Sociobiology, 8*, 251–259.

Sherman, P. W. (1985). Alarm calls of Belding's ground squirrels to aerial predators: Nepotism or self-preservation? *Behavioral Ecology and Sociobiology, 17*, 313–323.

Sherman, P. (1988). The levels of analysis. *Animal Behaviour, 36*, 616–619.

Sherman, P. W. (2001). Wood ducks: A model system for investigating conspecific parasitism in cavity-nesting birds. In L. A. Dugatkin (Ed.), *Model systems in behavioral ecology: Integrating conceptual, theoretical and empirical perspectives* (pp. 311–337). Princeton: Princeton University Press.

Sherman, P. W., & Billing, J. (1999). Darwinian gastronomy: Why we use spices. *Bioscience, 49*, 453–463.

Sherman, P. W., & Flaxman, S. M. (2001). Protecting ourselves from food. *American Scientist, 89*, 142–151.

Sherman, P., & Flaxman, M. (2002). Nausea and vomiting of pregnancy in an evolutionary perspective. *American Journal of Obstetrics and Gynecology, 186*, S109–S197.

Sherman, P. W., & Hash, G. A. (2001). Why vegetable recipes are not very spicy. *Evolution and Human Behavior, 22*, 147–163.

Sherman, P. W., & Holmes, W. (1985). Kin recognition: Issues and evidence. *Fortschritte der Zoologie, 31*, 437–460.

Sherman, P. W., Jarvis, J., & Alexander, R. (Eds.). (1991). *The biology of the naked mole-rat.* Princeton: Princeton University Press.

Sherry, D. F. (2006). Neuroecology. *Annual Review of Psychology, 57*, 167–197.

Sherry, D. F., & Vaccarino, A. (1989). Hippocampus and memory for food caches in black-capped chickadees. *Behavioral Neuroscience, 103*, 308–318.

Shettleworth, S. J. (1998). *Cognition, evolution and behavior.* New York: Oxford University Press.

Shettleworth, S. J. (2007). Animal behaviour: Planning for breakfast. *Nature, 445*, 825–826.

Shi, Y. S., Radlwimmer, F. B., & Yokoyama, S. (2001). Molecular genetics and the evolution of ultraviolet vision in vertebrates. *Proceedings of the National Academy of Sciences, U.S.A., 98*, 11731–11736.

Shi, Y. S., & Yokoyama, S. (2003). Molecular analysis of the evolutionary significance of ultraviolet vision in vertebrates. *Proceedings of the National Academy of Sciences, U.S.A., 100*, 8308–8313.

Shier, D. M., & Owings, D. H. (2006). Effects of predator training on behavior and post-release survival of captive prairie dogs (*Cynomys ludovicianus*). *Biological Conservation, 132*, 126–135.

Shuster, S. M., & Caldwell, R. (1989). Male defense of the breeding cavity and factors affecting the persistence of breeding pairs in the stomatopod, *Gonodactylus bredini* (Crustacea: Hoplocarida). *Ethology, 82,* 192–207.

Shutler, D., & Campbell, A. A. (2007). Experimental addition of greenery reduces flea loads in nests of a non-greenery using species, the tree swallow *Tachycineta bicolor. Journal of Avian Biology, 38,* 7–12.

Sigg, D., Thompson, C. M., & Mercer, A. R. (1997). Activity-dependent changes to the brain and behavior of the honey bee, *Apis mellifera* (L.). *Journal of Neuroscience, 17,* 7148–7156.

Sigmund, K. (1993). *Games of life: Explorations in ecology, evolution, and behaviour.* Oxford: Oxford University Press.

Sih, A., Bell, A., & Johnson, J. C. (2004a). Behavioral syndromes: An ecological and evolutionary overview. *Trends in Ecology and Evolution, 19,* 372–378.

Sih, A., Bell, A., Johnson, J. C., & Ziema, R. (2004b). Behavioral syndromes: An integrative approach. *Quarterly Review of Biology, 79,* 241–277.

Sih, A., Bell, A. M., & Johnson, J. C. (2004c). Reply to Neff and Sherman. Behavioral syndromes versus Darwinian algorithms. *Trends in Ecology & Evolution, 19,* 622–623.

Sih, A., & Christensen, B. (2001). Optimal diet theory: When does it work, and when it does it fail? *Animal Behaviour, 61,* 379–390.

Simmons, L. W. (2001). *Sperm competition and its evolutionary consequences.* Princeton: Princeton University Press.

Simmons, L. W., Tomkins, J. L., Kotiaho, J. S., & Hunt, J. (1999). Fluctuating paradigm. *Proceedings of the Royal Society of London, Series B, 266,* 593–595.

Singer, W. (1994). Putative functions of temporal correlations in neocorticol processing. In C. Koch & J. Davis (Eds.), *Large-scale neuronal theories of the brain* (pp. 201–237). Cambridge, MA: MIT Press.

Sinn, D. L., Apiolaza, L. A., & Moltschaniwskyj, N. A. (2006). Heritability and fitness-related consequences of squid personality traits. *Journal of Evolutionary Biology, 19,* 1437–1447.

Sinn, D. L., & Moltschaniwskyj, N. A. (2005). Personality traits in dumpling squid (*Euprymna tasmanica*): Context-specific traits and their correlation with biological characteristics. *Journal of Comparative Psychology, 119,* 99–110.

Siviy, S. (1998). Neurobiological substrates of play behavior: Glimpses into the structure and function of mammalian playfulness. In M. Bekoff & J. Byers (Eds.), *Animal play: Evolutionary, comparative and ecological perspectives* (pp. 221–242). Cambridge: Cambridge University Press.

Siviy, S., & Panksepp, J. (1985). Dorsomedial diencephalic involvement in the juvenile play of rats. *Behavioral Neuroscience, 99,* 1103–1113.

Siviy, S., & Panksepp, J. (1987). Juvenile play in the rat: Thalamic and brain stem involvement. *Physiology and Behavior, 41,* 103–114.

Skinner, B. F. (1938). *The behavior of organisms.* New York: Appleton-Century-Crofts.

Skinner, B. F. (1959). A case history in scientific method. In S. Koch (Ed.), *Psychology: A study of science* (pp. 359–379). New York: McGraw-Hill.

Slabbekoorn, H., & Smith, T. B. (2002). Bird song, ecology and speciation. *Philosophical Transactions of the Royal Society of London, Series B, 357,* 493–503.

Slansky, F., & Scriber, J. (1985). Food consumption and utilization. In G. A. Kerkut & L. I. Gilbert (Eds.), *Comprehensive insect physiology, biochemistry and pharmacology* (pp. 87–163). Oxford: Pergamon Press.

Slater, P. J. B. (1981). Individual differences in animal behavior. In P. Bateson & P. Klopfer (Eds.), *Perspectives in ethology* (pp. 35–49). New York: Plenum Press.

Slater, P. J. B. (2003). Fifty years of bird song research: A case study in animal behaviour. *Animal Behaviour, 65,* 633–639.

Slocombe, K. E., & Zuberbuhler, K. (2005). Agonistic screams in wild chimpanzees (*Pan troglodytes schweinfurthii*) vary as a function of social role. *Journal of Comparative Psychology, 119,* 67–77.

Slocombe, K., & Zuberbuhler, K. (2007). Chimpanzees modify recruitment screams as a function of audience composition. *Proceedings of the National Academy of Sciences, U.S.A., 104,* 17228–17233.

Sluyter, F., Bult, A., Lynch, C., Oortmerssen, G., & Koolhaus, J. (1995). A comparison between house mouse lines selected for attack latency or nest building: Evidence for genetic basis for alternative behavioral strategies. *Behavior Genetics, 25,* 247–252.

Smith, A. P., & Alcock, J. (1980). A comparative study of the mating systems of Australian eumenid wasps (Hymenoptera). *Zeitschrift fur Tierpsychologie, 53,* 41–60.

Smith, C., Barber, I., Wootton, R. J., & Chittka, L. (2004). A receiver bias in the origin of three-spined stickleback mate choice. *Proceedings of the Royal Society of London, Series B, 271,* 949–955.

Smith, D. G., Davis, R. J., Gehlert, D. R., & Nomikos, G. G. (2006). Exposure to predator odor stress increases efflux of frontal cortex acetylcholine and monoamines in mice: Comparisons with immobilization stress and reversal by chlordiazepoxide. *Brain Research, 1114,* 24–30.

Smith, D. R., & Hagen, R. H. (1996). Population structure and interdemic selection in the cooperative spider *Anelosimus eximius. Journal of Evolutionary Biology, 9,* 589–608.

Smith, I. C., Huntingford, F. A., Atkinson, R. J. A., & Taylor, A. C. (1994). Strategic decisions during agonistic behaviour in the velvet swimming crab, *Necora puber. Animal Behaviour, 47,* 885–894.

Smith, P. K. (1982). Does play matter? Functional and evolutionary aspects of animal and human play. *Behavioral and Brain Sciences, 5,* 139–184.

Smith, P. S. (1991). Ontogeny and adaptiveness of tail-flagging behavior in white-tailed deer. *American Naturalist, 138,* 190–200.

Smith, R. J. F. (1986). Evolution of alarm signals: Role of benefits of retaining group members or territorial neighbors. *American Naturalist, 128,* 604–610.

Smith, R. L. (1979). Paternity assurance and altered roles in the mating behavior of a giant water bug, *Abedus herberti* (Heteroptera: Belostomatidae). *Animal Behaviour, 27,* 716–725.

Smith, R. L. (Ed.). (1984). *Sperm competition and the evolution of animal mating systems.* New York: Academic Press.

Smith, W. J. (1968). Message meaning analysis. In T. Sebeok (Ed.), *Animal communications* (pp. 44–60). Bloomington: Indiana University Press.

Smith, W. J. (1977). *The behavior of communicating: An ethological approach.* Cambridge, MA: Harvard University Press.

Smits, C. J., & Visser, G. (1993). Effects of disturbance on shorebirds: A summary of existing knowledge from the Dutch Wadden sea and delta area. *Wader Study Group Bulletin, 68,* 6–19.

Smolker, R., Richards, A., Connor, R., Mann, J., & Berggren, P. (1997). Sponge carrying by dolphins (Delphinidae, Tursiops sp.): A foraging specialization involving tool use? *Ethology, 103,* 454–465.

Smuts, B. (1985). *Sex and friendship in baboons.* New York: Aldine.

Smythe, N. (1977). The function of mammalian alarm advertising: Social signals or pursuit invitation. *American Naturalist, 111,* 191–194.

Sober, E. (1987). What is adaptationism? In J. Dupre (Ed.), *The latest on the best: Essays on evolution and optimality* (pp. 105–118). Cambridge, MA: MIT Press.

Sober, E., & Wilson, D. S. (1998). *Unto others: The evolution and psychology of unselfish behavior.* Cambridge, MA: Harvard University Press.

Sol, D., Duncan, R. P., Blackburn, T., Cassey, P., & Lefebvre, L. (2005a). Big brains, enhanced cognition, and response of birds to novel environments. *Proceedings of the National Academy of Sciences, U.S.A., 102,* 5460–5465.

Sol, D., Lefebvre, L., & Rodriguez-Teijeiro, J. D. (2005b). Brain size, innovative propensity and migratory behaviour in temperate Palaearctic birds. *Proceedings of the Royal Society of London, Series B, 272,* 1433–1441.

Sol, D., & Lefebvre, L. (2006). Behavioral flexibility and response in birds to changes in the environment. *Journal of Ornithology, 147,* 34–34.

Sol, D., Szekely, T., Liker, A., & Lefebvre, L. (2006). Big-brained birds survive better in nature. *Journal of Ornithology, 147,* 254–254.

Sol, D., Szekely, T., Liker, A., & Lefebvre, L. (2007). Big-brained birds survive better in nature. *Proceedings of the Royal Society of London, Series B, 274,* 763–769.

Solberg, L. C., Valdar, W., Gauguier, D., Nunez, G., Taylor, A., Burnett, S., Arboledas-Hita, C., Hernandez-Pliego, P., Davidson, S., Burns, P., Bhattacharya, S., Hough, T., Higgs, D., Klenerman, P., Cookson, W. O., Zhang, Y. M., Deacon, R. M., Rawlins, J. N. P., Mott, R., & Flint, J. (2006). A protocol for high-throughput phenotyping, suitable for quantitative trait analysis in mice. *Mammalian Genome, 17,* 129–146.

Solomon, N. G., & French, J. A. (Eds.). (1996). *Cooperative breeding in mammals.* Cambridge: Cambridge University Press.

Sordahl, T. A. (1990). The risks of avian mobbing and distraction behavior: An anectodal review. *Wilson Bulletin, 102,* 349–352.

Sorrells, S. F. & Sapolsky, R. M. (2007). An inflammatory review of glucocorticoid actions in the CNS. *Brain Behavior and Immunity, 21,* 259–272.

Soti, C., Sreedhar, A. S., & Csermely, P. (2003). Apoptosis, necrosis and cellular senescence: Chaperone occupancy as a potential switch. *Aging Cell, 2,* 39–45.

Sparks, J. (1967). Allogrooming in primates: A review. In D. Morris (Ed.), *Primate ethology* (pp. 148–175). London: Weidenfeld and Nicolson.

Spencer, S. J., Buller, K. M., & Day, T. A. (2005). Medial prefrontal cortex control of the paraventricular hypothalamic nucleus response to psychological stress: Possible role of the bed nucleus of the stria terminalis. *Journal of Comparative Neurology, 481,* 363–376.

Spieth, H. T., & Ringo, J. M. (1983). Mating behavior and sexual selection in Drosophila. In M. Ashburn, H. Carson, & J. L. Thompson (Eds.), *The genetics and biology of drosophila* (pp. 224–284). London: Academic Press.

Spinka, M., Newberry, R., & Bekoff, M. (2001). Mammalian play: Training for the unexpected. *Quarterly Review of Biology, 76,* 141–168.

Spinks, A. C., O'Riain, M. J., & Polakow, D. A. (1998). Intercolonial encounters and xenophobia in the common mole rat, *Cryptomys hottentotus hottentotus* (Bathyergidae): The effects of aridity, sex and reproductive status. *Behavioral Ecology, 9,* 354–359.

Spoolder, H., Burbidge, J., Lawrence, A., Simmins, P., & Edwards, S. (1996). Individual behavioral differences in pigs: Intra- and inter-test consistency. *Applied Animal Behavior Science, 49,* 185–198.

Spooner, C. (1964). Observations on the use of the chick in pharmacological investigation of the cental nervous system. University of California at Los Angeles.

Stacey, P., & Koenig, W. (Eds.). (1990). *Cooperative beeding in birds: Long-term studies of ecology and behavior.* Cambridge: Cambridge University Press.

Stacey, P. B., & Ligon, J. D. (1987). Territory quality and dispersal options in the acorn woodpecker, and a challenge to the habitat-saturation model of cooperative breeding. *American Naturalist, 130,* 654–676.

Stammbach, E. (1988). Group responses to specially skilled individuals in a *Macaca fascicularis* group. *Behaviour, 107,* 687–705.

Stamps, J. A. (1987a). Conspecifics as cues to territory quality: A preference of juvenile lizards (*Anolis aeneus*) for previously used territories. *American Naturalist, 129,* 629–642.

Stamps, J. A. (1987b). The effect of familiarity with a neighborhood on territory acquisition. *Behavioral Ecology and Sociobiology, 21,* 273–277.

Stamps, J. (1995). Motor learning and the adaptive value of familiar space. *American Naturalist, 146,* 41–58.

Stamps, J. (2001). Learning from lizards. In L. A. Dugatkin (Ed.), *Model systems in behavioral ecology* (pp. 149–168). Princeton: Princeton University Press.

Stamps, J. (2003). Behavioural processes affecting development: Tinbergen's fourth question comes of age. *Animal Behaviour, 66,* 1–13.

Stamps, J. A. (2007). Growth-mortality tradeoffs and "personality traits" in animals. *Ecology Letters, 10,* 355–363.

Stamps, J., & Krishnan, V. V. (1999). A learning-based model of territorial assessment. *Quarterly Review of Biology, 74,* 291–318.

Stamps, J. A., & Krishnan, V. V. (2001). How territorial animals compete for divisible space: A learning-based model with unequal competitors. *American Naturalist, 157,* 154–169.

Stander, P. (1990). A suggested management strategy for stock raiding lions in Namibia. *South African Journal of Wildlife Research, 20,* 37–43.

Stankowich, T., & Blumstein, D. T. (2005). Fear in animals: A meta-analysis and review of risk assessment. *Proceedings of the Royal Society of London, Series B, 272,* 2627–2634.

Stankowich, T., & Sherman, P. W. (2002). Pup shoving by adult naked mole-rats. *Ethology, 108,* 975–992.

Stearns, S. (1989). The evolutionary significance of phenotypic plasticity. *BioScience, 39,* 436–444.

Stearns, S. C., & Ebert, D. (2001). Evolution in health and disease: Work in progress. *Quarterly Review of Biology, 76,* 417–432.

Stein, R. C. (1968). Modulation in bird sound. *Auk, 94,* 229–243.

Stephens, D. (1991). Change, regularity and value in the evolution of learning. *Behavioral Ecology, 2,* 77–89.

Stephens, D., & Krebs, J. (1986). *Foraging theory.* Princeton: Princeton University Press.

Stephens, D. W. (1993). Learning and behavioral ecology: Incomplete Information and environmental predictability. In D. Papaj (Ed.), *Insect learning* (pp. 195–218). New York: Chapman Hall.

Stephens, D. W., Anderson, J. P., & Benson, K. E. (1997). On the spurious occurrence of tit-for-tat in pairs of predator-approaching fish. *Animal Behaviour, 53,* 113–131.

Stevens, A., & Price, J. (1996). *Evolutionary psychiatry: A new beginning.* New York: Routledge.

Stevens, J. R., & Gilby, I. C. (2004). A conceptual, framework for nonkin food sharing: Timing and currency of benefits. *Animal Behaviour, 67,* 603–614.

Stevenson-Hinde, J., Stillwell-Barnes, R., & Zunz, M. (1980). Subjective assessment of rhesus monkeys over four successive years. *Primates, 21,* 66–82.

Stevenson-Hinde, J., & Zunz, M. (1978). Subjective assessment of individual rhesus monkeys. *Primates, 19,* 473–482.

Stockley, P., Gage, M., Parker, G., & Møller, A. (1997). Sperm competition in fishes: The evolution of testis size and ejaculate characteristics. *American Naturalist, 149,* 933–954.

Stoewe, M., Bugnyar, T., Heinrich, B., & Kotrschal, K. (2006). Effects of group size on approach to novel objects in ravens (*Corvus corax*). *Ethology, 112,* 1079–1088.

Strassmann, B. (1996). The evolution of endometrial cycles and menstruation. *Quarterly Review of Biology, 71,* 181–220.

Stratakis, C., & Chrousos, G. (1955). Neuroendocrinology and pathophysiology of the stress system. *Annals of the New York Academy of Sciences, 771,* 1–18.

Struhsaker, T. T. (1967). Auditory communication among vervet monkeys (*Cercopithecus aethiops*). In S. A. Altmann (Ed.), *Social communication among primates* (pp. 281–324). Chicago: University of Chicago Press.

Suboski, M. (1990). Releaser-induced recognition learning. *Psychological Review, 97,* 271–284.

Suboski, M., & Templeton, J. (1989). Life skills training for hatchery fish: Social learning and survival. *Fisheries Research, 7,* 343–352.

Suddendorf, T. (2006). Foresight and evolution of the human mind. *Science, 312,* 1006–1007.

Suddendorf, T., & Corballis, M. C. (1997). Mental time travel and the evolution of the human mind. *Genetic Social and General Psychology Monographs, 123,* 133–167.

Sugita, S., Baxter, D. A., & Byrne, J. H. (1994). Camp-independent effects of 8–(4–Parachlorophenylthio)-Cyclic Amp on spike duration and membrane currents in pleural sensory nmeurons of *Aplysia. Journal of Neurophysiology, 72,* 1250–1259.

Sullivan, J. P., Fahrbach, S. E., Harrison, J. F., Capaldi, E. A., Fewell, J. H., & Robinson, G. E. (2003). Juvenile hormone and division of labor in honey bee colonies: Effects of allatectomy on flight behavior and metabolism. *Journal of Experimental Biology, 206,* 2287–2296.

Sullivan, J., Jassim, O., Fahrbach, S., & Robinson, G. (2000). Juvenile hormone paces behavioral development in the adult worker honey bee. *Hormones and Behavior, 37,* 1–14.

Sullivan, K. (1984). The advantages of social foraging in downy woodpeckers. *Animal Behaviour, 32,* 16–32.

Sullivan, K. (1985). Selective alarm calling by downy woodpeckers in mixed-species flocks. *Auk, 102,* 184–187.

Summers, K., Weigt, L. A., Boag, P., & Bermingham, E. (1999). The evolution of female parental care in poison frogs of the genus Dendrobates: Evidence from mitochondrial DNA sequences. *Herpetologica, 55,* 254–270.

Summers-Smith, J. D. (1963). *The house sparrow.* London: Collins.

Sumner, F. B. (1929a). The analysis of a concrete case of intergradation between two subspecies. *Proceedings of the National Academy of Sciences, U.S.A., 15,* 110–120.

Sumner, F. B. (1929b). The analysis of a concrete case of intergradation between two subspecies: Additional data and interpretation. *Proceedings of the National Academy of Sciences, U.S.A., 15,* 481–493.

Sumner, P., & Mollon, J. D. (2000). Catarrhine photopigments are optimized for detecting targets against a foliage background. *Journal of Experimental Biology, 203,* 1963–1986.

Sumner, P., & Mollon, J. D. (2003). Colors of primate pelage and skin: Objective assessment of conspicuousness. *American Journal of Primatology, 59,* 67–91.

Sumner, S. (2006). Determining the molecular basis of sociality in insects: Progress, prospects and potential in sociogenomics. *Annales Zoologici Fennici, 43,* 423–442.

Sutherland, W. J. (1983). Aggregation and the "ideal free" distribution. *Journal of Animal Ecology, 52,* 821–828.

Sutherland, W. J., & Parker, G. (1985). Distribution of unequal competitors. In R. Sibly & R. Smith (Eds.), *Behavioural ecology* (pp. 255–274). Oxford: Blackwell Science.

Suthers, R. A. (1997). Peripheral control and lateralization of birdsong. *Journal of Neurobiology, 33,* 632–652.

Suthers, R. A. (1999). The motor basis of vocal performance in songbirds. In M. D. Hauser & M. Konishi (Eds.), *The design of animal communication* (pp. 37–62). Cambridge, MA: MIT Press.

Suthers, R. A., & Goller, F. (1996). Respiratory and syringeal dynamics of song production in northern cardinals. In M. Burrows, T. Matheson, P. Newland, & H. Schuppe (Eds.), *Nervous systems and behavior: Proceedings of the 4th international congress on neuroethology* (p. 333). Stuttgart: Georg Thieme Verlag.

Suthers, R. A., Goller, F., & Hartley, R. S. (1994). Motor dynamics of song production by mimic thrushes. *Journal of Neurobiology, 25,* 917–936.

Suthers, R. A., Goller, F., & Hartley, R. S. (1996). Motor stereotypy and diversity in songs of mimic thrushes. *Journal of Neurobiology, 30,* 231–245.

Suthers, R. A., & Hartley, R. S. (1990). Effect of unilateral denervation on the acoustic output from each side of the syrinx in the singing mimic thrushes. *Society for Neuroscience (Abst), 16,* 1249.

Suthers, R. A., Vallet, E., Tanvez, A., & Kreutzer, M. (2004). Bilateral song production in domestic canaries. *Journal of Neurobiology, 60,* 381–393.

Suthers, R. A., & Zollinger, S. A. (2004). Producing song: The vocal apparatus. In H. P. Zeigler & P. Marler (Eds.), *Behavioral neurobiology of bird song. Annals of the New York Academy of Sciences, 1016,* 109–129.

Swaddle, J. P. (2003). Fluctuating asymmetry, animal behavior, and evolution. *Advances in the Study of Behavior, 3,* 169–205.

Swaddle, J. P., & Cuthill, I. C. (1995). Asymmetry and human facial attractiveness: Symmetry may not always be beautiful. *Proceedings of the Royal Society of London, Series B, 261,* 111–116.

Symons, D. (1978). *Play and aggression: A study of rhesus monkeys.* New York: Columbia University Press.

Tai, Y. F., Scherfler, C., Brooks, D. J., Sawamoto, N., & Castiello, U. (2004). The human premotor cortex is "mirror" only for biological actions. *Current Biology, 14,* 117–120.

Talbot, C. J., Nicod, A., Cherny, S. S., Fulker, D. W., Collins, A. C., & Flint, J. (1999). High-resolution mapping of quantitative trait loci in outbred mice. *Nature Genetics, 21,* 305–308.

Tatar, M., Khazaeli, A., & Curtsinger, J. (1997). Chaperoning extended life. *Nature, 390,* 30.

Taub, D. (1980). Female choice and mating strategies among wild Barbary macaques. In D. Lindburg (Ed.), *The macaques: Studies in ecology, behavior and evolution.* New York: van Nostrand Reinhold.

Taub, D. (1984). Male caretaking behavior among wild Barbary macaques. In D. Taub (Ed.), *Primate paternalism.* New York: van Nostrand Reinhold.

Tautz, J., Maier, S., Groh, C., Rossler, W., & Brockmann, A. (2003). Behavioral performance in adult honey bees is influenced by the temperature experienced during their pupal development. *Proceedings of the National Academy of Sciences, U.S.A., 100,* 7343–7347.

Taylor, M. (1986). Receipt of support from family among black Americans: Demographic and familial differences. *Journal of Marriage and the Family, 48,* 67–77.

Telecki, G. (1973). *The predatory behavior of chimpanzees.* Lewisburg, PA: Bucknell University Press.

Templeton, A., Crease, T., & Shah, F. (1985). The molecular through ecological genetics of abnormal abdomen in *Drosophila mercatorum.* I. Basic genetics. *Genetics, 111,* 805–818.

Templeton, J. J., & Giraldeau, L.-A. (1996). Vicarious sampling: The use of personal and public information by starlings foraging in a simple patchy environment. *Behavioral Ecology and Sociobiology, 38,* 105–114.

Temrin, H., Buchmayer, S., & Enquist, M. (2000). Step-parents and infanticide: New data contradict evolutionary predictions. *Proceedings of the Royal Society of London, Series B, 267,* 943–945.

ten Cate, C., & Vos, D. R. (1999). Sexual imprinting and evolutionary processes in birds: A reassessment. *Advances in the Study of Behavior, 28,* 1–31.

Teramitsu, I., Kudo, L. C., London, S. E., Geschwind, D. H., & White, S. A. (2004). Parallel FoxP1 and FoxP2 expression in songbird and human brain predicts functional interaction. *Journal of Neuroscience, 24,* 3152–3163.

Terry, R. L. (1970). Primate grooming as a tension reduction mechanism. *Journal of Psychology, 76,* 129–136.

Thatch, W., Goodkin, H., & Keating, J. (1992). The cerebellum and adaptive coordination of movement. *Annual Review of Neuroscience, 15,* 403–442.

Thierry, B., Theraulaz, G., Gautier, J. Y., & Stiegler, B. (1995). Joint memory. *Behavioural Processes, 35,* 127–140.

Thiessen, D., & Yahr, P. (1977). *The gerbil in behavioral investigations.* Austin: University of Texas Press.

Thomas, K., & Shutler, D. (2001). Ectoparasites, nestling growth, parental feeding rates, and begging intensity of tree swallows. *Canadian Journal of Zoology, 79,* 346–353.

Thompson, J. N. (1982). *Interaction and coevolution.* New York: Wiley.

Thompson, K. V. (1996). Play-partner preferences and the function of social play in infant sable antelope, *Hippotragus niger. Animal Behaviour, 52,* 1143–1152.

Thorndike, E. L. (1898). Animal intelligence: An experimental study of the association processes in animals. *Psychological Review Monographs,* Whole (issue).

Thorndike, E. L. (1911). *Animal intelligence: Experimental studies.* New York: MacMillan.

Thornhill, R. (1976). Sexual selection and nuptial feeding behavior in *Bittacus apicalis. American Naturalist, 110,* 529–548.

Thornhill, R. (1979a). Adaptive female-mimicking in a scorpionfly. *Science, 295,* 412–414.

Thornhill, R. (1979b). Male and female sexual selection and the evolution of mating systems in insects. In M. Blum & N. Blum (Eds.), *Sexual selection and reproductive competition in insects.* New York: Academic Press.

Thornhill, R. (1980a). Mate choice in *Hylobittacus apicalis* and its relation to some models of female choice. *Evolution, 34,* 519–538.

Thornhill, R. (1980b). Sexual selection in the black-tipped hangingfly. *Scientific American, 242,* 162–172.

Thornhill, R., & Alcock, J. (1983). *The evolution of insect mating systems.* Cambridge, MA: Harvard University Press.

Thornton, A., & McAuliffe, K. (2006). Teaching in wild meerkats. *Science, 313,* 227–229.

Thorpe, W. H. (1956). *Learning and instinct in animals.* London: Methuen.

Thorpe, W. H. (1961). *Bird-song: The biology of vocal communication and expression in birds.* Cambridge: Cambridge University Press.

Thorpe, W. H. (1963). *Learning and instinct in animals* (2nd ed.) London: Methuen.

Tinbergen, L. (1960). The natural controls of insect in pinewoods. I. Factors influencing the intensity of predation by songbirds. *Archives Neerlandaises de Zoologie, 13*, 265–343.

Tinbergen, N. (1963). On aims and methods of ethology. *Zeitschrift fur Tierpsychologie, 20*, 410–440.

Tinbergen, N. (1964). The evolution of signalling devices. In W. Etkin (Ed.), *Social behavior and organization among vertebrates* (pp. 206–230). Chicago: University of Chicago Press.

Todt, D., & Naguib, M. (2000). Vocal interactions in birds: The use of song as a model in communication. *Advances in the Study of Behavior, 29*, 247–296.

Toivanen, P., & Toivanen, A. (Eds.). (1987). Avian immunology. Boca Raton, FL: CRC Press.

Tollrian, R., & Harvell, C. (Eds.). (1998). *The ecology and evolution of inducible defenses.* Princeton: Princeton University Press.

Toma, D., Bloch, G., Moore, D., & Robinson, G. (2000). Changes in *period* mRNA levels in the brain and division of labor in honey bee colonies. *Proceedings of the National Academy of Sciences, U.SA., 97*, 6914–6919.

Tomaru, M., & Oguma, Y. (1994). Genetic basis and evolution of species specific courtship song in the *Drosophila auraria* complex. *Genetical Research, 63*, 11–17.

Travasso, M., & Pierce, N. (2000). Acoustics, context and function of vibrational signalling in a lycaenid butterfly-ant mutualism. *Animal Behaviour, 60*, 13–26.

Trivers, R. L. (1971). The evolution of reciprocal altruism. *Quarterly Review of Biology, 46*, 189–226.

Trivers, R. L. (1974). Parent-offspring conflict. *American Zoologist, 14*, 249–265.

Trivers, R. (1985). *Social evolution.* Menlo Park, CA: Benjamin Cummings.

Turri, M. G., DeFries, J. C., Henderson, N. D., & Flint, J. (2004). Multivariate analysis of quantitative trait loci influencing variation in anxiety-related behavior in laboratory mice. *Mammalian Genome, 15*, 69–76.

Tyack, P. L., & Clark, C. W. (2000). Communication and acoustic behavior of dolphins and whales. In W. W. Au, A. Popper, & R. Ray (Eds.), *Hearing by whales and dolphins* (pp. 156–224). New York: Springer.

Udelsman, R., Blake, M., Stagg, C., Li, D., Putney, D., & Holbrook, N. (1993). Vascular heat shock protein expression in response to shock: Endocrine and autonomic regulation of this age-dependent response. *Journal of Clinical Investigations, 91*, 465–473.

Uehara, T., Iwasa, Y., & Ohtsuki, H. (2007). ESS distribution of display duration in animal contests to assess an opponent before fighting or fleeing. *Evolutionary Ecology Research, 9*, 395–408.

Uehara, S., Nishida, T., Hamai, M., Hasegawa, T., Hayaki, H., Huffman, M., Kawanaka, K., Kobayashi, S., Mitani, J., Takahata, Y., Takasaki, H., & Tsukahara, T. (1992). Characteristics of predation by the chimpanzees in the Mahale National Park, Tanzania. In T. Nishida, W. C. McGrew, P. Marler, M. Pickford, & F. de Waal, (Eds.), *Topics in primatology* (pp. 143–158). Tokyo: University of Tokyo Press.

Uetz, G. W. (1992). Foraging strategies of spiders. *Trends in Ecology & Evolution, 7*, 155–159.

Valone, T. J. (1989). Group foraging, public information and patch estimation. *Oikos, 56*, 357–363.

Valone, T. J., & Giraldeau, L.-A. (1993). Patch estimation by group foragers: What information is used? *Animal Behaviour, 45*, 721–728.

Valone, T., & Lima, S. (1987). Carrying food items to cover for consumption: The behavior of ten bird species under the risk of predation. *Oecologia, 71*, 286–294.

Valone, T. J., & Templeton, J. J. (2002). Public information for the assessment of quality: A widespread social phenomenon. *Philosophical Transactions of the Royal Society of London, Series B, 357*, 1549–1557.

van Baaren, J., Outreman, Y., & Boivin, G. (2005). Effect of low temperature exposure on oviposition behaviour and patch exploitation strategy in parasitic wasps. *Animal Behaviour, 70*, 153–163.

van den Berg, C., van Ree, J., Spruijt, B., & Kitchen, I. (1999). Effects of juvenile isolation and morphine treatment on social interactions and opioid receptors in adult rats: Behavioural and autoradiographic studies. *European Journal of Neuroscience, 11*, 3023 3032.

van Oers, K., Drent, P. J., de Jong, G., & van Noordwijk, A. J. (2004a). Additive and nonadditive genetic variation in avian personality traits. *Heredity, 93*, 496–503.

van Oers, K., Drent, P. J., de Goede, P., & van Noordwijk, A. J. (2004b). Realized heritability and repeatability of risk-taking behaviour in relation to avian personalities. *Proceedings of the Royal Society of London, Series B, 271*, 65–73.

van Oers, K., de Jong, G., van Noordwijk, A. J., Kempenaers, B., & Drent, P. J. (2005). Contribution of genetics to the study of animal personalities: A review of case studies. *Behaviour, 42*, 1185–1206.

van Oordt, G., & Junge, G. (1936). Die hormonal Wirkung der Gonaden auf Sommer and Prachtklied. III. Der Einfluss der kastration suf mannliche Kampflaufer (*Philomachus pugnax*). *Wilhem Roux' Arch. Entwicklungsmech Org., 134*, 112–121.

Vandermeer, J. (1984). The evolution of mutualism. In B. Shorrocks (Ed.), *Evolutionary ecology* (pp. 221–232). Oxford: Blackwell Science.

Vander Meer, R., Breed, M., Espelie, K., & Winston, M. (Eds.). (1997). *Pheromone communication in social insects.* Boulder, CO: Westview Press.

Veenema, A. H., de Kloet, E. R., de Wilde, M. C., Roelofs, A. J., Kawata, M., Buwalda, B., Neumann, I. D., Koolhaas, J. M., & Lucassen, P. J. (2007). Differential effects of stress on adult hippocampal cell proliferation in low and high aggressive mice. *Journal of Neuroendocrinology, 19*, 489–498.

Veenema, A. H., Koolhaas, J. M., & De Kloet, E. R. (2004). Basal and stress-induced differences in HPA axis, 5–HT responsiveness, and hippocampal cell proliferation in two mouse lines. *Stress: Current neuroendocrine and genetic approaches* (Vol. 1018, pp. 255–65). New York: Annals of the New York Academy of Sciences.

Vehrencamp, S. (1983). A model for the evolution of despotic versus egalitarian societies. *Animal Behaviour, 31*, 667–682.

Verbeek, M., Boone, A., & Drent, P. (1996). Exploration, agonistic behaviour and dominance in juvenile male great tits. *Behaviour, 133*, 945–963.

Verbeek, M., Drent, P., & Wiepkema, P. (1994). Consistent individual differences in early exploration behaviour of male great tits. *Animal Behaviour, 48*, 1113–1121.

Verbeek, M. E. M., De Goede, P., Drent, P. J., & Wiepkema, P. R. (1999). Individual behavioural characteristics and dominance in aviary groups of great tits. *Behaviour, 136*, 23–48.

Verderane, M. P., Falotico, T., Resende, B. D., Labruna, M. B., Izar, P., & Ottoni, E. B. (2007). Anting in a semifree-ranging group of *Cebus apella*. *International Journal of Primatology, 28*, 47–53.

Verrell, P. (1986). Wrestling in the red spotted newt: Resource value and contest asymmetry determine contest duration and outcome. *Animal Behaviour, 34*, 398–402.

Via, S., & Lande, R. (1985). Genotype-environment interaction and the evolution of phenotypic plasticity. *Evolution, 39*, 505–522.

Viitala, J., Korpimaki, E., Palokangas, P., & Koivula, M. (1995). Attraction of kestrels to vole scent marks visible in ultraviolet light. *Nature, 373*, 425–427.

Vila, C., Savolainen, P., Maldonado, J. E., Amorim, I. R., Rice, J. E., Honeycutt, R. L., Crandall, K. A., Lundeberg, J., & Wayne, R. K. (1997). Multiple and ancient origins of the domestic dog. *Science, 276*, 1687–1689.

Villarreal, R., & Domjan, M. (1998). Pavlovian conditioning of social-affiliative behavior in the Mongolian gerbil (*Meriones unguiculatus*). *Journal of Comparative Psychology, 112*, 26–35.

Visalberghi, E., & Addessi, E. (2000). Seeing group members eating a familiar food enhances the acceptance of novel foods in capuchin monkeys. *Animal Behaviour, 60*, 69–76.

Visscher, P. K., & Seeley, T. (1982). Foraging strategies of honeybee colonies in a temperate forest. *Ecology, 63*, 1790–1801.

vom Saal, F. (1989). Sexual differentiation in litter-bearing mammals: Influence of sex of adjacent fetuses in utero. *Journal of Animal Science, 67*, 1824–1840.

vom Saal, F. S., & Bronson, F. H. (1978). In utero proximity of female mouse fetuses to males: Effect on reproductive performance during later life. *Biology of Reproduction, 19*, 842–853.

vom Saal, F. S., Grant, W. M., McMullen, C. W., & Laves, K. S. (1983). High fetal estrogen concentrations: Correlation with increased adult sexual activity and decreased aggression in male mice *Science, 220*, 1306–1309.

von Frisch, K. (1967). *The dance language and orientation of bees.* Cambridge, MA: Harvard University Press.

Voultsiadou, E., & Tatolas, A. (2005). The fauna of Greece and adjacent areas in the Age of Homer: Evidence from the first written documents of Greek literature. *Journal of Biogeography, 32*, 1875–1882.

Wagener-Hulme, C., Kuehn, J. C., Schulz, D. J., & Robinson, G. E. (1999). Biogenic amines and division of labor in honey bee colonies. *Journal of Comparative Physiology A, 184*, 471–479.

Waldman, B. (1987). Mechanisms of kin recognition. *Journal of Theoretical Biology, 128*, 159–185.

Walker, P. (Ed). (1989). *Cambridge dictionary of biology.* Cambridge: Cambridge University Press.

Walters, J. R., Doerr, P. D., & Carter, J. H. I. (1992). Delayed dispersal and reproduction as a life-history tactic in cooperative breeders: Fitness calculations from red-cockaded woodpeckers. *American Naturalist, 139*, 623–643.

Ward, P., & Zahavi, A. (1973). The importance of certain assemblages of birds as "information centres" for finding food. *Ibis, 115*, 517–534.

Warkentin, K. (1995). Adaptive plasticity in hatching age: A response to predation risk trade-offs. *Proceedings of the National Academy of Sciences, U.S.A., 92*, 3507–3510.

Warkentin, K. (1999). The development of behavioral defenses: A mechanistic analysis of vulnerability in red-eyed tree frog hatchlings. *Behavioral Ecology, 10*, 251–262.

Warkentin, K. (2000). Wasp predation and wasp-induced hatching of red-eyed treefrog eggs. *Animal Behaviour, 60*, 503–510.

Warkentin, K. M. (2005). How do embryos assess risk? Vibrational cues in predator-induced hatching of red-eyed treefrogs. *Animal Behaviour, 70*, 59–71.

Warkentin, K. M., Caldwell, M. S., & McDaniel, J. G. (2006). Temporal pattern cues in vibrational risk assessment by embryos of the red-eyed treefrog, *Agalychnis callidryas*. *Journal of Experimental Biology, 209*, 1376–1384.

Warkentin, K. M., Caldwell, M. S., Siok, T. D., D'Amato, A. T. & McDaniel, J. G. (2007). Flexible information sampling in vibrational assessment of predation risk by red-eyed treefrog embryos. *Journal of Experimental Biology, 210*, 614–619.

Watson, J. D. (Ed). (2005). *Darwin: The indelible stamp: The evolution of an idea.* Philadelphia: Running Press Book Publishers.

Webster, M. M., & Hart, P. J. B. (2006). Subhabitat selection by foraging threespine stickleback (*Gasterosteus aculeatus*): Previous experience and social conformity. *Behavioral Ecology and Sociobiology, 60*, 77–86.

Webster, M. S., & Westneat, D. F. (1998). The use of molecular markers to study kinship in birds: Techniques and questions. In R. DeSalle & B. Schierwater (Eds.), *Molecular approaches to ecology and evolution* (pp. 7–35). Basel: Birkhauser.

Wedekind, C., & Furi, S. (1997). Body odour preferences in men and women: Do they aim for specific MHC combinations or simply heterozygosity? *Proceedings of the Royal Society of London, Series B, 264*, 1471–1479.

Wedekind, C., Seebeck, T., Bettens, F., & Paepke, A. J. (1995). MHC dependent mate preferences in humans. *Proceedings of the Royal Society of London, Series B, 260*, 245–249.

Wegner, K. M., Kalbe, M., Kurtz, J., Reusch, T. B. H., & Milinski, M. (2003a). Parasite selection for immunogenetic optimality. *Science, 301*, 1343–1343.

Wegner, K. M., Reusch, T. B. H., & Kalbe, M. (2003b). Multiple parasites are driving major histocompatibility complex polymorphism in the wild. *Journal of Evolutionary Biology, 16*, 224–232.

Weigensberg, I., & Roff, D. (1996). Natural heritabilities: Can they be reliably estimated in the laboratory? *Evolution, 50*, 2149–2157.

Weiner, J. (1995). *The beak of the finch: A story of evolution in our time.* New York: Vintage Books.

Weinstock, M. (1997). Does prenatal stress impair coping and regulation of hypothalamic-pituitary-adrenal axis? *Neuroscience and Biobehavioral Reviews, 21,* 1–10.

Weiss, D., Helmreich, S., Mostl, E., Dzidic, A., & Bruckmaier, R. M. (2004). Coping capacity of dairy cows during the change from conventional to automatic milking. *Journal of Animal Science, 82,* 563–570.

Weiss, J. (1972). Influence of psychological variables on stress-induced pathology. In R. Porter & J. Knight (Eds.), *Physiology, emotion and psychosomatic illness.* Amsterdam: Elsevier.

Wells, J. C. K. (2007). The thrifty phenotype as an adaptive maternal effect. *Biological Reviews, 82,* 143–172.

Wenegrat, B. (1984). *Sociobiology and mental disorders: A new view.* Menlo Park, CA: Addison/Wesley.

Wenseleers, T., & Ratnieks, F. L. W. (2006). Enforced altruism in insect societies. *Nature, 444,* 50–50.

Werner, E. E., & Hall, D. J. (1974). Optimal foraging and the size selection of prey by the bluegill sunfish *Lepomis macrochirus. Ecology, 55,* 1042–1055.

West, H., Clancy, A., & Michael, P. (1992). Enhanced responses of nucleus accumbens neurons in male rats to novel odors associated with sexually receptive males. *Brain Research, 585,* 49–55.

West, M. J., King, A. P., & Freeberg, T. M. (1998). Dual signaling during mating in brown-headed cowbirds (*Molothrus ater,* family Emberizidae/Icterinae). *Ethology, 104,* 250–267.

West, M. J., King, A. P., & White, D. J. (2003). The case for developmental ecology. *Animal Behaviour, 66,* 617–622.

West-Eberhard, M. J. (1975). The evolution of social behavior by kin selection. *Quarterly Review of Biology, 50,* 1–35.

West-Eberhard, M. J. (1979). Sexual selection, social competition and evolution. *Proceedings of the American Philosophical Society, 123,* 222–234.

West-Eberhard, M. J. (1981). Intragroup selection and the evolution of insect societies. In R. D. Alexander & D. W. Tinkle (Eds.), *Natural selection and social behavior* (pp. 3–17). New York: Chiron Press.

West-Eberhard, M. J. (1989). Phenotypic plasticity and the origins of diversity. *Annual Review of Ecology and Systematics, 20,* 249–278.

West-Eberhard, M. J. (2003). *Developmental plasticity and evolution.* New York: Oxford University Press.

Westneat, D. F. (1987a). Extra-pair copulations in a predominantly monogamous bird: Genetic evidence. *Animal Behaviour, 35,* 877–886.

Westneat, D. F. (1987b). Extra-pair copulations in a predominantly monogamous bird: Observations of behaviour. *Animal Behaviour, 35,* 865–876.

Westneat, D. F., Frederick, P. C., & Wiley, R. H. (1987). The use of genetic markers to estimate the frequency of successful alternative reproductive tactics. *Behavioral Ecology and Sociobiology, 21,* 35–45.

Westneat, D. F., Sherman, P. W., & Morton, M. L. (1990). The ecology and evolution of extra-pair copulations in birds. In D. Power (Ed.), *Current ornithology* (pp. 331–369). New York: Plenum Press.

Westneat, D. F., Walters, A., McCarthy, T., Hatch, M., & Hein, W. (2000). Alternative mechanisms of nonindependent mate choice. *Animal Behaviour, 59,* 467–476.

Wheeler, J., & Rissing, S. (1975). Natural history of *Veromessor pergandei* I. The nest. *Pan- Pacific Entomologist, 51,* 205–216.

White, L. (1994a). Coresidence and leaving home: Young adults and their parents. *Annual Review of Sociology, 20,* 81–102.

White, L. (1994b). Stepfamilies over the life course: Social support. In A. Booth & J. Dunn (Eds.), *Stepfamilies: Who benefits? Who does not?* (pp. 109–137). Hillsdale, NJ: Lawrence Erlbaum Associates.

White, L., & Reidmann, A. (1992). Ties among adult siblings. *Social Forces, 71,* 85–102.

Whitehead, H., & Connor, R. (2005). Alliances I. How large should alliances be? *Animal Behaviour, 69,* 117–126.

Whiten, A. (1992). On the nature and evolution of imitation in the animal kingdom: Reappraisal of a century of research. *Advances in the Study of Behavior, 21,* 239–283.

Whiten, A. (2005). The second inheritance system of chimpanzees and humans. *Nature, 437,* 52–55.

Whiten, A., & Boesch, C. (2001). The culture of chimpanzees. *Scientific American,* January 2001, 60–67.

Whiten, A., Goodall, J., McGrew, W., Nishida, T., Reynolds, V., Sugiyama, Y., Tutin, C., Wrangham, R., & Boesch, C. (1999). Cultures in chimpanzees. *Nature, 399,* 682–685.

Whiten, A., Horner, V., & de Waal, F. B. M. (2005). Conformity to cultural norms of tool use in chimpanzees. *Nature, 437,* 737–740.

Whitfield, C. W., Cziko, A. M., & Robinson, G. E. (2003). Gene expression profiles in the brain predict behavior in individual honey bees. *Science, 302,* 296–299.

Whiting, A. R. (1967). The biology of the parasitic wasp *Mormoniella vitripennis* (= *Nasonia brevicornis*) (*Walker*). *Quarterly Review of Biology, 42,* 333–406.

Whitten, P. L. (1987). Infants and adult males. In B. B. Smuts, D. L. Cheney, R. M. Seyfarth, R. Wrangham, & T. T. Struhsaker (Eds.), *Primate societies* (pp. 343–357). Chicago: University of Chicago Press.

Widemo, F. (1998). Alternative reproductive strategies in the ruff (*Philomachus pugnax*): A mixed ESS. *Animal Behaviour, 56,* 329–336.

Wilcox, R. S. (1972). Communication by surface waves: Mating behavior of a water strider (Gerridae). *Journal of Comparative Physiology, 80,* 255–266.

Wilcox, R. S. (1995). Ripple communication in aquatic and semi-aquatic Insects. *Ecoscience, 2,* 109–115.

Wilkinson, G. (1984). Reciprocal food sharing in vampire bats. *Nature, 308,* 181–184.

Wilkinson, G. (1985). The social organization of the common vampire bat. I. Patterns and causes of association. *Behavioral Ecology and Sociobiology, 17,* 111–121.

Wilkinson, G. S. (1990). Food sharing in vampire bats. *Scientific American,* February 1990, 76–82.

Wilkinson, G. S. (1993). Artificial sexual selection alters allometry in the stalk-eyed fly *Cyrtodiopsis dalmanni* (Diptera: Diopsidae). *Genetical Research, 62,* 213–222.

Wilkinson, G. S., Kahler, H., & Baker, R. H. (1998a). Evolution of female mating preferences in stalk-eyed flies. *Behavioral Ecology, 9,* 525–533.

Wilkinson, G. S., Presgraves, D. C., & Crymes, L. (1998b). Male eye span in stalk-eyed flies indicates genetic quality by meiotic drive suppression. *Nature, 391,* 276–279.

Wilkinson, G. S., & Reillo, P. R. (1994). Female choice response to artificial selection on an exaggerated ale trait in a stalk-eyed fly. *Proceedings of the Royal Society of London, Series B, 255,* 1–6.

Williams, G. (1957). Pleiotropy, natural selection, and the evolution of senescence. *Evolution, 11,* 398–411.

Williams, G. (1966). *Adaptation and natural selection.* Princeton: Princeton University Press.

Willmer, P. G., & Stone, G. N. (2004). Behavioral, ecological, and physiological determinants of the activity patterns of bees. *Advances in the Study of Behavior, 34,* 347–466.

Wills, C. (1991). Maintenance of multiallelic polymorphism at the MHC region. *Immunologica Reviews, 124,* 165–220.

Wilson, A. D. M., & McLaughlin, R. L. (2007). Behavioural syndromes in brook charr, *Salvelinus fontinalis*: Prey-search in the field corresponds with space use in novel laboratory situations. *Animal Behaviour, 74,* 689–698.

Wilson, A. D. M., & Stevens, E. D. (2005). Consistency in context-specific measures of shyness and boldness in rainbow trout, *Oncorhynchus mykiss. Ethology, 111,* 849–862.

Wilson, D., Coleman, K., Clark, A., & Biederman, L. (1993). Shy-bold continuum in pumpkinseed sunfish (*Lepomis gibbosus*): An ecological study of a psychological trait. *Journal of Comparative Psychology, 107,* 250–260.

Wilson, D. J., & Lefcort, H. (1993). The effects of predator diet on the alarm response of red-legged frog, *Rana aurora,* tadpoles. *Animal Behaviour, 46,* 1017–1019.

Wilson, D. S. (1980a). *The natural selection of populations and communities.* Menlo Park, CA: Benjamin Cummings.

Wilson, D. S. (1990). Weak altruism, strong group selection. *Oikos, 59,* 135–140.

Wilson, D. S., Clark, A. B., Coleman, K., & Dearstyne, T. (1994). Shyness and boldness in humans and other animals. *Trends in Ecology & Evolution, 9,* 442–446.

Wilson, D. S., Muzzall, P. M., & Ehlinger, T. J. (1996). Parasites, morphology, and habitat use in a bluegill sunfish (*Lepomis macrochirus*) population. *Copeia,* 348–354.

Wilson, D. S., & Wilson, E. O. (2007). Rethinking the theoretical foundation of sociobiology. *Quarterly Review of Biology, 82,* 327–348.

Wilson, E. O. (1971). *The insect societies.* Cambridge, MA: Harvard University Press.

Wilson, E. O. (1975). *Sociobiology: The new synthesis.* Cambridge, MA: Harvard University Press.

Wilson, E. O. (1980b). Caste and division of labor in leaf-cutter ants (Hymenoptera: Fromicidae: Atta). I. The ergonomic optimization of leaf cutting. *Behavioral Ecology and Sociobiology, 7,* 157–165.

Wilson, E. O. (1980c). Caste and division of labor in leaf-cutter ants (Hymenoptera: Fromicidae: Atta). I. The overall pattern in *A. sexdens. Behavioral Ecology and Sociobiology, 7,* 143–156.

Wilson, E. O. (Ed.). (2005). *From so simple a beginning: Darwin's four great books.* New York: Norton.

Wilson, E. O., & Holldobler, B. (2005a). Eusociality: Origin and consequences. *Proceedings of the National Academy of Sciences, U.S.A., 102,* 13367–13371.

Wilson, E. O., & Holldobler, B. (2005b). The rise of the ants: A phylogenetic and ecological explanation. *Proceedings of the National Academy of Sciences, U.SA., 102,* 7411–7414.

Wilsson, E. O., & Sundgren, P. E. (1997). The use of a behaviour test for selection of dogs for service and breeding. 2. Heritability for tested parameters and effect of selection based on service dog characteristics. *Applied Animal Behaviour Science, 54,* 235–241.

Wiltschko, R., & Wiltschko, W. (1995). *Magnetic orientation in animals.* Berlin: Springer-Verlag.

Wiltschko, R., & Wiltschko, W. (2003). Avian navigation: From historical to modern concepts. *Animal Behaviour, 65,* 257–272.

Wiltschko, W. (1968). Uber den Einflu-2 statischer Magentfelder auf die Zugorientierung der Rotkehlchen (*Erithacus rubecula*). *Zeitschrift fur Tierpsychologie, 65,* 257–272.

Wimberger, P. (1984). The use of green plant material in birds' nests to avoid ectoparasites. *Auk, 101,* 615–618.

Winberg, S., Nilsson, G., & Olsen, K. H. (1992). Changes in brain serotonergic activity during hierarchy behavior in Artic charr (*Savelinus alpinus L.*) are socially mediated. *Journal of Comparative Physiology, 170,* 93–99.

Winberg, S., Winberg, Y., & Fernald, R. (1997). Effect of social rank on brain monoaminergic activity in a cichlid fish. *Brain, Behavior and Evolution, 49,* 230–236.

Wingfield, J. C., Lynn, S. E., & Soma, K. K. (2001). Avoiding the "costs" of testosterone: Ecological bases of hormone-behavior interactions. *Brain, Behavior and Evolution, 57,* 239–251.

Withers, G., Fahrbach, S., & Robinson, G. (1993). Selective neuroanatomical plasticity and division of labour in the honeybee. *Nature, 354,* 238–240.

Witkin, S. R., & Ficken, M. S. (1979). Chickadee alarm calls: Does mate investment pay dividends. *Animal Behaviour, 27,* 1275–1276.

Witschi, E. (1961). Sex and secondary sexual characteristics. In A. Marshall (Ed.), *Biology and comparative physiology of birds* (pp. 115–168). New York: Academic Press.

Witte, K., Hirschler, U., & Curio, E. (2000). Sexual imprinting on a novel adornment influences mate preferences in the Javanese mannikin *Lonchura leucogastroides. Ethology, 106,* 349–363.

Wood-Gush, D. G. M., & Vestergaard, K. (1991). The seeking of novelty and its relation to play. *Animal Behaviour, 42,* 599–606.

Woodland, D. J., Jaafar, Z., & Knight, M.-L. (1980). The "pursuit deterrent" function of alarm calls. *American Naturalist, 115,* 748–753.

Woolfenden, G. E., & Fitzpatrick, J. W. (1978). Inheritance of territory in group-breeding birds. *Bioscience, 28,* 104–108.

Woolfenden, G. E., & Fitzpatrick, J. W. (1984). *The Florida scrub jay: Demography of a cooperative-breeding bird.* Princeton: Princeton University Press.

Woolfenden, G. E., & FitzPatrick, J. W. (1990). Florida scrub jays: A synopsis after 18 years. In P. B. Stacey & W. D. Koenig (Eds.), *Cooperative breeding in birds* (pp. 241–266). Cambridge: Cambridge University Press.

Wooton, R. J. (1976). *The biology of sticklebacks*. New York: Academic Press.

Wrangham, R. (1995). Relationship of chimpanzee leaf-swallowing to a tapeworm infection. *American Journal of Primatology, 37*, 297–303.

Wrangham, R., & Goodall, J. (1989). Chimpanzee use of medicinal leaves. In P. Heltne & L. Marquardt (Eds.), *Understanding chimpanzees* (pp. 22–37). Cambridge, MA: Harvard University Press.

Wright, W. G. (1998). Evolution of nonassociative learning: Behavioral analysis of a phylogenetic lesion. *Neurobiology of Learning and Memory, 69*, 326–337.

Wright, W. G. (2000). Neuronal and behavioral plasticity in evolution: Experiments in a model lineage. *Bioscience, 50*, 883–894.

Wright, W. G., Kirschman, D., Rozen, D., & Maynard, B. (1996). Phylogenetic analysis of learning-related neuromodulation in molluscan mechanosensory neurons. *Evolution, 50*, 2248–2263.

Wyatt, G., & Davey, K. (1996). Cellular and molecular action of juvenile hormones: II. Roles of juvenile hormone in adult insects. *Advances in Insect Physiology, 26*, 2–155.

Wyles, J., Kunkel, J., & Wilson, A. (1983). Birds, behaviour and anatomical evolution. *Proceedings of the National Academy of Sciences, 80*, 4394–4397.

Xitco, M. J., & Roitblat, H. L. (1996). Object recognition through eavesdropping: Passive echolocation in bottlenose dolphins. *Animal Learning & Behavior, 24*, 355–365.

Yalcin, B., Willis-Owen, S. A. G., Fullerton, J., Meesaq, A., Deacon, R. M., Rawlins, J. N. P., Copley, R. R., Morris, A. P., Flint, J., & Mott, R. (2004). Genetic dissection of a behavioral quantitative trait locus shows that Rgs2 modulates anxiety in mice. *Nature Genetics, 36*, 1197–1202.

Yamamoto, I. (1987). Male parental care in the raccoon dog (*Nyctereutes procyonoides*) during the early rearing stages. In Y. Eto, J. L. Brown, & J. Kikkawa (Eds.), *Animal societies* (Vol. 4, pp. 189–196). Tokyo: Japan Societies Scientific Press.

Yarbrough, W. G., Quarmby, V. E., Simental, J. A., Joseph, D. R., Sar, M., Lubahn, D. B., Olsen, K. L., French, F. S., & Wilson, E. M. (1990). A single base mutation in the androgen receptor gene causes androgen insensitivity in the testicular feminized rat. *Journal of Biological Chemistry, 265*, 8893–8900.

Ydenberg, R. C., & Dill, L. M. (1986). The economics of fleeing from predators. *Advances in the Study of Behavior, 16*, 229–249.

Yeh, S., Musolf, B., & Edward, D. (1997). Neuronal adaptations to changes in social dominance status in crayfish. *Journal of Neuroscience, 17*, 697–708.

Yoerg, S. I. (1991). Ecological frames of mind: The role of cognition in behavioral ecology. *Quarterly Review of Biology, 66*, 288–301.

Yokoyama, S. (2002). Molecular evolution of color vision in vertebrates. *Gene, 300*, 69–78.

Yokoyama, S., Radlwimmer, B., & Blow, N. (2000). Ultraviolet pigments in birds evolved from violet pigments by a single amino acid change. *Proceedings of the National Academy of Sciences, U.S.A., 97*, 7366–7371.

Young, H. (1987). Herring gull preying on rabbits. *British Birds, 80*, 363.

Young, L. J., Young, A. Z. M., & Hammock, E. A. D. (2005). Anatomy and neurochemistry of the pair bond. *Journal of Comparative Neurology, 493*, 51–57.

Zabel, C., Glickman, S., Frank, L., Woodmansee, K., & Keppel, G. (1992). Coalition formation in a colony of prepubertal spotted hyenas. In A. H. Harcourt & F. B. M. de Waal (Eds.), *Coalitions and alliances in humans and other animals* (pp. 112–135). Oxford: Oxford University Press.

Zahavi, A. (1975). Mate selection: A selection for a handicap. *Journal of Theoretical Biology, 53*, 205–214.

Zahavi, A. (1977). The cost of honesty (futher remarks on the handicap principle). *Journal of Theoretical Biology, 67*, 603–605.

Zahavi, A. (2003). Indirect selection and individual selection in sociobiology: My personal views on theories of social behaviour. *Animal Behaviour, 65*, 859–863.

Zahavi, A., & Zahavi, A. (1997). *The handicap principle*. New York: Oxford University Press.

Zajonc, R. B. (1965). Social facilitation. *Science, 269–274*.

Zak, P. J. (2004). Neuroeconomics. *Philosophical Transactions of the Royal Society of London, Series B, 359*, 1737–1748.

Zak, P. J., Kurzban, R., & Matzner, W. T. (2005). Oxytocin is associated with human trustworthiness. *Hormones and Behavior, 48*, 522–527.

Zamble, E., Hadad, G., Mitchell, J., & Cutmore, T. (1985). Pavlovian conditioning of sexual arousal: First- and second-order effects. *Journal of Experimental Psychology: Animal Behavior Processes, 11*, 598–610.

Zamble, E., Mitchell, J., & Findlay, H. (1986). Pavlovian conditioning of sexual arousal: Parametric and background manipulations. *Journal of Experimental Psychology: Animal Behavior Processes, 12*, 403–411.

Zentall, T. R. (2005). Selective and divided attention in animals. *Behavioural Processes, 69*, 1–15.

Zentall, T. R., & Galef, B. G. (1988). *Social learning: Psychological and biological perspectives*. Hillsdale, NJ: Lawrence Erlbaum Associates.

Zhang, S., Amstein, T., Shen, J., Brush, F. R., & Gershenfeld, H. K. (2005). Molecular correlates of emotional learning using genetically selected rat lines. *Genes, Brain and Behavior, 4*, 99–109.

Ziegler, A., Kentenich, H., & Uchanska-Ziegier, B. (2005). Female choice and the MHC. *Trends in Immunology, 26*, 496–502.

Zill, N. (1988). Behavior, achievement and health problems among children in stepfamilies: Findings from a national survey of child health. In E. M. Hetherington & J. D, Arasteh (Eds.), *Impact of divorce, single parenting and stepparenting on children* (pp. 325–368). Hillsdale, NJ: Lawrence Erlbaum Associates.

Zink, R. M. (2002). Towards a framework for understanding the evolution of avian migration. *Journal of Avian Biology, 33*, 433–436.

Zuckerman, M. (1979). *Sensation seeking.* Hillsdale, NJ: Lawrence Erlbaum Associates.

Zuckerman, M. (1991). *Psychobiology of personality.* Cambridge: Cambridge University Press.

Zuckerman, M. (1994). *Behavioral expressions and biosocial bases of sensation seeking.* Cambridge: Cambridge University Press.

Zuckerman, M. (1996). The psychobiological model for impulsive unsocialized sensation seeking: A comparative approach. *Neuropsycholobiology, 34*, 125–129.

Zuckerman, S. (1932). *The social life of monkeys and apes.* New York: Harcourt Brace.

Zuk, M., & Kolluru, G. R. (1998). Exploitation of sexual signals by predators and parasitoids. *Quarterly Review of Biology, 73*, 415–438.

Zuk, M., Rotenberry, J. T., & Tinghitella, R. M. (2006). Silent night: Adaptive disappearance of a sexual signal in a parasitized population of field crickets. *Biology Letters, 2*, 521–524.

Credits

Index

Page numbers in *italics* refer to illustrations; those in **bold** refer to figures.

migration of, 433, 443–44, 446–50, *446*, **449**

mobbing behavior in, 390, 392–93

offspring rule and, 268

personality in, 551–54, *551*, **552**, 553

play in, 491–93, *491*, **492**, 510–11

plumage coloration in, 76–80, *76*, *78*, *79*, *198*, *199*

polyandry in, 232

PTM in, 243–44, *243*

sibling rivalry in, 284–86, *284*, *285*, **287**

social learning in, 360–62, *360*, **361**, *361*, **363**

song learning and mate choice in, 214–15, 414–18

syrinx of, 416–17

territorial defense in, 440–41, *440*, *442*

territorial dispersion in, 271, *271*, *272*

ultraviolet vision in, 100, 102, *102*, 116

winner-loser effects and, *463*, 473–74, *473*, **474**

See also specific species

Birkhead, T. R., 249, 252, 253

Bischof, H., 210

Bishop, D. T., 468

Bitterman, M., 131–32, 135

blackbirds (*Turdus merula*), 392, 416–17, **416**

Blackburn, J., 506

blackcap (*Sylvia atricapilla*), 448, **449**

black-capped chickadee, 354–55, 420

black grouse, 212–13, *212*, **213**

black-tailed prairie dog, 263, *263*

Blaffer-Hrdy, S., 279

Blake, M., 526

Blanco, J., 558

Blaustein, A., 292, 527

blocking, 128–29, 154

blue-footed booby (*Sula nebouxii*), 473–74, *473*, **474**

bluegill sunfish, *220*, *342*, **342**
foraging by, 350–51, **350**, *350*, *351*

blue gourami (*Trichogaster trichopterus*), 143, *143*, 145–46, **145**

blue jay (*Cyanocitta cristata*), 314–15, **315**, *389*

blue tit (*Parus caeruleus*), 170, *170*

Blumstein, D. T., 378, 379–80

Boake, C., 64–65, **65**

"Bobo" doll experiment, 168, *169*

bobolink (*Dolichonyx oryzivorus*), 448

Boccia, M. L., 214

Boesch, C., 161, 351, 402, 554

Boesch, H., 351

boldness, 542–46
defined, 542

Bolig, R., 548

bombardier beetles, 391, *391*

Bonner, J. T., 158

Borgerhoff-Mulder, M., 243, 244

Bottger, K., 418, 419

bottle-nosed dolphin (*Tursiops truncatus*), 56, 176–77, *177*, 298, 321, 323, 373–75, *374*, **375**
coalition formation in, 321, *321*, 323

Boucher, D., 326

Boulton, M. J., 502

Boyd, R., 138, 158, 162–63, 164

Boyse, E., 288

Bradbury, J. W., 241

Braithwaite, V. A., 140

Brantley, R., 90

Brass, M., 170

Bray, J., 279

Brenowitz, E. A., 414, 416

Brick, O., 471

Brightsmith, D., 376

Bronstein, J. L., 326

brood parasitism, 50–53, *50*

brood raiding, 318

Brown, C. A., 42–44, **43**, 165, 178, 407–8, 464

Brown, J. H., 196

Brown, J. L., 18, 45, 143, 242, 268, **268**, 269, 273, 300, 313, 324, 441

Brown, J. S., 434

Brown, M., 42–44, **43**, 497

brown-headed cowbird (*Molothrus ater*), 214–15, *215*, 418

brown thrasher (*Toxostoma rufum*), 414, 418

Bruderer, B., 444

Brush, A., 77

bryozoan (*Membranipora membranacea*), 122, *122*

budding, territorial, 442, *442*

budgerigars, 170

Bufo bufo (toad), 406, **406**

bullfrog (*Rana catesbeiana*), 528–29, *528*

Burgess, J. W., 467

Burghardt, G., 491

Burke, T., 234–35

bursa of Fabricus, 450

Buss, A., 550

Busse, C., 351

Butcher, G., 77

Buteo jamaicensis (red-tailed hawk), 396

butterflies, 326–27, **327**, *327*, 330, **330**, 444–46, 466–67

Byers, J., 160, 197, 489–90, 496, 497

Bygott, J. D., 56

byproduct mutualism, 313–17, **315**, **317**, 331, 441
in blue jays, 314–15, **315**, **317**
food calls and, 316–17, **317**
reciprocity and, 313–15, **315**

Byrne, R. W., 356

bystander effects, 478–79, 482, 483–84

caching food:
learning and, 183, 356–58
memory and, 354–55
phylogeny and, 355–56

cactus finch (*Geospiza scandens*), 180–81

Cahan, S., 320

Calamospiza melanocorys (lark bunting), 243–44, *243*

Caldwell, R., 134–35

Callithrix jacchus (marmoset), 298

Callosobruchus chinensis (adzuki bean beetle), 386–87, **388**

camouflage, as antipredator behavior, 372–73

Campbell, C., 68, **68**

Campbell, T., 378

Canales, C., 473–74

canary (*Serinus canaria*), 418

Canis lupus (wolf), 56, 321

Cannon, W., 555

capuchin monkey (*Cebus paella*), *167*, 530

Caraco, T., 166, 347, 349, 351, 541

Carlier, P., 135–36

Caro, T., 173–74, 390, 491, 493–94, 540

Carpdacus mexicanus (house finch), 76–80, *76*, *78*, *79*

Carpenter, C. R., 299, 498

Carter, C. S., 231

Case, T. J., 318

Catchpole, C., 414

cave paintings, 4–5, *5*

Cebus paella (capuchin monkey), *167*, 530

Centrocercus urophasianus (sage grouse), 213, **213**

cephalopods, 372–73, 548–51
Cervus elaphus (red deer), 216, **217**, *217*
cetaceans. *See* bottle-nosed dolphins
c-fos gene, 507–8
Chapais, B., 56
Charnov, E., 343, 364, 390
Chase, I. D., 478
cheetah (*Actinonyx jubatus*), *19*, 56, *56*, *174*, *339*
    object play in, *491*, 493–94, **493**, *493*
    and predator inspection by gazelles, 383–84, *383*, **384**
chemical defense, 390, 391, *391*
Cheney, D. L., 402, 420, 422
Cherrett, J., 412
Chesser, R. T., 450
Chiel, H., 134
child abuse, 279, **280**
chimpanzees, *162*
    alarm calls in, 402
    between-group raiding in, 437–38
    cooperative hunting by, 351–52, *352*
    cultural transmission in, 554–55, 562
    learning in, *168*
    personality in, 540, 554–55, 562
    self-medication in, 531–32, **531**
    soil ingestion in, 535
    tricolor vision in, 207
    See also primates
Chivers, D., 120
chlordiazepoxide (Librium), 378
Choleris, E., 214
Christensen, B., 338
Church, S., 102
cichlid fish:
    Melanochromis auratus, 322
    Nannacara anomala, 471–72, *471*
circadian rhythm, 110
Cissa erythrorhyncha (red-billed blue magpie), 354, **354**
Cistothorus palustris (marsh wren), 414
Claar, J., 558
Clark, A., 37
Clark, A. B., 540
Clark, C. W., 374
Clark, M., 86–87
Clarke, J. A., 393
classical conditioning, *See* Pavlovian conditioning
Clayton, N. S., 210, 354, 355–56, 359
Cleland, J., 286
Clements, K. C., 314
Clethrionomys rufocanus (grey-sided vole), 241–42
Clever Hans, 403, *403*

cliff swallow (*Petrochelidon pyrrho-nota*), 42–44, *42*, **43**, 165
    food calling in, 407–8, **408**
Close, R., 497
clown anemonefish, *62*
Clunie, F., 530
Clutton-Brock, T., 216, **217**, 356, 522–23
coalition formation, 56–57, 299, 321–23
    alliances and, 321–323
    defined, 321, 331
    in mammals, 323
    in primates, 321–22, *321–22*
    reciprocal, 322–23
coati (*Nasua narica*), 56, 321
coho salmon (*Oncorhynchus kisutch*), 140–41
Coleman, K., 542, 543, 545
Coleman, R., 219
Columba livia. See pigeon
common crow, 357
common mole rat (*Cryptomys hotten-totus*), 9–10, *9*, **10**
common raven (*Corvus corax*), 408, **408**, *408*, 510–11
    object play in, 491–93, *491*, **492**
communication, 401–29, *403*, **406**, *407*, **408**, *408*, **409**, *410*, **412**, *413*, *414*, **418**, **423**, *423*
    alarm calls and, 419–23, *420*, **423**, *423*
    animal-human, 403
    "arms race" in, 405
    birdsong as, 414–17, **418**
    by chemical signaling, 412–13
    classical approach to, 405
    deceptive, 421–22, 427
    defined, 403
    foraging and, 406, 427
    handicap principle and, 406
    honesty in, 404–6, 427
    learning and, 408
    mate investment and, 420
    mating and, 418–19
    modes of, 404
    predation and, 419–23, *420*, **423**, *423*
    by ripples, 418–19, *419*, 427
    by vibrations, 412–13, 427
conditioned response (CR), 127, *127*
conditioned stimulus (CS), 126, *127*–28, 154
Conner, W. E., 389
Connor, R., 313, 323, 326
conspecific cueing hypothesis, 439

convergent evolution, 59, *60*
Cook, M., 179
Cooke, F., 209
cooperation, 295–333, *296*, *298–99*, **301–8**, *308–9*, *313*, **315**, **317**, **319**, **320**, *320*, *321–22*, **325**, *327*, *327*, *330*
    alliances and, 321, 323
    byproduct mutualism and, 300, **301**, 313–17, *313*, **315**, **317**, 331
    coalitions and, 56–57, 299, 321–23, *321–22*, 331
    cooperative breeding and, 324–25, **325**, 331
    definition of, 296–97, 331
    food sharing and, 308–9, *308–9*, **309**
    foraging and, 351–52, *352*
    game theory and, 301–2
    group selection and, 300, **301**, 317–20, **319**, **320**, *320*, 331
    group size and, 351–52, *352*
    and helping in birthing process, 297–98, *298*
    interspecific mutualism and, 326–27, **327**, *327*, *330*, **330**, 331
    learning and, 316–17
    phylogenetic component of, 324–26, **325**, 331
    play and, *501*
    reciprocity and, 300–313, **302–8**, 331
    social grooming and, 298–300, *299*
cooperative breeding, 17–18, 54–55, 105–6, 143–44, 175, 275–79, 324–25, 331, 441–44. *See also* helpers-at-the-nest
coping style, 555–57, **556**, 562
copperhead snake (*Agkistrodon contortrix*), 475–76, *476*
Corballis, M. C., 358
Cords, M., 300
Cordts, R., 524
corpora pedunculata (mushroom bodies), 109, *109*
corpus allatum, 112
correspondence problem, 170
corticosterone, 87–90, 148–49, 476, 525–26, 557
corticotropin-releasing hormone (CRH), 85
cortisol, 82, 85
Corvus:
    C. corax. See common raven
    C. corone (European crow), 354
    C. frugilegus (rook), 354, **354**
    C. monedula (jackdaw), 354, **354**

Holmes, W., 292
home range, 433
homicide, 263–64, **265**
homology, 59
homoplasy, 59
honeybee (*Apis mellifera*), **54**, 290
    foraging by, *108*, 110–13, **111**, *112*, 349
    "policing" by, 277–78, *277*, **278**
    spatial learning in, 109
    waggle dance of, 407, 410–11, *410*, **412**
Hoogland, J., 263, 293
Hopster, H., 557
horizontal cultural transmission, 176, *176*, 178
hormones, 116
    aging and, 525–26, 536
    aggression and, 460–62, 476, 482
    behavior and, 81–86
    helping-at-the-nest and, 86–87
    personality and, 552–53, **552**, 557
    placentally produced, 283
    play and, 504–6, 508, **509**
    proximate causation and, 81–87, **84**, *86*
    See also specific hormones
Hosoi, A., 415, **415**
Houde, A. E., 45, 46, 48, 181
    interview with, 222–23
house finch (*Carpdacus mexicanus*), 76–80, *76*, *78*, **79**
house mouse (*Mus musculus domesticus*), 289, 292
house sparrow (*Passer domesticus*), 316–17, **317**
Houston, A., 347, 440
Howe, N., 120
Hrdy, S., 279
Hsu, Y., 474–75, **475**
Huffman, M., 159–61, **161**, 530, 532, 535
Hughes, L., 330
Hugie, D. M., 551
humans:
    alliances and, 323
    child abuse in, 279, 280
    cultural transmission in, *163*, *165*, 168, *169*, 178
    disposable soma theory and longevity in, 521–22
    family stability in, 271–72
    homicide in, 263–64, **265**
    imitation in, *163*
    in-utero conflicts in, 282–84, 283

mate choice and, 223, 244–45
polygyny in, 244–45, *244*, **245**
PTM and mate choice in, 244–45, *244*, **245**
reciprocity in, 310–13
social play in, 503
stepfamily violence in, 278–79, **280**
wealth and kinship in, 274, **275**
Humphreys, A., 502, 506
Huntingford, F. A., 124, 137–38, 144, 458
Hutt, C., 490
Huxley, J., 6, 29, 192
Huxley, T. H., 66, 184, 458–59
Hyla versicolor (gray treefrog), 527, 528, **528**
Hylobittacus apicalis (scorpionfly), 194–96, *195*, **196**
hypothalamus, 84–85, 148, 507

Iacoboni, M., 171
ideal free distribution (IFD) model, 434–37
identical by descent, genes, 266
imitation (observational learning), *163*, 169–71, 186
    birdsong and, 180–81, 214–15
    brain activation and, 170–71
    communication and, 144, 214–15, 316–17, 420–21
    cross-fostering and, 43–44, 144, 214–15
    dolphins and, 176–77
    foraging and, 352–53, 360–63
    guppies and, 178, 181–82
    mate choice and, 171–72, 211–15
    mobbing and, 393–93
    rhesus monkeys and, 178–79
    social learning and, 144, 158–61, 167–73, 352–53, 360–63
    territory choice and, 438–39
    See also cultural transmission
Immelmann, K., 210
imperial blue butterfly (*Jalmenus evagoras*), 327, **327**, *327*, **330**
imprinting, 209–10
Ims, R. A., 241–42
inclusive fitness (kin selection) theory, 17–18, 264–68, 269, 271, 280, 290, 293
    calculating, 266–68
    relatedness and, 266–68
    See also family dynamics
Indian elephant (*Elephas maximus*), 298

indigo bunting (*Passerina cyanea*), 246–47, *246*, **247**
    stellar navigation in, 446, *446*
indirect fitness, *17*
infanticide, 279
information-center hypothesis, 14–15
innovations, and brain size, 182–83, 356–58
insects, 257, 290–91, 300, 331
    aggression in, *459*, 466–69, *467*, *468*, **470**
    antipredator behavior in, 381
    communication in, 410–14, *410*, **412**, *413*, *414*, 418–19, *419*
    cooperative breeding in, *270*, 276–78, **278**
    eusocial, **54**
    female defense polygyny in, 232–33
    foraging in, *108*, 110–13, **111**, *112*, 336–37, *337*, 412–14
    group selection in, 318–21, *319*, *320*
    haplodiploidy in, 276, 290
    learning in, 11–13, **11**, 109, *109*
    migration of, 433
    sperm competition in, 248–50, *249*, **250**
    sperm morphology of, 252, *252*
    See also specific species
instrumental (operant) conditioning, 130–31, *131*
intersexual selection, 190–95, 414. *See also* mate choice, sexual selection
interspecific mutualism, 326–27, **327**, *327*, 330, **330**, 331
intrasexual selection, 190–95, *192*, 414. *See also* mate choice, sexual selection
intrauterine position (IUP), 85, 86–87
in-utero conflict, 282–84, 283
Iridomyrmex anceps (ant), 326–27, **327**, *327*, 330
Irwin, D. E., 137
Iwaniuk, A., 509

Jablonski, P., 123
Jacana:
    J. jacana (wattled jacana), 232, *232*
    J. spinosa (American jacana), 215
jackdaw (*Corvus monedula*), 354, **354**
Jacobs, G. H., 100
Jacobson, M., 497
Jalmenus evagoras (imperial blue butterfly), 327, **327**, *327*, 330
Janik, V. M., 158, 374
Janzen, D., 529